AF823125

Swine Nutrition

Swine Nutrition

Edited by

Elwyn R. Miller
Duane E. Ullrey
Austin J. Lewis

With 54 Contributing Authors

Butterworth–Heinemann
Boston London Singapore Sydney Toronto Wellington

Copyright © 1991 by Butterworth–Heinemann, a division of Reed Publishing (USA) Inc. All rights reserved.

No part of this publication may be reproduced, stored in a retrieval system, or transmitted, in any form or by any means, electronic, mechanical, photocopying, recording, or otherwise, without the prior written permission of the publisher.

Recognizing the importance of preserving what has been written, it is the policy of Butterworth–Heinemann to have the books it publishes printed on acid-free paper, and we exert our best efforts to that end.

Library of Congress Cataloging-in-Publication Data

Swine nutrition / [edited by] Elwyn R. Miller, Duane E. Ullrey, Austin J. Lewis.
Includes bibliographical references and index.
ISBN 0-409-90095-8 (hard : alk. paper)
1. Swine—Nutrition. 2. Swine—Feeding and feeds. I. Miller, Elwyn R. II. Ullrey, Duane E. III. Lewis, Austin J.
SF396.5.S95 1991
636.4'0852—dc20 90-2504
CIP

British Library Cataloguing in Publication Data

Swine Nutrition.
1. Livestock : Pigs. Nutrition
I. Miller, Elwyn R. II. Ullrey, Duane E. III. Lewis, Austin J.
636.40852

ISBN 0-409-90095-8

Butterworth–Heinemann
80 Montvale Avenue
Stoneham, MA 02180

10 9 8 7 6 5 4 3 2 1

Printed in the United States of America

The editors and authors of *Swine Nutrition* dedicate this comprehensive text–reference to all of the scientists who have contributed to the current body of knowledge that comprises the science of swine nutrition. *Swine Nutrition* is especially dedicated to the scientists who have been members of, or administrative advisors to, NCR–42 since its genesis in 1964. A very special dedication goes to Dr. Jacob A. Hoefer, who was a charter member of, and later administrative advisor to, NCR–42, and was an inspiration to an entire generation of swine nutritionists.

Present and Past Members of NCR–42

G.L. Allee
D.E. Becker
C.C. Calvert
T.R. Cline
J.H. Conrad
S.G. Cornelius
J.D. Crenshaw
T.D. Crenshaw
G.L. Cromwell
W.E. Dinusson
R.A. Easter
R.C. Ewan
L.T. Frobish
R.H. Grummer
R.C. Hamilton
R.L. Harrold
V.W. Hays
J.A. Hoefer
A.H. Jensen
B.A. Koch
A.J. Lewis
D.C. Mahan
R.J. Meade
E.C. Miller
E.R. Miller
J.L. Nelssen
E.R. Peo, Jr.
J.E. Pettigrew
M.P. Plumlee
W.G. Pond
R.W. Seerley
V.C. Speer
N.C. Steele
J.W. Stephenson
H.S. Teague
L.F. Tribble
T.L. Veum
R.C. Wahlstrom
J.T. Yen

Present and Past Administrative Advisors

O.G. Bentley
J.A. Hoefer
F.E. Regnier
W.H. Pfander
M.E. Tumbleson

Contents

Contributing Authors

D.K. Aaron, PhD
Associate Professor
Department of Animal Sciences
University of Kentucky
Lexington, Kentucky

David H. Baker, PhD
Professor of Comparative Nutrition
Department of Animal Sciences
University of Illinois
Urbana, Illinois

Larry J. Bark, MS
Graduate Assistant
Department of Animal Sciences
University of Kentucky
Lexington, Kentucky

N.J. Benevenga, PhD
Professor
Department of Meat and Animal Science
University of Wisconsin
Madison, Wisconsin

Michael C. Brumm, PhD
Associate Professor
Animal Science Department
University of Nebraska
Concord, Nebraska

C.C. Calvert, PhD
Research Animal Scientist
USDA, Agricultural Research Service
Livestock and Poultry Science Institute
Nonruminant Animal Nutrition Laboratory
Beltsville, Maryland

T.R. Cline, PhD
Professor
Department of Animal Sciences
Purdue University
West Lafayette, Indiana

William H. Close, PhD, MI Biol
Head of Department
Pig Department
AFRC Institute for Grassland and Environmental Research
Shinfield, Reading, Berks.
United Kingdom

David A. Cook, MS
Research Assistant
Department of Animal Sciences
University of Illinois
Urbana, Illinois

J.D. Crenshaw, PhD
Associate Professor
Department of Animal and Range Science
North Dakota State University
Fargo, North Dakota

T.D. Crenshaw, PhD
Associate Professor
Department of Meat and
Animal Science
University of Wisconsin
Madison, Wisconsin

Gary L. Cromwell, PhD
Professor
Department of Animal Sciences
University of Kentucky
Lexington, Kentucky

Stanley E. Curtis, PhD
Professor and Head
Department of Dairy and
Animal Science
The Pennsylvania State University
University Park, Pennsylvania

D.M. Danielson, PhD
Professor
Department of Animal Science
University of Nebraska
Lincoln, Nebraska

David P. Dyer, Jr., PhD
Director of Research
Research Department
Moorman Manufacturing Company
Quincy, Illinois

Robert A. Easter, PhD
Professor of Swine Nutrition
Department of Animal Sciences
University of Illinois
Urbana, Illinois

K.E. Ekstrom, PhD
President
Cargill Taiwan Corporation
Taipei, Taiwan
Republic of China

Richard C. Ewan, PhD
Professor, Swine Nutrition
Department of Animal Science
Iowa State University
Ames, Iowa

Dale M. Forsyth, PhD
Associate Professor
Department of Animal Sciences
Purdue University
West Lafayette, Indiana

V.W. Hays, PhD
Professor
Department of Animal Sciences
University of Kentucky
Lexington, Kentucky

M.G. Hogberg, PhD
Professor
Department of Animal Science
Michigan State University
East Lansing, Michigan

Palmer J. Holden, PhD
Professor, Extension Swine Specialist
Department of Animal Science
Iowa State University
Ames, Iowa

Katherine A. Houpt, VMD, PhD
Professor of Veterinary Physiology
Department of Physiology
New York State College of
Veterinary Medicine
Cornell University
Ithaca, New York

T. Richard Houpt, VMD, PhD
Professor of Veterinary Physiology
Department of Physiology
New York State College of
Veterinary Medicine
Cornell University
Ithaca, New York

Aldon H. Jensen, PhD
Professor of Animal Nutrition, Emeritus
Department of Animal Sciences
University of Illinois
Urbana, Illinois

Keith W. Kelley, PhD
Professor of Immunophysiology
Department of Animal Sciences
University of Illinois
Urbana, Illinois

Darrell A. Knabe, PhD
Associate Professor
Department of Animal Science
Texas A & M University
College Station, Texas

Vernon D. Leibbrandt, PhD
Professor
Department of Meat and Animal Science
University of Wisconsin
Madison, Wisconsin

Austin J. Lewis, PhD
Professor
Department of Animal Science
University of Nebraska
Lincoln, Nebraska

George W. Libal, PhD
Professor of Animal Science
Department of Animal and Range Sciences
South Dakota State University
Brookings, South Dakota

Dennis O. Liptrap, PhD
Extension Swine Specialist
Department of Animal Sciences
University of Kentucky
Lexington, Kentucky

A.G. Low, PhD
Research Group Leader
Pig Department
AFRC Institute for Grassland and Environmental Research
Shinfield, Reading, Berks.
United Kingdom

Donald C. Mahan, PhD
Professor of Animal Nutrition
Department of Animal Science
The Ohio State University
Columbus, Ohio

Harry J. Mersmann, PhD
Department of Pediatrics
USDA/ARS Children's Nutrition Research Center
Baylor College of Medicine
Houston, Texas

Elwyn R. Miller, PhD
Professor
Department of Animal Science
Michigan State University
East Lansing, Michigan

Ronny L. Moser, PhD
Associate Professor
Department of Animal Science
University of Minnesota
St. Paul, Minnesota

Jerome C. Pekas, PhD
Research Physiologist
USDA, Agricultural Research Service
Roman L. Hruska U.S. Meat Animal Research Center
Clay Center, Nebraska

Ernest R. Peo, Jr., PhD
Professor Emeritus
Department of Animal Science
University of Nebraska–Lincoln
Lincoln, Nebraska

James E. Pettigrew, PhD
Associate Professor
Department of Animal Science
University of Minnesota
St. Paul, Minnesota

Wilson G. Pond, PhD
Adjunct Professor
Department of Pediatrics
Baylor College of Medicine
and
USDA-ARS Research Animal Scientist
Children's Nutrition Research Center
Houston, Texas

Steven V. Radecki, MS
Graduate Student (PhD)
Department of Animal Science
Michigan State University
East Lansing, Michigan

Robert W. Seerley, PhD
Professor
Department of Animal and
Dairy Science
University of Georgia
Athens, Georgia

Richard Graham Shields, Jr., PhD
Senior Nutritionalist, Swine and
Pet Products
Department of Market Services
Farmland Industries, Inc.
Kansas City, Missouri

Vaughn C. Speer, PhD
Professor, Swine Nutrition
Department of Animal Science
Iowa State University
Ames, Iowa

Tim S. Stahly, PhD
Professor
Department of Animal Sciences
University of Kentucky
Lexington, Kentucky

Andy J. Thulin, PhD
Associate Professor
Department of Animal Science
Michigan State University
East Lansing, Michigan

L.F. Tribble, PhD
Professor Emeritus
Department of Animal Science
Texas Tech University
Lubbock, Texas

Duane E. Ullrey, PhD
Professor
Department of Animal Science
Michigan State University
East Lansing, Michigan

Richard C. Wahlstrom, PhD
Distinguished Professor Emeritus
Department of Animal and
Range Sciences
South Dakota State University
Brookings, South Dakota

Trygve L. Veum, PhD
Professor
Department of Animal Sciences
University of Missouri
Columbia, Missouri

J.T. Yen, PhD
Research Animal Scientist
Roman L. Hruska U.S. Meat Animal
Research Center
U.S. Department of Agriculture
Clay Center, Nebraska

Melvin T. Yokoyama, PhD
Professor
Department of Animal Science
Michigan State University
East Lansing, Michigan

L.G. Young, PhD
Professor
Department of Animal and Poultry Science
University of Guelph
Guelph, Ontario, Canada

Dean R. Zimmerman, PhD
Professor of Animal Nutrition
Department of Animal Science
Iowa State University
Ames, Iowa

Preface

I became aware of the need for a comprehensive text-reference in swine nutrition as I have endeavored to teach an advanced swine nutrition course at Michigan State University biennially since 1969. During that period, more than 250 senior undergraduates, graduate students, and foreign visiting scholars have taken the course. I also taught the course in one intensive week to 63 persons in the Brazilian swine industry at the Federal University of Rio Grande do Sul in Porto Alegre, R.S., Brazil, in 1978. Again, the need for a text-reference was apparent.

I discussed this need with colleagues at Michigan State University and the NCR-42 committee (consisting of one swine nutrition scientist at each of the land grant universities of the 12 states in the North Central region of the United States). This committee meets annually to report on and plan for cooperative research, resulting in a number of publications in the *Journal of Animal Science.* A most worthwhile rapport also has developed among these scientists.

About 4 years ago, I became convinced that the NCR-42 scientists, each with their own specialty in swine research, would comprise an excellent core of authors for this book. Several of these scientists were also teaching an advanced swine nutrition course at their respective universities and expressed the need for a comprehensive book on the subject. At the 1985 meeting of NCR-42, the members were challenged to produce such a book. They were unanimous in their support of this project, provided I would serve as the editor. After issuing the challenge, I could hardly retreat from their stipulation.

I enlisted my long-time colleague at Michigan State University, Duane Ullrey, to serve as co-editor. Butterworth–Heinemann expressed an interest in publishing the book, which we had outlined and decided to call, simply, *Swine Nutrition.* We were fortunate also that the NCR-42 scientist from Nebraska, Austin Lewis (currently editor-in-chief of the *Journal of Animal Science*), volunteered to help Dr. Ullrey and me with the editing.

Swine Nutrition opens with a section on the interdependencies of swine and humans. This is followed by a section on the development of the digestive, absorptive, and metabolic capabilities of swine, and the maximization of lean tissue growth.

From a nutritional science standpoint, the section on nutrient utilization by swine is the core of the book. This is followed by an equally important section on factors influencing swine nutrition, including nutrient bioavailability, appetite and feeding behavior, physical forms of feed, environment and management, immunocompetence, genetic and sex considerations, mycotoxins, and intestinal microbiology.

The applied feeding section contains a chapter on major feedstuffs and chapters on feeding newborn pigs, 3-week-old pigs, growing and finishing pigs, developing gilts and boars, and gestating and lactating sows. This is followed by a section on utilizing unique feedstuffs, including milk by-products, raw soybeans, and grain by-products. The final section deals with techniques in swine nutrition research and their application to computer modeling, diet optimization, statistical methods, digestion and metabolism studies, body composition, and surgical techniques.

The publisher, authors, and editors have combined their efforts to make *Swine Nutrition* a uniquely comprehensive text-reference that should be useful as a text in advanced swine nutrition courses and as a reference for anyone seeking current information in swine nutrition.

Elwyn R. Miller
Senior Editor

PART I

Interdependencies of Swine and Humans

Chapter 1

Of Pigs and People

W.G. Pond

HISTORICAL PERSPECTIVE

Pig Domestication

The exact time and place of the domestication of the pig is lost in history. Evidence collected from several sources (Towne and Wentworth 1950; Mellen 1952; Zeuner 1963; Mersmann 1986) indicates that ancestors of the modern pig lived in China and Europe about 25 million years ago and somewhat more recently in India. Domestication probably occurred in several areas of the world, including China, Persia, Africa, and Europe 6000 to 8500 years ago; for example, one study suggests that the earliest domestication was in what is now Iraq in about 6750 B.C. Biblical reference to the pig appears in Genesis, and domesticated pigs are reported to have been found in China by 2900 B.C. The modern pig, which supplies pork throughout the world, remains genetically diverse. The contemporary pig in the United States, whose ancestry probably includes the European wild pig and the Far Eastern pig, has an appearance far different from that of the contemporary Chinese pig (Figure 1.1). Such a diverse germ plasm would be expected when one considers the results of thousands of years of natural selection and, more recently, the application of Mendelian genetic principles by animal breeders. Changes in such traits as body type, pork composition, and nutritional requirements depend on this genetic diversity.

Demographic Relationships

The partnership between pigs and humans throughout history has thrived based on the ability of the pig to respond favorably to widely different environments and to the changing needs and desires of humans. This plasticity must continue to be an essential attribute of the pig if this valuable historic partnership is to be sustained.

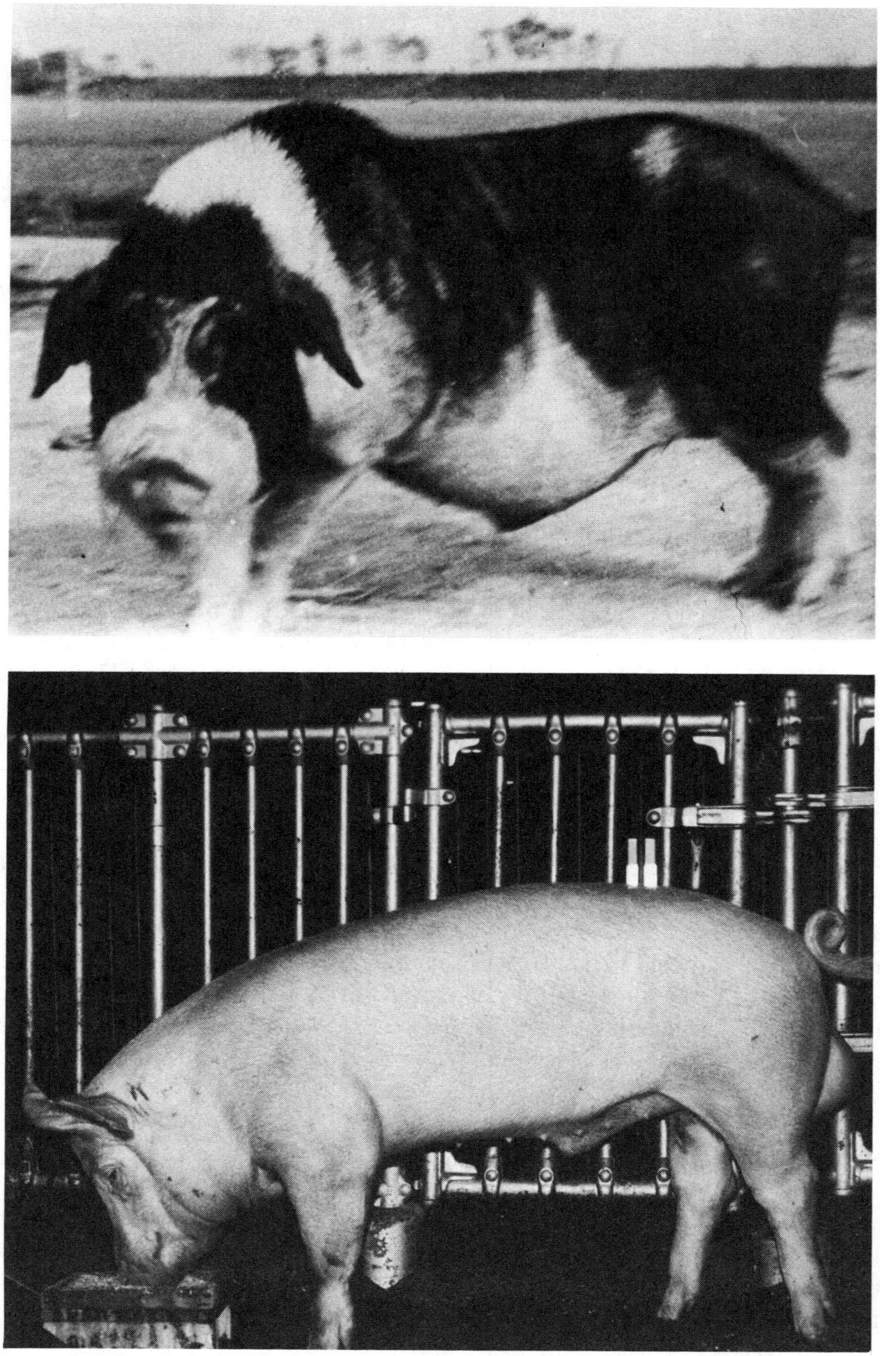

FIGURE 1.1 *(Top) Contemporary Chinese Ningxiang boar, Hunan Province, Republic of China; and (Bottom) contemporary Yorkshire boar, United States. Note the extreme difference in body shape and type.*

The pig converts low-quality plant and animal products and by-products to food and is an efficient storage depot for fat, proteins, vitamins, and minerals that, taken separately, would be very expensive. Pigs traditionally have been scavengers, and in early domestication they were raised as a means of utilizing food wastes. In many parts of the world, they still perform that function and, as such, are an integral part of the culture, as in Haiti and other developing countries where they are held in high esteem.

Most commercial production of swine in the United States and other developed countries occurs in areas where cereal grains, maize, and other high-energy feeds are grown in large quantities and are economically priced. An example is the maize belt of the United States, which has soil and climate ideal for the production of high-yielding maize and soybeans; the latter is an excellent protein supplement for swine. The abundance of favorably priced feedstuffs allows the farmer to market crops through swine at a greater profit than that available by selling them as cash crops. Profitability of swine production based on this method of marketing grain and other surplus feed resources and by-products has for many years been an alternative among farmers and, for this reason, the pig has been long known as "the mortgage lifter."

The world-wide demand for pork continues to grow, as evidenced by the faster growth rate of world swine numbers relative to the human population. This relationship is shown in Figure 1.2 (Pond and Maner 1984) with projections for the future. The extent of swine production in various countries is suggested by the comparison of human and pig populations (Figure 1.3; Pond 1983). This comparison has limitations because of variations in the "extraction rate," the ratio of pigs sent to market per year

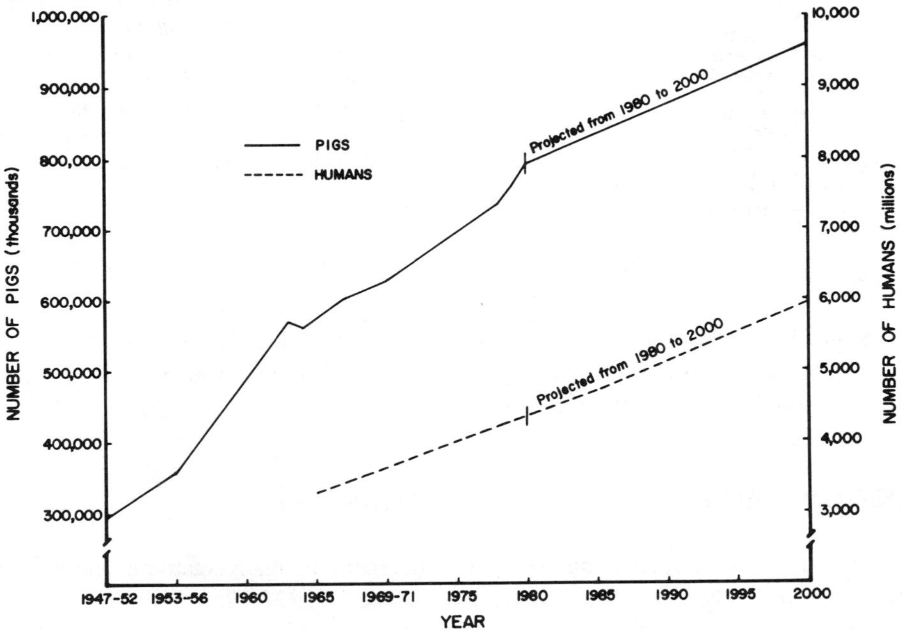

FIGURE 1.2 *World population of pigs and humans with projections to 2000 A.D.*

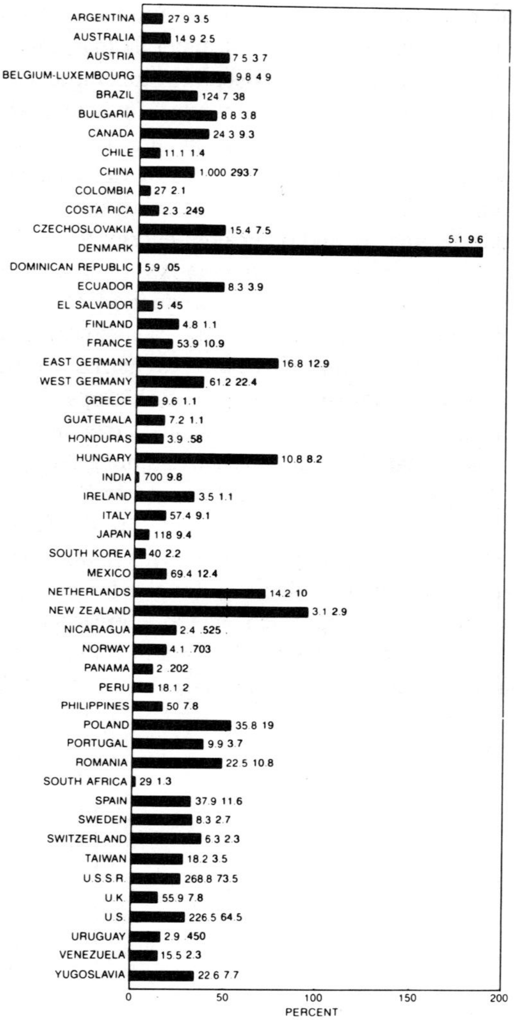

FIGURE 1.3 *Extent of pig production in various countries is suggested by this comparison of human and pig populations. For each country the first number represents human population, the second number, pig population, both in millions. The bar shows the number of pigs as a percentage of the human population. The comparison is inexact because of variations in "extraction rate," the ratio of the number of pigs marketed per year to the number on hand at any time. For example, in the United States, the rate is about 1.5 and, in Brazil it is about 0.4.*

to the number on hand at any one time. For example, in the United States the rate is about 1.5 while in Brazil it is about 0.4, reflecting differences in reproductive efficiency, growth rate, and other production traits.

ANATOMIC AND PHYSIOLOGIC SIMILARITIES

Several published summaries and symposia document the many anatomic and physiologic similarities between pigs and humans (Bustad and McClellan 1966; Pond and Houpt 1978; Roberts and Dodds 1982; Stanton and Mersmann 1986; Tumbleson 1986). Among the similarities most relevant to the use of the pig as an animal model for biomedical research are those of the skin (Montagna 1966); dental characteristics

(Weaver et al. 1962); kidney morphology and function (Nielson et al. 1966); eye structure and visual acuity (Prince et al. 1960); cardiovascular anatomy and physiology (Stanton and Mersmann 1986); gastrointestinal anatomy, physiology, and nutritional requirements (Pond and Houpt 1978; Miller and Ullrey 1987; Schummer et al. 1979); and body composition (Widdowson and Dickerson 1964). Of particular relevance to this discussion are the comparative aspects of the anatomy and physiology of the digestive tract and of body composition in swine and humans. Comparative nutrient requirements are discussed in a separate section of this chapter.

Digestive Tract Anatomy and Physiology

The general architecture of the gastrointestinal tracts of the pig and the human is similar. Notable differences are the higher proportion of cardiac mucosa lining the stomach of the pig, as compared with the human (Stevens 1977), and the presence of a cecum in the pig, as compared with only a vestige, the appendix, in the human. The digestive functions of each of the segments of the gastrointestinal tract of both species are similar, qualitatively; amylolytic, lipolytic, and proteolytic activities are similar, and the secretions of each digestive organ, including the stomach, small intestine, and pancreas, are comparable. Even the endocrine and paracrine control of gastrointestinal tract growth, motility, and overall function appear to be similar, particularly with respect to peptide hormones, some of which are found both in the brain and the intestinal tract, for example, cholecystokinin (Yalow and Straus 1977). Both pigs and humans are able to use some fiber as a source of energy because of fermentation that occurs in the large intestine.

Based on this increasing awareness of many parallels between pigs and humans regarding digestive tract function, it is not surprising that the pig is finding favor as a model animal for biomedical research (Tumbleson 1986). Details of digestive physiology in the pig are available (Kidder and Manners 1978; Low and Partridge 1980; Moran 1982).

Body Composition

The adult human and pig are similar in body composition, and both species tend to become obese during adulthood if eating is not restrained. Thus the pig is a favorable model for human obesity; furthermore, it allows the study of lipid metabolism in animals of contrasting body fat to lean ratios. The newborn pig contains less than 2% body fat, in contrast to the full-term human infant with an average fat content of more than 10%. Baker et al. (1970) observed that the newborn pig resembles the low–birth-weight human infant in fat content and suggested the pig as a model for studies of alimentation of premature infants. Mersmann (1986) reviewed lipid metabolism in swine and pointed out important differences between pigs and humans. The primary site of fatty acid biosynthesis is adipose tissue in swine and the liver in humans. Lipoprotein structure is similar in pigs and humans, but metabolism may differ because pigs must transport lipids from adipose tissue, where fatty acids are synthesized, to the liver, where lipoproteins are synthesized. Lipolysis in adipose tissue is stimulated by beta-adrenergic agonists and inhibited by alpha-adrenergic agonists. The specificity of these agonists for control of lipolysis is different in pigs and humans. The pig does not have alpha-adrenergic inhibition of lipolysis; this represents a distinct species difference in the metabolism of lipids. Despite these differences, the pig serves as an excellent animal model for humans leading a sedentary life and tending toward excessive calorie intake. Also, a wide range of body types occurs in swine, as in humans. Contemporary swine bred for leanness represent the major segment of the pig population in the United States. In contrast, some strains of pigs have been selectively bred for their small size (Hanford, Hormel, and Gottingen miniature swine) while others evolved naturally (Yucatan swine). Some swine display a tendency toward obesity (Ossabaw swine); still others have been selected for low or high backfat thickness over many generations (Hetzer and Harvey 1967). Ferrell and Cornelius (1984) determined the changes in body composition of pigs representing contemporary and obese (Hetzer and Harvey 1967) body types from age 4 to 24 weeks. These data are summarized in Table 1.1. Fat accumulated in the bodies of obese pigs much more rapidly than in lean contemporary pigs. By age 24 weeks, obese pigs contained 46.5% fat, as compared with 25.4% for lean pigs. Human infants compare roughly with 4-week-old pigs in body fat content (obese, 13.3%; contemporary, 9.7%) and normal adult humans are similar to 24-week-old contemporary swine, while obese adult humans compare favorably with 24-week-old obese swine. Direct measurements of body composition in living humans, of course, are not feasible, but estimates based on indirect procedures indicate that highly trained male athletes contain about 9% fat, while sedentary obese males may contain 40% to 50% or more fat; females in all categories are slightly fatter. Davidson et al. (1979) listed the normal chemical composition of a man weighing 65 kg as 17.0% protein, 13.8% fat, 1.5% carbohydrate, 6.1% minerals, and 61.6% water. This information was compiled from actual analyses of several cadavers. Table 1.2 summarizes literature data (Davidson et al. 1979) on fat content of adult men and women estimated from indirect measurements. For studies of swine nutrition and feeding, a knowledge of genetic background of the animal is important, for there is evidence of interactions between nutrition and genetic background as related to body composition. A similar relationship probably exists in humans, though it is not well documented.

NUTRIENT REQUIREMENTS OF PIGS AND PEOPLE

In more ways than any other nonprimate mammal, the pig's nutrient requirements resemble those of the human. Much has been written about the nutrition of the pig (Whitehair and Miller 1975; Cunha 1977; Kidder and Manners 1978; Low and Partridge 1980; Moran 1982; Pond and Maner 1974, 1984; Tumbleson 1987). Additionally, the National Research Council (1973, 1979, 1988), National Academy of Sciences, regularly publishes new information on quantitative nutrient requirements of swine during each phase of the life cycle. Table 1.3 lists the nutrients known to be required by swine. Humans are known to require the same nutrients plus vitamin C, chromium, and probably inositol and para-aminobenzoic acid. The National Research

Table 1.1 Least-Square Means for Live Weight, Empty Body Weight, and Weight of Gross Chemical Empty Body Components of Obese and Contemporary Pigs

			Empty Body Component (kg)					
Type	*Age (wk)*	*No. of Pigs*	*Total Weight*	*Water*	*Fat*	*Nitrogen*	*FFOM*	*Ash*
Obese	4	4	4.56	3.08	0.61	0.09	0.72	0.15
	8	3	9.78	6.53	1.39	0.19	1.76	0.33
	12	6	24.8	14.4	5.82	0.61	3.90	0.71
	18	6	50.5	25.2	16.7	1.17	7.25	1.38
	24	6	87.8	34.4	40.8	1.70	10.5	2.05
Contemporary	4	5	7.75	5.38	0.75	0.20	1.34	0.28
	8	6	13.3	9.31	1.36	0.34	2.19	0.40
	12	6	31.3	20.6	4.47	0.81	5.38	0.88
	18	6	63.2	37.9	12.2	1.80	11.1	1.96
	24	6	81.9	44.9	20.8	2.22	13.7	2.47
SE			0.79	0.47	0.33	0.020	0.13	0.026

Abbreviation: FFOM, fat-free organic matter.

(Reprinted, by permission, from Ferrell and Cornelius 1984.)

Table 1.2 Estimates of Fat Content Obtained by Underwater Weighing of Adult Men and Women (Fat as a Percentage of Body Weight)

Sex/Location	*Age (yr)*	*Mean*	*Range*
Males			
Prague, Czechoslovakia (trained runners)	22.5	6.3	
Edinburgh, Scotland	18–22	11	5–27
Tokyo, Japan	22	12	6–22
Minneapolis, MN	25	14	
Minneapolis, MN	55	26	
Females			
Prague, Czechoslovakia (Olympic gymnasts)		8	
Edinburgh, Scotland	18–22	26	18–35
Ithaca, NY	16–30	29	20–38
Tokyo, Japan	21	23	13–33
Minneapolis, MN	24	25	
Ithaca, NY	50–60	42	29–55
Minneapolis, MN	56	38	

(Reprinted, by permission, from Davidson et al. 1979.)

Council (1980b) provides recommended daily allowances (RDA) of all nutrients known to be required by humans.

The list of required mineral elements for both swine and humans may be expected to increase as more sensitive instrumentation and more complete control of environmental contamination (plastic instead of metal cages and utensils; highly purified air, water, and feed) become available. A large number of mineral elements are found in animal tissues, but no metabolic function has been assigned to some of them. Their significance in practical swine feeding remains unknown. Most are of more concern as toxic elements than as possible required nutrients. Others, including vanadium, chromium, and silicon, are required for specific animal species but have not yet been shown to be required for swine (National Research Council, 1988; Church and Pond 1982). Quantitative estimates of the requirements by swine in various phases of growth and productive function are discussed elsewhere in this book.

THE PIG AS AN ANIMAL MODEL FOR NUTRITION RESEARCH

General Considerations

The use of swine in biomedical research of nutrition and metabolic diseases has increased dramatically in recent years and can be expected to accelerate due to public sentiment against the use of dogs, the escalating cost of pound dogs, and their largely unknown genetic background and health. Research into chronic human diseases with nutritional implications, such as atherosclerosis, hypertension, cerebrovascular arteriosclerosis, gastric ulcers, obesity, alcoholism, osteoporosis, certain types of cancer, and protein-calorie malnutrition has increasingly involved the pig as the animal model

Table 1.3 Nutrients Known to Be Required by Swine

- Inorganic elements
  - Calcium
  - Chlorine
  - Cobalt (only as a component of vitamin B_{12})
  - Copper
  - Iron
  - Iodine
  - Magnesium
  - Manganese
  - Phosphorus
  - Potassium
  - Selenium
  - Sodium
  - Sulfur (as a component of thiamin, biotin, methionine, cystine, several other organic components, and sulfate)
  - Zinc
- Amino acids
  - Arginine (required for growth and probably lactation)
  - Histidine
  - Isoleucine
  - Leucine
  - Lysine
  - Methionine (50% can be replaced by cystine)
  - Phenylalanine (30% can be replaced by tyrosine)
  - Threonine
  - Tryptophan
  - Valine
- Vitamins
  - Fat-soluble
    - A
    - D
    - E
    - K
  - Water-soluble
    - Biotin
    - Choline
    - Folacin
    - Niacin (nicotinic acid, nicotinamide)
    - Pantothenic acid
    - Riboflavin
    - Thiamin
    - Vitamin B_{12}
    - Vitamin B_6 (pyridoxine, pyridoxamine, pyridoxal are all active forms)
- Fat
  - Essential fatty acids (linoleic and possibly alpha-linolenic, arachidonic)

(Pond and Houpt 1978; Roberts and Dodds 1982; Stanton and Mersmann 1986; Tumbleson 1987). An exhaustive review of the literature is beyond the scope of this chapter.

Diet and Cardiovascular Disease

A brief summary of how the pig is being used to study one group of chronic diseases, cardiovascular disease, may invoke a better appreciation of the great importance of swine in biomedical research. The role of nutritional factors in cardiovascular health is interrelated with age, sex, genetic background, exercise, drugs, and psychosocial conditions; the pig has been used to study each of these. There is clear documentation that the pig is a useful animal model for studies of human cardiovascular disease (Chapman and Goldstein 1976; Wissler and Vesselinovitch 1978; Pond 1982; Roberts et al. 1982; Stanton and Mersmann 1986).

As in humans, hypercholesterolemic diets produce aortic atherosclerosis in swine (Mahley et al. 1975; Goldsmith and Jacobi 1978). The evidence for an association between serum cholesterol and coronary artery disease in humans is persuasive and has led to recommendations (United States Department of Agriculture-Health, Education and Welfare [USDA-HEW] 1980) for decreased intake of red meat, increased consumption of fish and poultry, decreased intake of foods high in fat and cholesterol, and partial substitution of polyunsaturated fat for saturated fat in the diet. There is disagreement as to whether such recommendations should apply to the general population or just to individuals with the well-established forms of familial hyperlipidemia. Given the knowledge of wide genetic diversity in the United States, one might predict variable responses to particular diets. The genetic diversity of the pig offers the opportunity to explore the interrelationships between nutrition and genetic background in cardiovascular disease. Widespread occurrence of spontaneous atherosclerosis among many genotypes is reported in aged swine populations. Swine are generally fed diets containing cereals with little or no added fat, in contrast to humans, whose typical diet in the United States contains fat providing 30% to 40% of metabolizable energy. There is a large body of data showing nutritionally induced atherosclerosis in swine from an array of genetic backgrounds (Rowsell et al. 1960; Fuller et al. 1972; Mahley et al. 1975; Khan et al. 1977; Goldsmith and Jacobi 1978; Kummerow et al. 1978; Pownell et al. 1980). The literature is replete with reports of atherosclerosis induced in swine by high fat-high cholesterol diets (Pond 1986). Dietary fat source (Goldsmith and Jacobi 1978), protein level (Barnes et al. 1959; Baker et al. 1968; Pond et al. 1986), and protein source (Kim et al. 1978; Forsythe et al. 1980) have all been shown to affect plasma cholesterol. Saturated fatty acids, cholesterol, low-protein diets, and animal protein increase plasma cholesterol in swine and other species. The role of these factors in the development of atherosclerotic lesions in swine needs further clarification, but the response of plasma cholesterol to these dietary variables is striking. Oxidized cholesterol (Imai et al. 1976; Peng and Taylor 1984) and excess vitamin D (Huang et al. 1977) are both of concern as atherogenic agents.

Cholesterol is unstable and is easily oxidized when stored. These oxidized products of cholesterol, present in powdered eggs and powdered milk, increase aortic smooth muscle cell death and produce defects in arterial cell wall surfaces in animals. The possibility for nutritional intervention at the dietary or cellular level with antioxidants for control of atherosclerosis seems plausible, and the pig may be a good model for this exploration. Pigs fed diets supplemented with fat and high levels of vitamin

D have greater aortic atherosclerosis than pigs fed either one alone. Controlled long-term studies are needed to clarify these relationships between dietary vitamin D, fat, and atherosclerosis.

The role of dietary fiber in protecting against atherosclerosis has received some attention in swine. Kim et al. (1980) found an increase in fecal loss of bile acids in swine fed a grain-based diet compared with a semipurified diet and suggested that the mixed natural fibers in the former accounted for the loss.

The dynamics of cholesterol metabolism as related to the atherogenic process, which are so difficult to quantify in humans, can be addressed more readily in swine (Marsh et al. 1972; Arguepirse et al. 1983). The similarity in structure and physiology of the gastrointestinal tract to that of humans makes the pig an excellent animal model because of the role of the gut in cholesterol metabolism. The pathogenesis of diet-induced atherosclerotic lesions is still not firmly established. Lee et al. (1986) proposed that atherosclerosis is due to selective accumulation of lipids in the intimal cell masses that are present from birth in swine. The final answer to this question in humans may be derived from definitive studies in swine under carefully controlled nutritional conditions. The importance of genetic background, relative to response to diet, looms in atherogenesis as in many other chronic metabolic diseases, as exemplified by the observation (Pond et al. 1985) that obesity per se is not necessarily associated with the development of atherosclerosis in pigs and that an innate ability to metabolize high dietary cholesterol is of greater importance than body fatness in determining the response to diet.

Diet and Immunity

There are many examples in the literature of interactions between nutritional adequacy and immune responses (Good et al. 1980). Miller (1985) reviewed mineral and infectious disease interactions in animals including swine, and Blair and Newsome (1985) did so for swine. As the rapidly expanding field of immunology unfolds, there likely will be many interrelationships discovered between immune response and nutritional status. The pig has already become a well-accepted model animal for this type of research as evidenced by the activities of several biomedical research groups reporting work in pig immunology (Tumbleson 1986).

PORK IN THE HUMAN DIET

Pork is an excellent source of many nutrients not supplied abundantly by plant materials. It contains large amounts of vitamins and trace mineral elements, and its amino acid balance is much superior to that of most plant proteins. One might consider the pig as an efficient storage depot for fat, including essential fatty acids, and for protein, vitamins, and minerals. If one were to purchase each of the nutritional components of pork off the shelves of a health food store, that is, vitamins, minerals, and amino acids, the cost of the nutrients provided in a 3-ounce chop would be prohibitive. Of course, this is true of meat from other food animal species as well, but each has its own unique flavor and special eating qualities, and pork enjoys good acceptance by consumers world-wide, as discussed earlier in this chapter. The role of the pig as a scavenger in many places and as a family food bank or cash (piggy) bank in many cultures, for example, Haiti, speaks clearly in favor of its survival as an important food source for the foreseeable future. Some argue that pork production cannot be sustained in a world in which the pig competes directly with humans for food. This argument notwithstanding, there are both aesthetic and nutritional grounds for the pig to survive and flourish. No one has yet produced a synthetic ham or pork chop equal to the real thing at any price.

Pork Composition

The chemical composition of pork has been described by Leverton and Odell (1958), Watt and Merrill (1963), Kiernat et al. (1964), Rice (1971), Moss et al. (1983), and the USDA (1983). The fat content of pork has declined dramatically since the 1960s, as reflected by increases in protein and decreases in fat percentages in retail carcass weight, decreased carcass backfat thickness, and decreased kilocalories of metabolizable energy per 100 g of retail carcass (Pond and Maner 1984). The relationships between USDA grade, backfat, percentages of protein, fat, and water, and kilocalories of metabolizable energy per 100 g of retail cuts of pork (Ono 1982, cited by Pond and Maner 1984) are shown in Table 1.4. Note the marked decline in fat and calorie content of contemporary pork as compared with that reported in the 1960s (Kiernat et al. 1964). The relatively low fat content of most lean cuts of pork is noteworthy. The publication, Composition of Foods (USDA 1983), contains detailed information on composition of raw, cooked, and processed pork and pork products. Cooking reduces the water content so that percentages of protein, fat, and ash are increased appreciably. Roasted lean pork may contain as little as 82% of the water and up to 150% of the protein of raw pork (Kiernat et al. 1964). Cooking methods obviously affect fat losses, and any method that results in dripping losses of fat will reduce the percentage of fat as well as of water in the consumed product.

In addition to variations in composition related to processing and cooking, there may be variations associated with biological factors such as age, sex, nutritional background, and genetic make-up of the animal. Interactions between and among these factors are not well understood or documented; this void in information provides opportunities and challenges for scientists engaged in swine research, including those associated with nutrition. Now, more than ever before, consumers are conscious of nutritional attributes and liabilities of food products, and the knowledge to be gained through research associated with nutritional factors affecting pork composition will be especially valuable.

The composition of specific cuts of pork from contemporary swine is summarized in Table 1.5 from the USDA (1983). This information provides mean ± standard deviation for each nutrient. Pork is notable among other animal products in its high content of thiamin and unsaturated fatty acids. It is similar to lean beef, lamb, and poultry meat

Table 1.4 Water, Protein, Fat, and Metabolizable Energy Content of Retail Cuts of Pork

Retail Cut	*USDA Grade*	*Backfat (cm)*	*Protein (%)*	*Fat (%)*	*Water (%)*	*ME (kcal/100 g)*
Picnic	1	2.78	19.9	7.2	73.6	150
	2	4.01	19.4	7.4	73.3	150
	3	4.51	19.2(15.8)[a]	6.8(24.7)	74.0(58.9)	144(290)
Ham	1	2.78	20.0	5.5	74.0	140
	2	4.01	19.4	5.6	73.9	135
	3	4.51	20.5(15.9)	6.2(26.6)	73.6(56.5)	144(308)
Loin	1	3.00	20.7	6.9	71.5	151
	2	4.09	20.6	8.1	70.7	161
	3	4.74	20.2(17.1)	9.8(24.9)	69.2(57.2)	175(298)
Spare rib	1	2.49	17.8	26.2	57.7	312
	3	4.23	17.0(14.5)	25.2(33.2)	58.1(51.8)	300(361)

Abbreviation: ME, metabolizable energy.

[a]Values in parentheses are from Kiernat et al. 1964, based on data from pork produced in the 1950s and early 1960s. Note the dramatic decrease in fat content of picnic, ham, and loin, and the increase in protein content during the 20-year period. These dramatic changes have resulted from improved feeding and genetic selection for leanness.

(Data from United States Department of Agriculture. K. Ono. 1982. [Unpublished data.] Meat Science Research Laboratory, Agricultural Research Service. Beltsville, MD.)

Table 1.5 Composition of Selected Pork Cuts (Fresh, Whole, Separable Lean Only, Raw)

	Loin[a]			*Ham*[a]		
Nutrients (Units)	*Mean*	*Standard Error*	*No. of Samples*	*Mean*	*Standard Error*	*No. of Samples*
Proximate						
Water	70.55	0.159	77	72.90	0.177	51
Energy (kcal)	156			136		
(kJ)	654			570		
Protein (N × 6.25) (g)	20.68	0.077	78	20.48	0.139	53
Total lipid (fat)(g)	7.54	0.177	77	5.41	0.190	51
Carbohydrate, total (g)	0.00			0.00		
Fiber (g)	0.00			0.00		
Ash (g)	1.05	0.004	72	1.05	0.009	37
Minerals (mg)						
Calcium	7	0.121	36	6	0.339	38
Iron	0.85	0.015	115	1.01	0.024	167
Magnesium	23	0.171	72	25	0.431	25
Phosphorus	230	1.952	75	229	3.895	11
Potassium	353	1.672	60	369	3.071	149
Sodium	64	1.160	111	55	1.099	123
Zinc	2.14	0.025	60	2.27	0.105	27
Copper	0.075	0.001	96	0.075	0.002	51
Manganese	0.014	0.000	60	0.029		
Vitamins						
Ascorbic acid (mg)	0.9			0.9		
Thiamin (mg)	1.007	0.031	89	0.875	0.027	47
Riboflavin (mg)	0.300	0.019	87	0.228	0.010	46
Niacin (mg)	5.403	0.066	60	5.338	0.140	34
Pantothenic acid (mg)	0.814			0.805		
Vitamin B_6 (mg)	0.53	0.014	61	0.50		
Folacin (μg)	5			9	3.150	4
Vitamin B_{12} (μg)	0.86	0.009	60	0.71	0.056	11
Vitamin A (IU)	7			6		

Lipids						
Fatty acids						
Saturated, total (g)	2.61			1.88		
4:0						
6:0						
8:0						
10:0	0.01	0.000	73	0.01	0.000	73
12:0	0.01	0.001	75	0.01	0.000	75
14:0	0.09	0.003	377	0.07	0.002	377
16:0	1.67	0.040	377	1.20	0.042	377
18:0	0.82	0.020	377	0.59	0.021	377
Monounsaturated, total (g)	3.42			2.45		
16:1	0.24	0.007	377	0.17	0.006	377
18:1	3.11	0.075	377	2.23	0.079	377
20:1	0.05	0.002	71	0.04	0.001	71
22:1						
Polyunsaturated, total (g)	0.79			0.57		
18:2	0.66	0.020	377	0.47	0.018	377
18:3	0.04	0.003	112	0.03	0.002	112
18:4						
20:4	0.09	0.005	314	0.07	0.004	314
20:5						
22:5						
22:6						
Cholesterol (mg)	60	0.436	64	68	3.212	25
Amino acids (g)						
Tryptophan	0.278		14	0.275		14
Threonine	0.973		270	0.963		270
Isoleucine	0.999		277	0.989		277
Leucine	1.681		277	1.664		277
Lysine	2.038		285	2.018		285
Methionine	0.510		286	0.505		286

(*Table 1.5. continued*)

Nutrients (Units)	*Loin*[a]			*Ham*[a]		
	Mean	*Standard Error*	*No. of Samples*	*Mean*	*Standard Error*	*No. of Samples*
Amino acids (g)						
Cystine	0.268		48	0.265		48
Phenylalanine	0.827		285	0.819		285
Tyrosine	0.738		285	0.731		285
Valine	1.109		285	1.097		285
Arginine	1.436		285	1.422		285
Histidine	1.049		285	1.038		285
Alanine	1.224		282	1.212		282
Aspartic acid	1.919		284	1.900		284
Glutamic acid	3.213		285	3.181		285
Glycine	0.943		282	0.934		282
Proline	0.784		276	0.776		276
Serine	0.850		270	0.842		270

[a]Amount in 100 g, edible portion.

(Reprinted, by permission, from USDA 1983.)

in cholesterol and total fat. Potential changes in the concentration of any one nutrient in pork that might be possible through genetic selection, nutritional manipulation, or some combination, are currently unknown, but will depend on the nature of the components contributing to the variability for each constituent.

Pork Acceptability

In addition to the high nutritive value of pork discussed previously, there are aesthetic factors to be considered. The acceptability of pork in relation to other needs depends on aesthetic, economic, cultural, and religious constraints. Variations in palatability factors such as tenderness, juiciness, color, aroma, and flavor are less with pork than with beef and lamb so that differences in age, breed, and environment have relatively little effect on pork quality. Color, firmness, and water-holding capacity are included in a general appraisal of quality ranging from pale, soft exudative (PSE) pork to dark, firm, dry (DFD) pork; the most desirable is between these extremes. The amount of intermuscular fat is rather constant and no differences have been noted between PSE and normal muscle in their percentages of protein, fat, and water. The pale color and excessive exudation of PSE pork detracts from its marketability in the retail store. Some believe that undue selection for larger, bulging muscles resulted in an increased incidence of this syndrome; as a result, lean swine production has been moderated in the United States. The nutritional implications of this and other potential analogous syndromes in swine production are largely undetermined.

Other detracting influences on pork acceptability are the boar odor problem and trichinosis. Meat from mature boars has an objectionable odor and flavor when cooked, due to the presence of at least one fat-soluble substance, 5-alpha-androstenone. Because boars grow faster, require less feed per unit of body weight gain, and produce leaner carcasses than castrated males, it would be advantageous to producers and consumers if the boar odor could be removed without castration. Such a possibility is being explored in several laboratories using selection (Willeke et al. 1980), immunological, and hormone implant approaches (Schanbacher et al. 1985; Falvo et al. 1986). If these techniques reach commercial application, there will be a need for further quantification of nutritional requirements of boars for meat production.

The persistence of the parasite *Trichinella spiralis* has been a detriment to the consumption of pork in the United States and elsewhere. This is true despite the fact that in the United States the number of reported human cases of trichinosis has declined to less than 100 annually in recent years. Nevertheless, the perception of a threat of infection from eating raw pork continues to exist disproportionately to its actual importance. *Trichinella* organisms are destroyed by heating pork to an internal temperature of 77 °C, by freezing it for 20 days at −15 °C (Price and Schweigert 1971), and by gamma irradiation. Commercial application of irradiation of all pork marketed in the United States could eliminate the danger of trichinosis; the public perception of this method of control will probably determine its economic feasibility.

Table 1.6 Leading Pork-Consuming Countries (kg/Person/Year)

Rank	*1971*		*1981*[a]	
1	West Germany	(41)	Denmark	(56)
2	Austria	(38)	East Germany	(55)
3	Denmark	(36)	West Germany	(51)
4	United States	(33)	Austria	(48)
5	Switzerland	(32)	Switzerland	(46)
6	Hungary	(32)	Hungary	(46)
7	Bel-Lux	(31)	Bel-Lux	(42)
8	Canada	(30)	The Netherlands	(40)
9	France	(30)	Czechoslovakia	(49)
10	Republic of Ireland	(30)	China/Taiwan	(37)
11	United Kingdom	(30)	France	(36)
12	Sweden	(30)	Republic of Ireland	(34)

[a]Estimated.

Future of Pork Consumption

The future of swine in the United States and world-wide will depend on the adaptability of the industry to changing economic conditions and consumer needs and desires. Major challenges will be to promote the economic, educational, and cultural climate needed to enhance food production capabilities in developing countries. Such enhancement will stimulate economic incentives for pork production. Changes in per capita pork consumption are dynamic (Table 1.6), as shown by the changes in ranking among some of the countries in which pork is a major food item. Note that the United States, where per capita consumption of pork has remained nearly constant for many decades, was not among the top 12 countries in 1981. Eastern and Western European countries dominated in per capita pork consumed in 1981, with Denmark increasing by 20 kg (56%) and Hungary by 14 kg (44%) from 1971. Fitzhugh et al. (1978) projected the proportions of food energy and protein that humans will obtain from pigs, poultry, and ruminants by the year 2000. They predicted an increase of 23% for pigs, 23% for poultry (chickens, ducks, and turkeys), and 28% for ruminants (cattle, sheep, and goats) between 1970 and 2000. They projected that pigs will provide 215 billion megacalories of metabolizable energy and 3 million metric tons of protein in the year 2000. By their estimates, pork will provide 23% of the energy and 8% of the protein from animal sources, including milk, in the year 2000, as compared with 25% and 9%, respectively, in 1970. Thus, the production of pork is predicted to increase substantially, but the overall contribution of pork to human nutrition is predicted to decline slightly. The accuracy of this prediction obviously will be affected not only by advances in production technology, including feeding and nutrition, but also by economic, cultural, and political developments that transcend considerations of animal biology and human nutrient requirements.

REFERENCES

Arguepirse, J., J. Ferezou, and F. Chevallier. 1983. *Biochimie* 65:275.
Baker, D.H., R.R. Diller, and C.E. Jordan. 1968. *J. Anim. Sci.* 27:660.
Baker, G.L., D.W. Anderson, and S.A. Eash. 1970. *J. Clin. Nutr.* 23:926.
Barnes, R.H., et al. 1959. *J. Nutr.* 69:269.
Blair, R., and F. Newsome. 1985. *J. Anim. Sci.* 60:1508.
Bustad, L.K., and R.O. McClellan. 1966. *Swine in Biomedical Research.* Richland, WA: Pacific Northwest Laboratory.
Chapman, M.J., and S. Goldstein. 1976. *Atherosclerosis* 25:267.
Church, D.C., and W.G. Pond. 1982. *Basic Animal Nutrition and Feeding.* 2d ed. New York: John Wiley and Sons.
Cunha, T.J. 1977. *Swine Feeding and Nutrition.* New York: Academic Press.
Davidson, S., et al. 1979. *Human Nutrition and Dietetics.* New York: Churchill, Livingstone.
Falvo, R.E., et al. 1986. *J. Anim. Sci.* 63:986.
Ferrell, C.L., and S.G. Cornelius. 1984. *J. Anim. Sci.* 58:903.
Fitzhugh, H.A., et al. 1978. *The Role of Ruminants in Support of Man.* Morrilton, AR: Winrock International Livestock Research and Training Center.
Forsythe, W.A., et al. 1980. *J. Nutr.* 110:2467.
Fuller, G.C., et al. 1972. *Connect. Tissue Res.* 1:217.
Goldsmith, D.P.J., and H.P. Jacobi. 1978. *Lipids* 13:174.
Good, R.A., A. West, and G. Fernandez. 1980. *Fed. Proc.* 39:3098.
Hetzer, H.O., and W.R. Harvey. 1967. *J. Anim. Sci.* 26:1244.
Huang, W.Y., et al. 1977. *Artery* 3:439.
Imai, H., et al. 1976. *Arch. Pathol. Lab. Med.* 100:565.
Khan, M.A., et al. 1977. *Exp. Mol. Pathol.* 26:63.
Kidder, D.E., and M.J. Manners. 1978. *Digestion in the Pig.* Bath, England: Kingston Press.
Kiernat, B.H., J.A. Johnson, and A.J. Siedler. 1964. Chicago: *Am. Meat Inst. Found. Bull. No. 57.*
Kim, D.N., et al. 1978. *Exp. Mol. Pathol.* 29:385.
Kim, D.N., et al. 1980. *Exp. Mol. Pathol.* 33:25.
Kummerow, F.A., et al. 1978. *Artery* 4:360.
Lee, K.T., D.N. Kim, and W.A. Thomas. 1986. In: *The Use of Swine in Cardiovascular Research,* Vol. 2. Stanton, H.C., and H.J. Mersmann (Eds.). Boca Raton, FL: CRC Press.
Leverton, R.M., and G.V. Odell. 1958. *Oklahoma Agricultural Experiment Station Miscellaneous Publication No. MP-49.* Stillwater, OK: Oklahoma Agricultural Experiment Station.
Low, A.G., and I.G. Partridge. 1980. *Current Concepts of Digestion and Absorption in Pigs. Tech. Bull. 3.* Reading, U.K.: College of Estate Management.
Mahley, R.W., et al. 1975. *Biochemistry* 14:2817.
Marsh, A., et al. 1972. *J. Lipid Res.* 13:600.
Mellen, I.M. 1952. *The Natural History of the Pig.* New York: Exposition Press.
Mersmann, H.J. 1986. In: *Swine in Cardiovascular Research.* Stanton, H.C., and H.J. Mersmann (Eds.). Boca Raton, FL: CRC Press.
Miller, E.R. 1985. *J. Anim. Sci.* 60:1500.
Miller, E.R., and D.E. Ullrey. 1987. *Ann. Rev. Nutr.* 7:361.
Montagna, W. 1966. In: *Swine in Biomedical Research.* Bustad, L.K., and R.O. McClellan (Eds.). p. 285. Richland, WA: Pacific Northwest Laboratory.
Moran, E.T., Jr. 1982. *Comparative Nutrition of Fowl and Swine. The Gastrointestinal Systems.* Guelph, Ontario: Office for Educational Practice, University of Guelph.
Moss, M., et al. 1983. *J. Food Sci.* 48:1767.
National Research Council. 1973. *Nutrient Requirements of Swine.* Washington, DC: National Academy of Sciences.

National Research Council. 1979. *Nutrient Requirements of Swine.* Washington, DC: National Academy of Sciences.
National Research Council. 1980a. *Mineral Tolerance of Domestic Animals.* Washington, DC: National Academy of Sciences.
National Research Council. 1980b. *Recommended Daily Allowances.* Washington, DC: National Academy of Sciences.
National Research Council. 1988. *Nutrient Requirements of Swine.* Washington, DC: National Academy of Sciences.
Nielson, T.W., et al. 1966. In: *Swine in Biomedical Research.* Bustad, L.K., and R.O. McClellan (Eds.). p. 259. Richland, WA: Pacific Northwest Laboratory.
Peng, S.-K., and C.B. Taylor. 1984. *World Rev. Nutr. Diet* 44:117.
Pond, W.G. 1982. In: *Pig Model for Biomedical Research.* Roberts, H.R., and W.J. Dodds (Eds.). p. 43. Maoli, Taiwan, R.O.C.: Pig Research Institute of Taiwan.
Pond, W.G. 1983. *Scientific American* May, p. 96.
Pond, W.G. 1986. In: *Swine in Cardiovascular Research.* Stanton, H.C., and H.J. Mersmann (Eds.). Boca Raton, FL: CRC Press.
Pond, W.G., and K.A. Houpt. 1978. *Biology of the Pig.* Ithaca, NY: Cornell University Press.
Pond, W.G., and J.H. Maner. 1974. *Swine Production in Temperate and Tropical Environments.* San Francisco: W.H. Freeman and Co.
Pond, W.G., and J.H. Maner. 1984. *Swine Production and Nutrition.* Westport, CT: AVI Publishing Co., Inc.
Pond, W.G., H.J. Mersmann, and J.T. Yen. 1985. *Proc. Soc. Exp. Biol. Med.* 170:90.
Pond, W.G., H.J. Mersmann, and J.T. Yen. 1986. *J. Nutr.* 116:1116–1124.
Pownell, H.J., et al. 1980. *J. Lipid Res.* 21:1108.
Price, J.F., and B.S. Schweigert. 1971. *The Science of Meat and Meat Products.* 2d ed. San Francisco: W.H. Freeman and Co.
Prince, J.H., et al. 1960. *Anatomy and Histology of the Eye and Orbit in Domestic Animals.* Springfield, IL: Thomas.
Rice, E.E. 1971. In: *The Science of Meat and Meat Products.* 2d ed. Price, V.F., and B.S. Schweigert (Eds.). San Francisco: W.H. Freeman and Co.
Roberts, H.R., and W.J. Dodds. 1982. In: *Pig Model for Biomedical Research.* Roberts, H.R., and W.J. Dodds (Eds.). Maoli, Taiwan, R.O.C.: Pig Research Institute of Taiwan.
Roberts, H.R., T.R. Griggs, and K.M. Brinkhaus. 1982. In: *Pig Model for Biomedical Research.* Roberts, H.R., and W.J. Dodds (Eds.). p. 60. Maoli, Taiwan, R.O.C.: Pig Research Institute of Taiwan.
Rowsell, H.C., H.G. Downie, and J.F. Mustard. 1960. *Can. Med. Assoc. J.* 83:1175.
Schanbacher, B.D., J.T. Yen, and W.G. Pond. 1985. *Meat Sci.* 13:237.
Schummer, A., R. Nickel, and W.O. Sack. 1979. *The Viscera of Domestic Animals.* 2d ed. New York: Springer-Verlag.
Stanton, H.C., and H.J. Mersmann. 1986. *Swine in Cardiovascular Research.* Boca Raton, FL: CRC Press.
Stevens, C.E. 1977. In: *Duke's Physiology of Domestic Animals.* 9th ed. Sevenson, M.J. (Ed.). p. 216. Ithaca, NY: Cornell University Press.
Towne, C.W., and E.N. Wentworth. 1950. *Pigs from Cave to Cornbelt.* Norman, OK: University of Oklahoma Press.
Tumbleson, M.E. 1986. *Swine in Biomedical Research.* Vols. 1, 2, and 3. New York: Plenum Publishing Co.
USDA. 1983. *Composition of Foods. Pork Products. Agriculture Handbook No. 8-10.* Washington, DC: Consumer Nutrition Division, Human Nutrition Information Service, USDA.
USDA-HEW. 1980. *Nutrient Content of the National Food Supply, Publication No. NRF-9.* Washington, DC.
Watt, B.K., and A.L. Merrill. 1963. *Agriculture Handbook No. 8.* Washington, DC: Consumer and Food Economic Research Division, Agriculture Research Service, USDA.
Weaver, M.E., F.W. Sorenson, and E.B. Jump. 1962. *Arch. Oral Biol.* 7:17.

Whitehair, C.K., and E.R. Miller. 1975. In: *Diseases of Swine*. Dunne, H.W., and A.D. Leman (Eds.). p. 1087. Ames, IA: Iowa State University Press.

Widdowson, E.M., and J.W.T. Dickerson. 1964. In: *Mineral Metabolism*. Vol. 2, Part A. Comar, C.L., and F. Bronner (Eds.). pp. 1–247. New York: Academic Press.

Willeke, H., et al. 1980. "A selection experiment on boar taint." In: *Selection Experiments in Laboratory and Domestic Animals*. Robertson, A. (Ed.). pp. 31–33. Slough, UK: Commonwealth Agricultural Bureaux.

Wissler, R.W., and D. Vesselinovitch. 1978. In: *International Symposium State of Prevention and Therapy in Human Arteriosclerosis and in Animal Models*. Hauss, W.G., et al. (Eds.). p. 13. Opladen, West Germany: Westdeutscher Verlag.

Yalow, R.S., and E. Straus. 1977. *First International Symposium Hormonal Receptors in Digestive Tract Physiol.* INSERM Sympos. No. 3. p. 79. Amsterdam: Elsevier/North Holland Biomedical Press.

Zeuner, F.E. 1963. In: *A History of Domesticated Animals*. London: Hutchinson.

Chapter 2

Ethology: Pigs and People

S.E. Curtis

Pigs fascinate people. They always have. Forty thousand years ago pigs and people were already interacting with one another. Humans hunted pigs in those days; then about ten thousand years ago we started domesticating them. This entailed much consideration—not to mention tolerance—of the pig's behavioral nature, its potentials, and its limitations (Price 1984).

All the while, some people have regarded pigs with reverence, others with loathing (Towne and Wentworth 1950; Bustad and Horstman 1986). As Marvin Harris (1974) wrote: "The riddle of the pig . . . presents the challenge of having to explain why certain people should hate, while others love, the very same animal." Most swineherds throughout history have experienced both feelings, sometimes toward the same pig on the same day; a pig can be intriguing one minute, exasperating the next. As Joseph Harris (1870) wrote:

> A cross-grained man will soon spoil a lot of well-bred pigs. They know the tones of his voice, and it is amusing to see what tricks they will play on him. We have seen such a man trying to get the pigs into their respective pens, and it would seem as though he had brought with him a legion of imps, and that seven of them had entered each pig.

See also the Gospel of Mark, chapter 5, verses 1 through 20, from the New Testament of the Bible.

Originally, people erected fences not to keep the swine in, but rather to keep them out of the gardens and crop fields. As early as the 1500s, English farmers were ringing pigs' noses: "Ring him be sure when he goes in your Meadow or Pasture: for he will be ploughing for ground Nuts, to the great Damage of your Ground, and no great profit to himself" (Tusser 1984).

There is further evidence of a close association between pigs and people by the late Middle Ages. In 1386, a sow, having been found guilty of killing a child, was sentenced by a French tribunal to be dressed in a man's clothes and taken to the town square, where it was to be "mangled and maimed in the head and forelegs, and then to be hanged" (Evans 1987).

More recently, pigs have been highly favored grist for many a writer's mill. We have been treated to wonderful renditions of true stories about a pet gilt, by Robert Newton Peck (1972); a moribund pig, by E.B. White (1977); and a variety of beguiling porcine characters, in works by Kent Britt (1978), William Hedgepeth (1978), Stephen S. Hall (1985), and Karl Schwenke (1985), among many others.

The curious fact that some people relish pork as food while others abhor it has had new light shed upon it by Marvin Harris (1985). Pigs have caught numerous artists' fancies, too (Winfrey 1982). Certainly, few children who have read them have failed to be enchanted by dozens of stories about pigs, like the one about Wilbur, in *Charlotte's Web* (White 1952).

The most likely reason pigs fascinate people is that these beasts are anything but subtle. They behave in obvious and interesting ways. They are such unusual creatures that, to a greater extent than most animals, they capture and hold our attention. For as long as we have been sharing life with pigs, we have been observing them carefully and thoughtfully. Therefore, it sometimes surprises us when we realize how little we know for sure about the ways pigs behave.

Most of our observations of swine behavior up to now have been casual and have not been subjected to scientific rigor. We now know, for example, that pigs behave differently in the presence of people than when they are alone. Because most casual observations of pigs in the past have been made in the presence of human beings, many of our earlier conclusions undoubtedly were clouded by procedural artifacts.

During the 1970s and especially the 1980s, however, the pace of sound ethological and psychological research on all agricultural animals quickened (Curtis and McGlone 1982; Curtis and Houpt 1983; Stricklin 1983, 1985), particularly on the pig (Curtis 1983; D. Fraser 1984; Hartsock and Curtis 1984; A.F. Fraser, 1985; van Putten 1987). The new, more scientific approaches currently being employed in investigations of pig behavior have resulted from the increasing recognition in agriculture and academe that swine welfare and productivity may be limited by behavioral constraints, many of which probably could be reduced or even eliminated if we better understood animal behavior. Such knowledge is attainable only from systematic observations, formalized studies, and controlled experiments.

The purpose of this chapter is to provide a brief overview of our current knowledge of pig behavior. It is not intended to be a thorough review of the scientific literature on the subject; the excellent contribution by David Fraser (1984) and the swine portions of the compilation edited by Andrew F. Fraser (1985) can be consulted in that regard. In this chapter, reference is made to some selected aspects of pig behavior that are being investigated actively now.

EATING AND DRINKING AND MEANS OF FEEDING AND WATERING

One cause of variation in growth rate among pigs is variation in voluntary feed intake, so pigs' eating and drinking behaviors are important. When feed was infused directly into pigs' digestive tracts at a rate 20% faster than the ad libitum intake rate, the pigs' rate of body-weight gain increased by 40%, but carcass composition remained the same

(Pekas 1985). The physiological control of feed intake in the pig is not yet understood completely (Houpt 1984), but it appears that there ordinarily are factors that limit pigs' feed intake to less than that which would support maximal lean growth.

The means of offering pigs feed and water are important determinants of ingestion rates. Olsson (1983) studied valve drinking systems for growing-finishing hogs. Drinking schedules were characterized under several schemes of water availability and were related to water wastage, environmental conditions, productive performance, and carcass quality. Continuous access to water was not necessary under the experimental conditions, and it was beneficial only if there were no behavioral or technical problems.

The movements a sow makes while eating feed have been quantified by kinematic analysis of high-speed cinematographic records (Taylor et al. 1987, 1988). This information, as well as body dimension data, has been used to design a sow feeder with which feed wastage is negligible and injury to the sow nil (Taylor et al. 1988).

MATING BEHAVIOR AND REPRODUCTIVE PERFORMANCE

Total reproductive efficiency of the swine herd can be affected by numerous behavioral factors (Curtis and Gonyou 1984). Findings that boars can hardly discriminate between estrous and anestrous sows while estrous sows show a clear preference to associate with intact boars (Signoret 1976) have implications for the design of breeding facilities and mating-management schemes. Knowledge of the effects of prepubertal and postpubertal social environments on reproductive development and efficiency is important for designers. For example, isolating adult boars from gilts and sows can reduce their libido, and prepubertal isolation of gilts from boars can lead to behavioral problems at mating (Hemsworth 1982). However, gilts also may become habituated to stimuli from boars residing nearby (Hemsworth et al. 1987b, 1988).

Effects of housing and management practices on the behavior, performance, and welfare of pregnant gilts and sows have been studied extensively as well (e.g., Barnett et al. 1984, 1986, 1987; Clark et al. 1985; Jensen 1984; McFarlane et al. 1988).

Farrowing sows' adaptability to various farrowing systems has been investigated, too, in terms of both behavior (Hansen and Curtis 1981; Heckt et al. 1988; Jensen 1986; Jensen and Redbo 1987; Jensen et al. 1987; Lammers and De Lange 1986; McGlone and Blecha 1987; Rohde Parfet et al. 1989; Vestergaard and Hansen 1984) and performance (Collins et al. 1987; Curtis et al. 1989). The behavior of newborn piglets also is becoming better understood, both basically and in terms of environmental and management factors (Lewis and Hurnik 1985; Rohde and Gonyou 1987; Rohde Parfet et al. 1989; Welch and Baxter 1986).

MANAGING FRUSTRATION

Pigs quickly learn to press a lever to obtain a feed reward. Soon they expect feed every time they operate the lever. At this point, in one experiment, researchers stopped rewarding the pigs for lever pressing. This frustrated the pigs, and the resulting stress was reflected by a 50% increase in the concentration of corticosteroids in the blood (Dantzer et al. 1980). Later, hungry pigs were fed at 4-minute intervals, and it was found that plasma corticosteroid concentration rose in the impatient animals' blood (Dantzer and Mormede 1981). However, when a chain was hung near the feeder, the pigs nibbled on it during periods between feed deliveries. Displacement or adjunctive activities of this sort might ordinarily be considered anomalous, but it was found further that pigs having access to a chain did not have an increase in corticosteroids at feeding time. Apparently, the opportunity to nibble on a chain served a homeostatic function.

Offering swine objects to manipulate as means of stabilizing their activities, particularly aggression, has been practiced by some producers for a long time, but in the past these recommendations have been based on anecdotes. Recent experiments with young pigs (Grandin et al. 1988) and prepartum sows (Widowski and Curtis 1988) provided new information on the value of manipulanda to the pig.

ENVIRONMENTAL ENRICHMENT

Weanling pigs given a simple means of environmental enrichment (viz., a trough of soil in the pen with a group of pigs) used the soil in a variety of activities (Wood-Gush and Beilharz 1983). In fact, when presented new soil and new feed at the same time, the pigs invariably used the soil before eating any feed. It was concluded that the trough of soil reduced boredom because it elicited various behaviors, and the pigs with access to soil spent less time lying. Environmental complexity can affect the development of the pig's somatosensory cortical neurons as well as several aspects of its subsequent behavior, including investigatory activities, maladaptation to social situations, time to approach a novel object or person, ease of handling, and vulnerability to being startled (Schouten 1986; Grandin et al. 1988).

OPERANT CONTROL OF ENVIRONMENTAL FEATURES

As pointed out by Kilgour et al. (1982), operant conditioning is a potent tool not only for learning animals' preferences but also in production systems aimed at returning some environmental control—so important to the pig's sense of well-being (Wiepkema 1982, 1987)—to the pigs themselves.

OPERANT CONTROL OF PHOTOPERIOD

How many hours a day should the lights in a hog house be left on? In practice, the current range is from constantly on to almost always off. When individual pigs were given a means of turning the lights on and off for themselves, they kept the lights on around 75% of the time (Baldwin and Meese 1977). Also, they inserted some darkness into almost every hour, around the clock, but did not leave the lights off for hours on end during the night. In a recent experiment, pigs were motivated to operate a system that rewarded them with 40 seconds of light, but not 40 seconds of darkness (Baldwin and Start 1985).

OPERANT CONTROL OF ENVIRONMENTAL TEMPERATURE

Environmental temperature has widely recognized effects on the health and productivity of growing swine (Curtis 1985a,b). This is especially so for newly weaned pigs. Certain behaviors contribute to the pig's ability to regulate body temperature. Selecting a comfortable niche is one such strategy (Fraser 1985; Balsbaugh and Curtis 1986).

The temperature inside houses for weanling pigs is usually kept uniform over space and constant over time. Of course, this arrangement precludes the pigs' selecting an environment more comfortable than that chosen by the caretaker. During cold weather, pigs that can control environmental temperature themselves—by operating a switch-relay device substituted for the common thermostat—called in orderly fashion for an afternoon high averaging 26 °C and a nighttime low of 15 °C; grew and converted feed to body-weight gain at rates similar to those observed in pigs residing at approximately 27 °C around the clock; and on average called for the burning of only half as much fuel as in a constant-temperature environment (Curtis and Morris 1982).

PREFERENCE TESTS

The interpretation of preference tests is controversial (Dawkins 1977; Duncan 1978; Duncan and Dawkins 1983). The attractiveness of letting a pig express its numerous preferences encourages ethologists to continue to learn more about the interpretation per se of preference test results and to develop test situations likely to reduce the biases inherent in this approach.

One study, by Mwanjali et al. (1983), employed a hexagonal system in an attempt to reduce the effects of biasing factors such as location, outer walls versus inner, feeder and water locations, air distribution, light intensity, and environmental temperatures. Its wedge-shaped cubicles were identical. Interpretational problems such as the extent to which short-term choices are related to long-term benefits still remain.

AGGRESSION AMONG GROUPMATES

Another important behavioral problem with swine is the extreme aggressiveness that sometimes erupts within a group. Jensen (1983) focused not on aggressiveness in terms of a dominance order, but rather on an avoidance order among sows in the same group, and found that such avoidance orders exist so long as the sows have sufficient space in which to operate. Young pigs have been found to be attracted to pig blood (Fraser

1987), and it has been suggested that minor wounds could stimulate vicious attacks of one pig by another.

At the time of group formation, young pigs will hide their heads as a means of avoiding aggressive groupmates, and the result is a significant reduction in wounding (McGlone and Curtis 1985). Of course, many modern production facilities have few or no places for animals to get away from an aggressive groupmate.

Urine or blood plasma from pigs that are engaging in aggressive encounters can modulate the aggressive behavior of other pigs on which it is applied, and this effect can be mimicked by the pheromone 5α-androst-16-en-3-one (McGlone et al. 1987). Use of this compound to manage aggression among pigs on farms is being evaluated (McGlone and Morrow 1988). The potential of artificial compounds for controlling aggression and stress in swine is also being studied (Gonyou et al. 1988; Bjork et al. 1988).

CONTACT WITH HUMANS

With reference to relations between caretakers and swine and the impact of these on performance traits, recent research has documented scientifically what has been suspected for a long time: there is considerable correlation between the ways pigs are treated by humans and the way they grow and reproduce.

Early handling of piglets affects the way they interact behaviorally with other pigs (Schoen et al. 1974) and with humans (Hemsworth et al. 1986b). Gilts that were handled in some unpleasant or negative fashion acted more anxiously in the presence of humans, grew more slowly, and had higher plasma concentrations of corticosteroids both while at rest and while in the presence of a human than did their counterparts that were handled in a pleasant or positive manner (Hemsworth et al. 1981a, 1986a; Gonyou et al. 1986). Moreover, human handlers send specific signals to pigs by the way they approach the pigs, the posture they assume, and whether they are wearing gloves (Hemsworth et al. 1986c). When gilts were treated inconsistently, frequent pleasant encounters with humans did not compensate for the untoward effects of brief, infrequent unpleasant ones (Hemsworth et al. 1987). Sows that were more at ease with a human experimenter tended to have higher reproductive performances as well (Hemsworth et al. 1981b).

VOCALIZATIONS

If pigs can understand the tones of our voices (Hemsworth et al. 1986), then we should be able to understand theirs. Vocalizations of pigs are being scrutinized phonetically and semantically by ethologists (Klingholz and Meynhardt 1979; Klingholz et al. 1979). Twenty-two discrete calls have been identified in adult swine (Grauvogl 1958). Jensen and Algers (1984) have categorized into five classes the vocalizations of piglets while they were suckling. Jensen and Algers are analyzing the behavioral contexts in which certain vocalizations occur at inordinate frequencies in an attempt to correlate specific vocalizations with the pigs' actions. The Nebraska group (DeShazer et al. 1988) is analyzing pig vocalizations electronically as they search for patterns associated with accidents, discomfort, and the like, which could be detected by computer in the first step of a pig-activated alarm system.

CODA

The recent advances in our knowledge of the behavioral adaptation of the pig to its physical and social surroundings cited herein are but examples of the many that could have been discussed. Little has been said about the welfare of the pigs or the limits of their adaptability (van Putten 1987), and nothing about the effects of social stress on growth (McGlone et al. 1987) or immune status (Kelley 1990); the handling of pigs in transportation and marketing channels (Grandin 1983); the stunning of pigs for slaughter (Hoenderken 1983); the ways floor quality affects the pig's foothold and gait (Christison and de Gooijer 1986; Applegate et al. 1988); how unpredictable management practices can influence the performance of growing pigs (Carlstead 1986); or a dozen other important topics. However, it is hoped that the examples will serve to demonstrate how rigorous scientific investigation is being brought to bear on the pig and the ways it behaves so that new understanding is crystallizing regularly. The job is much like the peeling of an onion—layer by layer, the organism reveals itself. However, for most people—though not all, certainly—most pigs are much more fascinating than most onions.

REFERENCES

Applegate, A.L., et al. 1988. *J. Anim. Sci.* 66:334.
Baldwin, B.A., and G.B. Meese. 1977. *Anim. Behav.* 25:497.
Baldwin, B.A., and I.B. Start. 1985. *Appl. Anim. Behav. Sci.* 14:233.
Balsbaugh, R.K., and S.E. Curtis. 1986. *J. Anim. Sci.* 62:315.
Barnett, J.L., et al. 1984. *Appl. Anim. Behav. Sci.* 12:209.
Barnett, J.L., et al. 1986. *Appl. Anim. Behav. Sci.* 16:249.
Barnett, J.L., et al. 1987. *Appl. Anim. Behav. Sci.* 17:229.
Baxter, M. 1983. *Appl. Anim. Ethol.* 9:207.
Bjork, A., et al. 1988. *J. Anim. Sci.* 66:669.
Britt, K. 1978. *National Geographic* 154:398.
Bustad, L.K., and V.G. Horstman. 1986. "Pigs: from B.C. to 2000 A.D.: from outhouse to penthouse." In: *Swine in Biomedical Research.* Vol. 1. Tumbleson, M.E. (Ed.). pp. 3–16. New York: Plenum Press.
Carlstead, K. 1986. *Appl. Anim. Behav. Sci.* 16:25.
Christison, G.I., and J.A. de Gooijer. 1986. *Livestock Prod. Sci.* 15:191.
Clark, J.R., et al. 1985. *Appl. Anim. Behav. Sci.* 14:127.
Collins, E.R., Jr., E.T. Kornegay, and E.D. Bonnette. 1987. *Appl. Anim. Behav. Sci.* 17:51.
Curtis, S.E. 1983. "Review of research on management, behavior and well-being of swine." In: *Proceedings of the Conference on the Human-Animal Bond.* Hall, W.F. (Ed.). pp. 26–38. St. Paul, MN: University of Minnesota.
Curtis, S.E. 1985a. "Physiological responses and adaptations of swine (hot environments)." In:

Stress Physiology in Livestock. Vol. 2. Yousef, M.K. (Ed.). pp. 59–66. Boca Raton, FL: CRC Press.

Curtis, S.E. 1985b. "Physiological responses and adaptations of swine (cold environments)." In: *Stress Physiology in Livestock.* Vol. 2. Yousef, M.K. (Ed.). pp. 129–140. Boca Raton, FL: CRC Press.

Curtis, S.E., and H.W. Gonyou. 1984. "Swine behavior and how it affects total reproductive efficiency." In: *Proceedings of the 1984 Pork Industry Conference.* pp. 122–132. Urbana, IL: University of Illinois.

Curtis, S.E., and K.A. Houpt. 1983. *J. Anim. Sci.* 57(Suppl. 2):234.

Curtis, S.E., et al. 1989. *J. Anim. Sci.* (In press.)

Curtis, S.E., and J.J. McGlone. 1982. *J. Anim. Sci.* 54:450.

Curtis, S.E., and G.L. Morris. 1982. "Operant supplemental heat in swine nurseries." In: *Proceedings of the Second International Livestock Environment Symposium.* pp. 295–297. St. Joseph, MI: American Society of Agricultural Engineers.

Dantzer, R., and P. Mormede. 1981. *Horm. Behav.* 15:386.

Dantzer, R., M. Arnone, and P. Mormede. 1980. *Physiol. Behav.* 24:1–4.

Dawkins, M. 1977. *Anim. Behav.* 25:1034.

Duncan, I.J.H. 1978. *Appl. Anim. Ethol.* 4:197.

Duncan, I.J.H., and M.R. Dawkins. 1983. "The problem of assessing 'well-being' and 'suffering' in farm animals." In: *Indicators Relevant to Farm Animal Welfare.* Smidt, D. (Ed.). pp. 13–24. Boston: Martinus Nijhoff.

Evans, E.P. 1987. *The Criminal Prosecution and Capital Punishment of Animals: The Lost History of Europe's Animal Trials.* Boston: Faber and Faber.

Fraser, A.F. (Ed.). 1985. *Ethology of Farm Animals: A Comprehensive Study of the Behavioural Features of the Common Farm Animals.* New York: Elsevier.

Fraser, D. 1984. *Appl. Anim. Ethol.* 11:317.

Fraser, D. 1985. *Appl. Anim. Behav. Sci.* 14:117.

Fraser, D. 1987. *Appl. Anim. Behav. Sci.* 17:61.

Gonyou, H.W., et al. 1986. *Appl. Anim. Behav. Sci.* 16:269.

Gonyou, H.W., et al. 1988. *J. Anim. Sci.* 66:2856.

Grandin, T. 1983. "The human factor in livestock handling." In: *Proceedings of the Conference on the Human-Animal Bond.* Hall, W.F. (Ed.). St. Paul, MN: University of Minnesota.

Grandin, T., S.E. Curtis, and W.T. Greenough. 1988. "Environmental enrichment for pigs: Differences in somatosensory cortical neurons and subsequent behavior." In: *Proceedings of the 6th Congress of the International Society of Animal Hygiene.* pp. 692–695. Skara, Sweden: Swedish University of Agricultural Sciences.

Grauvogl, A. 1958. Ueber das Verhalten des Hausschwein unter besonderer Besucksichtung des Vortpflanzungsverhaltens. *Vet.-Med. Dissertation,* Freie Universitaet, Berlin.

Hall, S.S. 1985. *Smithsonian Magazine* Nov., 146.

Hansen, K.E., and S.E. Curtis. 1981. *J. Anim. Sci.* 51:456.

Harris, J. 1870. *Harris on the Pig.* New York: Orange Judd.

Harris, M. 1974. *Cows, Pigs, Wars and Witches: Riddles of Culture.* New York: Random House.

Harris, M. 1985. *Good to Eat: Riddles of Food and Culture.* New York: Simon and Schuster.

Hartsock, T.G., and S.E. Curtis. 1984. *Appl. Anim. Ethol.* 11:401.

Heckt, W.L., et al. 1988. *J. Anim. Sci.* 66:1378.

Hedgepeth, W. 1978. *The Hog Book.* Garden City, NY: Dolphin Books/Doubleday.

Hemsworth, P.H. 1982. Social environment and reproduction. In: *Control of Pig Reproduction.* Cole, D.J.A., and G.R. Foxcroft (Eds.). pp. 585–601. Boston: Butterworths.

Hemsworth, P.H., J.L. Barnett, and C. Hansen. 1981a. *Horm. Behav.* 15:396.

Hemsworth, P.H., A. Brand, and P. Willems. 1981b. *Livestock Prod. Sci.* 8:67.

Hemsworth, P.H., J.L. Barnett, and C. Hansen. 1986a. *Appl. Anim. Behav. Sci.* 15:303.

Hemsworth, P.H., et al. 1986b. *Appl. Anim. Behav. Sci.* 15:55.

Hemsworth, P.H., H.W. Gonyou, and P.J. Dziuk. 1986c. *Appl. Anim. Behav. Sci.* 15:45.

Hemsworth, P.H., J.L. Barnett, and C. Hansen. 1987a. *Appl. Anim. Behav. Sci.* 17:245.
Hemsworth, P.H., et al. 1987b. *Appl. Anim. Behav. Sci.* 19:81.
Hemsworth, P.H., et al. 1988. *Appl. Anim. Behav. Sci.* 19:255.
Hoenderken, R. 1983. "Electrical and carbon dioxide stunning of pigs for slaughter." In: *Stunning of Animals for Slaughter.* Eikelenboom, G. (Ed.). pp. 59–63. Boston: Martinus Nijhoff.
Houpt, T.R. 1984. *J. Anim. Sci.* 59:1345.
Jensen, P. 1983. *Appl. Anim. Ethol.* 9:47.
Jensen, P. 1984. *Appl. Anim. Behav. Sci.* 12:93.
Jensen, P. 1986. *Appl. Anim. Behav. Sci.* 16:131.
Jensen, P., and B. Algers. 1984. *Appl. Anim. Ethol.* 11:237.
Jensen, P., and I. Redbo. 1987. *Appl. Anim. Behav. Sci.* 18:355.
Jensen, P., K. Floren, and B. Hobroh. 1987. *Appl. Anim. Behav. Sci.* 17:69.
Kelley, K.W. 1990. "Stress, immunity and pig health." In: *Proc. Mtg. Amer. Assoc. Swine Practitioners,* Des Moines, IA.
Kilgour, R., T.M. Foster, and W. Temple. 1982. "Operant technology applied to solving farm animal problems." In: *Proc. Mtg. N. Z. Psychol. Soc.* Hamilton: New Zealand Psychological Society.
Klingholz, F., and H. Meynhardt. 1979. *Z. Tierpsychol.* 50:250.
Klingholz, F., C. Siegert, and H. Meynhardt. 1979. *Zool. Garten* 49:277.
Lammers, G.J., and A. De Lange. 1986. *Appl. Anim. Behav. Sci.* 15:31.
Lewis, N.J., and J.F. Hurnik. 1985. *Appl. Anim. Behav. Sci.* 14:225.
McFarlane, J.M., K.E. Boe, and S.E. Curtis. 1988. *J. Anim. Sci.* 66:326.
McGlone, J.J., and F. Blecha. 1987. *Appl. Anim. Behav. Sci.* 18:269.
McGlone, J.J., and S.E. Curtis. 1985. *J. Anim. Sci.* 60:20.
McGlone, J.J., and J.L. Morrow. 1988. *J. Anim. Sci.* 66:880.
McGlone, J.J., S.E. Curtis, and E.M. Banks. 1987. *Behav. Neural. Biol.* 47:27.
McGlone, J.J., W.F. Stansbury, and L.F. Tribble. 1987b. *J. Anim. Sci.* 65:456.
Mwanjali, S., D. Smidt, and F. Ellendorff. 1983. *Appl. Anim. Ethol.* 9:263.
Olsson, O. 1983. "Valve drinking systems for growing-finishing pigs: Effects on pig performance and behavior and biometric considerations for technical design." In: *Report 111.* Uppsala, Sweden: Swedish University of Agricultural Science.
Peck, R.N. 1972. *A Day No Pigs Would Die.* New York: Knopf.
Pekas, J.C. 1985. *Growth* 49:19.
Price, E.O. 1984. *Q. Rev. Biol.* 59:1.
Rohde, K.A., and H.W. Gonyou. 1987. *Appl. Anim. Behav. Sci.* 19:57.
Rohde Parfet, K.A., et al. 1989. *J. Anim. Sci.* 67:94–104.
Rosillon-Warnier, A., and R. Paquay. 1984. *Appl. Anim. Behav. Sci.* 13:47.
Schoen, A.M.S., S.E. Curtis, and E.M. Banks. 1974. *J. Anim. Sci.* 39:136. (Abstr.)
Schouten, W.G.P. 1986. *Rearing Conditions and Behaviour in Pigs.* Wageningen, The Netherlands: Proefschrift, Agricultural University.
Schwenke, K. 1985. *In a Pig's Eye.* Chelsea, VT: Chelsea Green.
Signoret, J.P. 1976. "Chemical communication and reproduction in domestic mammals." In: *Mammalian Olfaction, Reproductive Processes and Behavior.* Doty, R.L. (Ed.). pp. 243–256. New York: Academic Press.
Stricklin, W.R. 1983. *Int. J. Stud. Anim. Prob.* 4:279.
Stricklin, W.R. 1985. "Recent advances and developments in applied ethology." In: *Ethology of Farm Animals: A Comprehensive Study of the Behavioural Features of the Common Farm Animals.* Fraser, A.F. (Ed.). pp. 9–16. New York: Elsevier.
Taylor, I.A., J.L. Groppel, and S.E. Curtis. 1987. *J. Anim. Sci.* 65(Suppl. 1):233. (Abstr.)
Taylor, I.A., et al. 1988. "Design of feeders for swine: Kinematics, behavior, and individuality." In: *Proceedings of the Congress of the International Society of Animal Hygiene.* Skara, Sweden: Swedish University of Agricultural Sciences.

Towne, C.W., and E.N. Wentworth. 1950. *Pigs: From Cave to Corn Belt.* Norman, OK: University of Oklahoma Press.
Tusser, T. 1984. *Five Hundred Points of Good Husbandry.* New York: Oxford University Press.
van Putten, G. 1987. Farming beyond the ability of pigs to adapt. Paper presented at International Symposium on Bio-Ethics and Applied Ethology, 15–16 August, Montreal, Quebec.
Vestergaard, K., and L.L. Hansen. 1984. *Ann. Vet. Res.* 15:245.
Welch, A.R., and M.R. Baxter. 1986. *Appl. Anim. Behav. Sci.* 15:203.
White, E.B. 1952. *Charlotte's Web.* New York: Harper & Row.
White, E.B. 1977. "Death of a pig." In: *Essays of E.B. White.* pp. 17–24. New York: Harper Colophon Books.
Widowski, T.M., and S.E. Curtis. 1988. "Effects of access to straw, cloth tassel, or both on prepartum behavior of sows." In: *Proceedings of the 6th Congress of the International Society of Animal Hygiene.* pp. 696–699. Skara, Sweden: Swedish University of Agricultural Sciences.
Wiepkema, P.R. 1982. "On the identity and significance of disturbed behaviour in vertebrates." In: *Disturbed Behaviour in Farm Animals.* pp. 7–17. Stuttgart, FRG: Eugen Ulmer.
Wiepkema, P.R. 1987. "Behavioral aspects of stress." In: *Biology of Stress in Farm Animals: An Integrative Approach.* Wiepkema, P.R., and P.W.M. van Adrichem (Eds.). pp. 113–133. Boston: Martinus Nijhoff.
Winfrey, L.P. 1982. *Pig Appeal.* New York: Walker.
Wood-Gush, D.G.M., and R.G. Beilharz. 1983. *Appl. Anim. Ethol.* 10:209.

PART II

Development of Nutritional Capabilities

Chapter 3

Digestion and Absorption Capacity and Their Development

J.C. Pekas

Digestion and absorption are integrated functions. Digestion without absorption is futile. The capacity to absorb in excess of the capacity to digest is similarly futile. The emphasis of this chapter is on the extent that digestion-absorption compromise or delimit the rate or efficiency of growth and other performance of swine. ''Growth'' in meat animals should not be based solely on measurement of body-weight gain and should be redefined as net accretion of edible lean tissue. Accretion of carcass fat could be viewed as ''negative growth'' and accretion of viscera and other offal as ''undesirable growth.'' It is acknowledged that minimum amounts of these undesirable tissues are essential to the life of the animal and are salvaged for by-products that can be used as animal foods and to some extent as human food. Development of methods to improve ''meat growth'' might be accelerated by focusing on the rate and efficiency of life cycle production of animal protein, meat quality, and consumer acceptance of the product.

Research findings since 1980 are emphasized in this chapter. Several important monographs, bulletins, and proceedings should be considered important supplements to this chapter. These include Lucas and Lodge (1961), Kidder and Manners (1978), Low and Partridge (1980), Laplace et al. (1982), Moran (1982), and Just et al. (1985).

Factors within the digestive system that may delimit lean tissue accretion are discussed. Net extraction of nutrients from the diet is accomplished by thousands of molecular and cellular events, all operating and interacting simultaneously. Identification of a specific molecular event that controls extraction of the ''most limiting'' nutrient seems unlikely.

ANATOMY AND HISTOLOGY

Development of the gastrointestinal system after birth has been considered both in terms of physical size and physiological functions. Understanding each of these aspects requires some knowledge of the anatomy and histology of gastrointestinal organs and supporting tissues and vessels. Simplified sketches are provided. The stomach is illustrated in Figure 3.1; small and large intestine and a close-up of a region of jejunum in Figure 3.2; a magnified intestinal villus and epithelial cell (enterocyte) in Figure 3.3; the luminal surface created by the epithelium of the intestine in Figure 3.4; and details of the microvillus surface of an enterocyte in Figure 3.5. More detailed discussions and diagrams of the anatomy of the digestive system can be found in textbooks; examples of excellent general material are Schummer et al. (1979) and Sisson and Grossman (1975).

The physical dimensions and weight of the digestive system change with age and body weight, as illustrated in Table 3.1. The proportions of the length and volume represented by stomach, small intestine, cecum, and colon are summarized in Table 3.2. It is important to point out that the physiological capacities of the respective organs have no direct relationship to the absolute or relative physical size of the organ as measured postmortem. For example, the small intestine of an adult pig was shown to hold 9.2 L or 33.5% of the total volume capacity of the whole gastrointestinal tract. It is doubtful that the actual volume of ingesta recovered from the small intestine of living animals exceeds 5% to 10% of the postmortem volume capacity. For this reason, it is more reliable to measure functional capacity in terms of the quantity of nutrient substrate digested or absorbed, or in terms of the quantity of digestive enzymes synthesized or secreted. Such measurements are emphasized in later sections.

ENDOCRINOLOGY OF THE DIGESTIVE SYSTEM

Although endocrinology was born in the field of gastrointestinal physiology at the advent of the twentieth century (secretin was first described in 1902 by Bayliss and Starling [1902] and became the first substance to be named a "hormone"), endocrinology of the gastrointestinal system did not flourish until the 1970s. It is now known that digestive and absorptive functions are under intricate endocrine regulation, but many of these regulation mechanisms remain to be verified in swine and other domestic mammals. Recent textbooks of medical gastrointestinal physiology should be consulted (e.g., Glass 1980). Insulin, glucagon, gastrin, secretin, cholecystokinin, vasoactive intestinal polypeptide, gastric inhibitory polypeptide, motilin, chymodenin, enteroglucagon, bulbogastrone, pancreatic polypeptide, and somatostatin have been confirmed in gastrointestinal tissues of the pig (Kidder and Manners 1978).

Undoubtedly, most of these gastrointestinal hormones will eventually be shown to have an effect on digestion or absorption in swine. Other peptides and polypeptides probably will be discovered and shown to have a role in digestion and absorption.

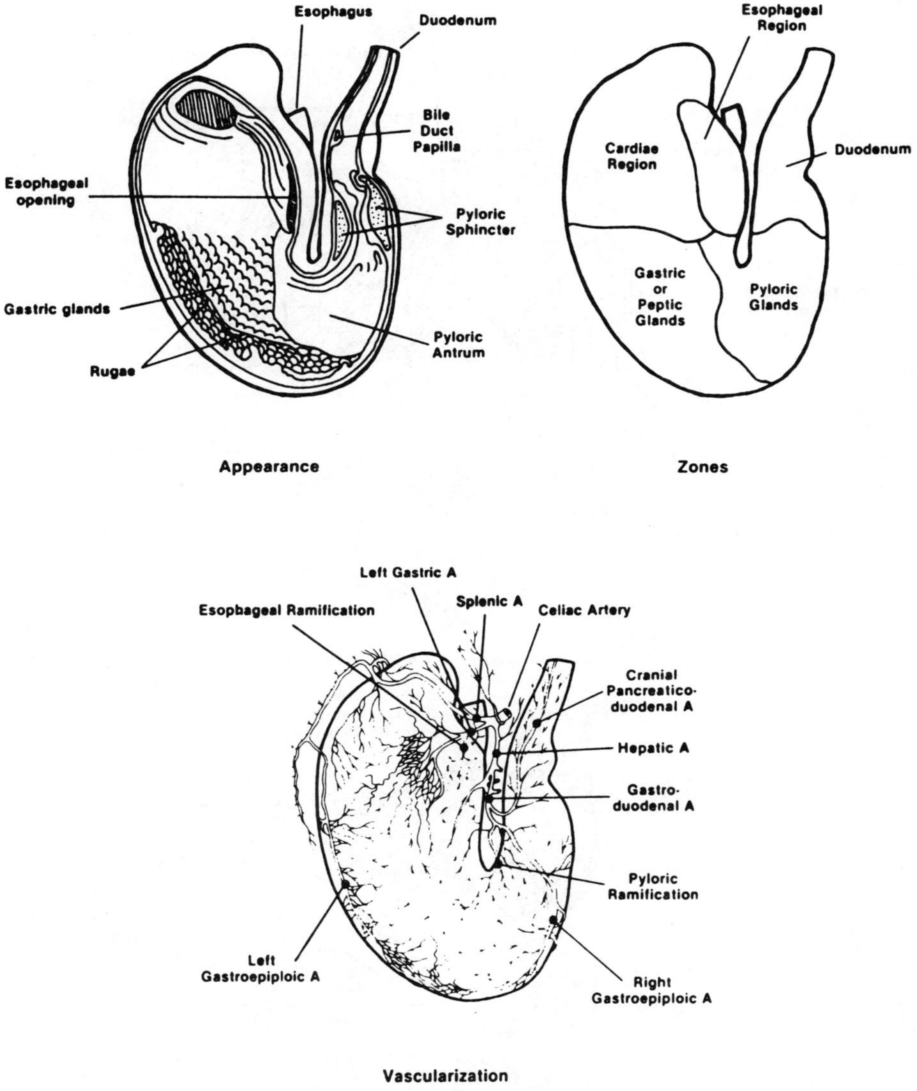

(Adapted by, and by permission of, Moran 1982.)

Figure 3.1 *Representations of the pig's stomach showing relative appearance, locations of the various type mucosa, and distribution of primary arterial vessels. Upon transit through the stomach, food passes through the cardiac, gastric, and pyloric areas before entering the small intestine. Mucus protects the surface from digestion. HCl and pepsin come from the gastric glands and are mixed to the greatest extent in the pylorus. Blood supply to each of these main areas is distinct from the others.*

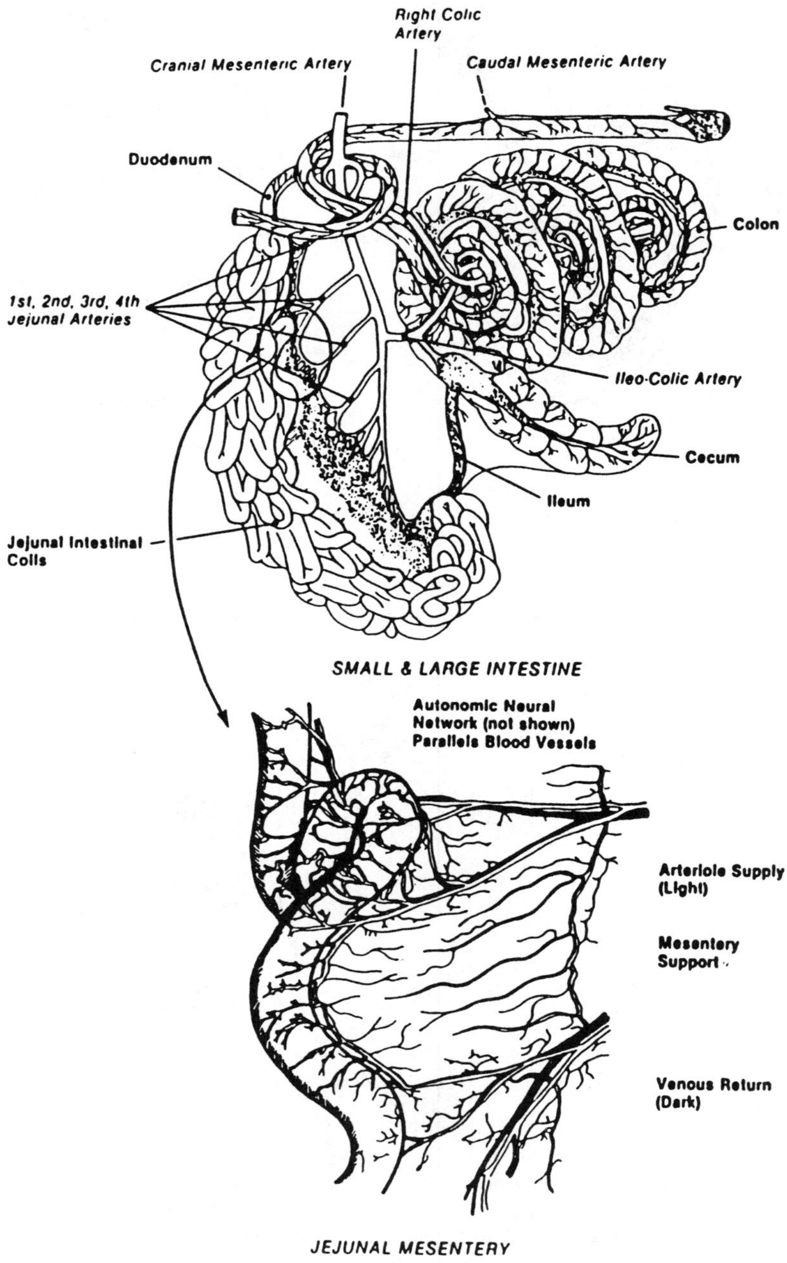

(Adapted [from Chatelain 1973b] by, and by permission of, Moran 1982.)

FIGURE 3.2 *Diagram of the intestines and mesenteric arterial system of the pig. The cranial part of the mesenteric artery supplies the overwhelming part of small and large intestine with blood.*

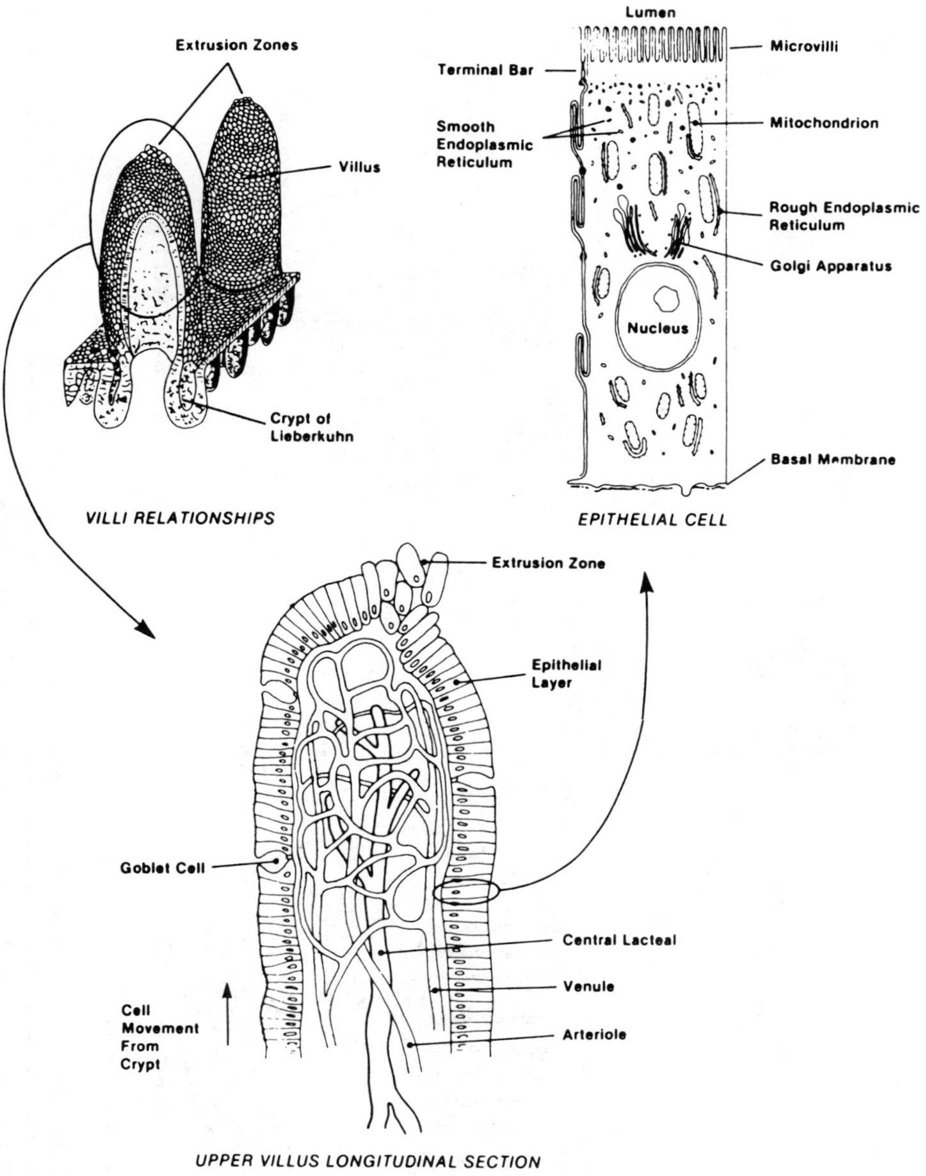

(Adapted by, and by permission of, Moran 1982.)

FIGURE 3.3 *Structure of the intestinal villus and its enterocyte.*

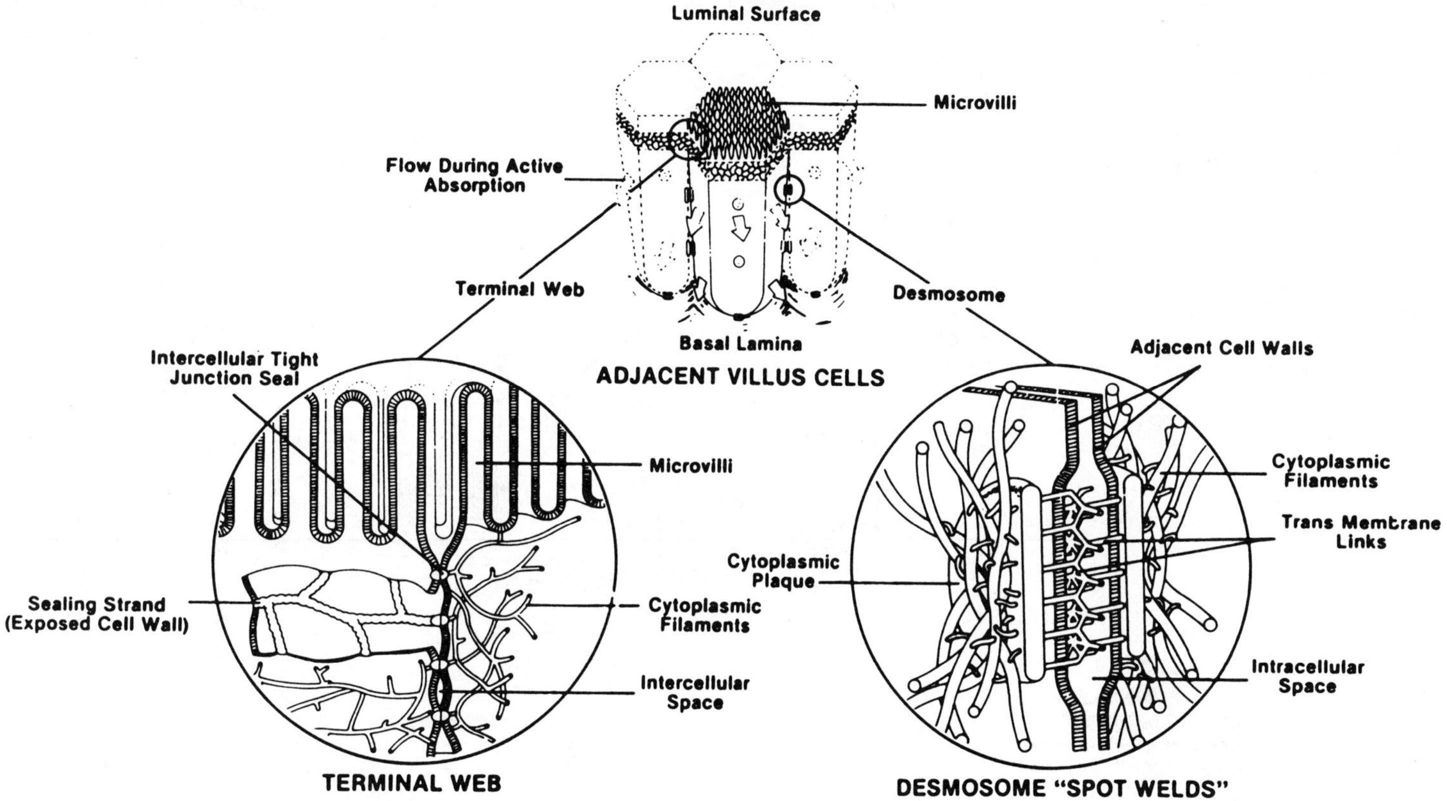

(Adapted by, and by permission of, Moran 1982.)

FIGURE 3.4 *Features of the epithelial surface of the intestine: intestinal epithelial cell binding. Tight junctions between cells prevent lumen contents from by-passing selective absorption. Desmosomes lend added integrity to the surface yet permit a maximal basal area for absorbed nutrients to pass into the lamina propria and to be carried away by the vascular and lymphatic systems.*

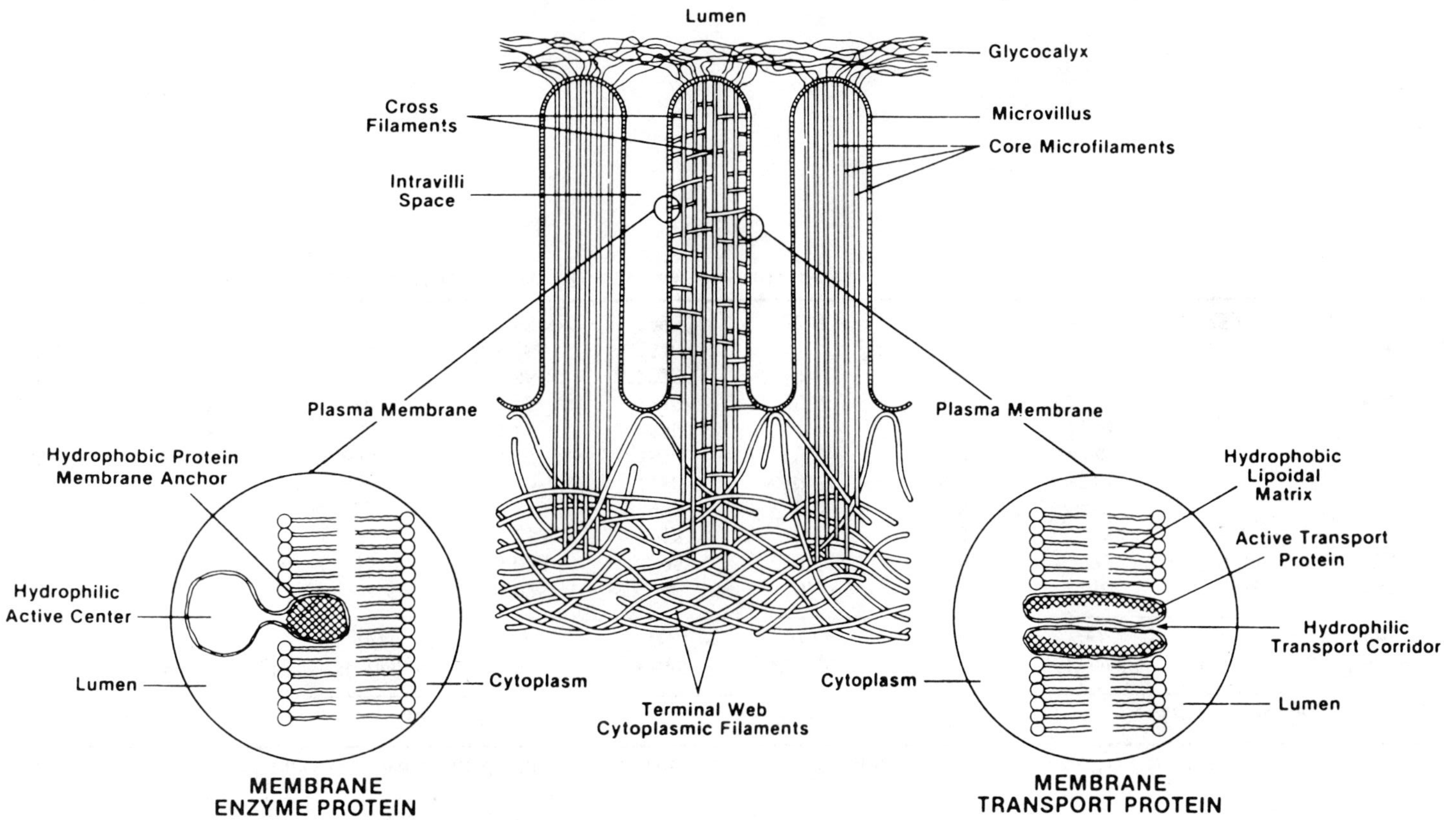

(Adapted by, and by permission of, Moran 1982.)

FIGURE 3.5 *Schematic representation of the enterocyte luminal surface. A greatly increased absorptive surface is presented by microvilli that are stabilized by filaments. Enzymes, such as the disaccharidases and peptidases, are envisaged as being held immobilized on the surface. Upon digestion, focal areas of concentration lead to improved absorptive efficiency by being near membrane proteins that facilitate their transport into the cell.*

Table 3.1 Mean Weights and Dimensions of the Stomach, Small Intestines, and Large Intestines of Pigs of Different Age Groups

Animal		*Stomach*		*Small Intestine*			*Large Intestine*		
Age	*Mean Weight (kg)*	*Weight (g)*	*Volume (L)*	*Weight (g)*	*Volume (L)*	*Length (m)*	*Weight (g)*	*Volume (L)*	*Length (m)*
1 d	1	4.5	0.025	40	0.1	3.8	10	0.04	0.8
10 d	2	15	0.073	95	0.2	5.6	22	0.09	1.2
20 d	3	24	0.213	115	0.7	7.3	36	0.1	1.2
70 d	18	232	1.815	996	6.0	16.5	458	2.1	3.1
115 d	32	360	2.50	1180	10.7	18.0	714	6.6	4.3
208 d	69	685	3.17	1670	13.3	18.8	1380	11.7	5.4
255 d	103	754	3.40	1530	14.1	18.8	1280	10.1	5.0
380 d	152	980	3.55	2510	20.6	23.7	2010	15.7	6.8
428 d	156	844	4.56	2323	19.1	22.4	2184	18.1	6.1
449 d	154	980	5.16	2310	17.4	21.2	1970	17.2	6.3
4 y	270	1430	12.68	1998	22.6	22.9	2790	25.6	7.5

(Reprinted, by permission, from Kidder and Manners 1978; originally from Kvasnitskii 1951.)

Table 3.2 Proportions of Length and Volume Capacity of Various Organs of the Gastro-Intestinal System of the Mature Pig

	Length		*Volume Capacity*	
Organ	*Meters*	*% of Total*	*Liters*	*% of Total*
Stomach	—	—	8.0	29.2
Small intestine	18.3	77.9	9.2	33.5
Cecum	0.2	0.9	1.6	5.6
Colon	5.0	21.2	8.7	31.7
Total	23.5	100.0	27.5	100.0

(Reprinted, by permission, from Moran 1982; originally from Stevens 1977.)

THE CONCEPT OF FIRST-LIMITING FACTORS

Quantitative information required to estimate digestive capacity is illustrated in Figure 3.6. Consideration of the critical elements of the model in Figure 3.6 leads to the concept of the "first-limiting digestive factor" theory and has guided this author's research activities over the last several years. The relationships outlined in Figure 3.6 require that k_I exceed k_D at all times if one is to measure the maximum rate of digestion, k_D MAX. Similarly, k_D, and thus k_I, must exceed k_A at all times to measure the maximum rate of absorption, k_A MAX. The true k_A MAX is that value that cannot be increased by further increases of k_D and k_I.

Rates of k_A and k_D are essentially impossible to distinguish without surgical intervention. Measurements of yield of carcass or of carcass lean are preferred in attempts to maximize performance of meat animals. This is based on the presumption that accretion of carcass can be accelerated because digestion-absorption functions are not limited, that is, when k_D and k_A are not at k_D MAX and k_A MAX.

The first-limiting digestive factor concept was derived from enzyme kinetics in which the rate of formation of the final chemical compound in a sequence of multiple enzyme reactions is determined by the "rate-limiting" enzyme. The rate-limiting enzyme is that enzyme, in the chain of enzymes, that regulates the rate of product formation. Similarly, the first-limiting digestive factor concept implies that there is one process in the complex array of processes (between nutrient ingestion and incorporation into tissue) that regulates the rate of lean tissue accretion. Identification of the first-limiting digestive factor in animal production requires measurement of the full range of biological activities depicted in Figure 3.6. Regardless of what aspect of animal performance we are considering, whether it be reproduction, lactation, or growth, the performance is derived from the sum of nutrients extracted by digestion-absorption. It may be that specific digestion-absorption processes operate, or have the potential to operate,

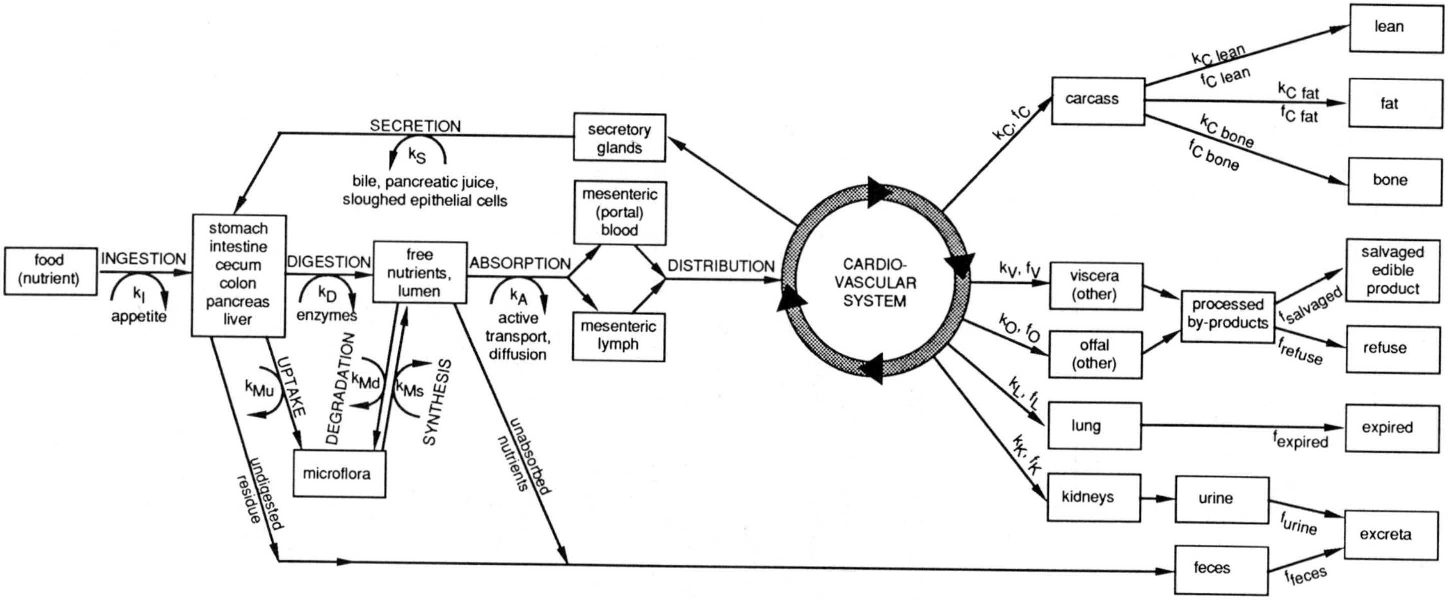

FIGURE 3.6 *Simplified diagram of the role of ingestion, digestion, and absorption and the effects of capacity or kinetics of these functions or availability of nutrients for production of meat. The diagram could be modified to include reproduction and lactation by adding these functions to the right side of the diagram to produce viable fetuses and milk. Processes that can be estimated or quantitated are indicated by capital letters. Rate processes within the digestive system that have a direct bearing on the capacity of digestion-absorption are indicated by a curved line; the rate constant is indicated by k. (k_I, rate constant for intake of food; k_D, rate constant for digestion of the ingested food; k_A, rate constant for absorption of ingested and digested food.) Measurement of the maximum rate of digestion, k_D MAX, requires that k_I MAX be greater than k_D MAX during measurement of k_D MAX. Similarly, to measure k_A MAX requires that k_D MAX and thus also k_I MAX be greater than k_A MAX during measurement of k_A MAX. k_C, k_V, k_O, k_L, k_K, k_S are rate constants for delivery of absorbed nutrient to the carcass, other viscera, other offal, lung, kidneys or secreted back into the lumen of the digestive system. Constants k_C, k_V, k_O, k_L, k_K, and k_S sum to k_A. Fractional distributions, f, are computed as ratios of the respective k constant to k_A; i.e., $f_C = k_C/k_A$. Fractional distributions f_C, f_V, f_O, f_L, f_K, f_S sum to a value of 1.000. The subset k_{CL}, k_{CF}, k_{CB} (carcass subset) sums to k_C (carcass); also f_{CL}, f_{CF}, f_{CB} sum to f_C.*

at an excessive level. Metabolism to support the physiological system in excess of that required for current nutrient intake may contribute to inefficiencies. It might be that specific digestion-absorption processes can be elevated to higher levels by specific challenges. The concept of first-limiting digestive factors is illustrated by examining studies that were specifically designed to identify first-limiting factors in the digestive-absorption process. In those situations, where appetite or digestion-absorption are not limiting factors, increasing nutrient intake, digestion, or absorption would not be expected to be beneficial.

EVIDENCE THAT FOOD INTAKE AND APPETITE ARE LIMITING FACTORS

Evidence indicates that appetite regulation may be such a first-limiting digestive factor. Appetite regulation in young swine is precise; food intake cannot be increased by natural ingestion (Pekas 1983c, 1983d). For this reason, research in this area is very complex.

Food administered through a gastric fistula has been increased to 120% of ad libitum intake (grams per kilogram of body weight; dry matter basis). Administration of a diet in excess of ad libitum intake has been called *superalimentation.* Superalimentation for 23 days increased rate of gain 40%, body weight 10.5%, and carcass weight 13.4% (6.4 kg); carcass lean increased 1.7 kg, fat 2.6 kg, undissected parts 2.1 kg, and bone decreased 0.1 kg (Pekas 1985). That superalimentation increased body-weight gain and lean gain demonstrated that ad libitum feed intake is not sufficient to obtain the full potential for growth inherent in these swine.

Either swine have a reserve capacity or the capacity for digestion-absorption was enhanced by superalimentation. This raises fundamental questions about observed versus real growth maxima. Voluntary ingestion has been increased in a recent preliminary study by manipulating a hormone thought to suppress appetite (Pekas et al. 1990). Voluntary ingestion was increased above ad libitum intake in pigs, and as with superalimentation, body-weight gain was increased but carcass composition was not affected.

DIGESTION-ABSORPTION CAPACITY: FIXED OR RESPONSIVE

Whether the functional capacity for digestion-absorption is fixed at each stage of development or is adaptive (responsive) to dietary factors is important to define. Greater growth from greater food intake, both by superalimentation and by appetite modulation, emphasizes the importance of this issue (Pekas 1985, 1990). Simply increasing food intake effected greater quantities of nutrients to be extracted by digestion-absorption and incorporated into carcass tissues. Additional growth from additional food intake could be explained either by a normal excess of capacity or by enhancement of digestive-absorption functions in response to the increased food intake. These findings indicate that the capacities for digestion-absorption and for tissue synthesis in pigs are either in excess of the capacity for ad libitum nutrient intake or are stimulated by ingestion at levels distinctly above ad libitum intake (Pekas 1985). Virtually every gastrointestinal organ increases in size during superalimentation (Pekas 1983b), indicating that functional capacities are enhanced (Table 3.3). Stomach and small intestine weight increase in greater proportion than body weight, thus confirming that gastric and small intestinal functions specifically were enhanced (Table 3.3).

Feed restriction, in contrast to superalimentation, reduces gastrointestinal organ size (Pekas 1986a, 1986b). Therefore the level of food intake appears to be a critical messenger in the regulation of digestion-absorption capacity. Future research, therefore, will require that food intake be enhanced and that the degree of enhancement be described.

More specifically, morphometric measurements involving the total cross section of the entire small intestinal wall, called a circumsection (Pekas 1986a), in feed-restricted pigs have been reported. Subnormal alimentation was enforced by three unique feed restriction schedules. The results showed that the responses were specific to the mucosa (Pekas 1986b). Mucosa accounted for 88% of the weight change of the small intestine, musculature accounted for 10%, and the remainder (of tissue) for 2% (Pekas 1986b). The mucosal responses were associated with responses of the villi and thus of the epithelial surface area (Pekas 1983a). These findings indicate that intestinal functions associated with the mucosa and epithelium were increased or decreased in proportion to the level of food intake (Table 3.4). In a concurrent experiment, using the same feed restriction schedules and the same genotype and source of pigs (Koong et al. 1982), basal metabolism (estimated by whole-body measurements of fasting heat production) was associated with the level of feed intake and the size of certain organs (Table 3.5), most notably the stomach, small intestine, large intestine, pancreas, liver, and kidneys.

POSTNATAL DEVELOPMENT OF DIGESTION-ABSORPTION CAPACITY

Development from Birth to Weaning

In the 1950s, several research groups conducted investigations into the development of the digestive system by assaying enzyme levels of tissues. Results from Iowa State University emphasizing the neonatal pig were summarized by Catron et al. (1957). General findings were reviewed by Lucas and Lodge (1961). Many of those early studies involved nonspecific assays, and the results were expressed in general terms of protease, amylase, and lipase activity instead of specific enzyme units. Definite changes with age were revealed. More recently, Corring et al. (1982) reviewed the development of digestive functions in the pig during the early postnatal period. This chapter extends beyond the early postnatal period, from about 4 weeks of age or 20 kg body weight, to 110 kg body weight, or that period in which the greatest mass of growth or of conversion of nutrient to lean pork occurs.

Table 3.3 Comparison of Actual and Relative Weights (Mean; N = 4) of Visceral Organs from Control (Ad Libitum Intake; 100%) and Superalimentated (120%) Swine (50 to 70 kg Body Weight)

	Actual Size (g)				*Relative Size (g/kg)*			
	Treatment				*Treatment*			
Organ	*C*	*SA*	*(SA−C)/C (%)*	*P*[a]	*C*	*SA*	*(SA−C)/C (%)*	*P*[a]
Stomach	432	571	+32.1	.005	5.60	6.75	+20.4	.01
Small intestine	1679	2301	+37.0	.01	21.9	27.3	+24.7	.01
Cecum	124	135	+ 8.9	NS	1.63	1.60	− 1.8	NS
Colon-rectum	1051	1124	+ 6.9	NS	13.6	13.3	− 2.5	NS
Pancreas	107	110	+ 2.6	NS	1.38	1.30	− 6.2	NS
Liver	1392	1672	+20.1	NS	18.2	19.8	+ 9.0	NS
Heart	248	255	+ 2.8	NS	3.22	3.03	− 5.9	NS
Spleen	84.3	85.8	+ 1.8	NS	1.10	1.02	− 6.6	NS
Kidneys	258	336	+30.2	.025	3.36	3.98	+18.5	NS

Abbreviations: C, control; SA, superalimentation.

[a] Probability of difference due to treatment in a two-way analysis of variance (treatment, litter).

(Adapted from data presented at the International Union of Physiological Sciences, Sydney, Australia [Pekas, 1983b].)

Table 3.4 Estimation of Mass (g) of Three Tissue Components of Small Intestine and the Effect of Level of Feed Intake (N = 2 for Each Treatment)

	Treatment			*Response*	
	HL	*MM*	*LH*	*(LH − HL)/HL (%)*	*P*
Total tissue[a]	639.5	869.0	1181.5	+ 84.8	<.05[b]
Muscle	111.8	129.1	167.1	+ 49.5	.340
Matrix	88.5	94.2	99.5	+ 12.4	.591
Mucosa	439.2	645.7	914.9	+108.3	.035

Abbreviations: HL, high-low; MM, medium-medium; LH, low-high. (All refer to plane of nutrition in two sequential periods.

[a]Total tissue (g) at each region was computed from the total small intestine weight and therefore was not tested statistically.

[b]Two-way analysis of variance (ANOVA) (treatment, litter); probability of greater treatment difference.

(Adapted, by permission of the publisher, from Pekas 1986b.)

Table 3.5 Summary of the Effects of Three Different Feeding Strategies[a] of Young Swine to Obtain Constant Live Weight Animals (40 kg) on Organ Size and Fasting Heat Production

	Treatment[a]		
	HL	*MM*	*LH*
Stomach	263[b]	287[c]	338[d]
Small intestine	699[b]	853[c]	1013[d]
Large intestine	451[b]	492[c]	588[d]
Pancreas	52[b]	63[c]	79[d]
Liver	447[b]	537[c]	646[d]
Heart	165	157	155
Kidneys	112[b]	120[c]	139[d]
Spleen	53	51	49
Fasting heat production (kcal/d)	1079[b]	1298[c]	1519[d]

[a]High-low (HL), medium-medium (MM), and low-high (LH) refer to plane of nutrition in two periods. All values are means stated in grams except for fasting heat production.

[b,c,d]Value in same horizontal row not sharing the same superscript are significantly different ($P < .01$).

(Adapted, by permission from the publisher, from Koong et al. 1982.)

It has been known for many years that piglets weaned during the first 2 weeks after birth tolerate diets based on milk protein better than diets based on soybean protein. This tendency has been confirmed by Newport (1980) and Newport and Keal (1982). Although most digestive enzymes are developing at this early stage, pancreatic enzymes are particularly insufficient; Pekas et al. (1964) demonstrated by elimination of exocrine pancreatic secretion (ligation of the pancreatic duct) that the pancreas played a greater role in digestion of soybean protein than of milk protein at 2 weeks of age and that the role of the pancreas diminished somewhat by 8 weeks of age when animals began to show improved tolerance of soybean protein.

Efird et al. (1982b) showed that gastric proteolytic activity and pancreatic trypsin and chymotrypsin activities are not consistently functional until about 3 weeks of age and that weaning tended to elicit greater activity of these enzymes. Lindemann et al. (1986) concluded that proteolytic enzymes in gastric mucosa and pancreatic tissue should not limit performance, with the possible exception of the first few days after weaning at 4 weeks of age. These workers suggested that digestion and performance may be more directly related to the release of enzymes into the lumen than to tissue levels of enzymes.

Measurement of age-dependent changes in nutrient digestibility is a dependable way to monitor functional development of the digestive system in postnatal pigs. Rodriguez and Young (1980) showed that as milk protein was replaced with increasing proportions of soybean protein, nutrient digestibility decreased. Furthermore, organ weight and enzyme levels in tissues were increased by early weaning in comparison with values in piglets reared on the sow. Kidder and Manners (1980a, 1980b) found that the levels of carbohydrate-hydrolyzing enzymes in intestinal mucosa of pigs undergo characteristic changes between 19 days and 8 years of age. Three patterns of development of mucosal brush-border enzymes (enzyme units per gram of mucosal protein) were proposed. The first pattern was a progressive increase throughout, as for sucrase and isomaltase. The second pattern was a progressive increase to near 200 days of age and then a plateau at that level, as for maltase 2, maltase 3, and trehalase. The third pattern was a continuous decline from the highest level at 3 weeks of age, as for lactase. In general, levels of brush-border carbohydrase enzymes were low at the cranial end, near the pylorus, increased to peak levels in the second or third quadrant, and declined in the caudal quadrant. Lactase and trehalase were exceptions and displayed peak levels in the cranial quadrant and decreased to the lowest levels in the caudal quadrant (Figure 3.7). Five-week-old piglets generally had higher levels of enzymes than did 3-week-old pigs. Weaned piglets generally had higher levels than suckled piglets the same age, except for lactase levels, which were always highest in suckled piglets. The brush-border content of these carbohydrase enzymes with age is illustrated in Figure 3.8.

Thus the quantity and composition of the diet before and after weaning induce responses of specific digestive enzymes, which can be referred to as substrate adaptations. It appears that digestive enzymes may be artificially induced by hormone administrations (Baintner and Nemeth 1982).

Attempts to predict quantitative and qualitative metabolism within gastrointestinal tissues in vivo using in vitro measurements can be misleading and must be carefully verified (Pekas 1980).

Development During Postweaning Period

Recent evidence affirms that development of digestive capacity in the postnatal pig is complex. Developmental responses are associated in varying degrees with chronologi-

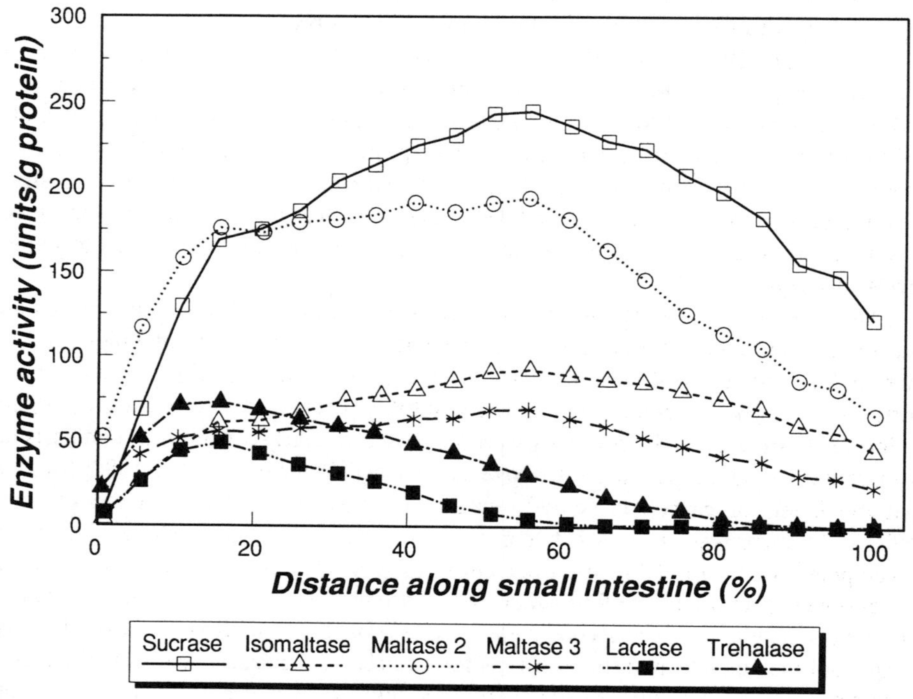

(Adapted, by permission of the publisher, from Kidder and Manners 1980b.)

FIGURE 3.7 *Illustration of gradients of brush-border carbohydrase enzymes in the mucosa of the small intestine of forty-nine pigs between 400 and 1500 days of age. Enzyme activity is the mMol substrate cleaved per minute per gram brush-border protein. Pylorus is 0% and ileocecal junction is 100% of distance along small intestine.*

cal age, age at weaning, and composition of the weaning diet. Each digestive or absorptive function tends to develop according to unique physiological and dietary signals. Thus each enzyme and transport function must be characterized in animals maintained within the range of normal diet, husbandry, and management practices.

Pancreatic duct ligation (Pekas et al. 1964) has been found to be a useful experimental model and has been used to distinguish gastrointestinal from pancreatic contributions to the normal digestion. Elimination of pancreatic secretion into the intestinal lumen of pigs 2 to 8 weeks of age suppressed protein and dry matter digestibilities for both the milk protein and soybean protein diets. Suppression of protein digestibility was greater for soybean protein (18% to 57% suppression) than for milk protein (5% to 39% suppression) and was greatest for 2- and 4-week-old pigs. Dry matter digestibility was suppressed 5% to 18% for soybean protein and milk protein diets and for all ages of pigs. Gastrointestinal digestion-absorption, without pancreatic secretion,

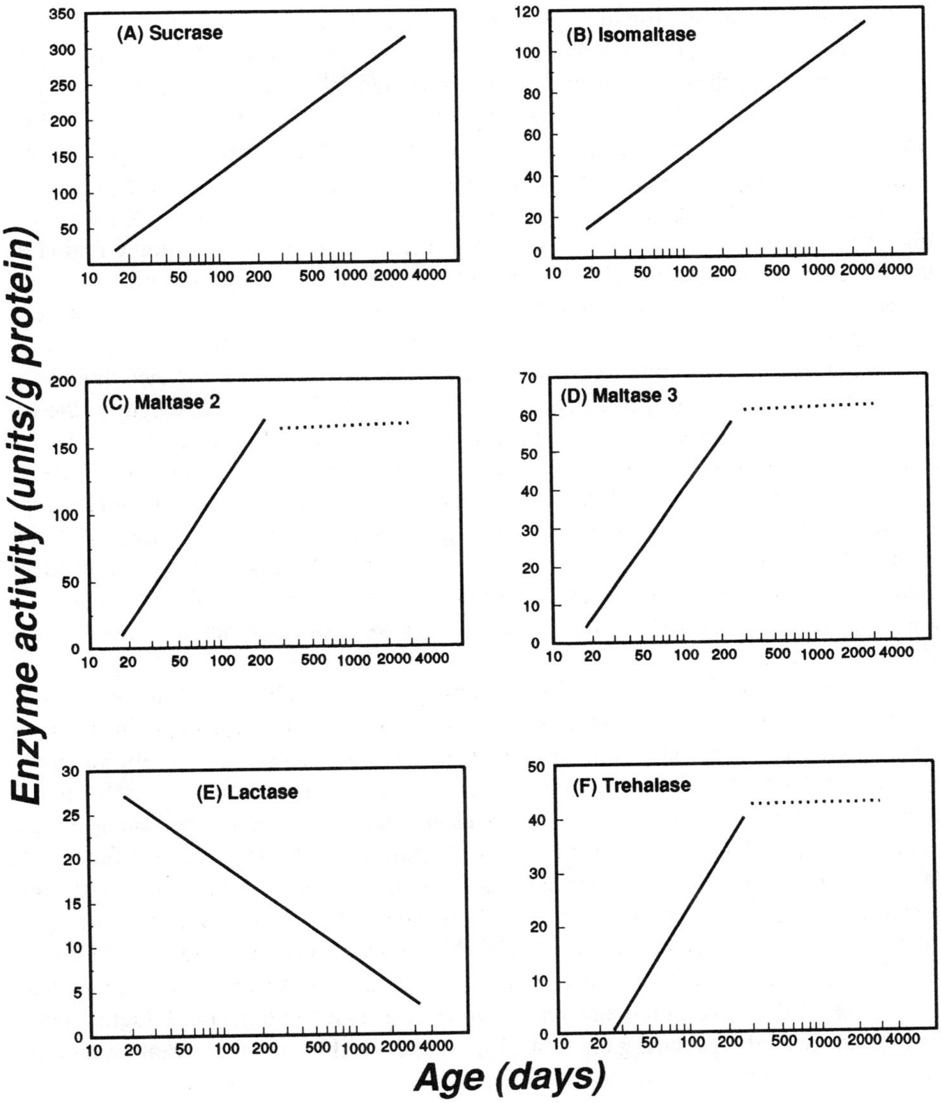

(Adapted, by permission of the publisher, from Kidder and Manners 1980b.)

FIGURE 3.8 *Illustration of age-dependent changes of activities for six carbohydrase enzymes in the brush-border of the small intestine mucosa of eighty-four pigs. Age is plotted on a logarithmic scale. Enzyme activity is presented as mMol substrate cleaved per minute per gram of brush-border protein. Only the resultant regression lines are presented for each enzyme. Suckled and weaned pigs tended to fit the same regression line. Broken lines (flat lines) represent the average values for those enzymes that appeared to reach maximum brush-border activity after pigs reached about 200 days of age.*

was greater for milk than for soybean protein and improved substantially with age for soybean protein but not for milk protein (Pekas et al. 1964).

Histology and morphology measurements of the gastrointestinal tract, particularly when combined with measurements of functional activities, have revealed that important changes occur with age and weaning. Smith (1984) has demonstrated that histological changes are induced in the mucosa of the small intestine of pigs by early weaning. Weaning at 2 weeks of age decreases villi length and increases crypt depth; weaning at 3 weeks of age increases crypt depth. Alanine transport, in vitro, was higher in 21- than in 15-day-old pigs and was confined to enterocytes in the region of the villus tip. Deprez et al. (1987) found that a liquid diet, compared with a dry diet, virtually eliminated the tendency for reduction of villi height in jejunal-ileal mucosa in early weaned piglets. The effects on digestion were not studied.

Weaning causes morphologic changes in the intestine that are associated more with enzymatic than with absorptive functions (Miller et al. 1986). Villus length in the intestine of 4- and 6-week-old suckled pigs was reduced to half that length within 5 days after weaning. Crypt depth normally increases in suckled pigs and is increased further by weaning. Lactase, which decreases with age, is suppressed by weaning, and the suppression is more severe than that of alpha-glucosidase (Figure 3.9). Maltase-2 and maltase-3 activities increase at weaning in 6-week-old pigs. Sodium-dependent transport of alanine by the intestinal enterocyte decreases from 4 to 6 weeks of age, and it is suppressed by the weaning of 4-week-old but not 6-week-old pigs (Figure 3.10).

Essentially the same morphological changes have been observed in the mucosa of the small intestine of piglets (Hampson 1986). Changes in crypt depth were most apparent in the caudal region and in villus height in the cranial region of the small intestine. Creep feeding before weaning had no obvious effect. These morphological responses indicate that important differences are likely to be found pertaining to the area of the epithelial surface, proliferation of epithelial cells, and mucosal functions. Weaning at 3 weeks of age causes large and rapid reductions in lactase activity, but temporary reduction of sucrase activity (Hampson and Kidder 1986). Brush-border enzyme activities are reduced and parallel the reduced capacity to absorb xylose.

Digestive enzyme activities in the stomach and pancreas also have been examined. Efird et al. (1982b) measured enzyme activities (expressed in units per kilogram body weight) in suckled pigs during the first 21 days after birth. They found that proteolytic activity in the stomach decreases and then recovers. Proteolytic activity in pancreatic tissue increases; however, secretion into the intestine is nil until about 22 days of age. Proteolytic activity in gastric and intestinal digesta increases sharply within 6 days after weaning, with both dry and liquid diets. Trypsin and chymotrypsin activities in intestinal digesta increase severalfold. Gastric, and especially pancreatic, proteolysis increases dramatically after weaning. Efird et al. (1982a) reported that the intestinal wall increases (weight per unit of intestinal length) during the first 7 days after weaning. Pancreas weight was not affected by age but was greater for pigs weaned onto a soybean than a milk diet. Trypsin activity in pancreatic tissue doubled in the 7-day period after weaning, but trypsin activity in intestinal digesta was not affected. Trypsin activity in intestinal digesta was greater in piglets weaned onto the soybean diet. Chymotrypsin activity did not behave as trypsin activity.

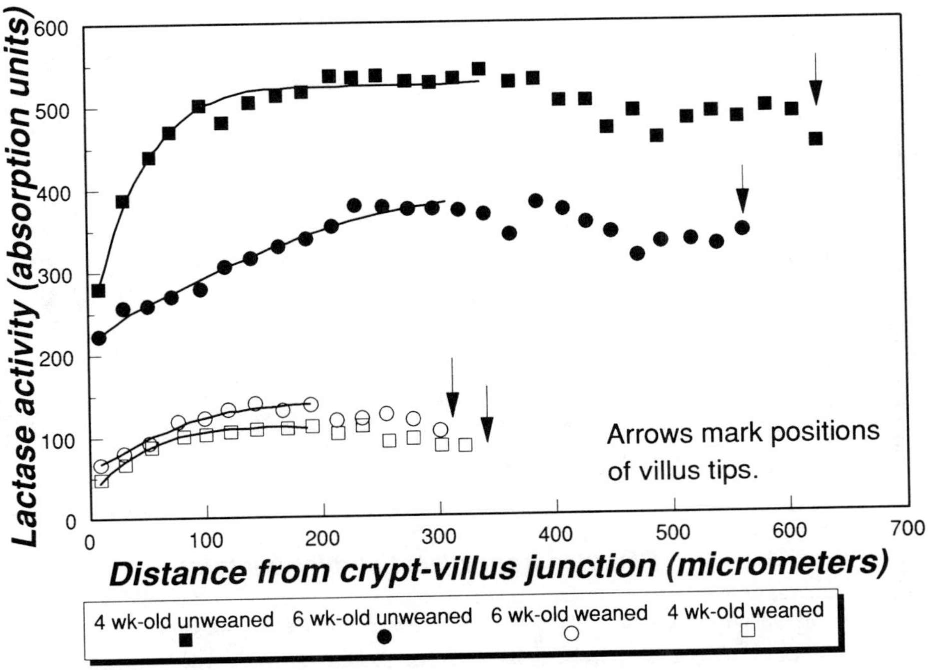

(Adapted, by permission of the publisher, from Miller et al. 1986.)

FIGURE 3.9 *The effect of enterocyte position on the villus on brush-border enzyme content illustrated with lactase. Position is the distance from the crypt-villus junction. Arrows mark the villus tip. Note that unweaned versus weaned piglets had villi about 600 and 300 mM, respectively; enterocytes from weaned pigs had greately reduced levels of the enzyme.*

The study by Efird et al. showed that intestinal weight per unit of intestinal length increased more in animals fed dry diets than in those fed a liquid milk diet. The pancreas is heavier in pigs fed a dry soybean diet than in pigs fed dry or liquid milk diets. Trypsin activity in pancreatic tissue is similar for all diets. Trypsin activity in intestinal digesta is higher for dry than for liquid diets, and it is considerably higher for a dry soybean diet than for a dry milk diet. Chymotrypsin activity in pancreatic tissue is lower in pigs fed soybean diets than in pigs fed milk diets. Chymotrypsin activity in intestinal digesta is higher for dry than for liquid diets, and higher for soybean than for milk diets.

Chemical modifications of dietary proteins have been shown to increase apparent digestibility and absorption of the amino acids contained therein (Liebert et al. 1981), but the mechanism of improvement was not suggested.

The relationship between animal performance and digestibility of diets has been measured in pigs weaned 4 days after birth (Leibholz 1981). Weight gain, gain efficiency, and nitrogen balance were greater for milk-protein than soybean-protein diets and were improved by partial hydrolysis with papain. Papain hydrolysis increases apparent nitrogen absorption and decreases the levels of trypsin and chymotrypsin activity in pancreatic tissues and duodenal digesta; however, performance was not

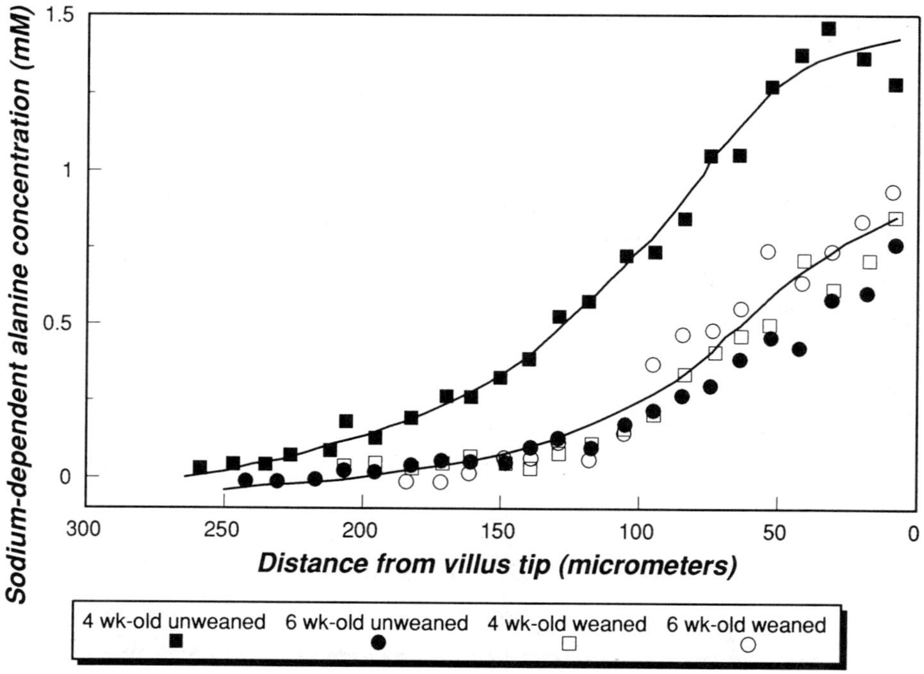

(Adapted, by permission of the publisher, from Miller et al. 1986.)

FIGURE 3.10 *The effect of enterocyte position on the villus on specific transport capabilities illustrated with Na-dependent alanine uptake by pig small intestine. Note that alanine uptake is greatest for enterocytes nearest the villus tip.*

improved. Perhaps papain or the products of papain hydrolysis of soybean protein are toxic.

Buraczewski (1980) used multiple re-entrant cannulas in the small intestine and obtained evidence that the capacity for digestion and absorption in swine might be improved. Although 84% of ingested nitrogen had been digested and absorbed cranial to the terminal ileum, 53% of the residual nitrogen was in nonprotein form. Digestion may have been still in progress or the capacity for digestion might have exceeded the capacity for absorption. The capacity to transport (absorb) specific amino acids has been characterized by perfusions of solutions of free amino acids. The proportion absorbed is greater for essential amino acids than for mixtures of essential and nonessential amino acids. Inclusion of hexose sugars in the perfusion solutions suppressed transport of essential amino acids and of some nonessential amino acids.

Total digestive capacity in pigs from birth to 10 weeks of age has been examined using general proteolytic and amylolytic assays and raw dietary substrates (Shields et al. 1980); the findings were reported as total enzyme activities per organ. In the period from birth to 10 weeks of age, body weight increased about 20-fold. Pancreas weight, intestinal length, and intestinal volume increased 23-fold, 3.5-fold, and 25-fold, respectively (Table 3.6). Total amylase (the sum of activities in pancreatic tissue,

Table 3.6 Mean Organ Size of Pigs between Birth and Ten Weeks of Age[a]

	Age (wk)					
Measurement	*0*	*2*	*4*	*6*	*8*	*10*
No. pigs	3	3	12	12	12	12
Body weight (kg)	1.31	3.78	6.71	9.07	15.61	26.04
Pancreas weight (g)	2.24	3.08	11.63	20.00	35.35	52.23
Intestine length (m)	4.09	5.99	9.20	10.86	13.18	14.61
Intestine volume (ml)	22.00	44.00	120.00	235.00	499.00	542.00

[a]The enzyme activities of these organs and contents are summarized in Table 3.7.
(Adapted, by permission of the publisher, from Shields et al. 1980.)

Table 3.7 Effect of Age and Source of Digestive Specimen on General Protease and Amylase Activites of Young Pigs[a]

	Age (wk)					
Measurement	*0*	*2*	*4*	*6*	*8*	*10*
No. pigs	3	3	12	12	12	12
Amylase activity[b]						
Total	15	52	98	208	540	1222
Pancreas	5	10	48	164	317	939
Intestinal contents	1	20	21	15	158	207
Intestinal mucosa	9	22	29	29	65	76
Protease activity[c]						
Total	6	12	49	84	166	338
Pancreas	5	9	38	57	77	169
Intestinal contents	1	3	11	27	89	169

[a]These enzyme activities were derived from the tissues and contents described in Table 3.6.
[b]Grams of starch hydrolyzed per minute.
[c]Milligram tyrosine equivalents produced per minute.
(Adapted, by permission of the publisher, from Shields et al. 1980.)

intestinal digesta, and intestinal mucosa) increased 82-fold, and total protease increased 56-fold. Amylase activity in pancreatic tissue increased 188-fold, while that in intestinal digesta increased 207-fold. Protease activity in pancreatic tissue increased 34-fold, and that in intestinal digesta increased 169-fold. Protease and amylase activities are summarized in Table 3.7 (Shields et al. 1980).

Development of Digestive Capacity in the Weanling Pig

Maximal secretory capacity of the stomach was evaluated in anesthetized pigs stimulated pharmacologically with betazole (Cranwell 1985). Stomach weight increases with body weight in both suckled and creep-fed piglets, but it increases at a faster rate in creep-fed pigs. Maximal pepsin output increases with stomach weight but increases faster in creep-fed pigs. Maximal output of acid per unit of stomach weight is similar for the suckled and creep-fed pig and remains constant with age. The digestive capacity of the stomach is increased by exposure to complex food before weaning.

Digestion and absorption of protein occur primarily in the cranial half of the small intestine (Zebrowska 1980), but continue at a decreasing rate as the digesta moves to the terminal ileum. The same multiple cannula method was used to show that 40- to 70-kg pigs secreted 20 to 27 g of endogenous nitrogen daily into the gastrointestinal tract (Zebrowska 1981). From 60% to 90% of dietary protein was absorbed in the small intestine and about 10% in the large intestine. The cecum and colon do not appear to be important in digestion and absorption of nitrogenous substances in the pig (Zebrowska 1982).

Strains of swine accustomed to a specialized diet might be expected to utilize the special nutrients more effectively than strains not so accustomed. However, Chel Guerrero (1983) reported that Pelon Mexicano pigs, accustomed to grazing for many generations, do not digest alfalfa diets any better than other pigs, nor did their gastrointestinal tract respond to the high-fiber diet. Pekas et al. (1983) found that the weight and length of the small intestine and the weight of the cecum-colon were increased in pigs fed high alfalfa meal diets; however, lean and obese genotypes of swine responded differently.

The rate of passage of digesta through the various regions of the digestive system may have important effects on the capacity to utilize the diet. However, measurements of the rate of digesta passage or of the time that digesta resides within each region are not precise or are not available. Difficulties derive from the fact that nonabsorbable markers used in such studies give differing values because of unique biophysical interactions of the markers with the digesta or epithelial surface. Chromium oxide and iron oxide have been used extensively to estimate elapsed time from ingestion to excretion because of the ease of visible identification of the markers in feces. Chromium oxide has also been used to estimate digestibility by the "index method," which requires measurement of the ratio of the nutrient per unit of marker in feed, excreta, or digesta. Suzuki et al. (1981) reported that 50% of chromium oxide in feed passed into the upper jejunum in 40 minutes, to the terminal ileum in 5 hours, and to the anus in 27.4 hours. If it is assumed that chromium oxide moves with the undigested residue without alteration of digestion, the mean residency period in the stomach and duodenum was little more than half an hour; in the jejunum and ileum, about 4.5 hours; and in the cecum-colon, about 22 hours. The chromium oxide marker spent most of its transit time in the cecum-colon. If the chromium oxide predicted transit with reasonable accuracy, it is evident that the undigested residue spent only about 20% of the time in that part where most digestion-absorption occurs and about 80% of the total transit time in that part of the gastrointestinal system where little digestion-absorption occurs.

It would seem then, theoretically, that digestion-absorption capacity in swine can be increased considerably by increasing the time spent in the small intestine, where most digestion and absorption takes place. It appears that considerably greater quantities of nutrient could be digested-absorbed if exposure of each meal to the stomach and small intestine could be sustained over a period considerably greater than the 5 hours reported by Suzuki et al. (1981).

The quality of dietary components, especially of dietary protein, has profound influences on the capacity to digest protein and on animal performance. Certain plant proteins have detrimental influences on digestion and growth of the young pig and compromise development of the digestive system. Development and exocrine function of the pancreas is of particular importance to efficient utilization of plant protein, as has been shown by complete elimination of exocrine pancreatic secretion of weanling pigs and measurement of digestibility of soybean protein versus milk protein (Pekas et al. 1964).

The superiority of milk versus soybean protein for baby pig diets was well documented in the 1950s and 1960s. Numerous studies have been conducted since that time with contemporary strains of swine and with similar findings. This has been illustrated by a series of reports by Wilson and Leibholz (1981a, 1981b, 1981c, 1981d, 1981e).

Different regions of the digestive system of the pig play greater or lesser roles for some diets than for others. Digestibility of amino acids was generally higher when measured at the rectum than at the ileum (Lin 1987), indicating that either absorption or degradation of amino acids occurred within the colon. In contrast, digestibilities of lysine, methionine, and phenylalanine were lower at the rectum than at the ileum, indicating that these amino acids were synthesized in the cecum-colon. About 7% of gross energy from corn, sorghum, wheat, and oat groats, 11% from barley, and 17% from wheat middlings is absorbed by the colon.

The small intestine is the principal digestive-absorptive organ. Carbohydrates are digested and absorbed primarily in the small intestine (Sambrook 1980); the cranial 2 to 3 m account for about half of the reducing substances absorbed. Lipid digestion and absorption in the small intestine are difficult to quantitate because of dietary effects and the substantial quantities of endogenous lipids. Most dietary and endogenous lipids enter the cranial and middle small intestine and are absorbed before they reach the ileal cannula. There remains considerable controversy about fiber digestion in the small intestine and the nutritional value of products of fermentation formed in the cecum-colon of the pig.

The output of gastric and pancreatic proteolytic enzymes has been examined in 40-kg pigs prepared with a single re-entrant cannula in either the duodenum, jejunum, or ileum (Low 1982). Output of pepsin, trypsin, and chymotrypsin combined in the digesta of the duodenum was between 6.2 and 7.1 g daily and accounted for only about 20% to 25% of endogenous protein secreted into this part of the intestine.

Development of Absorption Capacity in the Weanling Pig

As stated in the introduction, it is difficult to distinguish digestion from absorption. These processes are often viewed and measured as a single digestion-absorption process and referred to as "apparent digestibility." Quantitation of digestion requires measurement of the disappearance of the crude substrate. When the capacity for digestion exceeds absorption, the products of digestion accumulate in the digesta. Quantitation of digestion in this circumstance requires measurement of the degradation of the ingested substrate. Absorption in this circumstance is the difference between the rates of digestion and product accumulation. Thus the quantity of nutrient actually extracted is absorption. On the other hand, when the capacity for absorption exceeds digestion, the digested products are removed as rapidly as they are formed; the observed rates of digestion and absorption are equivalent. Absorption may be by simple diffusion of a free nutrient through the digesta to the epithelial surface and across the epithelial barriers.

Net absorption by simple diffusion occurs only when the diffusable substrate is present in the digesta at concentrations that exceed concentrations in the mesenteric blood plasma flowing through the intestinal villi. The opportunities for "down hill" diffusion are not common. For this reason most nutrients are absorbed by highly specialized cellular transport mechanisms that reside in membranes of the enterocyte (Figure 3.5). Active transport and facilitated transport are principally involved. Active transport is highly specific, requires energy, and is capable of transporting a substrate (nutrient) from a low concentration across the cellular membrane barrier to a higher concentration. Facilitated transport for the most part involves diffusion, but the process is facilitated by reduction of "back diffusion." Diffusion is generally considered not to be rate limiting. The capacity to absorb a specific nutrient by active transport therefore is determined by the maximum rate of the specific active transport system. Glucose and certain amino acids are known to be absorbed by active transport. Active transport is required for efficient glucose absorption from the intestine because plasma glucose concentrations are physiologically regulated at a relatively high level. The capacity of the pig intestine to transport glucose in vivo and kinetic characteristics of glucose transport have been observed by Pekas (1977) by perfusion of loops of intestine. Estimates of the kinetic coefficients, K_m (also called K_t in transport studies) and V_{max}, were derived from Lineweaver-Burk plots. K_m values for the pig ileum are similar to values for human and dog ileum; K_m values for the duodenum were not available for other domestic animals. The K_m, an estimate of the substrate concentration that would support transport at half the saturation rate (V_{max}), was about the same for duodenum and ileum (Figures 3.11 and 3.12). Phlorizin inhibition of glucose transport was demonstrated in perfused loops of pig intestine (Table 3.8); previously phlorizin inhibition had been demonstrated only in vitro.

ADAPTIVE RESPONSES OF DIGESTION-ABSORPTION CAPACITY

The capacities to digest and absorb nutrients from the diet are not fixed but are responsive to prevailing circumstances. In this regard, the digestive system is similar to other physiological systems. Knowledge about adaptive responses of the gastrointestinal system of swine is limited. This section emphasizes the effects of quantitative and qualitative dietary inputs on digestion-absorption. Environmental factors such as temperature

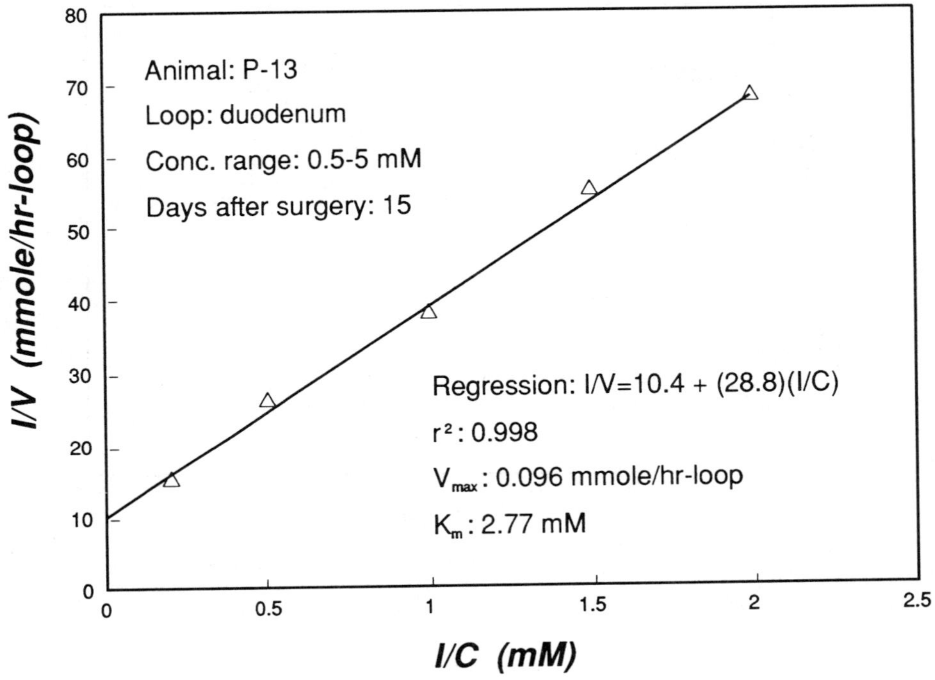

(Adapted, by permission of the publisher, from Pekas 1977.)

FIGURE 3.11 *Lineweaver-Burk plot of glucose transport data from an isolated loop of duodenum of a pig perfused with a series of solutions ranging from 0.5 to 5 mM glucose, thus below the glucose concentration of normal swine blood.*

and humidity may affect digestion-absorption by indirect influence on appetite and feed intake. The effects of diseases, parasites, and toxicants are not discussed.

Dietary Influences

The anatomical size (length, weight, area) and presumably the functional capacity of digestive organs is associated with performance in swine (Petersson and Hakansson 1979). Lean growth and lean gain efficiency are positively correlated with the length of the small intestine and the specific area (area per meter of length) but are negatively correlated with specific weight (weight per meter of length). The correlations tended to be strongest for the middle part of the small intestine. It is important that these measurements be made immediately after slaughter while the tissues are as near normal as attainable.

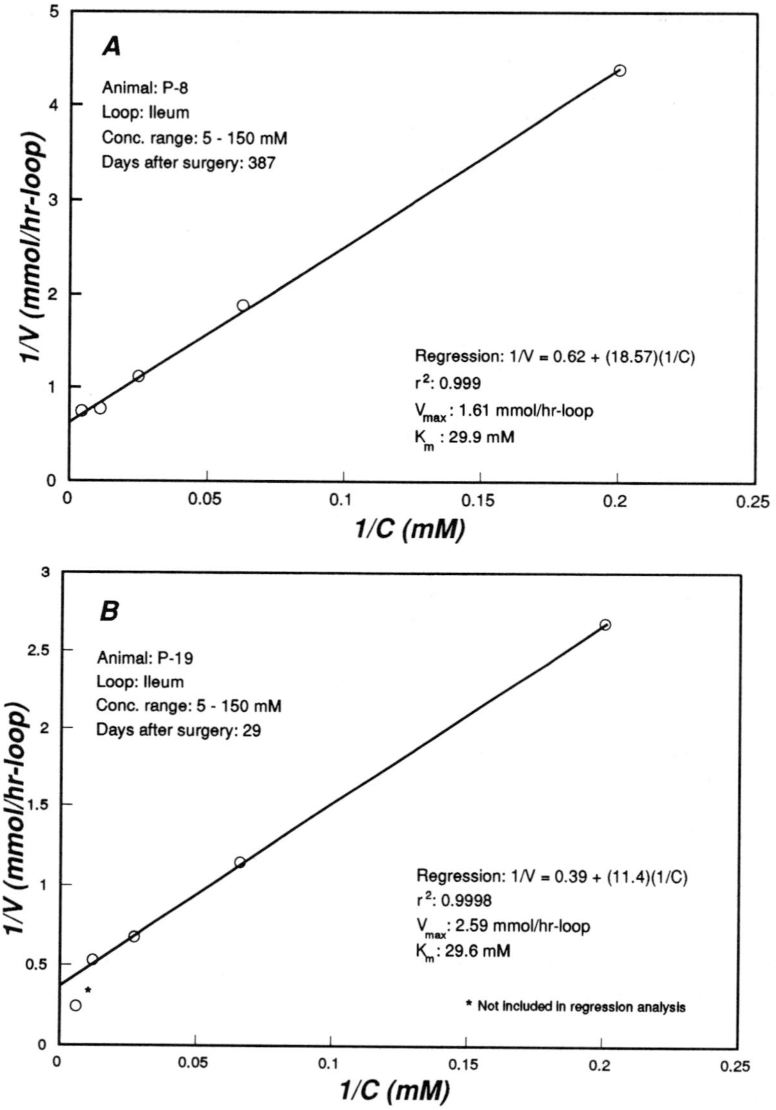

(Adapted, by permission of the publisher, from Pekas 1977.)

FIGURE 3.12 *Lineweaver-Burk plots of glucose transport data from two isolated loops of ileum; one prepared in a domestic pig (animal P-8), the other prepared in a miniature pig (animal P-19). The loops were perfused with a series of solutions ranging from 5 to 150 mM glucose, thus greater than the glucose concentration of normal swine blood.*

The average performance is associated with gastrointestinal organ measurements of lean and obese genotype swine (Pekas et al. 1983). Average daily gain is correlated with the weight of the small intestine, stomach, and pancreas, but not with the

Table 3.8 Demonstration of Phlorizin Inhibition of Glucose Transport in an In Vivo Perfused Loop of Ileum of a Pig[a]

Phlorizin Concentration (mM)	*Glucose ^{14}C Concentration (mM)*	*Absorption Rate*		*Degree of Inhibition (%)*
		Without Phlorizin (mmol/h)	*With Phlorizin (mmol/h)*	
0.1	0.05	0.0039	0.0019	51.2
0.1	5.0	0.281	0.098	65.8
1.0	150.0	1.27	0.0[a]	100.0[a]

[a]Loop was perfused with 150 mM nonlabeled glucose and 1.0 mM phlorizin immediately before the glucose ^{14}C absorption test.

(Adapted, by permission of the publisher, from Pekas 1977.)

weight of the cecum or colon. Feed consumption is correlated with stomach weight, and gain efficiency is correlated with small intestine weight.

Influences of Quantity of Diet

The quantity of dietary intake appears to have a profound effect on digestion-absorption capacity in swine, as has been observed using both undernutrition (restricted feeding) and overnutrition (superalimentation), as discussed above (Pekas 1983a, 1985, 1986a, 1986b).

The volume (L), lipid (g), protein (g), and mineral (g) secreted into the lumen of the gut of 35- to 100-kg gilts were measured by Tkachev (1983). The secretions accounted for about 70% of the total volume of about 32 L of chyme that enter the gastrointestinal tract daily; amounting to about 22.5 L of secretions, or 9 L for each kilogram of dietary dry matter ingested. Gastric, pancreatic, and bile output was about 6, 2, and 1 L/kg of dry matter ingested, respectively. Saliva output was variable but virtually ceased when a wet mash was fed. About 120 g of nitrogenous substances were secreted daily, which was nearly 30% of dietary nitrogen ingested.

There is a linear relationship between the quantity of nitrogen ingested and the quantity of endogenous nitrogen flow to the stomach and to each of three regions of the small intestine of early-weaned piglets (Leibholz 1982). This linear relationship has been confirmed in the intestine of older swine by use of the ^{15}N isotope dilution method (Souffrant et al. 1981b). The quantity of endogenous nitrogen secreted in the digesta of the small intestine was dependent on the quantity of dietary protein ingested. Similar results were obtained by use of modified dietary protein (Gebhardt et al. 1981).

Myoelectric complexes of the small intestine are altered by feed intake (Laplace 1978). True versus apparent digestibilities of protein have been estimated based on rates of endogenous nitrogen flow. The level of casein intake did not influence apparent digestibilities of protein or of amino acids measured at the ileum of 30-kg male pigs (Kies et al. 1986). Apparent digestibilities were in the range 67% to 98%; true digestibilities were in the range 92% to 104%.

As the quantity of intake of a barley-soybean diet is increased, the weight of digesta, dry matter, and nitrogen emptied from the stomach is increased proportionately but only in the first 1 to 2 hours (Low et al. 1985). Maize oil suppressed gastric emptying; water increased the volume of gastric emptying but had no effect on dry matter or nitrogen emptying.

The influence of the quantity of dietary intake on gastrointestinal functions is short-lived: about 30 to 60 minutes after each meal or about 3 to 4 hours of each day. The influence of the quantity ingested lasts less than 20% of the time, thus there appears to be ample opportunity to increase digestive-absorptive capacity. Evidence from superalimentation (Pekas 1985) confirmed that pigs either have an excess capacity or that their capacity can be increased substantially; the evidence is discussed in a later section.

Any attempt to increase the capacity of digestion-absorption simply by increasing crude feed intake immediately engages the mechanisms of appetite regulation. Appetite has been studied for centuries but little is known about the physiological mechanisms that influence food intake. A debated theory of appetite regulation at present involves the hormone cholecystokinin. Gibbs and Smith (1986) recently reviewed the role of various biologically active peptides, including cholecystokinin, in appetite regulation. No progress has been noted in consistently increasing voluntary feed intake over a sustained period in swine or any other animal. Recently, the author of this chapter conceived a hypothesis to obtain the benefits demonstrated by superalimentation. The results of a preliminary study demonstrated that pigs immunized against cholecystokinin consumed more feed and gained more weight than nonimmunized pigs (Pekas and Trout 1990).

Specific Influences of Nutrient Deprivation or Feed Restriction. The specific influences of the quantity of intake of feed or of a specific nutrient have been studied most often using restriction or deprivation. A recent study by Tullis and Whittemore (1986) with 51-kg pigs demonstrated that after a period of nitrogen deprivation, nitrogen retention was increased without an increase of protein digestibility, and thus was apparently obtained without affecting digestion-absorption capacity. Total parenteral nutrition causes retardation of growth and of development of the entire gastrointestinal tract, most notably the cranial small intestine. Such retardation indicates that digestion-absorption capacity of the small intestine is dependent on enteral exposure to dietary components (Morgan et al. 1987).

Specific Influences of Excess Food Intake or Superalimentation. One of each of four pairs of littermates of growing swine was fed through a gastric fistula at 120% of the rate (dry matter per kilogram body weight) of ad libitum intake (100%) by the other littermate. Gain over a 23-day test was profoundly increased to 140% of the gain of the ad libitum control, thus demonstrating that the inherent potential for growth in swine is much greater than that expressed during ad libitum intake of the same diet (Table 3.9). Such a profound increase in growth without loss of gain efficiency is evidence that digestion-absorption capacity in swine either is grossly in excess of that required during ad libitum intake or is somehow enhanced by the substantial increase in the rate of alimentation. Stomach, small intestine, pancreas, liver, and kidneys were

Table 3.9 Mean Body Weight Gain and Gain Efficiency and Responses to Superalimentation Over a 23-Day Period (N = 4)

Parameter	*C*	*SA*	*Response*[a] (*% of C*)	*P*[b]
Body weight (kg)				
Day 1	48.3	45.2	− 6.4	NS
Day 8[c]	56.4	56.1	− 0.4	NS
Day 31	77.3	85.5	+10.5	.05
Alimentation-dry matter; 23 d (kg)	70.9	93.1	+31.3	.025
Gain; 23 d (kg)	21.0	29.3	+40.0	.005
Gain efficiency; 23 d (kg/kg)	0.30	0.32	+ 7.3	NS

Abbreviation: C, control, SA, superalimentation; NS, not significant.

[a] $\frac{SA - C}{C} \times 100.$

[b]Two-way (treatment versus litter) analysis of variance.

[c]Day 8 was the first day of superalimentation at 120% of control intake.

(Adapted, by permission of the publisher, from Pekas 1985.)

enlarged, but the cecum, colon, rectum, spleen, heart, and lungs were not affected (Pekas 1983b); these responses confirmed that most digestion-absorption functions were enhanced by the superalimentation procedure. These findings are all the more important because the composition of the carcasses of the heavier superalimentated pigs was found to be virtually the same as would be expected if the same body weight were attained by continued ad libitum feeding (Pekas 1985). The results of a recent preliminary study indicated that voluntary feed intake, carcass weight, and carcass lean weight were each increased by immunization against cholecystokinin (Pekas et al. 1990).

Qualitative Aspects of Dietary Intake

Mere ingestion of food has an effect on intestinal motility (Laplace 1978); characteristics of the myoelectric complexes of the small intestine of Large White pigs before and after feed intake have been described. These myoelectric activities regulate motility and may have important influence on intestinal functions.

The composition of the diet has an effect on the composition of digesta. The composition of six diets, including a protein-free diet, was found to have an effect on the protein and amino acid content of intestinal chyme (Borgmann and Kreienbring 1979). The effects were seen in the supernatant and precipitate fractions and also in the trichloroacetic acid (TCA)-soluble fraction of supernatant. Composition of the TCA-insoluble fraction of the supernatant was not affected, probably because the TCA-insoluble fraction consisted largely of endogenous protein.

The composition of the diet has an effect on the output of digestive enzymes of young growing pigs (Zebrowska et al. 1983). The composition of digesta collected from a duodenal re-entrant fistula was directly related to the composition of two different diets. Total daily output of digesta, pepsin, combined salivary and gastric secretion volume, and pancreatic juice volume were each increased approximately twofold by a barley-soybean diet, as compared with a wheat starch-sucrose-casein diet. However, daily pancreatic outputs of trypsin, chymotrypsin, carboxypeptidase A, carboxypeptidase B, and amylase were not noticeably affected. Specific effects of three isonitrogenous diets on total daily enzyme output in swine were found (Low 1982). Pepsin output was found to be about 20% greater for the barley, fine wheat offal, white fish meal (BWF) diet than for the starch, sucrose, maize oil, cellulose, and groundnut (SSG) or the starch, sucrose, maize oil, cellulose, and casein (SSC) diets. Chymotrypsin output (recovered) was highest for the SSG diet, less for the SSC diet, and lowest for the BWF diet (84% of SSG). In contrast, trypsin output (recovery) was highest for the SSC diet, less for the BWF diet, and lowest for the SSG diet (60% of SSC). Adaptive responses of gastrointestinal secretions to the quality and quantity of the diet in swine and other simple-stomached animals have revealed interesting effects (Corring and Rerat 1983), particularly those of the pancreas.

Sambrook (1979b) examined the flow of total lipid, acid-detergent fiber (ADF), and volatile fatty acids from re-entrant fistulas of the duodenum, mid jejunum, and terminal ileum in swine. The BWF, SSG, and SSC diets, as described above, were used. There was substantial secretion of lipids into the cranial small intestine and reabsorption in the caudal intestine. Absorption of lipids in the large intestine was not apparent with diets SSG or SSC; net synthesis or secretion of lipid was evident with the BWF diet. ADF was not extracted in the cranial small intestine with any of the diets but was absorbed between the mid jejunum and the terminal ileum; the quantity absorbed was greatest for the SSG diet, less for the BWF diet, and very small for the SSC diet. Disappearance of ADF in the large intestine, between the terminal ileum and the rectum (feces), occurred only with the SSC diet but was not explained. The disappearance of carbohydrate substances from various regions of the digestive tract has been examined using a similar approach (Sambrook 1979a).

Digestive capacity is limited to some extent by the size of feed particles. Small (fine) particles tend to be associated with higher digestibilities of nutrients, indicating that a fine mesh hastens solution or improves enzyme attack of the particle. Digestibilities at the ileum of dry matter, starch, gross energy, and nitrogen are highest with fine particles of milled sorghum-casein diets (Owsley et al. 1981). Digestibilities of amino acids, lysine being an exception, are higher for fine than for coarse feed particles, both at the ileum and over the total digestive tract. Lawrence et al. (1980) reported gastric abnormalities in growing swine that may be related to particle size of barley diets.

Effects of Dietary Protein. Perhaps the most important issue in the consideration of digestive capacity of meat animals is the extent of utilization of dietary protein. This is because protein is the most expensive dietary ingredient, and carcass protein, derived from the dietary protein, is the primary product of meat production. The conversion of plant foodstuff protein to animal carcass protein is the ultimate goal of animal production. However, economic forces in the various meat markets of the world have not encouraged optimization of the plant protein to animal protein conversion. Nevertheless, protein digestibility and nitrogen retention are critical factors in the efficiency of conversion of plant to animal protein.

Performance of pigs weaned at 2 days of age onto liquid diets was not impaired if single-cell protein replaced no more than 40% of dried skim milk protein (Newport and Keal 1980). Greater substitutions with single-cell protein suppressed body-weight gain and gain efficiency. Skim milk protein and mixtures of skim milk and soybean protein appeared to be equivalent based on nonprotein nitrogen and total nitrogen in digesta of 2-day-old pigs (Newport and Keal 1982). The rate and efficiency of gain were greatly reduced by 75% substitution of milk protein with soybean protein in diets for 7- to 14-day-old piglets and were reduced about 30% for 21- to 28-day-old piglets (Wilson and Leibholz 1981a). Apparent digestibilities of dry matter and protein improved with advancing piglet age for the soybean diet but not for the milk diet. As the pigs aged, nitrogen retention increased from 57% to 67% in the case of the soybean diet, but it remained stable at 85% for the milk diet. These results are in general agreement with studies conducted in the 1950s and 1960s and confirm that the digestive capacity of early-weaned piglets improves considerably with age.

Wilson and Leibholz (1981a) used the same milk-protein– and soybean-protein–substituted diets to observe a variety of digestive events in a series of studies. Gastrointestinal retention time was found to be equivalent for the two diets and increased with age for the pelleted diets but not for the liquid diets. Stomach retention time was twofold longer for the pelleted than for the liquid milk diet. Restricted feeding reduced endogenous secretions into the small intestine. Dry matter digestibility to the ileum was similar for milk and purified soybean protein diets but was reduced for a crude soybean protein diet. Dry matter digestibility improved somewhat with age of pigs fed the purified soybean protein diet but not for the milk protein diet (Wilson and Leibholz 1981b). Apparent nitrogen digestibility to the ileum improved with age of early-weaned piglets fed purified or crude soybean protein but not of piglets fed milk protein (Wilson and Leibholz 1981c). Amino acid digestibility to the ileum was greater for milk protein than soybean protein. Soybean protein digestibility increased from 82% at 14 days of age to 87% at 35 days (Wilson and Leibholz 1981d). Apparent digestibility of essential amino acids was found to be 79% and 69% for essential and nonessential amino acids, respectively. True digestibility was 82% for both essential and nonessential amino acids. Digestion of plant proteins was marginal in the early-weaned piglet and improved substantially with age.

Nitrogen retention is more important than nitrogen digestibility in explaining lean meat production. Net protein accretion is the difference between protein synthesis and protein degradation; this issue is vitally debated and researched at present. The amino acid composition of empty bodies was not different for pigs fed milk versus soybean protein diets or among ages of young pigs (Wilson and Leibholz 1981e). Retention of absorbed nitrogen was greater for crude soybean protein than for either milk protein or purified soybean protein, and it was greater for pelleted than for liquid diets. These nitrogen retentions are not generally consistent with previous findings. The authors propose that methionine and threonine are limiting amino acids in crude soybean protein, whereas methionine and lysine are limiting in the purified soybean protein.

The composition of dietary proteins has important effects on digestive functions. Wheat gluten tends to suppress gastric emptying rate as compared with that of fish meal, and the effect is greater in combination with wheat starch than with maize starch

(Laplace et al. 1983). Emptying of digesta volume was found to be more involved than of digesta dry matter. Fevrier and Aumaitre (1979) examined the effects of dietary proteins on intestinal and pancreatic enzymes. The studies were initiated when pigs were 5 weeks old, but the measurements were made when the pigs reached 100 kg body weight. The complex experimental design involved three levels of whey (0%, 10%, and 20%) in weaning diets fed to 25 kg body weight. Thereafter a factorial design involving three growing diets (0%, 30%, and 60% whey) on each of the three weaning diets was used. Small intestine weight was not affected, but large intestine weight was always greater for pigs fed the whey diets. Lactase activity in the small intestine was not affected, but lactase in the cecum and large intestine increased when the growing diet contained 60% whey. It was proposed that lactase in the cecum and large intestine is of bacterial origin. Newport (1980) compared three protein sources using piglets weaned at 2 days of age onto liquid diets. One diet was based on dried skim milk protein; the second diet on purified soybean protein, whey, and methionine; and the third diet was an equal mixture of the other two. The purified soybean protein diet caused severe scours and a high mortality rate. Nitrogen retention was greater for the milk protein diet than for the mixed diet and decreased with age for both diets. Rate and efficiency of gain were not different for the two diets. Although pancreatic tissue content of chymotrypsin was reduced by the mixed diet, the quantities of trypsin and chymotrypsin recovered from the intestinal digesta were not different, indicating that total pancreatic output was not different. Rodriquez and Young (1980) have reported evidence pertaining to the effects of milk and soybean proteins on the development of 7-day-old pigs and included some observations of the effects of corn.

It has become common practice to measure digestibility at the ileocecal junction. Measurements at the ileum give an estimate of digestibility of the nutrient in the stomach and small intestine and thus provide an estimate of digestion-absorption that occurs before the microflora of the cecum and colon are involved. This is especially important in consideration of protein digestion because the microflora degrade and synthesize nitrogenous substances and confound measurements of net digestion and absorption. Darcy et al. (1983) concluded that measurements at the terminal ileum were more meaningful and reliable than measurements based on fecal output. They found that the amino acid composition of the ileal digesta was strongly influenced by the amino acid composition of the dietary protein, apparently due in part to the presence of undigested dietary protein in the digesta. This was apparent even in the case of gluten protein, which is highly digestible.

There is much interest in the relationship between the rate of digestion-absorption and the rate of growth of agricultural animals. One study involving an in vitro technique indicated that the rate of amino acid uptake into the small intestinal tissue was not necessarily associated with the rate of growth (Rothschild 1983).

There is also interest in the associations between compensatory growth, compensatory nitrogen retention, and protein digestion. Tullis and Whittemore (1986) demonstrated with young Large White barrows that after a period of nitrogen deprivation, nitrogen retention was increased without an increase of protein digestibility.

Buraczewski (1980) wrote an excellent review pertaining to estimations of the sites within the small intestine where ingested versus endogenous proteins appear and disappear. The Institute of Animal Physiology and Nutrition, Jablonna, Poland, has a long history of innovative research into these important questions. The reader is referred to that review. However, a few remarks about digestive-absorptive capacity would be appropriate. From one point of view, it appears that the capacity for digestion-absorption is excessive; the predominance of some substrates is absorbed in the cranial region, leaving very little to be accomplished in the major part caudal. There is convincing evidence, however, that protein hydrolysis is still active at the terminal ileum where high percentages of the nitrogen recovered were in a nonprotein form. Apparent digestibilities of essential amino acids measured at the rectum are higher than at the terminal ileum, indicating that some essential amino acids are either absorbed or degraded in the colon. Transport of amino acids from perfused intestinal loops has shown that rate-limiting transport is more readily demonstrable for essential than for nonessential amino acids. Inclusion of sugars in the perfusion medium suppressed the transport of essential more than that of nonessential amino acids.

Effects of Dietary Starch and Fat. There is evidence that digestive functions of the pig are adaptable to the composition of the diet. The dietary content of energetic foodstuffs has an effect on digestion-absorption functions and capacities. For example, Laplace et al. (1983) found that some mixtures of purified starches and proteins had an effect on gastric emptying. The effect seemed greater on the rate of emptying of digesta volume than of dry matter. High dietary lactose had no effect on average daily gains of three breeds of swine (Engstrom and Ekstrom 1979); however, levels of lactase enzyme in the cecum and colon were increased in all breeds.

Dietary fat has been shown to have specific effects. Juste et al. (1983) reported that bile secretions of young growing Large White males responded to the level of dietary fat. As the level of lard in the diet was increased from 2% to 20%, the rate of bile flow and the composition of bile changed. The concentration of bile acids, phospholipids, and cholesterol increased; digestibility of protein was not affected; digestibility of organic matter and energy was suppressed; and digestibility of lipids was increased. Ozimek et al. (1983) demonstrated that 15% of canola oil in the diet of 35-kg crossbred barrows caused a threefold increase of pancreatic output of lipase enzyme; heat-deteriorated oil increased the output nearly ninefold. The effect of canola oil on other pancreatic enzymes such as trypsin, chymotrypsin, and amylase was negligible as compared with that on lipase.

Effects of Dietary Fiber. The debate continues about the extent to which swine utilize dietary fiber. The reader is referred to recent reviews of the role of dietary fiber in swine feeding (Kaufmann 1982; Partridge 1982) for a bibliography of pertinent literature. Partridge (1982) proposed that the energy recovered from dietary fiber by swine contributes little or nothing toward metabolizable energy requirements. It is known that fiber degradation occurs in the colon with the aid of microorganisms. Varel et al. (1984) isolated two anaerobic cellulose-degrading bacteria from feces of swine; these have been identified as *Bacteroides succinogenes* and *Ruminococcus flavefaciens.* The numbers of xylanolytic and cellulolytic bacteria in the feces of 8-month-old barrows increased severalfold when the barrows were fed a 40% alfalfa meal diet (Varel et al. 1987). Eggum et al. (1982) reported that fecal excretions of numerous substances were clearly altered by the addition of grass meal to young, 22- to 26-kg body weight Landrace swine. The additions of a mixture of bacitracin and neomycin caused alterations of the microflora.

The influence of fiber on the digestibility of nutrients is important. Ehle et al. (1982) compared four sources of fiber in mature Yorkshire swine. Apparent protein digestibility was highest for the cellulose diet; true protein digestibility was highest for the coarse and fine bran diets; energy digestibility was not affected by fiber source; dry matter digestibility was highest for the cellulose diet; cell wall digestibility was highest for the coarse bran diet; cellulose digestibility was highest for alfalfa and cellulose diets; and hemicellulose digestibility was highest for the cellulose diet. Argenzio (1982) reported evidence that microbial degradation of residues that escape the small intestine must proceed to volatile fatty acids before nutritional value can be recovered by the pig. Bardon and Fioramanti (1983) demonstrated that the addition of bran to a milk diet for pigs weighing approximately 90 kg decreased retention time and increased fecal excretion of volatile fatty acids. Oral and intracecal neomycin reduced fecal excretion of volatile fatty acids nearly 50%, but retention time was not affected. Direct infusion of volatile fatty acids into the cecum increased retention time, indicating that bran and other poorly digested fibers decrease retention time by some method that does not involve fermentation products.

The utilization of energy from dietary fiber is of common interest. Kass et al. (1980) examined utilization of fiber from alfalfa meal by Yorkshire barrows weighing between approximately 20 and 90 kg with emphasis on the rates of formation and disappearance of volatile fatty acids from the colon. Although alfalfa meal was incorporated into the diets at rates up to 60%, the maximum formation of volatile fatty acids was observed with 20% alfalfa meal. The sum caloric content of acetic, proprionic, and butyric acids formed and absorbed from the digestive tract accounted for 5% to 7% of the maintenance energy requirement with no alfalfa meal in the diet; the proportion increased to 11% to 14% when alfalfa meal was 20% of the diet but did not increase further when alfalfa meal was 40% or 60% of the diet. The incremental increase of about 6 percentage points of the maintenance requirement should be considered of questionable importance. This small contribution to the energy requirements at maintenance is null for young animals capable of rapid growth. Young growing animals artificially held to zero gain or at maintenance are not productive animals. Moreover, the same caloric contribution, measured against the energy intake of similar animals on full feed, would represent less than 2 percentage points. It is debatable if such a small contribution falls outside the range of measurement error. The capacity to utilize dietary fiber to an economic advantage in growing swine is very limited.

Chel Guerrero et al. (1983) demonstrated that the Pelon Mexicano pig, which has a long history of grazing, appears not to digest diets containing a high proportion of alfalfa meal any better than other strains of pigs; furthermore, the weight of the gastrointestinal tract did not respond to the dietary fiber. This evidence indicates that the Pelon Mexicano did not adapt to fiber. Pond et al. (1981) compared the effects of 20% alfalfa meal in diets of three genotypes of swine; lean and obese genotypes, derived from the same parental stock by selection for backfat thickness, and a contemporary crossbred strain. Alfalfa meal decreased gain and gain efficiency in all three genotypes but had no effect on gastrointestinal organ measurements, carcass measurements, or on blood metabolites. This is in contrast to a later study involving the same three genotypes of pigs and a 50% alfalfa meal diet, in which it was found that the size of the gastrointestinal tract was increased by alfalfa in the lean but not in the obese strain (Pekas et al. 1983); the small intestine and colon-rectum each enlarged in the lean strain.

REFERENCES

Argenzio, R.A. 1982. *Les Colloques de l'I.N.R.A.* 12:207–216.
Bardon, T., and J. Fioramonti. 1983. *Br. J. Nutr.* 50:685.
Bayliss, W.M., and E.H. Starling. 1902. *J. Physiol.* (Lond.) 28:325.
Borgmann, E., and F. Kreienbring. 1979. *Arch. Tierernahr.* 29:419.
Buraczewski, S. 1980. *Arch. Anim. Nutr.* 30:29.
Catron, D.V., et al. 1957. *Proceedings of the 9th Research Conference, American Meat Institute.* p. 23.
Chel Guerrero, L., et al. 1983. *Tecnica Percuaria Mexico* 44:27.
Corring, T., and A. Rerat. 1983. *Int. J. Vitamin Nutr. Res.* 25:9.
Corring, T., et al. 1982. *World Rev. Nutr. Diet* 39:124.
Cranwell, P.D. 1985. *Br. J. Nutr.* 54:305.
Darcy, B., et al. 1983. *Ann. Zootechnie* 32:315.
Deprez, P., et al. 1987. *J. Vet. Med.* 34:254.
Efird, R.C., et al. 1982a. *J. Anim. Sci.* 55:1370.
Efird, R.C., et al. 1982b. *J. Anim. Sci.* 55:1380.
Eggum, B.O., et al. 1982. *Acta Agri. Scand.* 32:145.
Ehle, F.R., et al. 1982. *J. Anim. Sci.* 55:1071.
Engstrom, M.A., and K.E. Ekstrom. 1979. *J. Anim. Sci.* 48:1349.
Fevrier, C., and A. Aumaitre. 1979. *Ann. Zootechnie* 28:19.
Gebhardt, G., et al. 1981. *Arch. Anim. Nutr.* 31:763.
Gibbs, J., and G.P. Smith. 1986. *Fed. Proc.* 45:1391.
Glass, G.B. 1980. *Gastrointestinal Hormones.* New York: Raven Press.
Hampson, D.J. 1986. *Res. Vet. Sci.* 40:32.
Hampson, D.J., and D.E. Kidder. 1986. *Res. Vet. Sci.* 40:24.
Just, A., et al. 1985. *Proceedings of the 3rd International Seminar on Digestive Physiology in the Pig.* Copenhagen, Denmark.
Juste, C., et al. 1983. *J. Nutr.* 113:1691.
Kass, M.L., et al. 1980. *J. Anim. Sci.* 50:192.
Kaufmann, W. 1982. *Les Colloques l'I.N.R.A.* 12:295.
Kidder, D.E., and M.J. Manners. 1980a. In: *Current Concepts of Digestion and Absorption in Pigs.* Proceedings of the National Institute for Research in Dairying. Technical Bull. 3. Reading, England: College of Estate Management, p. 94.
Kidder, D.E., and M.J. Manners. 1980b. *Br. J. Nutr.* 43:141.
Kiles, A.K., et al. 1986. *Anim. Feed Sci. Technol.* 16:169.
Koong, L., et al. 1982. *J. Nutr.* 112:1638.
Kvasnitskii, A.V. 1951. Voprosy fiziologii pishchevareniya u svine. Sel'khozgiz, Moscow.
LaPlace, J.P. 1978. *Ann. Zootechnie* 27:377.
LaPlace, J.P., et al. 1982. *Les Colloques de l'I.N.R.A.* 12:27–29.
LaPlace, J.P., et al. 1983. *Ann. Zootechnie* 32:507.
Lawrence, T.L.J., et al. 1980. *Anim. Prod.* 31:93.
Leibholz, J. 1981. *Br. J. Nutr.* 46:59.
Leibholz, J. 1982. *Br. J. Nutr.* 48:509.

Liebert, F., et al. 1981. *Arch. Anim. Nutr.* 31:461.
Lin, F.D., et al. 1987. *J. Anim. Sci.* 64:1655.
Lindemann, M.D., et al. 1986. *J. Anim. Sci.* 62:1298.
Low, A.G. 1982. *Br. J. Nutr.* 48:147.
Low, A.G., and I.G. Partridge. 1980. In: *Current Concepts of Digestion and Absorption in Pigs.* Tech. Bull. 3. Proceedings of the National Institute for Research in Dairying. Reading, England: College of Estate Management.
Low, A.G., et al. 1985. *Br. J. Nutr.* 54:437.
Lucas, I.A.M., and G.A. Lodge. 1961. *The Nutrition of the Young Pig. A Review.* Tech. Comm. No. 22. Commonwealth Bureau of Animal Nutrition, Rowett Institute, Bucksburn, Aberdeen, Scotland. Reading, England: Lamport Gilbert & Co.
Miller, B.G., et al. 1986. *J. Agric. Sci. Cambridge* 107:579.
Moran, E.T., Jr., 1982. *Comparative Nutrition of Fowl and Swine: The Gastrointestinal Systems.* Guelph, Ontario, Canada: Office of Educational Practice, University of Guelph.
Morgan, W., III, et al. 1987. *J. Pediatr. Surg.* 22:541.
Newport, M.J. 1980. *Br. J. Nutr.* 44:171.
Newport, M.J., and H.D. Keal. 1980. *Br. J. Nutr.* 44:161.
Newport, M.J., and H.D. Keal. 1982. *Br. J. Nutr.* 48:89.
Owsley, W.F., et al. 1981. *J. Anim. Sci.* 52:557.
Ozimek, L., et al. 1983. *Bull. Alberta Univ. Faculty Ext.* 140.
Partridge, I.G. 1982. *Les Colloques L'I.N.R.A.* 12:217.
Pekas, J.C. 1977. *J. Anim. Sci.* 46:729.
Pekas, J.C. 1980. *Critical Reviews in Toxicology.* 7:37.
Pekas, J.C. 1983a. *Am. Phys. Soc.* (Abstr.).
Pekas, J.C. 1983b. *Proceedings of the International Union of Physiological Sciences.* The XXIX Congress Int. Union Phys. Sci. 15:302 (Abstr.).
Pekas, J.C. 1983c. *J. Intake Res.* 4:23.
Pekas, J.C. 1983d. *J. Intake Res.* 4:87.
Pekas, J.C. 1985. *Growth* 49:19.
Pekas, J.C. 1986a. *Digest. Dis. Sci.* 31:79.
Pekas, J.C. 1986b. *Digest. Dis. Sci.* 31:90.
Pekas, J.C., et al. 1964. *J. Nutr.* 82:277.
Pekas, J.C., et al. 1983. *Nutr. Rep. Int.* 27:259.
Pekas, J.C., and W.E. Trout. 1990. *Growth, Develop. Aging,* 54:51.
Petersson, H., and J. Hakansson. 1979. *Swedish J. Agric. Res.* 9:75.
Pond, W.G., et al. 1981. *J. Anim. Sci.* 51:367.
Rodriguez, J.P., and L.G. Young. 1980. *Proceedings of the 16th Annual Nutrition Conference of Feed Manufacturers.* p. 91.
Rothschild, B., and J.R. Reichl. 1983. *J. Anim. Physiol. Anim. Nutr.* 50:208.
Sambrook, I.E. 1979a. *Br. J. Nutr.* 42:267.
Sambrook, I.E. 1979b. *Br. J. Nutr.* 42:279.
Sambrook, I.E. 1980. In: *Current Concepts of Digestion and Absorption in Pigs.* Proceedings of the National Institute for Research in Dairying. Reading, England: College of Estate Management, p. 91.
Schummer, A., et al. 1979. *The Viscera of the Domestic Mammals.* 2d ed. New York: Springer-Verlag.
Shields, R.G., Jr., et al. 1980. *J. Anim. Sci.* 50:257.
Sisson, S., and J.D. Grossman. 1975. "Porcine Digestive System." In: *The Anatomy of the Domestic Animal.* Vol. 2. 5th ed. Getty, R. (Ed.). Philadelphia: W.B. Saunders Co.
Smith, M.W. 1984. *J. Agric. Sci.* 102:625.
Souffrant, W.B., et al. 1981a. *Arch. Anim. Nutr.* 31:35.
Suzuki, T., et al. 1981. *Jpn. J. Zootech. Sci.* 52:354.
Tkachev, E.Z. 1983. *Soviet Agric. Sci.* 7:53.
Tullis, J.B., and C.T. Whittemore. 1986. *Br. J. Nutr.* 56:259.
Varel, V.H., et al. 1984. *Appl. Environ. Microb.* 47:219.

Varel, V.H., et al. 1987. *Appl. Environ. Microb.* 53:22.
Wilson, R.H., and J. Leibholz. 1981a. *Br. J. Nutr.* 45:301.
Wilson, R.H., and J. Leibholz. 1981b. *Br. J. Nutr.* 45:321.
Wilson, R.H., and J. Leibholz. 1981c. *Br. J. Nutr.* 45:337.
Wilson, R.H., and J. Leibholz. 1981d. *Br. J. Nutr.* 45:347.
Wilson, R.H., and J. Leibholz. 1981e. *Br. J. Nutr.* 45:359.
Zebrowska, T. 1980. In: *Current Concepts of Digestion and Absorption in Pigs.* Proceedings of the National Institute for Research in Dairying. Reading, England: College of Estate Management, p. 52.
Zebrowska, T. 1981. In: Proceedings of the Nutrition in Health and Disease and International Development Symposia. New York: Alan R. Liss, p. 909.
Zebrowska, T. 1982. *Les Colloques l'I.N.R.A.* 12:225.
Zebrowska, T., et al. 1983. *Br. J. Nutr.* 49:401.

Chapter 4

Characteristics of Obese and Lean Swine

H.J. Mersmann

Obesity in pigs is a normal consequence of nineteenth and twentieth century husbandry practices. The genetic potential for the hog to become obese appears to be readily expressed as the result of a sedentary life under domestication coupled with excessive availability of food (Mersmann 1986a). It is only in the last 30 to 40 years that selection has been used to change the pig commercially raised in Europe and North America to a leaner body type (Fredeen and Harmon 1983; Topel 1986).

Obese pigs serve two major purposes in biological research: they provide a model for extremes in porcine growth, especially regarding accretion of carcass fat and muscle mass, and they provide a model, other than rodent models, to study the physiology of obesity.

TYPES OF PIGS

There are three types of obese pig models. The first is the contrast between a relatively lean and a relatively obese modern breed. For example, the smaller and more muscular Pietrain breed may be compared with contemporary pigs (Wood et al. 1975; Gregory et al. 1977; Moody et al. 1978) or a leaner breed may be compared with a fatter contemporary breed (Hood and Allen 1977). The diversity of body composition between obese and lean pigs in this type of model is less than in other models.

The second model is the Ossabaw pig, an inhabitant of an island off the coast of Georgia (Martin et al. 1972). It is not clear why this isolated population of feral pigs is obese when other feral populations are not obese (reviewed in Mersmann 1986a), but temperate climate and relatively lush vegetation on this island may not have provided selection pressure against the obese state. Graves (1984) has provided an excellent review on the behavior of the Ossabaw pig in its natural habitat.

The third model is the pig genetically selected for obesity. To this author's knowledge, there have been two major selection projects, one in the United States and one in Norway. The U.S. pigs were developed by Hetzer (Hetzer and Harvey 1967). Selection was for thick (obese) and thin (lean) backfat only in a purebred Duroc population for about 18 generations and in a purebred Yorkshire population for about 14 generations. Currently, descendants of the Hetzer selection project are maintained as lines of obese pigs established by crossing obese Duroc with obese Yorkshire and of lean pigs established by crossing lean Duroc with lean Yorkshire. The effect of crossbreeding the purebred Duroc and Yorkshire obese and lean pigs from the U.S. selection experiment is documented (Bereskin et al. 1974; Bereskin and Hetzer 1986). The Norwegian pigs were developed by Standal (Standal et al. 1973) and were selected from thin backfat coupled with high rate of gain (lean) and thick backfat coupled with low rate of gain (obese). For both U.S. and Norwegian pigs, the lean pigs provide a proper control group, selected at the same time, to which the obese pigs can be contrasted. Comparison of obese pigs to contemporary pigs broadens the scope for contrasts because it involves the multiplicity of traits for which contemporary pigs have been selected and thus is of limited value in many cases.

GROWTH

The U.S. obese and lean pigs were not selected for rate of gain, so when compared with contemporary pigs both lean and obese pigs have a lower rate of gain (Pond et al. 1980; Mersmann et al. 1982; Steele et al. 1982; Tess et al. 1984a). The postweaning growth rate of the current, crossbred U.S. obese pigs is usually less than (Pond et al. 1980b; Mersmann et al. 1982; Tess et al. 1984a), but in an occasional experiment with small animal numbers, sometimes is equal to (Scott et al. 1981a; Pekas et al. 1983; Yen and Pond 1985) that of lean pigs.

Genetically obese pigs are fatter and less muscular than lean pigs. In the U.S. pigs, considerable divergence in backfat thickness between obese and lean pigs was evident after only a few generations of selection (Hetzer and Harvey 1967; Hetzer and Miller 1972a,b). Lean pigs became more muscular than obese pigs even though there was no selection for this trait; divergence was slower in muscularity than in backfat thickness (Hetzer and Miller 1973). Carcass measurements made on these pigs (Hetzer and Harvey 1967; Davey et al. 1969; Hetzer and Miller 1972a,b, 1973; Steele et al. 1974; Bereskin and Davey 1976; Davey and Bereskin 1978; Pond et al. 1980a,b; Pekas et al. 1983; Mersmann et al. 1984b; Yen and Pond 1985) and chemical composition of the carcass detail the divergence in composition (Bereskin et al. 1978; Davey and Bereskin 1978). The current crossbred obese and lean pigs maintain the divergent characteristics in chemical carcass composition (Ferrell and Cornelius 1984; Tess et al. 1984a,b, 1986).

The Norwegian obese and lean pigs were selected for both rate of gain and backfat thickness; divergence between the lines in backfat thickness developed rapidly but divergence in rate of gain developed more slowly (Vangen 1974b, 1977, 1979, 1980a,b). In the obese line, selection resulted in little change in growth rate whereas in the lean line, growth rate was increased to a large extent with little decrease in backfat thickness (Vangen 1979). Norwegian obese pigs are fatter and less muscular than lean pigs (Trygstad et al. 1972; Standal et al. 1973; Bakke and Standal 1975; Vangen 1979, 1980a,b).

The U.S. and Norwegian obese pigs that resulted from two different selection schemes are similar in growth and body composition characteristics. The obese pig reaches compositional maturity at a younger age than the lean pig, that is, muscle deposition decelerates and fat deposition accelerates much earlier in obese than in lean pigs. For example, the U.S. obese pigs have greater carcass fatness but also have similar or even greater muscle mass than lean pigs at 9 to 10 weeks of age (Davey and Bereskin 1977; Mersmann et al. 1984b).

The Ossabaw pig is a unique animal with no appropriate control, therefore, it is usually compared with a contemporary pig. The Ossabaw pig grows slowly, reaches a body weight of less than 100 kg, is short, and can become excessively fat for its size, for example, 40% carcass fat at 45 kg body weight (Martin et al. 1972; Buhlinger et al. 1978; Etherton et al. 1982). When compared with contemporary pigs at constant weight (45 kg), the Ossabaw pig has smaller skeletal mass, greater backfat thickness, and less muscle mass (Buhlinger et al. 1978).

Studies of early growth establish that the divergence between obese and lean pigs is observable at young ages. The U.S. pigs are quite different in body composition at 9 to 10 weeks of age (Davey and Bereskin 1977; Mersmann et al. 1984b), at 4 or 8 weeks of age (Ferrell and Cornelius 1984) if body fat is adjusted for body weight, and even at 100 to 110 days of gestation (McNamara and Martin 1982; Stone et al. 1985). Thus, the obese state is expressed even before birth in the U.S. pigs. Ossabaw pigs are fatter than contemporary pigs at 3 days and at 6 to 8 weeks of age (Cote and Wangsness 1978; Wangsness and Soroka 1978; Kasser et al. 1981) and during late stages of gestation (Hoffman et al. 1983). Ossabaw pigs differ from contemporary pigs much as genetically obese and lean pigs differ with early expression of fatness and later divergence of muscle mass.

REPRODUCTION

The U.S. obese and lean pigs are divergent in reproductive traits (Hetzer and Miller 1970, 1972a; Mersmann et al. 1984a). Obese sows have a slightly shorter gestation period (113 versus 115 days), lose much less weight during lactation, and have a smaller number of fetal and live born pigs that weigh less at 110 days of gestation (Hausman et al. 1983b), at birth, or at weaning (Mersmann et al. 1984a). A striking difference is observed in piglet survival to weaning, wherein the percentage is 93 and 76 for obese and lean sows, respectively. In the Norwegian selection experiment, obese pigs weigh less at birth but have only slightly greater survival than lean pigs; the number of live born pigs is the same in both strains (Vangen 1972, 1974a, 1980c,d).

Ossabaw pigs have a low number of corpora lutea as compared with contemporary pigs (9 versus 15) and display similar survival rates at 80 to 110 days of gestation so that fetal number is about six and ten in Ossabaw and contemporary pigs, respectively (Hagen and Kephart 1980). Litter size in Ossabaw pigs is not limited by uterine size in late gestation (Hagen et al. 1980) but is limited in early gestation (Hagen et al. 1984). Ossabaw fetuses weigh considerably less than contemporary pig fetuses at 70 to 110 days of gestation (Hagen et al. 1980; Hausman et al. 1983b, 1985) and at 1 to 3 days postpartum (Cote and Wangsness 1978; Hausman and Martin 1981; Kasser et al. 1981). Although newborn Ossabaw pigs have greater survival during fasting than contemporary pigs (Kasser et al. 1981), there is no documentation of postweaning survival in fed Ossabaw pigs.

NUTRITION

Feed Consumption

The Ossabaw pig has been carefully studied to determine whether excessive feed intake is a major contributor to the obesity. Ossabaw pigs have the same number of eating bouts per day but spend 50% more time eating each day and consume about 9% more feed per unit of body weight than do contemporary pigs (Wangsness et al. 1980a). At 4 to 22 days of age, Ossabaw pigs eat 25% more energy from a purified diet than crossbred pigs when expressed on a body weight basis (Wangsness and Soroka 1978). Thus, excessive feed intake could contribute to the obesity during suckling, depending on milk composition and quantity, and certainly contributes to the obesity after weaning.

The U.S. obese pigs have not been studied intensively regarding feeding behavior, but they probably eat more than lean pigs. For example, in obese and lean strains the reported respective gain per feed is 0.28 and 0.34 (Bereskin et al. 1975) or 0.24 and 0.28 (Pond et al. 1980). Results of many experiments (all with small numbers of pigs) indicate these same trends (Davey et al. 1969; Scott et al. 1981; Pekas et al. 1983; Tess et al. 1984b; Yen and Pond 1985). The contribution of excessive feed intake in these pigs appears to be less than in the Ossabaw pigs, but the studies are not as complete as with Ossabaw pigs.

The Norwegian obese pigs eat somewhat more than do the lean pigs; after about 4 years of selection, the obese and lean pigs had gain per feed ratios of about 0.30 and 0.33, respectively (Vangen 1974b; 1977; 1980a,b). The divergence appears to be about the same as that in the U.S. pigs in spite of the additional selection for rate of gain in the Norwegian pigs.

Maintenance

The basal metabolic rate, estimated as fasting heat production, is lower in U.S. obese than lean pigs (Koong et al. 1983; Tess et al. 1984a). The lower rate seems to be associated with less muscle mass and smaller digestive organs (Davey and Bereskin 1978;

Pond et al. 1980b; Koong et al. 1983; Pekas et al. 1983; Tess et al. 1984a, 1986). Lower maintenance requirements coupled with similar or slightly greater feed consumption would contribute in great part to the observed obesity in U.S. pigs.

The Norwegian obese pigs have a lower fasting heat production than do lean pigs (Sundstol et al. 1979). In contrast, the maintenance energy of obese pigs, observed in feeding trials, is greater than that of lean pigs (Vangen 1980b); the author does not resolve the divergence between this work and that of Sundstol et al. (1979) on the same lines of pigs. To this author's knowledge, gut organ size has not been measured in the Norwegian obese and lean pigs.

Dietary Energy

The earliest postnatal nutritional variation between obese and lean pigs could be the milk produced by sows. Milk from Norwegian obese pigs has similar composition to that from lean pigs (Bakke and Vold 1975). Milk composition has not been determined in Ossabaw pigs. Milk from U.S. obese pigs has more fat for the first 2 weeks of lactation than milk from U.S. lean pigs (Mersmann et al. 1984a). Thus, the greater energy in milk from U.S. obese pigs could contribute to the obesity. Milk consumption or output has not been measured in Ossabaw or U.S. or Norwegian obese and lean pigs. Although milk production might be deduced from growth rate in suckling pigs, comparison of two different strains of pigs with unequal growth potential does not seem appropriate. Cross-fostering of U.S. and obese pigs did not clarify the role of milk production because obese and lean pigs suckling their respective sows and lean pigs suckling obese sows all grew at the same rate, whereas obese pigs suckling lean sows grew at a greater rate than any other group (Mersmann et al. 1984a).

There does not appear to be any difference in U.S. obese and lean pigs regarding the ability to utilize dietary carbohydrate and fat (Steele and Frobish 1976); both strains deposit more carcass fat when fed isoenergetic-isonitrogenous diets with high-fat as compared with high-carbohydrate content (Mersmann et al. 1984b). Obese pigs and crossbred contemporary pigs both have depressed gain when 1,3-butylene glycol is substituted for glucose in the diet (Steele et al. 1982). Obese and lean pigs have the same digestibilities for energy when fed a high-carbohydrate diet (Yen et al. 1983).

It might be presumed that obese pigs would be more susceptible to atherogenesis than lean pigs; this is not demonstrable for U.S. obese and lean pigs fed high fat-high cholesterol diets (Pond et al. 1985). When obese and lean pigs are fed high fat-high cholesterol diets low in protein content, lean pigs have higher plasma cholesterol concentration than do obese pigs (Pond et al. 1986).

Dietary Protein

The primary nutritional difference in U.S. obese and lean pigs is the requirement for dietary protein. This is not due to nitrogen digestibility (Yen et al. 1983). Lean but not obese pigs have retarded growth when fed lower (e.g., 12% versus 20%) dietary protein as a result of the greater muscle and gut mass in lean than in obese pigs (Davey and Morgan 1969; Davey 1976; Pond et al. 1980a; Pond et al. 1983b; Pond and Yen 1984). The lower protein requirement is reflected in higher blood urea nitrogen concentrations in obese than in lean pigs when fed isonitrogenous diets because more of the dietary amino acids are deaminated and used as carbon skeletons in obese pigs (Mersmann et al. 1984b). Lean pigs fed protein-deficient diets also have lower serum protein and albumin concentrations than do obese pigs (Pond and Yen 1984). Obese and lean pigs are not differentially affected when fed a 14% protein diet (Bereskin et al. 1975; Bereskin and Davey 1976; Davey and Bereskin 1978).

Dietary Restriction

If feed intake is a major contributor to the obesity, dietary restrictions could eliminate the obesity. Restriction in dietary energy reduces the carcass weight and the weight of carcass fat in both U.S. obese and lean pigs (Davey et al. 1969; Pond et al. 1980b; Pekas et al. 1983). A modest restriction of the energy content of the diet does not markedly affect gain, feed conversion, or carcass traits in U.S. obese or lean pigs (Bereskin et al. 1975; Bereskin and Davey 1976; Davey and Bereskin 1978). Severe restriction of dietary intake reduces backfat thickness, mostly in the middle layer, to a lesser extent in U.S. obese than in contemporary pigs (Mersmann and Leymaster 1984). Although no differential growth responses are observed between lean and obese pigs, the adaptation of cecal cellulolytic bacteria appears greater in lean than in obese pigs fed a 50% alfalfa diet (Varel et al. 1982). As in U.S. obese pigs, restriction to 65% of ad libitum intake does not affect Ossabaw pigs as severely as contemporary pigs (Etherton et al. 1982).

Diet restriction from 1.8 to 0.6 kg/d during the last 75% of pregnancy causes U.S. lean sows to lose backfat depth but maintain body weight, whereas U.S. obese sows lose backfat depth but gain weight (Pond et al. 1983a). Preweaning growth and piglet survival of progeny of either strain of pigs are not affected by dietary intake. Maternal feed restriction causes retarded growth in lean but not in obese progeny to 10 weeks of age (Pond et al. 1983b). Thus, obese pigs or sows are less severely affected by dietary restriction than lean pigs or sows, probably as a consequence of greater endogenous energy stores coupled with lower amino acid requirements resulting from reduced muscle and gut organ mass in obese as compared with lean pigs.

ENDOCRINE AND METABOLITE STATUS

Metabolic differences between obese and lean pigs may be expressed in plasma concentrations of hormones and metabolites. Measurement of concentrations does not distinguish between primary events that could be crucial to decipher the genetic lesions that give rise to the obesity and secondary events that represent adaptation of the organism to altered metabolism. Regardless, altered hormone or metabolite concentrations in the fetus or early neonate suggest that these are primary, not secondary, events because the obesity has expressed itself to only a small degree at these stages of development.

In Ossabaw as compared with contemporary pigs in late fetal life or at birth, plasma concentration of growth hormone is low, triiodothyronine is high, and there is no difference in insulin, thyroxine, cortisol, glucagon, glucose, or free fatty acid concentrations (Kasser et al. 1981; Hoffman et al. 1983; Martin et al. 1985). During fasting, newborn Ossabaw pigs mobilize more free fatty acids and survive longer than contemporary pigs (Kasser et al. 1981). At 1, 3, and 6 months of age, plasma concentration of growth hormone is lower and insulin, glucose, and free fatty acid concentrations are similar in Ossabaw as compared with contemporary pigs (Wangsness et al. 1977, 1981; McCusker et al. 1985). Although growth hormone concentrations are lower and pigs are not hyperglycemic at 5 to 6 months of age (Martin et al. 1972; Wangsness et al. 1977), glucose- or insulin-induced release of growth hormone is greater in Ossabaw than in contemporary pigs (Wangsness et al. 1977, 1980b). As compared with contemporary pigs, Ossabaw pigs appear to have a greater rate of fasting glucose production (Cote et al. 1982), probably a result of greater capacity for hepatic gluconeogenesis (Martin et al. 1972; Martin and Herbein 1976). Fasted Ossabaw pigs have greater glucose clearance than do contemporary pigs (Cote et al. 1982), but they have impaired glucose clearance when confronted with a glucose load (Wangsness et al. 1977). The Ossabaw pigs are somewhat hyperinsulinemic when studied in detail (Wangsness et al. 1977, 1981; McCusker et al. 1985) and may be somewhat insensitive to insulin as indicated by lower insulin binding to liver in Ossabaw than in contemporary pigs (Meserole and Etherton 1984). At 10 to 12 months of age, Ossabaw pigs are hypercholesterolemic and hypertriglyceridemic with alterations in lipoprotein composition (Etherton and Kris-Etherton 1980).

In late prenatal life, plasma concentrations of growth hormone are lower, albumin and triiodothyronine are higher, and cortisol is similar in U.S. genetically obese as compared with lean pigs (Stone et al. 1985). Plasma concentration of albumin is greater and alpha-fetoprotein less in obese than in lean fetuses from 60 days of gestation (Stone 1984). The development of albumin synthesis and secretion to the plasma may be an indicator of physiological maturity, indicating obese pigs are more mature at this stage of development. Other indications of maturity are the higher hemoglobin, hematocrit, plasma protein, and albumin at birth in obese than in lean pigs (Mersmann et al. 1984a).

There are some differences observed between obese and lean pigs during postweaning growth to maturity. At weaning and at 95 kg body weight, plasma growth hormone concentration is lower in U.S. obese than in lean pigs (Althen and Gerrits 1976a); the U.S. pigs have similar metabolic clearance and secretion rates for growth hormone (Althen and Gerrits 1976b). Obese pigs have lower plasma triiodothyronine but not thyroxine than do lean pigs (Yen and Pond 1985). The U.S. obese pigs are not hyperglycemic, hypertriglyceridemic, hypercholesterolemic, or hyperinsulinemic from birth to 5.5 months of age (Mersmann et al. 1982); they also have normal glucose tolerance curves. Some studies indicate obese pigs are hypercholesterolemic and hypertriglyceridemic as compared with lean pigs (Pekas et al. 1983; Pond et al. 1985) but the plasma concentrations are all very low, i.e., cholesterol <200 and triglyceride <100 mg/dl. The U.S. obese as compared with lean pigs have elevated plasma free fatty acid concentrations in the fed state and depressed concentrations when fasted (Pekas et al. 1983; Mersmann and MacNeil 1985). In the Norwegian obese as compared with lean pigs, plasma growth hormone and somatomedin (sulfation factor) concentrations are lower at 90 kg (Lund-Larsen and Bakke 1975). Norwegian obese as compared with lean pigs have higher concentrations of plasma cortisol and cortisol-binding protein, and equal plasma testosterone concentrations (Lundstrom et al. 1983). Fed Norwegian obese and lean pigs have similar plasma glucose and free fatty acid concentrations, but glucose is elevated and free fatty acids are lowered during fasting in obese as compared with lean pigs (Bakke 1975b). Norwegian lean pigs have marginally greater serum cholesterol concentrations than do obese pigs, and triglyceride concentration is similar in the two strains (Bakke 1975a).

Each of the obese models is different from genetically lean or contemporary pigs regarding plasma hormone and metabolite concentrations. Although insulin might be expected to be a major endocrine influence on the development of these obesities (Martin et al. 1984), there is little evidence for hyperinsulinemia or alterations in carbohydrate metabolism in obese pigs except for the Ossabaw pigs. Carbohydrate and lipid metabolism in vivo have not been investigated except for the studies in Ossabaw pigs. Common to each obese pig model is lower growth hormone concentration at several stages of growth.

ADIPOSE TISSUE

The greater carcass fat mass is expressed as larger adipocytes in U.S. obese (Steele et al. 1974; Scott et al. 1981a; Mersmann and Koong 1984; Mersmann 1985, 1986) and in Ossabaw (Etherton 1980; Etherton et al. 1982) pigs as compared with U.S. lean or contemporary pigs, respectively. The obesities are evident in late gestation or shortly after birth by examination of body composition in Ossabaw (Cote and Wangsness 1978; Hoffman et al. 1983) and in U.S. pigs (McNamara and Martin 1982; Stone et al. 1985). Adipose tissue fatty acids are more saturated in obese than in lean pigs (Scott et al. 1981b).

Adipocyte size is slightly larger in U.S. obese than in lean pigs in late gestation, at birth, and during the neonatal period (Hausman et al. 1983; Mersmann 1986). In Ossabaw as compared with contemporary pigs, adipocytes are larger and develop earlier after 70 days of gestation (Hausman et al. 1983a; Hausman 1985; Hausman and Thomas 1985). Lipoprotein lipase activity is greater in adipocytes from Ossabaw than from contemporary pigs and in adipocytes from obese than from lean pigs at 110 days of gestation (McNamara and Martin 1982; Hausman et al. 1983a). This enzyme may be a marker by which differentiation of precursor cells into adipocytes capable of accreting considerable amounts of depot lipid may be judged. The enzyme allows utilization of circulating lipid as a source of fatty acids for tissue synthesis into triacylglycerol. One study indicates smaller adipocytes in Ossabaw than in contemporary pigs at 1 to 2 days postpartum but larger adipocytes by 2 to 3 weeks of age (Hausman and

Martin 1981); the slow-developing innermost backfat layer has similar adipocyte size and morphology at 110 days of gestation in Ossabaw and in U.S. obese and lean pigs (Hausman and Thomas 1984).

Adipose tissue lipogenic rates, that is, de novo fatty acid synthesis, measured by glucose incorporation into total lipids, are low and similar in obese and lean pigs before weaning when pigs convert dietary lipid to depot lipid via adipose tissue lipoprotein lipase coupled with triacylglycerol biosynthesis (Mersmann 1986b). Although not measured, the greater lipoprotein lipase activity observed in obese than in lean pigs at late gestational ages (McNamara and Martin 1982; Hausman et al. 1983) probably prevails during the suckling period. Lipogenic rates expressed per adipocyte accelerate markedly after weaning and are much greater in obese than in lean pigs 2 weeks postweaning (Mersmann 1986); these rates and lipogenic enzyme activities are greater in obese than in lean growing and finishing pigs (Steele et al. 1974; Steele and Frobish 1976; Scott et al. 1981a) even when pigs are fed isoenergetically (Mersmann et al. 1984b) or less than ad libitum (Mersmann and Koong 1984). Adipose tissue lipogenic rates and associated enzyme activities are greater in older Ossabaw than in contemporary pigs even when they are pair-fed; liver lipogenic rates and enzyme activities are similar in both strains (Martin et al. 1972; Martin and Herbein 1976; Buhlinger et al. 1978). It is not clear whether elevated lipogenic rates contribute to these obesities or are the result of excess energy intake in the obese strains.

The role of lipid degradation on adipose tissue accretion in obese pigs is not clear. Norwegian and U.S. obese pigs both have lower plasma free fatty acid concentrations during fasting than do lean pigs (Standal et al. 1973; Bakke 1975; Mersmann and MacNeil 1985). Another selection experiment indicated that lean pigs have greater plasma free fatty acid concentrations during fasting than do contemporary pigs (Gregory et al. 1980). The physiological contribution of fat accretion of this apparent decrease in lipolysis in vivo is questioned because pigs usually eat many meals distributed throughout the day (Gregory et al. 1980). However, in contemporary pigs, plasma free fatty acid concentration increases between 6 and 12 hours after removal of feed (Wangsness et al. 1981; Mersmann and MacNeil 1985), so this time may be long enough to allow mobilization rates to contribute to the obesity. Detailed time courses have not been generated for obese and lean pigs. Ossabaw pigs have plasma free fatty acid concentrations similar to contemporary pigs during the 24-hour period after feed removal (Wangsness et al. 1981).

Examination of adipose tissue lipolytic rates in vitro does not indicate a lower rate in U.S. obese than in lean pigs (Scott et al. 1981a; Mersmann and Koong 1984; Mersmann 1985, 1986). Data to indicate decreased lipolytic rates in obese as compared with lean Norwegian pigs were not expressed on a cell basis and probably are an indication of divergent adipocyte size rather than divergent metabolic activity (Trygstad et al. 1972; Standal et al. 1973). The sensitivity of lipolysis to adrenergic stimulation in vitro is slightly greater in adipose tissue from U.S. lean than from obese pigs (Mersmann 1985); if operable in vivo, this observation may indicate a role for lipolytic rates to contribute to adiposity and would be compatible with lower free fatty acid release to plasma during fasting. In Ossabaw as compared with contemporary pigs of equal weight, the basal lipolytic rate in vitro, expressed per total body fat, is similar, whereas the dibutyryl cyclic adenosine monophosphate (cAMP) stimulated rate is greater in the obese pigs (Buhlinger et al. 1978). Therefore, the lipolytic rate, as measured in vitro, does not appear to be a factor in this obesity.

MUSCLE

As indicated previously, there is much less muscle mass in obese than in lean pigs. Analysis of skeletal muscle protein, DNA and RNA content, and concentration in fetuses at 45 kg body weight and at 6 months of age suggests that semitendinosus muscle cell size is greater in contemporary than in Ossabaw pigs (Ezekwe and Martin 1975; Buhlinger et al. 1978; Hoffman et al. 1983). Fiber diameters are larger in Ossabaw than in contemporary pigs but fiber number is diminished, whereas the fiber types are similar in the two strains of pigs (Hausman et al. 1983b). Muscle enzyme development is similar in the two strains during the last third of gestation (Hausman et al. 1985). Muscles from U.S. lean and obese pigs have similar fiber size at 100 days of gestation, but both are larger than those from contemporary pigs (Hausman et al. 1983b). At 14 days of age, semitendinosus muscle weight is greater in U.S. obese than in lean pigs (Hausman and Campion 1986). The greater weight is accompanied not only by greater fiber diameter, dry matter, percentage protein, and protein/DNA, but also by a lower DNA concentration. The observations support greater muscle maturity in obese than in lean pigs at 14 days of age, but the depressed DNA concentration implies that muscle development will be less in the obese than in the lean pigs. The Norwegian obese pigs also have a lower muscle DNA concentration than do lean pigs (Lundstrom et al. 1983). Lower blood plasma cortisol and plasma corticosteroid-binding globulin concentrations in lean than in obese pigs suggest more glucocorticoid activity in obese than in lean pigs, which would contribute to less muscle deposition (Lundstrom et al. 1983).

A few selected aspects of muscle metabolism have been studied in U.S. obese and lean pigs. There is no difference in skeletal muscle lipoprotein lipase activity between lean and obese pigs at late gestation or at 14 days postpartum (McNamara and Martin 1982). Muscle from 14-day-old lean pigs has similar glucose oxidation and palmitate esterification rates but greater glycolytic flux and palmitate oxidation rates when compared with that from obese pigs (Campion et al. 1983). Glucose oxidation and glycolytic flux are greater in muscle from lean than from obese pigs at 110 days of gestation; divergence in palmitate metabolism or muscle lipid content is not evident at this stage of development (Darnton et al. 1983). These initial studies do not indicate a metabolic state leading to lesser muscle development in obese as compared with lean pigs. The higher circulating cortisol and cortisol-binding protein in Norwegian obese than in lean pigs could lead to greater catabolic rates in muscle from the former compared with the latter pigs. There are no studies on skeletal muscle protein synthesis or degradation in any of these obese models.

CONCLUSION

The increased fat deposition in growing obese pigs provides a model in which metabolic processes and endocrine secretions involved in adipose tissue hypertrophy, and possibly hyperplasia, are accentuated. We know little about metabolic rates, kinetics, or tissue turnover in whole animal muscle or adipose tissue in vivo in any of these models. A few studies on glucose and insulin metabolism have been done in Ossabaw pigs (Wangsness et al. 1977; Cote et al. 1982). Given continued interest, these various models may yield information that ultimately will be useful to alter fat accretion by genetic selection for a specific metabolic trait, by targeted nutritional change or by endocrinological or pharmacological manipulation. The U.S. and Norwegian obese and lean pigs present interesting models because in each case selection for both strains was in the same experiment and thus the lean pigs serve as controls for the obese pigs. The obese pigs with diminished muscle development may serve as a model for muscle hypertrophy, albeit in a negative manner. Finally, the lean pigs may supply information on factors involved in increased muscle development; because the U.S. and Norwegian lean pigs are not particularly well muscled and grow more slowly than contemporary pigs, little attention has been paid to these pigs that were selected not only for less backfat but indirectly for greater muscle mass.

Obese pigs also may serve as models for human obesity (Houpt et al. 1979). The pig models are not complicated by major defects in carbohydrate and/or lipid metabolism, as are most rodent obesity models (Hunt et al. 1976; Herberg and Coleman 1977; York 1985). The pig models express the obesity early without extraneous metabolic and endocrine abnormalities. Thus, the pig models represent an alternative and less complex but little used model for early-onset human obesity. It remains to be determined if the obese pig is a valuable model to decipher some of the defects leading to human obesity.

ADDENDUM

Several contributions to the literature have appeared since the completion of this chapter (October 1986 to February 1989). The usefulness of obese pigs as a biomedical model has been discussed (Mersmann 1986c). Pigs from obese and lean sows (U.S.) mated to Hampshire boars were fed complete diets at restricted intakes (Dickerson and Teague 1987). Lean pigs respond more favorably to feed restriction than obese pigs; total cost for production of lean mass is not reduced by any of the restricted feeding approaches. Obese pigs (U.S.) fed diets with high alfalfa content have smaller gut organ weights than lean pigs (Pond et al. 1988). Obese pigs have a faster rate of passage of digesta and possibly fewer cellulolytic bacteria, explaining the lower fiber digestibility in obese than lean pigs (Varel et al. 1988). U.S. obese dams do not mobilize more energy than in lean dams when subjected to restricted intake during gestation (Pond and Mersmann 1988). Serum lipids and lipoprotein lipids generally are more abundant in U.S. obese compared with contemporary sows and fetuses (Walsh-Hentges and Martin 1988). Thus, a small but significant increase in serum lipids is evident in the fetus before gross development of the obesity. U.S. obese pigs become hypercholesterolemic when fed a high-fat, high-cholesterol diet, and the effect is accentuated by low dietary protein; the response is less in obese than in lean pigs (Pond et al. 1986).

Reciprocal crosses between U.S. obese and lean pigs reveal no heterotic effect and the maternal obesity has little influence on fetal development to 110 days of gestation

(Campion et al. 1988); obese fetuses have more lipoprotein lipase in skeletal muscle and adipose tissue and are generally more mature than lean fetuses. Fetal development of the perirenal fat depot has been described in Ossabaw and U.S. obese and lean pigs by using morphological and histochemical techniques; Ossabaw and U.S. obese 110-day fetuses have larger adipocytes than fetuses from the lean strains (Hausman and Thomas 1987). Development of adipose tissue in the porcine fetus has been summarized (Hausman 1985b; Hausman et al. 1986); U.S. obese fetuses have greater adipose tissue fatty acid synthetic and esterification rates in vitro than lean fetuses at 110-day gestation. Triacylglycerol biosynthesis is greater in adipose tissue from U.S. obese than lean pigs at postweaning ages (Rule et al. 1989). Lipid mobilization in vivo is not different in U.S. obese compared with lean pigs (Mersmann and MacNeil 1989).

Sera from U.S. obese and lean fetuses stimulate proliferation of rat preadipocytes equally, but sera from obese fetuses and postnatal pigs stimulate differentiation to a greater extent than sera from lean fetuses and pigs (Jewell and Hausman 1988). Sera from Ossabaw crossbred pigs stimulate myogenic cell proliferation to a lesser extent than sera from lean crossbred pigs (Allen et al. 1982). Thus, factors in serum may be important in both the lesser muscle and greater adipose tissue development in obese than in lean pigs.

ACKNOWLEDGMENT

The opportunity to become associated with one of the obese strains of pigs was afforded by my location at the Meat Animal Research Center. I am grateful for the cooperation and help provided by many persons, especially W.G. Pond, with whom many studies were done. I thank M.M. Bierman for secretarial assistance. I have attempted to make this review of obese pigs as comprehensive as possible to October 1986.

REFERENCES

Allen, R.E., et al. 1982. *J. Anim. Sci.* 54:763.
Althen, T.G., and R.J. Gerrits. 1976a. *J. Anim. Sci.* 42:1490.
Althen, T.G., and R.J. Gerrits. 1976b. *Endocrinology* 99:511.
Bakke, H. 1975a. *Acta Agric. Scand.* 25:14.
Bakke, H. 1975b. *Acta Agric. Scand.* 25:113.
Bakke, H., and N. Standal. 1975. *Acta Agric. Scand.* 25:221.
Bakke, H., and E. Vold. 1975. *Acta Agric. Scand.* 25:325.
Bereskin, B., and R.J. Davey. 1976. *J. Anim. Sci.* 42:43.
Bereskin, B., and H.O. Hetzer. 1986. *J. Anim. Sci.* 63:395.
Bereskin, B., D.K. Rough, and R.J. Davey. 1978. *J. Anim. Sci.* 47:389.
Bereskin, B., et al. 1974. *J. Anim. Sci.* 39:1.
Bereskin, B., et al. 1975. *J. Anim. Sci.* 40:53.
Buhlinger, C.A., et al. 1978. *Growth* 42:225.
Campion, D.R., G.J. Hausman, and F.I. Meredith. 1983. *J. Anim. Sci.* 57:26.
Campion, D.R., et al. 1988. *J. Anim. Sci.* 66:28.
Cote, P.J. Jr., and P.J. Wangsness. 1978. *J. Anim. Sci.* 47:441.
Cote, P.J. Jr., et al. 1982. *J. Anim. Sci.* 54:89.
Darnton, S.M., et al. 1983. *J. Anim. Sci.* 56:838.

Davey, R.J. 1976. *J. Anim. Sci.* 43:598.
Davey, R.J., and B. Bereskin. 1977. *J. Anim. Sci.* 45:59.
Davey, R.J., and B. Bereskin. 1978. *J. Anim. Sci.* 46:992.
Davey R.J., and D.P. Morgan. 1969. *J. Anim. Sci.* 28:831.
Davey, R.J., D.P. Morgan and C.M. Kincaid. 1969. *J. Anim. Sci.* 28:197.
Dickerson, G.E., and H.S. Teague. 1987. *J. Anim. Breed. Genet.* 104:82.
Etherton, T.D. 1980. *Growth* 44:182.
Etherton, T.D., and P.M. Kris-Etherton. 1980. *Lipids* 15:823.
Etherton, T.D., et al. 1982. *J. Nutr.* 112:2314.
Ezekwe, M.O., and R.J. Martin. 1975. *Growth* 39:95.
Ferrell, C.L., and S.G. Cornelius. 1984. *J. Anim. Sci.* 58:903.
Fredeen, H.T., and B.G. Harmon. 1983. *J. Anim. Sci.* 57:100.
Graves, H.B. 1984. *J. Anim. Sci.* 58:482.
Gregory, N.G., et al. 1977. *J. Agric. Sci. Cambridge* 89:407.
Hagen, D.R., and K.B. Kephart. 1980. *Biol. Reprod.* 22:550.
Hagen, D.R., K.B. Kephart, and P.J. Wangsness. 1980. *Biol. Reprod.* 23:929.
Hagen, D.R., et al. 1984. *Biol. Reprod.* 30:423.
Hausman, G.J. 1985a. *J. Anim. Sci.* 60:1539.
Hausman, G.J. 1985b. In: *New Perspectives in Adipose Tissue: Structure, Function and Development.* Cryer, A., and R.L.R. Van (Eds.). pp. 1–21. London: Butterworths.
Hausman, G.J., and D.R. Campion. 1986. *Growth* 50:287.
Hausman, G.J., D.R. Campion, and G.B. Thomas. 1983a. *J. Lipid Res.* 24:223.
Hausman, G.J., D.R. Campion, and G.B. Thomas. 1983b. *J. Anim. Sci.* 57:1608.
Hausman, G.J., D.R. Campion, and G.B. Thomas. 1985. *J. Anim. Sci.* 60:1562.
Hausman, G.J., and R.J. Martin. 1981. *J. Anim. Sci.* 52:1442.
Hausman, G.J., and G.B. Thomas. 1984. *J. Anim. Sci.* 58:1550.
Hausman, G.J., and G.B. Thomas. 1985. *Acta Anat.* 123:137.
Hausman, G.J., and G.B. Thomas. 1987. *Int'l. J. Obesity* 11:545.
Hausman, G.J., R.J. Martin, and D.R. Campion. 1986. In: *Swine in Biomedical Research, Vol. 2.* Tumbleson, M.E. (Ed.). pp. 997–1006. New York: Plenum.
Herberg, L., and D.L. Coleman. 1977. *Metabolism* 26:59.
Hetzer, H.O., and W.R. Harvey. 1967. *J. Anim. Sci.* 26:1244.
Hetzer, H.O., and R.H. Miller. 1970. *J. Anim. Sci.* 30:481.
Hetzer, H.O., and R.H. Miller. 1972a. *J. Anim. Sci.* 35:730.
Hetzer, H.O., and R.H. Miller. 1972b. *J. Anim. Sci.* 35:743.
Hetzer, H.O., and R.H. Miller. 1973. *J. Anim. Sci.* 37:1289.
Hoffman, E.C., et al. 1983. *J. Anim. Sci.* 57:609.
Hood, R.L., and C.E. Allen. 1977. *J. Lipid Res.* 18:275.
Houpt, K.A., T.R. Houpt, and W.G. Pond. 1979. *Yale J. Biol. Med.* 52:307.
Hunt, C.E., J.R. Lindsey, and S.U. Walkley. 1976. *Fed. Proc.* 35:1206.
Jewell, D.E., and G.J. Hausman. 1988. *J. Anim. Sci.* 66:2393.
Kasser, T.R., et al. 1981. *J. Anim. Sci.* 53:420.
Koong, L.J., J.A. Nienaber, and H.J. Mersmann. 1983. *J. Nutr.* 113:1626.
Lund-Larsen, T.R., and H. Bakke. 1975. *Acta Agric. Scand.* 25:231.
Lundstrom, K., et al. 1983. *J. Anim. Sci.* 56:401.
McCusker, R.H., et al. 1985. *Physiol. Behav.* 35:383.
McNamara, J.P., and R.J. Martin. 1982. *J. Anim. Sci.* 55:1057.
Martin, R.J., and J.H. Herbein. 1976. *Proc. Soc. Exp. Biol. Med.* 151:231.
Martin, R.J., T.G. Ramsay, and R.B.S. Harris. 1984. *Domestic Anim. Endocrinol.* 1:89.
Martin, R.J., et al. 1972. *Proc. Soc. Exp. Biol. Med.* 143:198.
Martin, R.J., et al. 1985. *Growth* 49:400.
Mersmann, H.J. 1985. *J. Anim. Sci.* 60:131.
Mersmann, H.J. 1986a. In: *Swine in Cardiovascular Research.* Stanton, H.C., and H.J. Mersmann (Eds.). pp. 2–7. Boca Raton, FL: CRC Press.

Mersmann, H.J. 1986b. *J. Anim. Sci.* 63:741.
Mersmann, H.J. 1986c. In: *Swine in Biomedical Research, Vol. 2.* Tumbleson, M.E. (Ed.). pp. 981–995. New York: Plenum Press.
Mersmann, H.J., and L-J Koong. 1984. *J. Nutr.* 114:862.
Mersmann, H.J., and K.A. Leymaster. 1984. *Growth* 48:321.
Mersmann, H.J., and M.D. MacNeil. 1985. *J. Anim. Sci.* 61:122.
Mersmann, H.J., and M.D. MacNeil. 1989. *J. Anim. Sci.* 67:(1992)
Mersmann, H.J., W.G. Pond, and J.T. Yen. 1982. *Growth* 46:189.
Mersmann, H.J., W.G. Pond, and J.T. Yen. 1984b. *J. Anim. Sci.* 58:894.
Mersmann, H.J., et al. 1984a. *Growth* 48:209.
Meserole, V.K., and T.D. Etherton. 1984. *J. Anim. Sci.* 59:650.
Moody, W.G., et al. 1978. *J. Anim. Sci.* 46:618.
Pekas, J.C., J.T. Yen, and W.G. Pond. 1983. *Nutr. Rep. Int.* 27:259.
Pond, W.G., and J.H. Mersmann. 1988. *J. Nutr.* 118:1223.
Pond, W.G., and J.T. Yen. 1984. *J. Anim. Sci.* 59:710.
Pond, W.G., J.T. Yen, and R.N. Lindvall. 1980a. *J. Nutr.* 110:2506.
Pond, W.G., et al. 1980b. *J. Anim. Sci.* 51:367.
Pond, W.G., et al. 1983a. *J. Nutr.* 113:436.
Pond, W.G., et al. 1983b. *Nutr. Rep. Int.* 27:315.
Pond, W.G., et al. 1985. *Proc. Soc. Exp. Biol. Med.* 179:90.
Pond, W.G., et al. 1986. *J. Nutr.* 116:1116.
Pond, W.G., et al. 1988. *J. Anim. Sci.* 66:699.
Rule, D.C., S.B. Smith, and H.J. Mersmann. 1989. *J. Anim. Sci.* 67:364.
Scott, R.A., S.G. Cornelius, and H.J. Mersmann. 1981a. *J. Anim. Sci.* 52:505.
Scott, R.A., S.G. Cornelius, and H.J. Mersmann. 1981b. *J. Anim. Sci.* 53:977.
Standal, N., et al. 1973. *Anim. Prod.* 16:37.
Steele, N.C., and L.T. Frobish. 1976. *Growth* 40:369.
Steele, N.C., et al. 1974. *J. Anim. Sci.* 39:712.
Steele, N.C., et al. 1982. *J. Anim. Sci.* 54:116.
Stone, R.T. 1984. *Biol. Neonate* 46:122.
Stone, R.T., et al. 1985. *Proc. Soc. Exp. Biol. Med.* 180:191.
Sundstol, F., et al. 1979. *Acta Agric. Scand.* 29:337.
Tess, M.W., et al. 1984a. *J. Anim. Sci.* 58:99.
Tess, M.W., et al. 1984b. *J. Anim. Sci.* 58:111.
Tess, M.W., et al. 1986. *J. Anim. Sci.* 62:968.
Topel, D.G. 1986. *J. Anim. Sci.* 63:633.
Trygstad, O., et al. 1972. *FEBS Lett.* 26:311.
Vangen, O. 1972. *Acta Agric. Scand.* 22:238.
Vangen, O. 1974a. *Acta Agric. Scand.* 24:195.
Vangen, O. 1974b. *Acta Agric. Scand.* 24:309.
Vangen, O. 1977. *Acta Agric. Scand.* 27:331.
Vangen, O. 1979. *Acta Agric. Scand.* 29:305.
Vangen, O. 1980a. *Acta Agric. Scand.* 30:125.
Vangen, O. 1980b. *Acta Agric. Scand.* 30:142.
Vangen, O. 1980c. *Acta Agric. Scand.* 30:309.
Vangen, O. 1980d. *Acta Agric. Scand.* 30:320.
Varel, V.H., H.G. Jung, and W.G. Pond. 1988. *J. Anim. Sci.* 66:707.
Varel, V.H., et al. 1982. *Appl. Environ. Microbiol.* 44:107.
Walsh-Hentges, L.S., and R.J. Martin. 1988. *Int'l. J. Obesity* 12:49.
Wangsness, P.J., and G.H. Soroka. 1978. *J. Nutr.* 108:595.
Wangsness, P.J., R.J. Martin, and J.H. Gahagan. 1977. *Am. J. Physiol.* 233:E104.
Wangsness, P.J., et al. 1980a. *Physiol. Behav.* 24:407.
Wangsness, P.J., R.J. Martin, and B.B. Gatchel. 1980b. *Growth* 44:318.

Wangsness, P.J., et al. 1981. *J. Anim. Sci.* 52:69.
Wood, J.D., M.B. Enser, and D.J. Restall. 1975. *J. Agric. Sci. Cambridge* 84:221.
Yen, J.T., and W.G. Pond. 1985. *J. Anim. Sci.* 61:566.
Yen, J.T., et al. 1983. *J. Anim. Sci.* 56:426.
York, D.A. 1985. In: *New Perspectives in Adipose Tissue: Structure, Function and Development.* Cryer, A., and R.L.R. Van (Eds.). pp. 407–445. London: Butterworths.

Chapter 5

Maximizing Lean Tissue Growth: Genetic, Nutritional, and Environmental Factors

V.C. Speer

Muscle development as a most desirable feature of meat animals was recognized very early by the swine industry. Improvements in cutability and the reduction of external fat in the U.S. pig population beginning in the late 1940s have led to a number of revisions in the United States Department of Agriculture (USDA) grading standards. Objective measurements as guides to grades for pork carcasses were adopted in 1952. The standards were amended in 1955, and again in 1968, to reflect the improvements made in pork carcasses. Periodic surveys by the USDA Economic Research Service, the most recent in 1980 (Table 5.1), found over 70% of the pork carcasses were U.S. No. 1 grade. The USDA responded to their latest survey with another revision in grading standards that became effective in 1985. Briefly, the present USDA grading standards for barrow and gilt carcasses are based upon cutability, that is, expected lean meat yield, and quality of the lean and fat. There are four cutability grades: Nos. 1, 2, 3, or 4. Three degrees of muscling are considered in grading—thick, average, and thin—which, interacting with the backfat, determine the final cutability grade. A No. 1 carcass would be expected to yield 60.4% or more of the carcass as four lean cuts (ham, loin, picnic shoulder, and Boston butt). A No. 1 carcass would have less than 2.5 cm of backfat over the last rib and average muscling, or less than 3.2 cm of backfat over the last rib and thick muscling. There are only two quality attributes recognized in USDA pork grading: (1) acceptable, designated "U.S.," and (2) unacceptable, designated "U.S. Utility."

Realizing the need to stress the continued improvement in the lean content of pork carcasses, the National Pork Producers Council (NPPC) (1982) developed a "Pork Value" program based on last-rib backfat depth, carcass weight, and degree of muscling. The program emphasized economic incentives to encourage pork producers to produce lean, meaty hogs. Using one processor's grade and yield buying program that is similar to the NPPC "Pork Value" program (Hormel Farmer Magazine 1987),

Table 5.1 Comparison of Distribution of Barrow and Gilt Carcasses Among Cutability Grades from 1960 to 1961, 1967 to 1968, and 1980 Surveys Using 1968 Grading Standards

	1968 Standards (%)				
Year Surveyed	*U.S. No. 1*	*U.S. No. 2*	*U.S. No. 3*	*U.S. No. 4*	*U.S. Utility*
1960–61[a,b]	—	33.0[c]	38.8	25.9	2.2
1967–68[a]	8.1	42.1	35.7	12.2	1.8
1980[d]	71.7	24.2	3.7	0.3	0.1

[a] The 1960 to 1961 survey included about 45,000 head, and the 1967 to 1968 survey included about 57,000 head.

[b] Pigs in the 1960 to 1961 survey would have been one grade higher according to the 1955 grading standards.

[c] Some of these pigs would probably have been graded U.S. No. 1 using the 1968 grading standards.

[d] The 1980 survey included about 36,000 head.

(Data for years 1960 to 1961 and 1967 to 1968 are from Agnew 1969. Data from 1980 are from Parkham and Agnew 1982.)

carcass price spread can be as much as \$0.26/kg (assuming an average carcass price of \$1.65/kg) for a thick-muscled carcass with 2 cm or less tenth rib backfat as compared with a similar weight carcass with 4.6 cm or more of backfat and thin muscling.

GENETICS

Backfat depth and muscling in the pig are highly heritable characteristics, with a coefficient of 0.50 generally accepted as an average estimate (Craft 1958; Omtvedt 1968). Between 1955 and 1970, swine breeders and seed stock producers made rapid progress using genetic principles of selection to improve the breeding stock that was offered to commercial producers. Carcass information from the barrows submitted by breeders to the Iowa Swine Testing Station show the reduction in backfat and the increase in muscling that was occurring in the breeders' herds in the state of Iowa (Evans 1985). In the late 1960s, porcine stress syndrome (PSS) became an acute problem among pigs that had been intensely selected for thick muscling. In some herds, the incidence of sudden pig deaths was quite high. The economic loss was high because the problem generally emerged when sorting, loading, or transporting pigs for market (Bicknell 1968; Cassens et al. 1972). Additional economic loss was experienced by the processor when the carcasses of stress-susceptible pigs developed pale, soft, exudative (PSE) muscles (Briskey and Lister 1968). Beginning in the early 1970s, carcass cutability improvement seemed to reach a plateau; in fact, there is evidence that breeding stock actually became fatter from 1970 to 1985 (Table 5.2; Evans 1985) as breeders became suspicious that thick muscling and PSS were genetically linked. However, cutability improvement should now resume, because halothane testing, measurement of plasma

Table 5.2 Summary of Carcass Information on Barrows from Iowa Swine Testing Station

Year	*Backfat (cm)*	*Loin eye area (cm^2)*
1956	4.11	21.7
1960	3.86	24.9
1965	3.43	28.8
1970	3.07	33.0
1975	3.15	34.8
1980	3.35	32.0
1985	3.71	29.3

(Data from Evans 1985.)

creatine phosphokinase (CPK), and blood typing techniques have been developed to identify stress-positive, carrier, and normal animals (Christian 1977). Mating studies have provided substantial evidence for simple autosomal inheritance of the PSS. Pigs with this syndrome nearly always produce PSE carcasses (Christian 1981), so the opportunity exists for correction of two major problems.

SEX

Generally, intact males (boars) will yield carcasses with the least fat and most lean, females (gilts) will be intermediate in fat and lean, whereas castrates (barrows) will yield carcasses with the most fat and least amount of lean. Although gilts gain more slowly than barrows, they are more efficient (Wallace 1968). An example of these performance and carcass differences is presented in Table 5.3, from an article by Siers (1975). Until male aggressiveness (ranting) develops, boars usually gain most rapidly and most efficiently in comparison with the other sexes. There is, however, a potential off-flavor or odor problem that can occur in boar carcasses when slaughtered at typical U.S. market weights (100 to 115 kg) (Plimpton and Teague 1972). Major processors may not allow boar pigs to enter their plants, because of possible consumer complaints arising from the meat. Boar carcasses are acceptable in some other countries, such as

Table 5.3 Performance and Carcass Measurements of Boars, Barrows, and Gilts[a]

Item	*Boars*	*Barrows*	*Gilts*
No. animals	36	33	45
Daily gain (kg)	0.92	0.89	0.81
Feed/gain	2.85	3.10	3.08
Backfat (cm)	3.04	3.44	3.12
Ham and loin (%)	40.5	39.4	41.2
Loin eye area (cm^2)	33.1	28.6	34.0

[a] Individually fed from 27 to 99.5 kg.

(Data from Siers 1975.)

England and Australia, but in these countries the boars are slaughtered at light weights. This reduces the possibility of taint or off-flavors that might be detected by consumers in the meat products from boar carcasses.

WEIGHT

As pigs reach a live weight of about 90 kg, the rate of fat deposition begins to exceed lean tissue deposition. The rate of lean tissue deposition may or may not be decreasing, depending on the genetic background of the pigs as they reach about 90 kg. Optimum marketing weight can be influenced by several factors such as the following: (1) projected price trend; (2) carcass value relative to feed prices; (3) whether carcass grades for lightweight pigs are maintained as they reach heavy weight; and (4) price discounts for carcasses outside the optimum weight range (Grimes and Carlisle 1977). Currently, the optimum live weights specified by many packers fall in the 100- to 115-kg weight range, and market discounts can be more severe for lighter weight pigs than for heavier weight pigs outside of the optimum range. The current optimum weight range is a departure from the historical optimum range of 90- to 100-kg live weight. The major reasons for the shift include the unit labor cost in processing and the trend toward fabrication of value-added products from the heavier carcass cuts at the processing plant.

A comparison of performance, efficiency, and lean tissue deposition among pigs weighing about 60, 90, and 120 kg was summarized by the Agricultural Research Council (1981). The daily gain from representative pigs from ten breeding companies in Great Britain was most rapid for pigs slaughtered at 90 kg and decreased for pigs slaughtered at 120 kg. The rate of lean tissue gain followed a pattern similar to growth rate. Feed requirement increased as slaughter weights increased, and the increase was greater for pigs that were depositing less lean tissue (and presumably more fat) as their slaughter weight increased.

NUTRITION

Given acceptable management, housing, and nutrition, the genetic potential of the pig will have the greatest impact on carcass muscling. However, to attain maximum carcass muscling, the pig must be properly fed and managed. There are several nutrients that will affect carcass measurements either positively or negatively.

Protein

Increasing the corn and decreasing the soybean meal in a recommended diet will adversely affect rate of gain, feed efficiency, and carcass composition. The magnitude of the response to protein on carcass measurements depends on the type or genetic potential of the pig. The pig with the genetic potential for heavier muscling is more sensitive to dietary protein level than is a fat-type pig. Examples of this differential

Table 5.4 Effect of Protein Level on Carcass Measurements of Unimproved (1950s) and Improved (1960s) Growing-Finishing Pigs

	Protein Level (%)					
	10	*12*	*14*	*16*	*18*	*20*
Year	*Backfat Depth (cm)*					
1955[a]	4.06	3.94	4.06	3.81	3.81	3.81
1965[b]	3.94	3.71	3.66	3.61	3.56	3.50
	Trimmed Ham and Loin (% of Carcass)					
1955[a]	31.9	32.2	32.5	33.0	32.5	33.2
1965[b]	35.8	37.1	37.7	38.1	37.9	38.6

[a] (Data from Ashton et al. 1955.)
[b] (Data from Johnson 1965.)

Table 5.5 Effect of Protein Level on Fat- and Lean-Type Pigs

		Carcass Component (%)	
Carcass Type[a]	*Protein Level (%)*	*Lean*	*Fat*
Fat strain	20	46.8	37.8
	12	44.6	39.8
Lean strain	20	58.4	28.6
	12	50.9	31.3

[a] Pigs were selected for ten or twelve generations.
(Data from Davey and Morgan 1969.)

response are presented in Tables 5.4 and 5.5. In the examples (Ashton et al. 1955; Johnson 1965; Davey and Morgan 1969), the increase in percentage units of muscling as dietary protein increased was greater for the lean pigs as compared with the fat pigs. The lean-type pig is metabolically more efficient in lean tissue (nitrogen) deposition than is the fat-type pig as reported by McConnell et al. (1972) (Table 5.6).

Table 5.6 Effect of Body Type on Nitrogen Metabolism

	Weight (kg)		
	31	*53*	*91*
Body Type	*Retained N/Absorbed (%)*		
Fat	45.8	29.4	18.5
Lean	51.5	39.1	30.4

(Data from McConnell et al. 1972.)

Table 5.7 Effect of Lysine Level on Carcass Measurements of Growing-Finishing Pigs

Factor	*% Dietary Lysine*			
Growth stage				
Growing	0.60	0.65	0.70	0.75
Finishing	0.45	0.50	0.55	0.60
Backfat (cm)	3.84	3.88	3.70	3.63
Loin eye area (cm^2)	31.3	33.0	34.6	35.3
Estimated carcass lean (%)	51.8	52.7	54.0	54.6

(Data from Asche et al. 1985.)

Amino Acids

Adjusting corn and soybean meal proportions in a series of diets to study different levels of protein also changes the ratio of the essential amino acids. As dietary protein level is decreased, lysine becomes the first limiting amino acid. In some cases, it is possible that the response to increasing levels of protein is simply a response to increasing levels of dietary lysine. A definite response in carcass measurements and percentage lean to increasing levels of lysine was reported by Brown et al. (1973). Carcass responses to lysine levels from a recent report by Asche et al. (1985) are shown in Table 5.7.

Energy

The addition of fats or oils to diets fed to growing-finishing pigs usually improves feed efficiency. Daily gain may or may not be improved. Carcass measurements, however, generally have been adversely affected. An example of the effects of adding about 10% choice white grease to a corn-soybean meal diet fed to growing-finishing pigs is presented in Table 5.8. Formulating high-energy diets (added fat) to an equal calorie: protein ratio as compared with a control corn-soybean meal diet will likely improve daily gain, as well as improve feed efficiency. Although the protein level of the high-energy diet is proportionately increased, carcass measurements may be adversely affected. As shown in Table 5.9, daily gain and feed efficiency were improved when the protein level in the high-energy diet was adjusted to the same calorie:protein ratio as in the control diet. Carcass backfat, however, was increased when the high-energy diet was fed (3.4 versus 3.1 cm). Daily intake of energy by the pigs fed the diet with both higher energy and protein concentrations would contribute to a greater fat deposition. Also, it is well known that energy from fat is metabolized more efficiently with a lower heat increment than is energy from either protein or carbohydrate, thereby contributing additionally to fat deposition. Formulating diets and calorie:protein ratios using net energy values for the ingredients may overcome the adverse effects of dietary fat on carcass measurements.

The high-heat increment coefficients associated with dietary fiber and the concomitant reduction in net energy should reduce the potential for deposition of fat in

Table 5.8 Effect of Dietary Energy Levels on Performance, Carcass Measurements, and Lean Tissue Composition of Growing-Finishing Pigs

	ME (kcal/kg)	
Diets	*3185*	*3660*
Daily gain (kg)	0.70	0.75
Feed/gain	3.32	2.64
Daily ME intake (kcal)	7390	7250
Backfat (cm)	3.2	3.6
Lean cuts (%)	53.6	52.1
Fat content of longissimus muscle dry matter (%)[a]	9.9	13.2

[a] Lean tissue samples from the tenth to twelfth rib section.
(Data from Wagner et al. 1963.)

Table 5.9 Effect of Fat and Calorie:Protein Ratio on Performance and Carcass Measurements of Finishing Pigs

Dietary protein (%)	13.1	14.7	12.3
Added fat (%)	0	9	9
Calorie:protein ratio	24:1	24:1	29:1
ME (kcal/kg)	3145	3555	3560
Daily gain (kg)	0.69	0.78	0.72
Daily feed (kg)	2.47	2.28	2.38
Daily ME (Kcal)	7770	8105	8475
Feed/gain	3.65	2.92	3.31
Backfat (cm)	3.1	3.4	3.4
Loin eye area (cm^2)	31.3	34.2	30.0
Ham (% of carcass)	23.4	23.8	23.3

(Data from Allee 1976 and Allee et al. 1976.)

growing-finishing pigs. The inclusion of fiber in corn-soybean meal diets, however, has yielded varied carcass responses (Kennelly and Aherne 1980). Depending on the source and level of fiber in the diet, growing-finishing pigs will increase their daily feed intake to equal or exceed the energy intake of pigs fed corn-soybean meal diets with minimal effects on carcass measurements. If the fiber source is included at high enough levels, for example 30% oat hulls, or if the fiber source is unpalatable, for example, 10% alfalfa, daily digestible or metabolizable energy intake may be reduced, as will both weight gain and the deposition of fat.

FEEDING SYSTEM

"Restricted" or "controlled" feeding of growing-finishing pigs has been a common practice in Europe. A major reason for such a feeding system is carcass pricing that

Table 5.10 Effect of Feed Restriction on Performance and Carcass Measurements of Growing-Finishing Pigs

Trial	*Daily Gain (kg) (R/AL)*	*Daily Feed (kg) (R/AL)*	*Feed/Gain (R/AL)*	*Carcass Backfat (cm) (R/AL)*	*% Graded No. 1 (R/AL)*
I[a]	0.69/0.75	2.32/2.42	3.39/3.22	3.5/3.7	93/84
II[b]	0.77/0.84	2.55/2.75	3.34/3.28	3.5/3.7	90/71

Abbreviations: R, restricted feeding method; AL, ad libitum feeding method.

[a]Pigs (120) fed from 21 to 93 kg.

[b]Pigs (192) fed from 44 to 93 kg.

(Data from Speer 1966.)

imposes severe penalties on pigs that have excess backfat. Other advantages claimed for restricted feeding over ad libitum feeding include an improved feed efficiency and a reduction of feed wastage. A summary of 89 European experiments reported by Braude (1972) compared restricted versus ad libitum feeding of growing-finishing pigs and recorded the following information: (1) average daily gain was improved by ad libitum feeding in 88 of the trials; (2) feed efficiency was adversely affected in 60 of the 89 trials when the pigs were fed ad libitum; and (3) carcass measurements were adversely affected in 72 of the 89 trials by ad libitum feeding as compared with restricted feeding. Two trials reported by Speer (1966) follow a pattern similar to the European experience, except feed efficiency between the two feeding systems showed no difference (Table 5.10). Feed was restricted to about 94% of the daily intake of the ad libitum-fed pigs. The fact that these trials (Speer 1966) were conducted under production conditions, that is, 20 pigs per pen and the restricted-fed pigs were floor-fed, may explain why similar feed efficiency was found between the two systems. Producers in the United States would object to any reduction in growth rate of market pigs. Further, they would question whether the improvement in carcass measurements would result in enough additional income to offset the additional time to market and the increased management time imposed by a restricted feeding versus an ad libitum feeding system.

ENVIRONMENT

The effects of temperature on performance and carcass measurements are better defined than are other environmental effects that might be imposed on the pig. A summary of three experiments conducted in cold, thermoneutral, and warm environments with growing-finishing pigs is presented in Table 5.11 (Stahly and Cromwell 1979). Clearly, the environmental temperature had an effect on feed intake. Daily gain was severely depressed in the hot environment. Pigs housed in either a cold or hot environment required more feed (metabolizable energy [ME]) per unit of gain. The reduction of body fat among pigs fed in the hot environment can be directly attributable to a marked reduction in feed intake. Pigs in the cold environment increased their feed intake as compared with pigs fed in the neutral environment, but minimal effects were

Table 5.11 Relative Performance of Pigs Fed Supplemental Fat and Maintained in Three Environmental Temperatures[a]

	% Added Fat					
	0	*5*	*0*	*5*	*0*	*5*
	10°C		*22.5°C*		*35°C*	
Daily gain	99	98	100	109	66	75
Daily ME intake	114	112	100	103	72	77
Gain:ME	86	86	100	106	88	94
Backfat	93	97	100	106	85	92
Lean cuts	99	99	100	99	101	99
Body fat[b]	102	105	100	104	84	99

[a]Pigs fed ad libitum at 22.5 °C and a diet with no added fat were assigned values of 100%.
[b]Percent ether extract in the carcass.
(Data from Stahly and Cromwell 1979.)

Table 5.12 Relative Performance of Pigs Fed Alfalfa Meal and Maintained in Three Environmental Temperatures[a]

	Added Dehydrated Alfalfa Meal (17%CP)					
	0	*10*	*0*	*10*	*0*	*1C*
	10°C		*22.5°C*		*35°C*	
Daily gain	92	91	100	97	87	82
Gain:feed	80	79	100	93	104	94
Daily ME intake	115	113	100	102	85	86
Gain:ME	79	81	100	95	103	97
Backfat	93	90	100	102	97	92
Lean cuts	100	99	100	101	103	98

[a]Pigs fed ad libitum at 22.5 °C and a diet with no dehydrated alfalfa meal were assigned values of 100%.
(Data from Stahly and Cromwell 1986.)

observed on their carcass composition. Their increased energy intake was counteracted by an increased heat loss to the environment, and it was not available for carcass deposition. Dietary fat had no effect on daily gain or efficiency at low environmental temperatures, but at neutral and high temperatures, fat addition improved daily gain and efficiency. Dietary fat increased backfat and carcass fat to a greater extent at neutral and high temperatures than at the cold temperature. The increased fat deposition by pigs fed diets containing supplemental fat is related to efficiency of synthesizing or deposition of carcass fat from dietary fat, along with the reduced heat increment associated with fat. In another study by Stahly and Cromwell (1986), the effects of temperature on pigs fed to about 55 kg were similar to those found in their earlier study (Stahly and Cromwell 1979). Backfat was reduced by both the cold and hot temperatures as compared with the backfat of pigs fed in the neutral temperature (Table 5.12).

The addition of 10% dehydrated alfalfa meal to a control diet reduced the daily gain of pigs and feed efficiency to a greater extent in the hot environment than in either the neutral or cold environment. These effects were attributable to the high-heat increment of the fibrous ingredients used in the study. The reduction in backfat for pigs fed the alfalfa diets was not consistent among the three temperatures, nor were the percentages of lean cuts consistent with the relative backfat measurements. The expectation for the pigs fed the high-fiber diet would be an increase in fat deposition at the low temperature and less fat deposition at the high temperature. The pigs in this experiment were fed to only 55 kg and not to market weight, which may explain the lack of an interaction between dietary fiber and environmental temperature on the carcass measurements.

Dry Lot Versus Pasture Feeding

Hudman and Peo (1960) reported that pasture-fed pigs had less backfat than pigs fed in dry lot. The pigs fed in dry lot gained significantly more than did those pigs fed on pasture. One would expect the activity level of the pasture-fed pigs to be greater than that of the dry lot-fed pigs, and their reduced gains (and probably reduced energy intake) would account for the reduced fat deposition.

Exercise Versus No Exercise

Carcass responses have been variable in experiments employing a treadmill to force pigs to exercise. In reports by Weiss et al. (1975) and Hale et al. (1986), no differences were found between pigs that were exercised versus not exercised for carcass length, backfat thickness, loin muscle area, or lean cuts percentage. Seemingly, in these experiments the activity level was not intense enough to increase the energy expenditure significantly and thereby reduce fat deposition.

Space Allowance

In general, a reduction in daily feed or energy intake will decrease the amount of fat deposition in the growing-finishing pig. Decreasing the floor space allowance per pig has been shown to decrease daily gain, increase the feed requirement, and decrease daily feed intake (NCR-89 1986). Pigs housed in crowded conditions would probably have less carcass fat deposition than pigs housed with recommended floor space.

IMMUNOLOGY

There have been several recent developments in the field of immunology with the potential for decreasing the fat composition of pig carcasses. One of these capitalizes on the positive carcass attributes of growing boars by immunizing them against androstene steroids, those compounds responsible for boar taint and odor. Vaccination improved sensory scores and reduction of androstenes among boars as reported by Williamson et al. (1985) and Brooks et al. (1986). A reduction of the odor and taint compounds could also be attained through selection (Booth et al. 1986), which might make boar carcasses acceptable to the American consumer.

Encouraging results employing autoimmunization against somatostatin among lambs has been reported by Spencer and Garssen (1983). Circulating somatomedin concentrations were increased (nonsignificantly) and growth rate was improved among the vaccinated lambs as compared with the controls, and muscle growth was expected to be stimulated.

Another approach that might have application for swine has been reported by Flint and Futter (1986) in which rats were immunized against their fat cells. Upon postmortem examination, it was found that the immunized rats had about 30% less carcass fat than untreated rats.

SUMMARY

The reduction of carcass fat in pigs that are marketed today began as an industry effort in the late 1940s. It has been a remarkable accomplishment, with genetic changes in the pigs being the major component effecting the improvement. Of course, good nutrition and management have allowed the genetic potential for increased muscling to be fully expressed. Further improvements are possible through diet, feeding management, and environmental modifications, but to be implemented, the cost effectiveness must be considered. Physiological, anatomical, and immunological modifications also are potential approaches that can lead to further reductions in carcass fat and increased muscling.

REFERENCES

Agnew, D.B. 1969. United States Department of Agriculture. Economic Research Service Marketing Report No. 849. Washington, DC.

Agricultural Research Council. 1981. *The Nutrient Requirements of the Pig.* Slough, England: Commonwealth Agricultural Bureaux.

Allee, G.L. 1976. Swine Day '76. *Progress Report 283.* p. 26. Manhattan, KS: Agriculture Experimental Station, Kansas State University.

Allee, G.L., B.A. Koch, and R.H. Hines. 1976. *J. Anim. Sci.* 42:1349.

Asche, G.L., et al. 1985. *J. Anim. Sci.* 60:1412.

Ashton, G.C., et al. 1955. *J. Anim. Sci.* 14:82.

Bicknell, E.J. 1968. In: *The Pork Industry: Problems and Progress.* Topel, D.G. (Ed.). p. 206. Ames, IA: Iowa State University Press.

Booth, W.D., E.D. Williamson, and R.L.S. Patterson. 1986. *Anim. Prod.* 42:145.

Braude, R. 1972. In: *Pig Production.* Cole, D.J.A. (Ed.). p. 279. London: Butterworths.

Briskey, E.J., and D. Lister. 1968. In: *The Pork Industry: Problems and Progress.* Topel, D.G. (Ed.). p. 177. Ames, IA: Iowa State University Press.

Brooks, R.I., et al. 1986. *J. Anim. Sci.* 62:1279.

Brown, H.W., B.G. Harmon, and A.H. Jensen. 1973. *J. Anim. Sci.* 37:1159.

Cassens, R., F. Giesler, and Q. Kolb. 1972. *Proceedings of the Pork Quality Symposium.* Madison, WI: Cooperative Extension Service, University of Wisconsin.

Christian, L.L. 1977. *Proceedings of Pork Producers Day. AS-447D.* Ames, IA: Cooperative Extension Service, Iowa State University.

Christian, L.L. 1981. *Proceedings of Pork Producers Day. AS-528-F.* Ames, IA: Cooperative Extension Service, Iowa State University.

Craft, W.A. 1958. *J. Anim. Sci.* 17:960.

Davey, R.J., and D.P. Morgan. 1969. *J. Anim. Sci.* 28:831.

Evans, R. 1985. *Fall Summary Iowa Swine Testing Station,* Ames, IA.

Flint, D.J., and D.E. Futter. 1986. *Immunological Manipulation of Body Fat. Hannah Research 1985.* p. 123. Ayr, Scotland: Hannah Research Institute, University of Glasgow.

Grimes, G., and G.R. Carlisle. 1977. *Pork Industry Handbook. AS-452.* Ames, IA: Cooperative Extension Service, Iowa State University.

Hale, O.M., G.L. Newton, and K.D. Haydon. 1986. *J. Anim. Sci.* 62:665.

Hormel Farmer Magazine. 1987. 40:10.

Hudman, D.B., and E.R. Peo, Jr. 1960. *J. Anim. Sci.* 19:943.

Johnson, R.A. 1965. Ph.D. thesis. Iowa State University, Ames.

Kennelly, J.J., and F.X. Aherne. 1980. *Can. J. Anim. Sci.* 60:385.

NCR-89 Committee on Confinement Management of Swine. 1986. *J. Anim. Sci.* 62:871.

NPPC. 1982. *The Pork Value Approach.* Des Moines, IA: National Pork Producers Council.

Omtvedt, I.T. 1968. In: *The Pork Industry: Problems and Progress.* Topel, D.G. (Ed.). p. 128. Ames, IA: Iowa State University Press.

Parkham, K.D., and D.B. Agnew. 1982. United States Department of Agriculture, *Economic Research Service-675.* Washington, DC.

Plimpton, R.F., Jr., and H.S. Teague. 1972. *J. Anim. Sci.* 35:1166.

Siers, D.G. 1975. *J. Anim. Sci.* 41:522.

Speer, V.C. 1966. *Hog Farm Management* 3:13.

Spencer, G.S.G., and G.J. Garssen. 1983. *Livestock Prod. Sci.* 10:25.

Stahly, T.S., and G.L. Cromwell. 1979. *J. Anim. Sci.* 49:1478.

Stahly, T.S., and G.L. Cromwell. 1986. *J. Anim. Sci.* 63:1870.

Wagner, G.R., et al. 1963. *J. Anim. Sci.* 22:202.

Wallace, H.D. 1968. In: *The Pork Industry: Problems and Progress.* Topel, D.G. (Ed.). p. 77. Ames, IA: Iowa State University Press.

Weiss, G.M., et al. 1975. *J. Anim. Sci.* 40:457.

Williamson, E.D., et al. 1985. *Livestock Prod. Sci.* 12:251.

Chapter 6

Impact of Porcine Somatotropin and Beta-Adrenergic Agonists in Swine

T.S. Stahly and L.J. Bark

Major changes in pork production, processing, and utilization have occurred in the last half of the twentieth century. Many of these changes have been made to reduce the costs of pork production as well as to meet the demands of both the institutional food trade and health-conscious consumers for acceptable pork products. Recently, technologies have been developed that allow the economical synthesis of biologically active compounds that alter the rate and efficiency of pork production as well as the composition of the products produced. In this chapter, two modifiers (somatotropin and beta-adrenergic agonists) of the neural-endocrine system that have been evaluated most extensively in the pig will be characterized, their known biological effects identified, and their potential influences on the optimum dietary regimen, thermal environment, and genetic make-up of the pig discussed.

PORCINE SOMATOTROPIN

Somatotropin (ST) and growth hormone (GH) are synonyms for a protein of approximately 191 amino acid residues that is synthesized and secreted by the anterior pituitary gland. Somatotropin has a molecular mass of about 21,500 daltons and contains two disulfide bonds, which are necessary for the hormone's biological activity. The pituitary glands of the adult porcine and human are estimated to contain 5 to 15 mg of somatotropin (Etherton et al. 1986; Bechtel 1987).

Somatotropin synthesis and release are under the dual control of two neurohormones: a stimulatory factor, growth hormone releasing factor (GRF), and an inhibitory agent, somatostatin, both of which are produced in the hypothalamus. A variety of neurotransmitters, neuropeptides, opiates, and other compounds located in supra-hypothalamic centers controls the release of GRF and somatostatin (Berdu and Diamond 1986). In most animals, somatotropin is secreted in a pulsatile manner with circulating blood levels decreasing with age. Pigs at market weight (100 to 110 kg) normally exhibit low, baseline blood levels of less than 2 ng/ml of ST with three to five peaks daily of 3 to 15 ng/ml (ArGona et al. 1988; Bechtel 1987).

Somatotropin is thought to elicit its metabolic effects via (1) a direct effect on target tissues (i.e., tissue receptors, metabolic pathways, cell number) and (2) the stimulation of the synthesis and release of insulin-like growth factors (IGF) also called somatomedins, which in turn elicit various responses in target tissues. Metabolically, somatotropin inhibits the synthesis of lipids from glucose and accelerates the mobilization of fat from adipose tissue to the liver. In turn, oxidation of fatty acids in the liver as well as muscle tissue is increased. Glucose availability in blood and muscle also is increased, likely as a result of the increased oxidation of fatty acids. Body protein accretion is increased by somatotropin as a result of an elevated level of protein synthesis. Tissue metabolism and growth also are influenced by somatomedins. Somatomedins have insulin-like properties that include the ability to stimulate lipogenesis in adipose tissue and protein synthesis in muscle tissue. Somatomedins also have been shown to stimulate DNA accumulation in tissues, which results in hyperplastic growth.

In recent years, technologies have been developed that allow synthetic forms of porcine somatotropin (PST), commonly called recombinant porcine somatotropin, to be produced by genetically altered bacteria (Seeburg et al. 1983). The natural and recombinant forms of somatotropins are similar in molecular structure, but small differences do exist, such as in the formation of the two disulfide bonds and the presence of an additional methionine at the terminal N. As a result, the bioactivity and potency of the various somatotropin products differ and must be individually defined.

Effects of Exogenous PST in Swine

Body Growth and Composition

In growing pigs, the administration of PST depresses voluntary feed intake of pigs but enhances the rate and efficiency of body growth (Table 6.1). PST appears to be effective in stimulating growth in pigs during both the peak (30 to 60 kg) and declining (60 to 110 kg) stages of body protein accretion. Daily administration of 70 to 130 μg of PST/kg body weight has resulted in about a 0.44 kg (14%) reduction in daily feed intake, a 0.14 kg (15%) increase in daily weight gain, and a 0.79 kg (24%) reduction in feed per kilogram of live weight gain in finishing pigs (54 to 96 kg). The accelerated growth of PST-treated pigs is associated with an elevated rate of protein and mineral accretion and a reduction in fat accretion in the empty body (Table 6.2). PST stimulates the growth of skeletal muscles as well as internal organs such as the liver, kidneys, and gastrointestinal tract (Grebner et al. 1987). In contrast, the amount of fat in subcutaneous depots (Boyd et al. 1986; Etherton et al. 1987), skeletal muscle (Bechtel 1987), as well as the abdominal cavity (i.e., perirenal fat; Grebner et al. 1987) is reduced by PST administration. The PST-induced changes in body protein accretion and lipolysis result in significant changes in standard carcass measures such as in-

Table 6.1 Influence of Porcine Somatotropin Administration on Growth Rate and Efficiency of Feed Utilization in Pigs

	PST		*Pig*		*Daily Feed (kg)*			*Daily Gain (kg)*			*Feed/Gain*		
Stage (Reference)[a]	*Source*	*Dose (μg/kg)*	*Weight (kg)*	*Sex*	*Control*	*PST*	*%*[b]	*Control*	*PST*	*%*[b]	*Control*	*PST*	*%*[b]
Growing													
1	Nat.	100	25–55	C, G	2.32	2.06	−11	0.90	1.05	+17	2.56	1.96	−23
1	Nat.	100	30–60	C	1.98	1.94	− 2	0.76	1.04	+37	2.59	1.86	−28
Weighted means[c]					2.15	2.00	− 7	0.83	1.04	+25	2.58	1.91	−26
Finishing													
2	Nat.	132	53–95	C, G	2.87	2.61	− 9	0.77	0.83	+ 8	3.73	3.14	−16
2	Nat.	130	45–95	C, G	2.62	2.51	− 4	0.75	0.86	+15	3.50	2.92	−17
3	Nat.	120	45–100	C, G	2.87	2.39	−17	0.95	1.10	+16	3.02	2.18	−28
4	Recomb.	60	55–105	C, G	2.84	2.67	− 6	0.82	0.82	0	3.45	3.25	− 6
5	Nat.	70	45–76	C	2.57	2.43	− 5	0.90	1.03	+14	2.86	2.36	−17
6	Recomb.	85	57–103	C, G	2.93	2.28	−22	0.77	0.89	+16	3.74	2.67	−29
1	Nat.	100	60–100	B	3.21	2.96	− 8	1.19	1.34	+13	2.72	2.21	−19
1	Nat.	100	60–96	C	3.67	2.84	−23	1.06	1.22	+15	3.46	2.33	−33
1	Nat.	100	60–96	G	3.38	2.73	−19	1.01	1.24	+23	3.34	2.21	−34
Weighted means[c]					3.04	2.60	−14	.94	1.08	+15	3.26	2.47	−24

Abbreviations: PST, porcine somatotropin; Nat., natural PST; Recomb., recombinant PST; C, male castrated; G, gilt; B, boar.
[a]References as follows: 1, Steele et al. 1987; 2, Machlin et al. 1972; 3, Boyd et al. 1986; 4, Kraft et al. 1986; 5, Etherton et al. 1987; 6, McLaren et al. 1987.
[b]Percentage change from the values of the control treatment group.
[c]Means weighted on the basis of the number of replicates per treatment.

Table 6.2 Influence of Porcine Somatotropin Administration on Nutrient Accretion in Pigs[a]

	Nutrient Accretion (g/d)[b]								
	Protein			*Fat*			*Minerals*		
Animal	*Control*	*PST*	*%*[c]	*Control*	*PST*	*%*[c]	*Control*	*PST*	*%*[c]
Boar	196	238	+21	317	203	−36	23.6	29.9	+27
Gilt	148	235	+59	411	185	−55	24.1	37.8	+57
Barrow	139	225	+62	462	235	−49	27.4	29.2	+ 6
Weighted mean	161	233	47	397	208	−48	25.0	32.3	29

Abbreviation: PST, porcine somatotropin.

[a] Pigs administered 0 or 100 mg of natural PST daily per kilogram body weight from 60 to 97 kg body weight.

[b] Nutrient accretion rate in empty body.

[c] Percentage change in response criterion due to PST.

(Adapted, by permission, from Steele et al. 1987.)

creased loin eye area, reduced backfat thickness, and reduced carcass yield (Machlin 1972; Boyd et al. 1986; McLaren et al. 1987).

The administration of PST also has been shown to increase the energy maintenance requirement of growing pigs by 24% (Steele et al. 1987). The elevated energy expenditure is likely due in part to the increased metabolic activity of the liver and associated metabolic organs.

Lactation

Milk yield of sows has been reported to be increased by PST administration (Table 6.3); however, the response has not been observed consistently (Cromwell et al. 1989; Crenshaw et al. 1989). As observed in growing pigs, voluntary feed intake of the sow also is reduced by PST treatment. The reduction in energy and nutrient intake causes the sow to mobilize a substantial quantity of its body stores (i.e., fat and likely protein; Brendemuhl et al. 1986) to meet its elevated metabolic demand for milk production. The effects of this tissue catabolism on subsequent reproductive efficiency and the longevity of the PST-treated sow is currently unknown. However, large losses of body tissues in lactating sows have been associated with a reduction in the subsequent rebreeding efficiency of the sow (Reese et al. 1982a,b; Nelssen et al. 1985; Brendemuhl et al. 1987). Consequently, feeding-management programs must be utilized that allow or stimulate the PST-treated sow to consume sufficient nutrients to meet the elevated demands for milk production to prevent excessive loss of tissue reserves. Based on the assumption that PST administration would increase daily milk yield by 2 kg milk/day (Table 6.3) without altering the sow's maintenance requirement or metabolic efficiency of milk synthesis ($k_l = 0.68$), the additional energy needs of the PST-treated sow can be approximated. Consumption of an additional 1.0 kg of a fortified corn-soybean meal diet (3225 kcal metabolizable energy [ME]/kg) daily would be needed to produce an additional 2 kg of sow's milk containing 1100 kcal gross

Table 6.3 Influence of Porcine Somatotropin Administration on the Lactation Performance of Sows[a]

	PST (mg/sow/d)		
Criteria	*0*	*8.22*	*% Change*
Sow feed (kg/d)	5.8	4.7	−19
Sow weight change (kg)	−7.0	−13.6	−94
Sow backfat change (cm)	−0.12	−0.37	−208
Sow milk yield (kg/d)			
Milk	9.0	11.0	+22
Solids	1.6	2.0	+25
Pig weight gain (kg)	3.39	3.73	+10

Abbreviation: PST, porcine somatotropin.

[a] Multiparous sows administered 0 or 8.22 mg recombinant PST daily from day 12 to 28 of lactation. Sow feed intake, sow weight and backfat change, and pig weight gain for days 12 to 28 of lactation and sow milk yield for day 28 of lactation.

(Adapted, by permission, from Boyd 1987.)

energy/kg in midlactation (days 14 to 24). If feed intake were not increased, a 0.3-kg daily body weight loss (assuming only body fat was mobilized) would need to occur to supply the sow sufficient energy to synthetize the additional 2 kg of daily milk output.

In terms of dietary amino acid needs, the synthesis of two more kilograms of milk is estimated to require an additional dietary intake of 12 g of lysine/day. For sows consuming 5 to 6 kg/day of a corn-soybean meal diet, the dietary lysine concentration would need to be increased by 0.2 to 0.25 percentage units to minimize the catabolism of the sow's proteinaceous tissues. Mobilization of 0.68 kg/day of muscle tissue would be required to supply the needed amino acids if the sow's dietary intake was not altered.

Influence of Management Practices on Response to PST

The responses of pigs to PST administration are hypothesized to be influenced by the animal's genetic make-up, climatic environment, dietary regimen, and health status as well as the source and dosage of PST utilized. The efficacy of natural and recombinant sources of PST appears to be equal in swine when products of a high degree of purity are utilized (Boyd et al. 1986; Etherton et al. 1987). Linear improvements in weight gain and carcass leanness have been observed in pigs as the daily dosage of PST increased from 0 to about 100 μg/kg body weight (Boyd et al. 1986; Etherton et al. 1987).

The circulating concentrations of endogenous ST in pigs appear to be greater in animals with a high versus low genetic capacity for lean tissue growth (Wangsness et al. 1977; ArGona et al. 1988; Bark et al. 1988). These elevated concentrations of endogenous ST are hypothesized to enhance lean tissue accretion. However, the magnitude of response to exogenous PST administration has been shown to be similar in genotypes differing substantially in their genetic capacity for lean tissue accretion

Table 6.4 Influence of Genetic Capacity for Lean Tissue Growth on Responses of Pigs to Recombinant Somatotropin[a]

	Lean Growth Genotype					
	Medium			*High*		
Criteria	*Control*	*PST*	*Units of Change*	*Control*	*PST*	*Units of Change*
Growth performance						
Daily feed (kg)	2.97	2.65	−0.32	2.60	2.34	−0.26
Daily gain (kg)	0.88	0.98	+0.10	0.92	1.03	+0.11
Feed/gain	3.41	2.72	−0.69	2.83	2.29	−0.54
Carcass traits						
Backfat-10th rib (cm)	3.70	2.32	−1.38	2.47	1.29	−1.18
Est. muscle (kg)	39.9	44.0	+4.1	48.0	52.4	+4.4
Lean gain (kg/d)	0.30	0.38	+0.08	0.39	0.48	+0.09

Abbreviations: PST, porcine somatotropin; Est., estimated.
[a] Each genotype consisted of two genetic sources of pigs with nine sets of two littermates represented per source. Pigs (barrows) administered daily 0 or 70 μg PST/kg body weight from 23 to 115 kg body weight.
(Adapted, by permission, from Bark et al. 1989b.)

(Bark et al. 1989b; Table 6.4). Within a genotype, bones apparently exhibit a smaller response to PST than do gilts or barrows (Steele et al. 1987).

As the body fat content, particularly subcutaneous fat, is reduced in PST-treated pigs, the insulative properties of this fat covering are minimized. Consequently, the PST-treated pig potentially is more susceptible to cold exposure. The lower critical temperature (LCT) of a 75-kg pig treated with PST has been estimated to be raised by 12 °C due to the loss of 0.5 cm of subcutaneous fat (Curtis 1987). A lower rate of body fat accretion also reduces the amount of body heat produced as a result of the biochemical processes associated with fat accretion. However, this reduction in body insulation and body heat production associated with fat deposition may be partially offset by an increased level of heat production associated with the elevated maintenance requirement and body protein accretion induced by PST administration. Based on the nutrient accretion levels (78-kg pigs; Table 6.2) reported by Steele et al. (1987) and the energetic efficiencies of protein and fat accretion reported by Stahly (1985), daily heat production is estimated to be increased by about 350 kcal in animals administered 100 μg PST/kg of body weight. Ignoring the changes in the insulative coat of the pig, this elevated level of body heat production would lower the pig's LCT by about 3 °C. The combined result of these two effects of PST would be estimated to be a 9 °C increase in the LCT of a 75-kg pig. However, these interrelationships of PST treatment and thermal environment on pigs have not been experimentally evaluated.

The elevated body protein and mineral accretion in PST-treated pigs also alter the dietary nutrient needs of the pig. If PST does not alter the biological mechanisms (and thus efficiency) of protein accretion, but only the rate of accretion, the amino acid needs for these animals can be approximated. Work by Campbell et al. (1989) indicates that PST administration alters protein synthesis and degradation by an equal magnitude. Thus, the partial efficiency of incorporating amino acids and energy into proteinaceous tissue would be hypothesized to be unchanged. Furthermore, PST appears to stimulate the accretion of all major proteinaceous tissues (carcass muscle, bone, skin, and offal) by a similar magnitude (Bark et al. 1989; unpublished data). Thus, the relative pattern of amino acids needed for body protein accretion should be largely independent of PST administration.

The nutrient needs of barrows and gilts administered 100 μg PST/kg of body weight/day have been estimated in Table 6.5. It has been assumed that the pigs were housed in a thermoneutral environment and allowed to consume a corn-soybean meal diet ad libitum from 60 to 96 kg. The levels of nutrient accretion in the body represent actual data from Steele et al. (1987), whereas the magnitude of the difference in voluntary food intake between the two groups is based on data summarized in Table 6.1.

Table 6.5 Estimated Dietary Needs of Porcine Somatotropin-Treated Pigs

	PST (μg/kg/d)	
Item	*0*	*100*
Mean body weights (kg)	78	78
Nutrient accretion[a] (g/d)		
Protein	144	230
Fat	436	210
Ash	26	34
Daily lysine needs[b]		
Maintenance (0.065 g/kg$^{.75}$)	1.7	2.0
Lysine accretion (7.1% of protein)	10.2	16.3
Biological lysine needs (g)	11.9	18.3
Utilization of lysine	0.70	0.70
Digestible lysine (g)	17.0	26.1
Digestibility of lysine	0.82	0.82
Dietary lysine (g)	20.7	31.8
Daily ME needs[b]		
Maintenance (110 kcal/kg$^{.75}$)	2888	3580
Protein accretion (10.5 kcal/g)	1512	2415
Fat accretion (12.8 kcal/g)	5581	2688
Dietary ME needs (kcal)	9981	8683
Estimated feed intake (122 g/kg$^{.75}$/d) (kg)	3.20	2.78
Lysine needed (% of diet)	0.69	1.19
ME needed (Kcal/kg)	3119	3123

Abbreviations: PST, porcine somatotropin; ME, metabolizable energy.

[a] Adapted, with permission, from Steele et al. 1987.

[b] Assumptions: Pigs (50:50 barrows:gilts) possess a medium to high genetic capacity for lean tissue growth, are housed in a warm thermal environment, and are allowed to consume a fortified, corn-soybean meal diet ad libitum from 60 to 96 kg body weight. Maintenance needs for ME and lysine were assumed to be increased by 24% in the PST-treated pigs. The magnitude of the depression in feed intake in the PST-treated pigs was assumed to be equivalent to that in Table 6.1.

The efficiencies of dietary energy and amino acid conversion into body fat and protein stores are based on summaries of data in the literature (Stahly 1985; Stahly 1986).

From these calculations, the dietary need for lysine, the limiting amino acid, is increased by about 11 g daily for pigs treated with PST even though the daily demand for energy is reduced. In this instance, formulation of a corn-soybean meal diet containing 1.19% versus 0.69% lysine is estimated to be needed to meet the biological demand for amino acids created by PST administration in 78-kg pigs. The above calculations represent estimates of the nutritional needs of one set of pigs administered a particular dosage of PST. Obviously, the optimum dietary regimen for PST-treated pigs will be highly dependent on the dosage of PST administered, the pigs' genetic capacity for lean tissue growth, as well as the dietary level of ME consumed.

Less information is available for the estimation of mineral and vitamin requirements of PST-treated animals. However, the 50% to 60% increase in mineral accumulation (Table 6.2) resulting from PST administration indicates that the biological demand for these nutrients would also be substantially elevated.

BETA-ADRENERGIC AGONISTS

Two endogenous adrenergic agonists, epinephrine and norepinephrine (commonly referred to as catecholamines), are released regularly in small quantities by the adrenal medulla where concentrations of each are approximately 1 mg/g of tissue in pigs (Althen et al. 1977). Norepinephrine is also produced and secreted by sympathetic nerve endings (Martin 1985). Plasma concentrations of epinephrine and norepinephrine each range from 0.1 to 0.8 ng/ml in relaxed, catheterized pigs (Althen et al. 1977; Sharman et al. 1986). However, plasma concentrations can increase to 2 to 300 ng/ml when pigs are subjected to physical trauma (Althen et al. 1977). Once released, these agonists exert a variety of effects depending largely on the type and number of adrenergic receptors present in the respective target tissues and organs (Mersmann 1987). Adrenergic receptors were originally classified as alpha or beta based on their responsiveness to structurally different catecholamines (Ahlquist 1948). In subsequent studies, beta receptors were characterized by their role in smooth muscle relaxation, lipolysis, and glycolysis (Martin 1985). The presence of beta-adrenergic receptors has been verified in porcine adipose tissue and muscle membranes (Bocklen 1986).

Recently, several synthetic analogues of norepinephrine, called beta-adrenergic agonists, have been identified. When fed to swine these compounds have the ability to accelerate skeletal muscle accretion and reduce fat deposition (Mersmann 1987). The biological effects of natural or synthetic beta-adrenergic agonists on body fat metabolism are currently believed to be mediated via a second-messenger cyclic adenosine monophosphate (cAMP) (Fain and Garcia-Sainz 1983; Mersmann 1987). Stimulation of the beta receptors results in a cascade of intracellular events beginning with an increase in activity of adenylate cyclase, which subsequently increases intracellular cAMP (Minneman et al. 1981; Fain and Garcia-Sainz 1983). cAMP is responsible for the phosphorylation of protein kinase, which in turn activates or inactivates a variety of intracellular enzymes. Active protein kinase has at least two roles in adipose tissue metabolism. It activates hormone-sensitive lipase, which initiates triglyceride catabolism. It also inactivates acetyl CoA carboxylase (Martin and Makula 1987), which is believed to be the rate-limiting enzyme in mammalian lipogenesis (Bortz et al. 1965). Synthetic adrenergic agonists have been shown to increase glycerol release as well as decrease fatty acid synthesis in adipose tissue of pigs in vitro (Merkel et al. 1987; Williams et al. 1987a).

The mechanisms by which beta-adrenergic agonists increase body muscle accretion have not been clearly elucidated, particularly in meat-producing animals. It has been suggested but not documented that beta agonists may interfere with arachidonic acid metabolism and hence depress the protein degradation cascade postulated to be mediated by prostaglandin E_2 (PGE_2) (Reeds and Palmer 1986; Reeds 1987). However, the influence of synthetic beta agonists on protein synthesis and degradation in meat animals has been inconsistent in studies reported in the literature. For example, in vivo protein synthesis has been reported to be increased and protein degradation decreased in pigs fed ractopamine (Bergen et al. 1989). However, in vivo measures of protein synthesis and degradation were not affected in pigs fed ractopamine for 1 week (Johnson et al. 1987).

Effects of Exogenous Beta-Adrenergic Agonists in Swine

Work with exogenous catecholamines as potential modifiers of swine growth dates back to the early 1960s. Research performed by Cunningham et al. (1963) showed that subcutaneous injections of epinephrine increased body-weight gain and nitrogen retention. In recent years, several analogues of epinephrine and norepinephrine have been produced that appear to repartition nutrients in pigs fed the agonist in later stages (60 to 110 kg) of growth. Clenbuterol was the first synthetic agonist extensively evaluated in pigs (Ricks et al. 1984). Since then, research reported in the literature has centered on the use of either cimaterol or ractopamine (Figure 6.1) with less extensive evaluation of beta agonists L-644,969 (Wallace et al. 1987) and salbutamol (Wood and Brown 1987).

The ingestion of beta agonists has been shown to alter the voluntary feed intake and the rate, efficiency, and composition of growth in pigs (Tables 6.6 and 6.7). The magnitude of the responses to the agonists is at least partially dependent on the dosage level and type of beta agonist fed. Voluntary feed intake of pigs appears to be depressed in a dose-related manner in pigs fed either cimaterol or ractopamine. Live weight gains have not been consistently improved by the dietary inclusion of beta agonists, particularly at the higher levels of inclusion. The lack of a consistent growth response to beta agonists in some studies, particularly in the earlier trials (1985 and 1986), may have been due to insufficient levels of dietary amino acids in relationship to the animals' increased capacity for body protein accretion (Anderson et al. 1987a; Easter 1987). The efficiency of feed utilization for weight gain has been shown to be improved by 5% to 12% in pigs fed from about 60 to 105 kg body weight. Again, the availability of amino acids may have restricted the magnitude of improvement in feed utilization in certain trials.

The feeding of beta agonists depresses fat deposition and enhances muscle accretion consistently in finishing pigs. Beta agonists have been shown to reduce subcutaneous fat as measured at the tenth rib (Tables 6.6 and 6.7), perirenal fat, and intra-

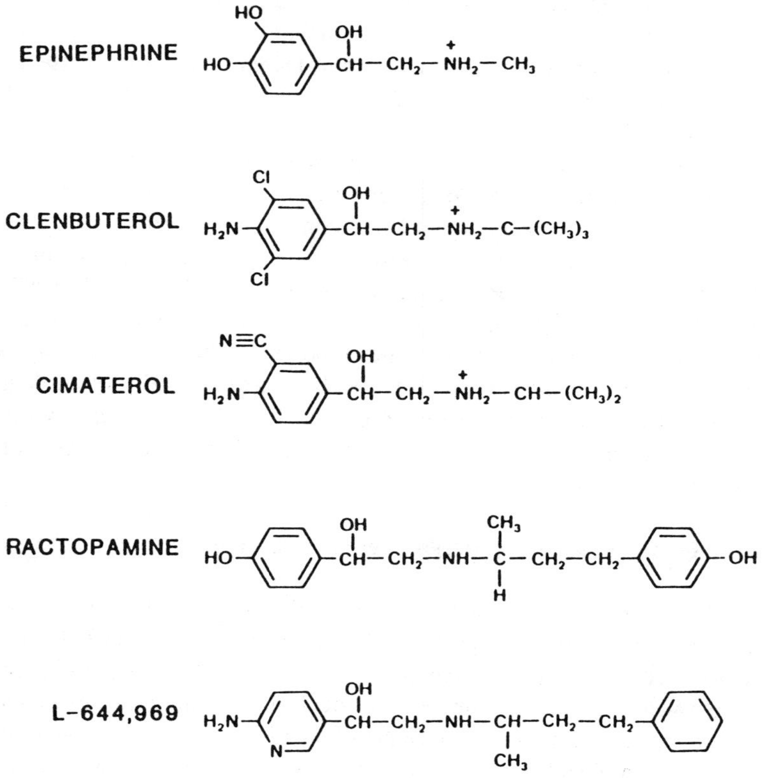

FIGURE 6.1 *Synthetic agonists evaluated in pigs.*

muscular fat (Cromwell et al. 1987; Novakofski 1987). Like growth parameters, changes in body fat measures appear to be dose-related. Total carcass fat (separable tissue) has been reported to be lowered by 2 and 4 percentage units in pigs fed 5 to 20 ppm ractopamine, respectively (Table 6.8). Muscle accretion, as estimated by loin eye area, increased by 6% to 15% in a series of studies involving cimaterol and ractopamine (Tables 6.6 and 6.7). Hypertrophy of the semitendinosus muscle also has been observed in response to beta agonist feeding (Jones et al. 1985; Bergen et al. 1989). Dissected muscle tissue, expressed as a percentage of the carcass, has been shown to be increased by 2 to 4 percentage units in pigs fed a beta agonist (Table 6.8).

Beta agonists also appear to have some influence on the distribution of nutrients to the carcass versus internal organs and gastrointestinal tract. The portion of the pig's body weight represented by organs such as liver (Moser et al. 1986; Cromwell et al. 1987) and heart (Jones et al. 1985) tend to be reduced. Consequently, the dressing percentage of pigs tends to be improved in pigs fed beta agonists (Tables 6.6 and 6.7).

Limited information is available on the effect of beta-adrenergic agonists on bone deposition and development in swine. Beta agonists have been reported to lower the

Table 6.6 Effects of Dietary Cimaterol on Growth and Carcass Characteristics in Swine[a]

	Dietary Cimaterol (ppm)		
	0.25	*0.50*	*1.00*
Criteria	*% Change from Controls*[b]		
Growth performance			
Daily feed	−1	−4	−7
Daily gain	+4	0	0
Gain/feed	+5	+4	+7
Carcass traits			
Backfat thickness	−9	−12	−14
Loin eye area	+6	+9	+9
Dressing %	+1	+1	+1

[a] Summary of five studies (means weighted by replicates/treatment): Jones et al. 1985; Prince et al. 1985; Moser et al. 1986; Cromwell et al. 1987; Walker et al. 1987; Williams et al. 1987b.

[b] Pig weights averaged 59 and 105 kg at the initiation and termination of the trials, respectively. The levels of performance for the pigs in the control treatment were as follows: 0.78 kg/d weight gain, 2.85 kg feed/d, 2.76 cm backfat, 32.6 cm^2 LEA, and 74.5% carcass yield.

Table 6.7 Effect of Dietary Ractopamine on Growth and Carcass Characteristics in Swine[a]

	Dietary Ractopamine (ppm)				
	2.5	*5.0*	*10.0*	*20.0*	*30.0*
Criteria	*% Change from Control*[b]				
Growth performance					
Daily feed	−2	−3	−3	−4	−7
Daily gain	+6	+6	+8	+8	+3
Gain/feed	+8	+9	+12	+12	+10
Carcass traits					
Backfat thickness	−9	−6	−11	−12	−13
Loin eye area	+6	+8	+11	+15	+15
Dressing %	0	+1	+1	+2	+2

[a] Summary of six studies (means weighted by replicates/treatment): Anderson et al. 1987a; Cline and Forrest 1987; Crenshaw et al. 1987; Hancock et al. 1987; Prince et al. 1987; Veenhuizen et al. 1987.

[b] Pig weights averaged 64 and 105 kg at the initiation and termination of the trials, respectively. The levels of performance for the pigs in the control treatment were as follows: 0.78 kg/d weight gain, 2.87 kg feed/d, 2.43 cm backfat, 32.3 cm^2 LEA, and 71.4% carcass yield.

bone content of pigs, expressed as an individual bone weight (Jones et al. 1985) or as a percentage of the carcass (Cline and Forrest 1987). The incidence of leg unsoundness or hoof cracks-abrasions has been observed to be increased as a result of feeding certain beta agonists in some studies (Jones et al. 1985; Cromwell et al. 1987) but not in others (Moser et al. 1986; Hill and Dalrymple 1987).

Table 6.8 Effect of Ractopamine on Carcass Fat and Lean Tissue Content[a,b]

	Dietary Ractopamine (ppm)		
Carcass Composition (%)[c]	*0*	*5*	*20*
Fat	27.3	25.4	23.0
Lean	53.1	55.5	57.9

[a] Summary of four studies (means weighted by replicates/treatment): Cline and Forrest 1987; Crenshaw et al. 1987; Hancock et al. 1987; Prince et al. 1987.

[b] Pig weights averaged 65 and 105 kg at the initiation and termination of the trials, respectively.

[c] Carcasses were physically dissected into fat and lean tissues.

Influence of Management Practices on Response to Beta-Adrenergic Agonists

The responses of pigs to beta agonists appear to be influenced by the genetic capacity for lean growth. Pigs with medium to high genetic capacity for lean tissue growth have exhibited greater improvements in lean tissue accretion rate and total carcass muscle than pigs with low lean tissue growth capacity when fed ractopamine (Bark et al. 1989a; Table 6.9). This response may be due to greater cell numbers in muscle found in lean strains of pigs (Staun 1972; Harbison et al. 1976), thus allowing a greater number of target cells for beta agonists to act upon in the high lean tissue growth genotype.

Table 6.9 Influence of Genetic Capacity for Lean Tissue Growth on Responses of Pigs to Ractopamine[a]

	Lean Growth Genotype					
	Low			*Medium*		
Criteria	*Control*	*RAC*	*Units of Change*	*Control*	*RAC*	*Units of Change*
Growth performance						
Daily feed (kg)	2.69	2.62	−0.07	2.89	2.71	−0.18
Daily gain (kg)	0.63	0.68	+0.05	0.89	0.98	+0.09
Feed/gain	4.28	3.88	−0.40	3.25	2.77	−0.48
Carcass traits						
Backfat-10th rib (cm)	7.15	6.52	−0.63	2.76	2.00	−0.76
Est. muscle (kg)	29.2	32.2	+3.0	39.5	45.0	+5.5
Lean gain (kg/d)	0.13	0.17	+0.04	0.28	0.40	+0.12

Abbreviations: RAC, ractopamine; Est., estimated.

[a] Each genotype consisted of eight sets of two littermate barrows. Pigs were self-fed corn-soybean meal diets containing 0 or 20 ppm of RAC from 63 to 104 kg body weight.

(Adapted, by permission, from Bark et al. 1989a.)

Table 6.10 Influence of Dietary Protein Level on the Response of Pigs to Ractopamine[a]

	Daily Gain (kg)			*Backfat (cm)*			*Loin Area (cm^2)*		
Dietary Protein (%)	*0*	*RAC*	*%*[b]	*0*	*RAC*	*%*[b]	*0*	*RAC*	*%*[b]
12	0.75	0.72	−4	3.15	2.84	−10	29.4	31.2	+ 6
15	0.78	0.79	+1	2.87	2.54	−11	32.3	35.0	+ 8
18	0.75	0.82	+9	2.69	2.26	−16	32.3	36.8	+14

Abbreviation: RAC, ractopamine.
[a] Pigs were self-fed corn-soybean meal diets containing 0 or 20 ppm RAC.
[b] Percentage change in value from the control treatment group.
(Adapted, by permission, from Anderson et al. 1987b.)

Like PST, the responses of pigs to beta agonists are also thought to be influenced by climatic environment, dietary regimen, and health status of the animal as well as source and level of the agonist utilized. For example, dietary amino acid levels needed to maximize performance have been shown to be increased in pigs administered a beta agonist (Table 6.10). However, the quantitative interrelationships of these factors have not been delineated.

SUMMARY

Recombinant PST and beta-adrenergic agonists allow unique opportunities for improvement in economical production of lean pork products. However, the metabolic changes induced by these compounds will alter the optimal dietary regimen of pigs. Specific dietary needs will be highly dependent on the type and level of the compounds utilized as well as on the animal's genetic capacity for lean tissue growth.

REFERENCES

Ahlquist, R.P. 1948. *Am. J. Physiol.* 153:586.
Althen, T.G., et al. 1977. *J. Anim. Sci.* 44:985.
Anderson, D.B., et al. 1987a. *J. Anim. Sci.* 65 (Suppl. 1):130.
Anderson, D.B., et al. 1987b. *Fed. Proc.* 46:1021 (Abstr).
ArGona, J.R., et al. 1988. J. Anim. Sci. 66:3068.
Bark, L.J., et al. 1988. *J. Anim. Sci.* 66 (Suppl. 1):270.
Bark, L.J., et al. 1989a. *J. Anim. Sci.* 67 (Suppl. 1):212.
Bark, L.J., et al. 1989b. *J. Anim. Sci.* 67 (Suppl. 2):122.
Bechtel, P.J. 1987. "Primer on somatotropins and their effects on finishing and lactating swine." In: *Proceedings of the University of Illinois Pork Industry Conference.* pp. 46–54. Champaign, IL: University of Illinois.
Berdu, B.B., and F.B. Diamond, Jr. 1986. *Adv. Pediatr.* 33:331.
Bergen, W.G., et al. 1989. *J. Anim. Sci.* 67:2255.
Bocklen, E., et al. 1986. *Anim. Prod.* 43:335.
Bortz, W.M., et al. 1965. *Adv. Enzym. Reg.* 3:407.

Boyd, R.D., et al. 1986. *Proceedings of Cornell Nutrition Conference.* p. 25. Ithaca, NY: Cornell University.

Boyd, R.D. 1987. *Proceedings of Cornell Nutrition Conference.* pp. 10–19. Ithaca, NY: Cornell University.

Brendemuhl, J.H., et al. 1986. *J. Anim. Sci.* 63(Suppl. 1):263.

Brendemuhl, J.H., et al. 1987. *J. Anim. Sci.* 64:1060.

Campbell, R.J., et al. 1989. In: *Biotechnology for Control of Growth and Product Quality in Swine—Implications and Acceptability.* Van der Wal, P., G.J. Nieuwhal, R.D. Politick (Eds.). pp. 137–145. Wageningen, The Netherlands: Pudoc Wageningen.

Cline, T.R., and J.C. Forrest. 1987. "Repartitioning agents and somatotropin for finishing swine." In: *Proceedings of Purdue Swine Day.* West Lafayette, IN: Purdue University.

Crenshaw, J.D., et al. 1987. *J. Anim. Sci.* 65(Suppl. 1):308.

Crenshaw, J.D., et al. 1989. *J. Anim. Sci.* 72(Suppl. 1):288.

Cromwell, G.L., et al. 1987. *J. Anim. Sci.* 65(Suppl. 1):300.

Cromwell, G.L., et al. 1989. *J. Anim. Sci.* 72(Suppl. 1):258.

Cunningham, H.M., et al. 1963. *J. Anim. Sci.* 23:623.

Curtis, S.E., 1987. "Management and environment considerations for successful use of repartitioning agents." In: *Proceedings of the University of Illinois Pork Industry Conference.* pp. 64–65. Champaign, IL: University of Illinois.

Easter, R.A. 1987. "Nutritional requirements and repartitioning agents." In: *Proceedings of the University of Illinois Pork Industry Conference.* pp. 193–199. Champaign, IL: University of Illinois.

Etherton, T.D., et al. 1986. *J. Anim. Sci.* 63:1389.

Etherton, T.D., et al. 1987. *J. Anim. Sci.* 64:433.

Fain, J.N., and J.A. Garcia-Sainz. 1983. *J. Lipid Res.* 24:945.

Grebner, G.L., et al. 1987. *J. Anim. Sci.* 65(Suppl. 1):245.

Hancock, J.D., et al. 1987. *J. Anim. Sci.* 65(Suppl. 1):309.

Harbison, S.A., et al. 1976. *Growth* 40:253.

Hill, M.A., and R.H. Dalrymple. 1987. *Can. J. Vet. Res.* 51:217.

Johnson, S.E., et al. 1987. *J. Anim. Sci.* 65(Suppl. 1):277.

Jones, R.W., et al. 1985. *J. Anim. Sci.* 61:905.

Kraft, L.A., et al. 1986. *J. Anim. Sci.* 63(Suppl. 1):218.

Machlin, L.J. 1972. *J. Anim. Sci.* 35:794.

Martin, C.R. 1985. *Endocrine Physiology.* New York: Oxford University Press.

Martin, R.J., and A. Makula. 1987. "Enzymology of adipocytes." In: *Biology of the Adipocyte: Research Approaches.* Hausman, G.J., and R.J. Martin (Eds.). pp. 86–119. New York: Van Nostrand Reinhold Co.

McLaren, D.G., et al. 1987. *J. Anim. Sci.* 65(Suppl. 1):245.

Merkel, R.A., et al. 1987. *Fed. Proc.* 46:1021.

Mersmann, H.J. 1987. "Primer on beta adrenergic agonists and their effect on the biology of swine." In: *Proceedings of the Illinois Pork Industry Conference.* pp. 19–45. Champaign, IL: University of Illinois.

Minneman, K.P., et al. 1981. *Ann. Rev. Neurosci.* 4:419.

Moser, R.L., et al. 1986. *J. Anim. Sci.* 62:21.

Nelssen, J.L., et al. 1985. *J. Anim. Sci.* 61:1164.

Novakofski, J. 1987. "Repartitioned pork: Sensory quality and consumer preference." In: *Proceedings of the University of Illinois Pork Industry Conference.* pp. 84–92. Champaign, IL: University of Illinois.

Prince, T.J., et al. 1985. *J. Anim. Sci.* 61(Suppl. 1):301.

Prince, T.J., et al. 1987. *J. Anim. Sci.* 65(Suppl. 1):309.

Reeds, P.J. 1987. *Anim. Prod.* 45:149.

Reeds, P.J., and R.M. Palmer. 1986. "The role of prostaglandins in the control of muscle protein turnover." In: *Control and Manipulation of Animal Growth.* Buttery, P.J., N.B. Haynes, and D.B. Lindsay (Eds.). London: Butterworths.

Reese, D.E., et al. 1982a. *J. Anim. Sci.* 55:590.
Reese, D.E., et al. 1982b. *J. Anim. Sci.* 55:867.
Ricks, C.A., et al. 1984. *Fed. Proc.* 43:857.
Seeburg, P.H. 1983. *DNA.* 2:37.
Sharman, D.F., et al. 1986. *Horm. Metabol. Res.* 18:145.
Stahly, T.S. 1985. *Anim. Nutr. Health.* August, pp. 22–26.
Stahly, T.S. 1986. Energy metabolism—A review of the Tenth International Symposium on energy metabolism. Paper presented at the Animal Nutrition Seminar, Leipzig, East Germany, July, 1986.
Staun, H. 1972. *World Rev. Anim. Prod.* 8:18.
Steele, N.C., et al. 1987. "Update of porcine growth hormone research: Practical and biological implications." In: *Proceedings of the Cornell Nutrition Conference.* p. 15. Ithaca, NY: Cornell University.
Veenhuizen, E.L., et al. 1987. *J. Anim. Sci.* 65(Suppl. 1):130.
Walker, W.R., et al. 1987. *J. Anim. Sci.* 65(Suppl. 1):31.
Wallace, D.H., et al. 1987. "Growth and efficiency of feed utilization of swine fed a beta-adrenergic agonist (L-644,969)." In: *Beta-Agonists and Their Effects on Animal Growth and Carcass Quality.* Hanrahan, J.P. (Ed.). p. 143. Essex, England: Elsevier Science Publishers.
Wangsness, P.J., et al. 1977. *Am. J. Physiol.* 233:E104.
Williams, A.C., et al. 1987a. *J. Anim. Sci.* 65(Suppl. 1):249.
Williams, L.T., and R.J. Lefkowitz. 1978. *Receptor Binding Studies in Adrenergic Pharmacology.* New York: Raven Press.
Williams, S.E., et al. 1987b. *J. Anim. Sci.* 65(Suppl. 1):31.
Wood, J.D., and A.J. Brown. 1987. *Anim. Prod.* 44:477.

PART III

Nutrient Utilization by Swine

Chapter 7

Energy Utilization in Swine Nutrition

R.C. Ewan

Feed accounts for about two thirds of the cost of producing market-weight swine. Through the years, efforts have been made to optimize feed efficiency so that feed costs might be minimized. Such efforts depend on a knowledge of nutrient availability in feed ingredients and the requirements of the pig for those nutrients for various physiological states.

The total digestible nutrient (TDN) system allows comparisons, roughly equivalent to digestible energy concentration, between feed ingredients. TDN is the sum of digestible protein, digestible ether extract, and digestible carbohydrate. Ether extract is multiplied by 2.25 to adjust for the greater energy concentration of fat. The system has been criticized because it gives protein the same weight as carbohydrates, and because it is the sum of several digestibility measurements; the errors associated with each of the individual measurements would reduce the accuracy of the value.

While the TDN system was used for many years, it has gradually been replaced by measures of energy to describe the value of feed ingredients. The heat of combustion is the maximum amount of energy that is available for use by animals and is defined as gross energy (GE). The GE concentration of a feed ingredient is dependent on the proportions of carbohydrate, fat, protein, minerals, and water present in the ingredient. Water and minerals contribute no energy while carbohydrates provide 3.7 (glucose) to 4.2 (starch) kcal/g. Protein provides 5.6 kcal and fat, 9.4 kcal/g. If the composition of a feed is known, GE can be predicted fairly accurately. Measurement of GE is generally done with an adiabatic bomb calorimeter.

The utilization of the energy of a feed by the pig is illustrated in Figure 7.1. Digestible energy (DE) is the GE of the feed minus the heat of combustion of the fecal material (FE). Indigestible energy is a major variable in evaluation of feed ingredients. Metabolizable energy (ME) is DE minus the heat of combustion of the urine (UE) and of gases produced in the intestinal tract. Energy losses in the urine are small and generally associated with the excretion of nitrogenous products of metabolism. Energy lost as gas is generally less than 1% of GE intake of pigs and is often ignored. In com-

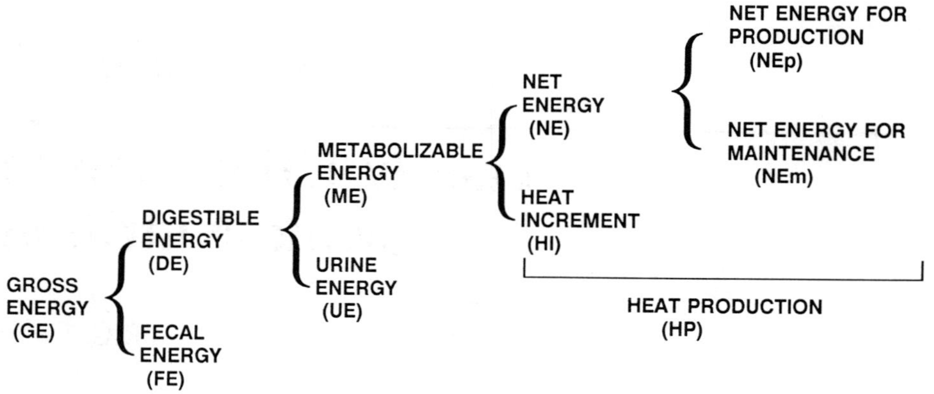

FIGURE 7.1 *Utilization of energy by pigs.*

plete feeds fed to pigs, ME is about 96% of DE but will decrease as the protein content of the diet increases.

ME is divided further into net energy (NE) and heat increment (HI). Heat increment is the heat produced by the digestion and metabolism of nutrients and fermentation in the intestinal tract. Normally, HI is waste energy, but HI can be used to maintain body temperature. The remaining energy is used to meet the requirement for maintenance (NE_m). The NE_m includes the energy needed to sustain life and to maintain body temperature. If the supply of NE is greater than the energy required for maintenance, it is used for production (NE_p). Productive processes include the synthesis of new tissue (protein, fat, or fetal development) or milk. Heat production (HP) is the sum of the HI and NE_m.

In nutrition, the joule is the basic unit used for energy in most of the world and the calorie is used in the United States. A joule is 10^7 ergs where 1 erg is the amount of energy expended in accelerating a mass of 1 g by 1 cm/s. A calorie is the amount of energy required to raise the temperature of 1 g of water from 16.5 °C to 17.5 °C and is equivalent to 4.184 J. Both joules and calories are more commonly expressed in multiples of 1000 so that a kilocalorie is 10^3 calories, and a megacalorie is 10^6 calories or 1000 kilocalories. Corresponding units for the joule are the kilojoule and the megajoule. The basic unit that will be used in this chapter is the kilocalorie.

In European countries, energy systems have been developed that are related to energy content of a common feed ingredient and expressed as feeding units. These have been reviewed by Henry et al. (1988).

ENERGY EVALUATION OF FEED INGREDIENTS

Pigs are normally fed diets containing several ingredients, complicating the determination of energy values of individual ingredients. The determination of DE and ME of a diet fed to pigs requires the completion of a metabolism study with total collection of feces and urine. The energy contents of the diet, feces, and urine are determined and DE (GE − FE) and ME (DE − UE) can be calculated.

Further evaluation to determine NE requires a measurement of energy retained or of HP. Energy retention can be determined in a comparative slaughter experiment in which the energy content of pigs slaughtered at the start of the experiment is subtracted from the energy content of the pigs at the end of the experiment to obtain the retained energy. Retained energy can also be determined by carbon-nitrogen balance in which nitrogen gain is attributed to protein gain and carbon retention after subtraction of the carbon in the protein gain is attributed to fat deposition. Retained energy is obtained by applying standard values for the energy concentrations of fat and protein.

Direct or indirect calorimetry can be used to measure HP. In direct calorimetry, the HP of the pig is measured by physical methods and requires complex equipment. Indirect calorimetry uses measurement of oxygen uptake, expired carbon dioxide, and methane loss. These measures are used with standard conversion factors to give HP (Brouwer 1965).

The maintenance requirement of the pig is necessary to complete the evaluation of NE. The maintenance requirement is generally expressed as an exponential function of body weight. The exponent that is generally used is 0.75 (Kleiber 1965) but values from 0.56 (Breirem 1939) to 1 (Kielanowski 1972) have been suggested. With the measurement of retained energy (RE) either by comparative slaughter or by carbon-nitrogen balance, the maintenance requirement can be estimated from the regression of ME intake and RE (ME intake = a + b RE). In this relationship, the intercept is a measure of NE_m and regression coefficient is a measure of the efficiency of conversion of ME to RE. The maintenance requirement in terms of ME is the intercept divided by the efficiency.

With direct or indirect calorimetry, the HP of the conscious animal in a fasting state is used as the maintenance requirement. This is based on the assumption that HI is zero in the fasted state so that relationship, $HP = HI + NE_m$, becomes $HP = NE_m$. The length of fast has to be standardized because HP declines as the length of the fast increases.

To determine the energy value of individual ingredients in a mixed diet, some means of partitioning the energy among the ingredients is necessary. In short-term studies, diets containing essentially one ingredient have been used, but this is not satisfactory for long-term studies and may be confounded by nutrient excesses or deficiencies. Substitution of one ingredient for another with observation of the change in energy values has been used. Regression techniques are used to determine the values of 100% intake of each individual component (Kromann et al. 1976). In some studies, a basal diet is fed at a constant level and the individual ingredient is fed in addition to the basal diet to determine the response to additional energy from the test ingredient (Diggs et al. 1965).

Ingredients in nylon bags have been placed into the duodenum of surgically prepared pigs. The bags allow digested nutrients to diffuse out but retain the undigested residue. Recovery of the bag allows measurement of the nutrient concentration of the residue. This technique has been used with protein (Sauer et al. 1983) and may provide an alternative to conventional metabolism studies for DE estimates.

Table 7.1 Energy Concentration of Feed Ingredients

Ingredient	*DM (air dry) (%)*	*GE*	*DE*	*ME*	*NE*
		kcal/kg air dry			
Alfalfa meal, dehy., 17% protein	92	3830	1880	1705	540
Barley	89	4395	3120	3040	1980
Beet pulp, dried	91	3785	2830	2560	1560
Blood meal, spray- or ring-dried	93	4965[a]	3225	2520	1740[a]
Brewers' dried grains	92	5015	2090	1900	750[a]
Corn, yellow dent	88	3945	3490	3380	2270
Corn and cob meal	87	3860[a]	3140	2680	1760[a]
Corn gluten feed	91	4215	3190	2725	1795
Corn gluten meal, 41% protein	91	5185	4290	3880	2440[a]
Corn, distillers' grains with solubles	91	4495	3560	3265	1900[a]
Corn, distillers' solubles, dehy.	91	4535	3295	2915	1770[a]
Corn, hominy feed	90	4215	3495	3310	2065
Cottonseed meal, exp. ext.	93	4510	2980	2730	1495[a]
Cottonseed meal, sol. ext.	92	4330	2670	2555	1410[a]
Feather meal	93	5030[a]	2755	2240	1670[a]
Fish meal, anchovy	92	4180[a]	3050	2465	1360[a]
Fish meal, herring	92	4605	3805	3095	1865[a]
Fish meal, menhaden	92	4495	3780	3370	2315
Lard	100	9320	7860	7750	4970[a]
Meat and bone meal	94	3970	2570	2305	1140
Meat meal, 55% protein	93	3965	2540	2385	950[a]
Molasses, beet	78	2990	2480	2350	1500
Molasses, cane	74	2655	2210	2005	955
Oats	89	4130	2760	2735	1490
Oat groats (dehulled oats)	87	4080	3590	3265	2225
Peas	89	3655	3360	3130	1855
Peanut meal, exp. ext.	93	4680	4190	3835	2725
Peanut meal, sol. ext.	93	4505	3245	3005	1865[a]
Rapeseed meal, sol. ext.	93	4470	3050	2805	1580
Rice bran	91	4320	3175	3065	1845
Rice, broken	89	3830	3505	3290	2240
Rice, polishings	90	4285[a]	3860	3215	2030[a]
Rye, grain	87	3800	3210	2935	1975
Safflower meal, sol. ext.	92	4035[a]	2720	2460	1070[a]
Sesame meal, exp. ext.	93	4335	3385	2975	1535[a]
Skim milk, dried	94	4010	3930	3650	2290

Sorghum, grain (milo)	89	3970	3415	3280	2070
Soybeans, full-fat, cooked	90	4720	4035	3625	2655
Soybean meal, dehulled, sol. ext.	90	4260	3680	3385	1760
Soybean meal, exp. ext.	90	4505	3490	3220	1870
Soybean meal, sol. ext.	90	4220	3530	3255	1805
Soybean oil	100	9395	7560	7280	5500
Sunflower meal, dehulled, sol. ext.	93	4575	2990	2650	1610
Tallow	100	9360	8200	7885	4180
Wheat bran	90	4020	2370	2155	1580
Wheat shorts	88	4060	3025	2835	1795[a]
Wheat middlings	89	4070	3115	3000	1390
Wheat	88	3965	3360	3200	2215
Whey, dried	93	3560	3215	3090	2045
Whey, low lactose	93	3550[a]	3055	2760	1750[a]
Yeast, dried, brewers'	93	4375	3360	3045	2245

Abbreviations: DM, dry matter; GE, gross energy; DE, digestible energy; ME, metabolizable energy; NE, net energy; dehy., dehydrated; exp. ext., expeller extracted; sol. ext., solvent extracted.

[a]Value was estimated from the following relationships:

$$\text{GE, kcal/g} = (\%\text{CP} \times 5.6 + \%\text{EE} \times 9.4 + \%\text{CHO} \times 4.2) \times .01$$

$$\text{NE, kcal/g} = \text{ME(kcal/g)} \times .599 - \%\text{ASH} \times .015 - \%\text{ADF} \times .030 + .328$$

(Reprinted, by permission, from Ewan 1989.)

Suggested values for GE, DE, ME, and NE for ingredients normally used in swine diets are listed in Table 7.1 (Ewan 1986).

EFFICIENCY OF ENERGY UTILIZATION

Growth

Growth or an increase in body mass results from the accumulation of protein, fat, and ash and the associated energy. The deposition of 1 g of protein increases energy stores by 5.67 kcal while 1 g of fat results in the storage of 9.46 kcal of energy. The total cost of deposition of fat (FD) and protein (PD) can be estimated from one of the following relationships:

$$\text{ME intake} = a + b\ \text{FD} + c\ \text{PD}$$

$$\text{NE}_p = b\ \text{FD} + c\ \text{PD}$$

A summary of estimates of the regression coefficients of these relationships by the Agriculture Research Council (ARC) (1981) resulted in the conclusion that the coefficient for protein was 10.5 kcal/g and for fat, 12.8 kcal/g. These values correspond to efficiencies of utilization of 0.54 for protein (k_p) and 0.74 for fat (k_f). The energy lost as heat during protein synthesis is much greater than the biochemical cost of protein synthesis (Millward et al. 1976). Protein turnover or the need to synthesize enough protein to equal the protein degraded plus the protein retained is one cause of the lower efficiency of protein deposition as compared with fat deposition.

The efficiency of energy utilization by the pig is determined by the amounts of fat and protein that are deposited in the gain. The deposition of 1 g of protein is accompanied by the deposition of about 4 g of water and results in the deposition of 5 g of tissue. Thus, the energy required per gram of tissue gain is 1.12 kcal. The deposition of 1 g of fat is associated with the deposition of about 0.2 g of water so that the energy required per gram of tissue gain is 7.83 kcal. The deposition of fat therefore requires more energy per unit of tissue gain than does protein. The composition of daily gain changes from primarily protein and minimal fat by the young pig to a maximum of protein and increasing amounts of fat by the finishing pig. Thus, the energy requirements per unit of gain increase during the growth period.

Gestation

During gestation, energy is required for the maintenance of the sow, some growth of the sow, and development of the conceptus (fetus and maternal tissue). Development of the conceptus takes priority and will develop at the expense of maternal tissue if nutrient intake is severely restricted (Walach-Janiak et al. 1986). Nutrient demands for the conceptus are greatest during the last third of gestation when fetal growth is at a maximum. Energy intake of the sow during gestation is restricted to prevent excessive growth and fattening (Verstegen et al. 1987).

Close et al. (1985) have reported that the efficiency of energy utilization for k_p by the pregnant gilt was 0.69 and for k_f, 0.88. The efficiency of protein deposition was greater in pregnant gilts than in nonpregnant littermate gilts (0.49). The efficiency of energy deposition in the reproductive tissue was 0.72. The study by Close et al. allowed partitioning of the energy deposition between maternal and conceptus energy gain and the workers concluded that the efficiency of maternal gain was 0.87 and of conceptus gain, 0.72.

Lactation

During lactation, after maintenance requirements are met, nutrients are utilized for milk production. If insufficient energy is available, energy will be mobilized from the maternal tissues to sustain milk production and weight loss will occur. Generally, lactating sows are allowed ad libitum access to feed, and feed intake will determine if weight is gained or lost during lactation. Noblet and Etienne (1986) reported that restriction of energy intake reduced milk yield slightly, but the concentration of fat, energy, and nitrogen in the milk from energy-restricted gilts was greater than in the milk from gilts fed a high level of energy.

Noblet and Etienne (1987) have reported that the efficiency of utilization of dietary energy for milk production was 0.72 and that the efficiency of utilization of energy from body stores for milk production was 0.88. They concluded that the overall efficiency of energy storage during pregnancy and mobilization during lactation was similar to the efficiency of utilization of dietary energy for milk production.

NUTRIENT:ENERGY RATIOS

Nutrient:energy ratios may be important because the pig, as other animals, eats to satisfy a demand for energy so that the actual amount of feed consumed depends on the energy density of the diet fed. Protein is the nutrient that is most frequently adjusted as energy density is changed, but the same logic can be applied to all nutrients. Nutrient requirements as established by the National Research Council (NRC 1988) are not, however, expressed per unit of energy, so that optimal nutrient:calorie ratios must be derived from the recommendations for energy density and the concentration of other nutrients. For protein, the current recommendations (NRC 1988) decrease from 59 g/1000 kcal of DE for the 5- to 10-kg pig to 38 g/1000 kcal of DE for the 50- to 110-kg pig. The values for lysine decrease from 3.39 g/1000 kcal of DE for the 5- to 10-kg pig to 1.76 g/1000 kcal of DE for the 50- to 110-kg pig.

FACTORS AFFECTING ENERGY UTILIZATION

Feed Composition

Amino acids absorbed in excess of the demands for amino acids for protein synthesis are deaminated. The nitrogen is excreted as urea, and the carbon skeleton is metabolized to yield energy. Energy is required for the synthesis of urea, and urea also contains 2.52 kcal/g (5.45 kcal/g of nitrogen). Thus, diets containing excess protein or protein with improper ratios of amino acids are utilized less efficiently than diets that contain adequate amounts of balanced protein. Diets that contain inadequate amounts of balanced protein limit protein retention and result in energy being diverted to fat synthesis.

Addition of fat to the diet increases energy density and results in a reduction in feed intake to maintain a constant DE intake. Fatty acids are liberated during digestion and are absorbed. They are generally deposited as fat and increase the efficiency of energy utilization. Added fat also has a lower heat increment than carbohydrate and can be beneficial at high environmental temperatures by maintaining energy intake to support maximal growth rate (Stahly and Cromwell 1979). In pigs weaned at 3 weeks of age, additional fat is not well utilized for 10 to 14 days after weaning and can result in depression of growth rate (Cera et al. 1988a,b).

Feed ingredients that contain fiber result in a reduction in energy density. Pigs have a limited ability to utilize fiber, and feed intake increases in an attempt to maintain a constant DE intake. The digestive tract enlarges to accommodate a larger volume of feed, and the rate of passage of ingesta increases, resulting in a small depression in digestibility of nutrients. Fiber is indigestible and passes to the cecum and large intestine. The cecum and large intestine have a microbial population that is similar to that in the rumen, and fiber is degraded with the production of volatile fatty acids. It has been estimated that volatile fatty acid production may provide as much as 30% of the maintenance energy requirement (Rérat et al. 1987).

Environment

Effective environmental temperature is the major factor that affects energy utilization by the pig. The pig has an upper and lower critical temperature bounding the thermoneutral zone, and if the effective environmental temperature is above the upper critical temperature, energy is required to dissipate heat from the body. Below the lower critical temperature, energy is diverted from productive processes to provide heat to maintain body temperature. Effective environmental temperature is the temperature that the pig experiences and is influenced by air temperature, building insulation and flooring, air movement, number of pigs per pen, size of pen, and level of DE intake (NRC 1981).

The effective environmental temperature will alter feed intake by reducing DE intake linearly as temperature increases between 5 °C and 30 °C (NCR 1986). Below 5 °C, feed intake increases markedly while above 30 °C, a marked reduction in feed intake occurs.

ENERGY REQUIREMENTS OF PIGS

The energy requirements of pigs have been estimated by empirical or factorial methods. The empirical method establishes the requirements based on maximizing performance in response to varying energy intake. The factorial method is based on the amount of energy required for a specific function (e.g., maintenance, growth, or milk production) and the efficiency of utilization of ME for the specific function. The empirical approach was used by NRC (1979), while the factorial approach was used by ARC (1981) and NRC (1988). Close and Fowler (1985) summarized the factorial approach used by ARC (1981). The following discussion describes the factorial approach with comparison to the empirical estimates of energy requirements.

Maintenance Requirements

Maintenance requirements have been estimated from measurements of HP following periods of fasting. The ME can be estimated by assuming an efficiency of conversion of energy to meet maintenance (k_m). Measurements of fasting HP vary with the length of fast, previous nutritional history, and the difference in activity between fasted and fed animals; it may not relate to the maintenance requirement of the normal animal.

Maintenance requirements have been estimated from the relationship between retained energy and ME intake. Maintenance requirements are calculated as the ME intake that is necessary for zero energy retention. At zero energy retention, however, the growing animal will continue to deposit protein and mobilize fat.

A third method that has been used is to determine the multiple regression between ME intake and retention of fat and protein. This relationship provides an estimate of the ME required when no fat or protein are retained and is an estimate of maintenance requirements.

ARC (1981) reported the results of the logarithmic analysis of data for pigs between 5 and 90 kg and derived the following relationship for the ME requirement at maintenance:

$$172\ W^{.63}\ (\text{kcal/d})$$

The derived exponent differs from the interspecies exponent of .75, but if the data were constrained to the exponent of .75, the following relationship was obtained:

$$109\ W^{.75}\ (\text{kcal/d})$$

Energy Requirements for Growth

Energy requirements per unit of live weight gain will vary because the amounts of protein and fat in the gain will depend on the stage of growth and the available amino acids and energy. Daily protein deposition increases to a maximum at a body weight of about 60 kg and is relatively constant from 60 kg to market weight. Daily energy intake continues to increase from 60 kg to market weight so that a constant amount of energy is required for protein deposition, and the additional available energy is deposited as fat. The maximum amount of protein deposition varies with genetic strain and sex, suggesting that energy requirements for growth also vary with these factors.

Factorial estimates of energy requirements for growth are presented in Table 7.2 based on the efficiencies noted in the previous sections. The factorial method gives lower estimates of the total ME intake required for the respective level of performance than are suggested by NRC (1979). The factorial estimates do not include any allowance for environmental factors that reduce the efficiency of utilization of energy and increase the ME required for a given level of performance.

Energy Requirements for Gestation

Energy intake during gestation is generally limited to control weight gain and maintain an appropriate condition of the sow. NRC (1979) recommends an intake of 1.8 kg of

Table 7.2 Factorial Estimates of Energy Requirements for Growth

	Daily Gain (g)			*Daily ME (kcal)*			
Body Weight (kg)	*Weight*	*Protein*[a]	*Fat*[b]	*Gain*[c]	*Maintenance*[d]	*Total*	*NRC 1988 Daily ME*
15	450	69	72	1650	831	2480	3090
35	700	106	143	2949	1291	4518	6200
80	820	118	253	4477	2916	7392	10185

[a]Protein gain = 2.012 W − 0.0156 W^2 + 0.161 ADG − 0.0000954 ADG^2 − 10.843. Lean gain = protein gain/dry matter of lean tissue. (ADG = average daily gain.)

[b]Fat gain = (ADG − lean gain)/dry matter of fat tissue.

[c]ME for gain = protein gain × 10.5 kcal/g + fat gain × 12.8 kcal/g.

[d]ME for maintenance = 109 $W^{.75}$.

air-dry feed containing 3200 kcal of ME/kg or an intake of 5760 kcal of ME daily. A protein level of 12% is recommended, providing 216 g of protein daily (34.56 g of nitrogen). Williams et al. (1985) described nitrogen retention as a linear function of protein intake and use of this function would predict a retention of 10.32 g of nitrogen daily ($0.37 \times 34.56 - 2.47$). Close et al. (1985) reported that the efficiency of deposition of energy in protein by the gestating sow was 0.69 so that retention of 10.32 g of nitrogen would result in the deposition of 366 kcal as protein ($10.32 \times 6.25 \times 5.67$) and would require 530 kcal of ME (366/0.69). Close et al. (1985) also reported that the maintenance requirement during gestation was 100 kcal of ME per unit of metabolic weight. The ME requirement of a sow averaging 160 kg during gestation would be 4499 kcal ($100 \times 160^{.75}$). The remaining energy would be used for fat deposition with an efficiency of 0.88 resulting in deposition of 67.9 g of fat.

$$[5760 - 4499 - 530 = 731;\ (731 \times 0.88)/9.47 = 67.9]$$

The fat and protein gain can be converted to fat and lean tissue by dividing by their dry-matter concentration to give a tissue gain of 356 g.

$$[(10.32 \times 6.25)/0.23 + 67.9/0.9]$$

Williams et al. (1985) concluded that fat and lean gain were 90% of live weight gain and that the balance was ash and fill. Total daily live weight gain would be 396 g (356/0.9). Total weight gain during gestation would be about 45 kg (396×114), and from the data of Shields and Mahan (1983), about 18 kg would be the fetuses and associated fluids so that maternal gain would be about 27 kg.

Energy Requirements for Lactation

Energy is required during lactation for maintenance of the sow and for production of milk. Noblet and Etienne (1987) reported that the maintenance requirement of the lactating sow was 109 kcal ME/kg$^{.75}$ so that a 150-kg sow would require 4672 kcal of ME daily for maintenance. Noblet and Etienne (1986) reported that the GE energy concentration of sow's milk was 1200 kcal/kg, and Noblet and Etienne (1987) reported that the efficiency of producing milk GE from dietary ME was 0.72. Therefore, a sow producing 7 kg of milk would require 11,667 kcal of ME for milk production [(7×1200)/0.72]. A total ME intake of 16,339 kcal (4672 + 11,667) would be required to maintain the sow in energy balance and is similar to the ad libitum intake suggested by NRC (1986).

REFERENCES

Agriculture Research Council. 1981. *The Nutrient Requirements of Pigs.* Slough, England: Commonwealth Agriculture Bureaux.

Breirem, K. 1939. *Tierernahrung* 11:487.
Brouwer, E. 1965. In: *Energy Metabolism.* EAAP No. 11. Blaxter, K.L. (Ed.). p. 441. London: Academic Press.
Close, W.H., and V.R. Fowler. 1985. In: *Recent Advances in Pig Nutrition.* Cole, D.J.A. and W. Haresign (Eds.). p. 1. London: Butterworths.
Close, W.J., J. Noblet, and R.P. Heavens. 1985. *Br. J. Nutr.* 53:267.
Cera, K.R., D.C. Mahan, and G.A. Reinhart. 1988a. *J. Anim. Sci.* 66:1430.
Cera, K.R., D.C. Mahan, and G.A. Reinhart. 1988b. *J. Anim. Sci.* 66:1438.
Diggs, B.G., et al. 1965. *J. Anim. Sci.* 24:555.
Ewan, R.C. 1986. Energy Values of Feed Ingredients. Iowa State University, Ames. (Unpublished.)
Ewan, R.C. 1989. In: *Energy Metabolism of Farm Animals.* EAAP Pub. No. 43. van der Honing, Y, and W.H. Close (Eds.). p. 215. Pudoc Wageningen. The Netherlands: Centre for Agricultural Publishing and Documentation.
Henry, Y., H. Vogt, and P.E. Zoiopoulos. 1988. *Livest. Prod. Sci.* 19:299.
Kielanowski, J. 1972. In: *Pig Production.* Cole, D.J.A. (Ed.). p. 183. London: Butterworths.
Kleiber, M. 1965. In: *Energy Metabolism,* EAAP No. 11. Blaxter, K.L. (Ed.). p. 427. London: Academic Press.
Kromann, R.P., J.A. Froseth, and W.E. Meiser. 1976. *J. Anim. Sci.* 42:1451.
Millward, D.J., et al. 1976. In: *Protein Metabolism and Nutrition,* EAAP No. 16. Cole, D.J.A. et al. (Eds.). p. 49. London: Butterworths.
Noblet, J., and M. Etienne. 1986. *J. Anim. Sci.* 63:1888.
Noblet, J., and M. Etienne. 1987. *J. Anim. Sci.* 64:774.
NRC. 1979. *Nutrient Requirements of Swine.* Washington, DC: National Research Council, National Academy of Sciences.
NRC. 1981. *Effect of Environment on Nutrient Requirements of Domestic Animals.* Washington, DC: National Research Council, National Academy of Sciences.
NRC. 1986. *Predicting Feed Intake of Food-Producing Animals.* Washington, DC: National Research Council, National Academy of Sciences.
NRC. 1988. *Nutrient Requirements of Swine.* Washington, DC: National Research Council, National Academy of Sciences.
Rérat, A., et al. 1987. *J. Anim. Sci.* 64:448.
Sauer, W.C., H. Jorgenson, and R. Berzins. 1983. *Can. J. Anim. Sci.* 63:233.
Shields, R.G., Jr., and D.C. Mahan. 1983. *J. Anim. Sci.* 57:594.
Stahly, T.S., and G.L. Cromwell. 1979. *J. Anim. Sci.* 49:1478.
Walach-Janiak, M., S. Raj, and H. Fandrejewski. 1986. *Livest. Prod. Sci.* 15:249.
Williams, I.H., W.H. Close, and D.J.A. Cole. 1985. In: *Recent Advances in Animal Nutrition.* Haresign, W., and D.J.A. Cole (Eds.). p. 133. Boston: Butterworths.
Verstegen, M.W.A., J.M.F. Verhagen, and L.A. den Hartog. 1987. *Livest. Prod. Sci.* 16:75.

Chapter 8

Fat in Swine Nutrition

J.E. Pettigrew and R.L. Moser

Lipids, including fats, are a family of chemical compounds with certain unifying chemical and physical characteristics. They are poorly soluble in water, but soluble in various organic solvents. Fats are collectively a major component of the pig's body and an important part of swine diets. Fats are found in various concentrations in major feedstuffs that are provided primarily as sources of amino acids and/or carbohydrates. Fats can also be added to the diet in the form of several commercially available products that are nearly 100% fat. This chapter deals primarily with the effects of these added-fat products.

Most of the lipid in swine diets is in the form of triacylglycerols (triglycerides), the true fats. These compounds consist of three fatty acid molecules attached by ester bonds to a single glycerol moiety. The three fatty acids may differ in chain length and/or degree of saturation. Other types of lipid in swine diets include diacyglycerides and monoacylglycerides (two or one fatty acids on a glycerol) and phospholipids, which are similar to a triacylglycerol except one fatty acid is replaced by orthophosphate and a nitrogenous base. Cholesterol and the fat-soluble vitamins (and their precursors) are lipids that do not contain fatty acids, but share solubility and other characteristics with the acylglycerols.

Fats can be in either liquid or solid state at room temperature, the melting point depending on both degree of saturation and chain length. The primary factor is saturation. When unsaturation is increased the melting point is decreased, making the fat softer. Thus, very unsaturated fats, such as corn oil, are liquid at room temperature. Fats containing shorter-chain fatty acids have lower melting points than longer-chain ones. The hardest fats (those with highest melting points) are long-chain saturated fats, such as beef tallow. Fats that are liquid at room temperature are often referred to as oils.

Fats are of special importance in energy nutrition because they are more energy-dense than other classes of nutrients. Animals obtain energy from nutrients by oxidizing carbon and hydrogen. These elements are in a more reduced state in fats than in carbohydrates or proteins, so there is the potential for more oxidation and therefore a greater yield of energy. In fact, according to Atwater's Physiological Fuel Values (Maynard et al. 1979), fats contribute about 2.25 times as much energy per gram as do carbohydrates or proteins.

There are physical effects of fat in swine diets that are of practical importance. First, inclusion of supplemental fat reduces the amount of airborne dust in the pig building (Chiba et al. 1985), because much of the airborne dust is derived from feed, and the added fat makes the feed less dusty. This is of considerable value to workers in swine buildings because long-term exposure to a dusty environment produces serious health problems in humans (Cermak and Ross 1978). Inclusion of supplemental fat also reduces flowability of feed. In fact, more than 6% to 7% added fat makes feed susceptible to bridging in bulk bins and self-feeders, causing difficulty in retrieval of the feed (see Chapter 2). There are special difficulties in handling fat and in mixing it with other ingredients (Atkinson 1984). In bagged feed, added fat causes unlined bags to become oily. Pellets made from a high-fat feed are usually soft and susceptible to disintegration.

BIOLOGICAL EFFECTS

Quantitatively, most of the fat in the pig's body serves as a long-term store of energy. The membranes that envelop cells or intracellular organelles are composed largely of phospholipids. The steroid hormones and the prostaglandins are lipids important in regulation of physiological and metabolic events. Vitamins A, D, E, and K are also lipids.

Specific polyunsaturated fatty acids must be provided in the diet because they are required in the synthesis of prostaglandins and phospholipids. There is metabolic capacity for interconversion of fatty acids, but with limitations. In particular, swine have no mechanism to form double bonds within six carbon atoms of the methyl end of a fatty acid. Some of the required fatty acids contain double bonds in this area, and because they cannot be produced in the tissues they must be provided in the diet. They are referred to as essential fatty acids.

There are two families of essential fatty acids, classified by the location of the double bond closest to the methyl end of the chain. In one family this double bond is at the third carbon from the methyl end ($\omega3$), in the other it is at the sixth carbon ($\omega6$). The $\omega3$ family is provided primarily by alpha-linolenic acid (18:3ω3), the $\omega6$ family by linoleic acid (18:2ω6) and arachidonic acid (20:4ω6). A recent series of studies has shown that the requirement for essential fatty acids is satisfied when they supply 0.26% of the dietary metabolizable energy (ME) (Christensen 1985).

The most significant difficulty in digestion and absorption of fat is handling water-insoluble materials in a water medium. This problem does not occur with other classes of nutrients and requires special mechanisms, described in Chapter 3.

The thoroughness of digestion and absorption of any nutrient depends on the rate at which these processes occur and the time available. Digesta containing a high concentration of fat move through the gastrointestinal tract more slowly than do digesta with lower fat concentrations, allowing more time for digestion and absorption of other nutrients. Thus, adding fat to a swine diet improves the digestion of carbohydrates and proteins in the small intestine (Sauer et al. 1980; Just 1982). Efficiency of use of proteins and carbohydrates is greater if they are digested in the small intestine rather than in the large intestine (Sauer et al. 1980; Just 1982). The result is greater-than-expected total energetic gain from added fat, sometimes referred to as an "extracaloric" or "extrametabolic" effect.

Growing or lactating animals store or secrete considerable quantities of fat, which is produced more efficiently from dietary fat than from carbohydrates or protein. This greater efficiency means that less energy escapes as heat (i.e., the heat increment of fat is lower). This lower heat increment is particularly important when animals are subjected to heat stress. Consumption of a high-fat diet, with its lower heat increment, is restricted less by heat stress than is consumption of a low-fat diet (Stahly 1984). Thus, fat supplementation appears more advantageous in thermoneutral or hot environments than in cold ones. The basis and practical ramifications of this interaction between fat and the thermal environment have been discussed by Stahly (1984).

SPECIFIC USES OF FAT IN SWINE DIETS

In growing pigs, the ability to utilize supplemental fat is influenced by the age of the pig and the types of fat added. Pigs can efficiently utilize large quantities of supplemental fat in their diets. In practice, however, the amount of fat added to diets is limited by physical problems of mixing and handling and the cost effectiveness of added fat in least-cost formulations. Supplemental fat can be used to increase the energy density of the diet because it contains 2.25 times the energy concentration of carbohydrates. Because pigs that are offered ad libitum consumption of feed tend to eat to meet their energy requirement, the addition of fat results in a reduction in feed intake. Even though feed intake is decreased, ME intake of the pig is increased. It is assumed that concentrations of other nutrients must be increased in diets containing added fat to compensate for the expected reduction in feed intake. Protein:energy ratio becomes an important consideration when formulating growing-finishing pig diets with added fat. The reduction in feed intake results in poorer gains and feed efficiency and a fatter carcass unless nutrient concentrations are increased to compensate for the reduction in feed intake. Because the nutrient requirements (particularly essential amino acids) are assumed to be greater for optimum carcass leanness than for maximum rate of body weight gain, it is expected that carcass leanness would be more greatly affected by diets containing added fats that do not have an adequate protein:energy ratio. The importance of adjusting diets to the appropriate protein:energy ratio appears to be influenced by the age of the pig (Allee 1985).

The effects of supplemental fat on performance of growing pigs have been investigated for several years. Hillier (1950) was one of the earliest researchers to report improved gain and feed efficiency of growing pigs fed supplemental fat. Moser (1977) conducted an extensive review of the research on feeding animal fat to growing-finishing pigs. To date, a similar review on feeding fat to starting pigs has not been conducted.

FAT IN STARTING PIG DIETS

Interest in the use of supplemental fat in starting pig (5- to 20-kg) diets has centered on two concerns: (1) improved gain and feed efficiency and (2) improved palatability.

We have examined published reports to determine the effects of supplemental fat on average daily gain, average daily feed intake, and gain:feed ratio of starting pigs. The numbers of positive and negative responses were counted, without regard to statistical significance within the experiment. Some comparisons showed identical performance between treatments, so they do not appear as either positive or negative responses. Also, we calculated means across trials weighted by the numbers of replicates for each treatment within each trial. A conservative statistical evaluation, a *t* test of the weighted responses, was applied.

A summary of the analysis is shown in Table 8.1. Average daily gain of starting pigs was reduced ($P < .05$) by the addition of supplemental fat. However, the reduction in gain was small (0.01 kg), and the number of positive and negative responses was similar. The reduction in gain occurred primarily in diets not adjusted to a constant protein:energy ratio. Adjustment to a constant protein:energy ratio resulted in zero response to added dietary fat. The number of positive responses was higher than negative responses when the diets were adjusted. As expected, daily feed intake was reduced ($P < .01$) for pigs fed supplemental fat, with negative responses outnumbering positive responses by almost 3:1. The reduction in daily feed intake was similar with or without adjustment to a constant protein:energy ratio. The level of added fat did not significantly affect feed intake. However, a trend toward greater reduction of feed intake with increasing levels of dietary fat was observed. The addition of fat to the diet improved ($P < .01$) gain:feed ratio, with greater improvement observed in

Table 8.1 Summary of Responses to Supplemental Fat in Starting Pig Diets

	No. of Responses			
Category	*Positive*	*Negative*	*Responses*	*Total No. of Comparisons*
Daily gain (kg)	37	39	-0.01 ± 0.005[a]	92
No adjustment	25	32	-0.01 ± 0.006[b]	71
Constant protein:energy ratio	12	7	0.00 ± 0.010	21
Daily feed intake (kg)	20	59	-0.05 ± 0.010[c]	92
No adjustment	18	44	-0.04 ± 0.011[c]	71
Constant protein:energy ratio	2	15	-0.07 ± 0.027[a]	21
Gain:feed ratio	66	20	0.04 ± 0.008[c]	92
No adjustment	47	19	0.03 ± 0.007[c]	71
Constant protein:energy ratio	19	1	0.07 ± 0.028[c]	21

[a] $P < .05$.
[b] $P < .10$.
[c] $P < .01$.

diets adjusted to a constant protein:energy ratio. Gain:feed ratio improved as the level of fat increased in the diet ($P < .01$) ($R^2 = .25$).

The addition of fat to diets of starting pigs will not improve gain greatly, but the reduction of feed intake without affecting gain will result in significantly improved feed efficiency. Although biologically important, the practical significance of improved feed efficiency is not great because pigs consume much less feed during the starting phase than later in life.

Palatability

It is assumed that the reduction in feed consumption associated with added fat is caused by the feed's increased energy concentration. However, the extent of the reduction is lessened by starting pigs' preference for a fat-supplemented diet. Leibbrandt et al. (1975) reported that pigs preferred diets containing fat over diets containing no fat. Furthermore, animal fats (lard and tallow) were preferred over hydrolyzed fat.

FAT IN GROWING-FINISHING PIG DIETS

Interest in the use of supplemental fat in growing-finishing (20- to 100-kg) pig diets has centered on two concerns: (1) improved gain and feed efficiency and (2) effects on backfat of pigs at market weight.

Moser (1977) examined the published data to evaluate the effects of fat on performance and backfat thickness. Specific effects of added fat levels were sought. We have updated that review, using the statistical techniques described earlier (Table 8.2). The addition of fat improved ($P < .01$) average daily gain as indicated by the overall positive response (0.04 kg) and the overwhelming number of positive responses as compared with negative responses. The response to fat does not seem to be affected greatly by whether or not the diets were adjusted to a constant protein:energy ratio. The effects of fat levels on daily gain were similar to results reported by Moser (1977). In our summary, daily gain improved up to approximately 5% added fat. At higher fat levels, gain decreased. As expected, daily feed intake was reduced ($P < .01$) in pigs fed supplemental fat. Negative responses outnumbered positive responses 5:1. The response to fat did not seem to be greatly affected by whether or not the diets were adjusted to a constant protein:energy ratio. Daily feed intake was related to fat level in the diet. At low added fat levels ($\leq 3\%$), feed intake increased slightly. As fat level increased above 3%, feed intake decreased. Moser (1977) reported similar results.

The addition of fat to the diet improved ($P < .01$) gain:feed ratio as indicated by the positive responses of added fat and the absence of reported negative responses. Adjusting for protein:energy ratio did not greatly affect the pig's response to supplemental fat. Gain:feed ratio improved consistently as the level of added fat increased. These data are similar to those reported by Moser (1977). Average backfat was greater ($P < .01$) for pigs fed added fat. The response in increased backfat was similar with or without adjustment to a constant protein:energy ratio. Average backfat increased

Table 8.2 Summary of Responses to Supplemental Fat in Growing-Finishing Pig Diets

	No. of Responses			
Category	*Positive*	*Negative*	*Responses*	*Total No. of Comparisons*
Daily gain (kg)	72	10	0.04 ± 0.007^a	92
No adjustment	39	4	0.04 ± 0.008^a	50
Constant protein:energy ratio	33	6	0.05 ± 0.012^a	42
Daily feed intake (kg)	15	75	-0.10 ± 0.021^a	92
No adjustment	7	41	-0.09 ± 0.023^a	50
Constant protein:energy ratio	8	34	-0.13 ± 0.043^a	42
Gain:feed ratio	87	0	0.04 ± 0.007^a	92
No adjustment	47	0	0.03 ± 0.006^a	50
Constant protein:energy ratio	40	0	0.04 ± 0.008^a	42
Average backfat (cm)	61	16	0.17 ± 0.034^a	90
No adjustment	32	11	0.12 ± 0.036^a	50
Constant protein:energy ratio	29	5	0.27 ± 0.072^a	40

$^a P < .05$.

consistently with increasing level of added fat. Moser (1977) reported little, if any, effect on backfat if low levels of supplemental fat ($\leq 3\%$) were used, and only slight increases of backfat at higher levels. Our results are more consistent, showing increased backfat with each increment of supplemental fat.

FAT IN SOW DIETS

Interest in the use of supplemental fat in sow diets has centered on two distinct objectives: (1) improving pig survival and (2) reducing the nutrient drain experienced by lactating sows.

We have examined and summarized the published empirical data describing the effects of supplemental dietary fat on sow performance. The data were summarized as described for starting pigs. Many of these summaries carry a positive bias to the extent that some studies failing to show a positive response are not published, and therefore are not available for our review. This problem is encountered in any review of the literature.

Seerley et al. (1974) first suggested that supplemental fat in the sows' diet during late pregnancy could improve the preweaning survival of the offspring by improving their energy status. Pigs are born with very small lipid energy reserves. They have large energy reserves in the form of glycogen, but much of this glycogen is depleted during the first 2 days after birth. Supplemental dietary fat for the sow before farrowing increases the fat content of the pigs at birth, but this increase is so small that it is likely to be of only limited importance (Pettigrew 1981). However, such supplementation increases the fat content of colostrum and milk, and in this way markedly increases the amount of energy available to the pigs. Seerley (1984) has recently reviewed the physiology and metabolism of the newborn pig, including the effects of fat supplementation of the dam's diet.

Moser and Lewis (1981) and Pettigrew (1981) examined the available literature to determine whether or not the increased mammary transfer of energy to the pigs resulted in an increase in pig survival from birth to weaning. The data suggested strongly that there was such a response. Pettigrew (1981) noted that the response was largest and most consistent when the lower treatment mean survival was ≤80% and when an adequate fat dose (>1 kg of supplemental fat before farrowing) was administered to the sow. Under those conditions, supplemental fat appeared to increase the proportion of pigs that survived weaning by 6.2 percentage units ($P < .01$), with positive responses in 14 of 18 comparisons. We have updated that summary, using the same techniques reported by Pettigrew (1981). Our present findings are somewhat less positive than those reported earlier. Under the conditions described above, survival to weaning was improved by 2.7 percentage units ($P > .10$), with positive responses in 14 of 20 cases (Table 8.3). The response was larger when the lower survival was from 70.1% to 80% than when it was ≤70%.

We are unable to identify a set of conditions under which a stronger positive response could be expected. There was little difference in response between vegetable fats and animal fats. The response was greater when mean birth weight was low, presumably related to the effect of overall survival.

Pettigrew (1981) stated that his estimates of response were probably exaggerated because results that fail to show a positive response may not be published, and that may explain the smaller responses we now find. Perhaps the tendency since publication of the earlier reviews has been that studies showing the "expected" positive response have not been published, neutralizing the earlier bias.

Pig survival is closely related to birth weight (Pettigrew et al. 1986). Fat supplementation during late pregnancy appears to have no effect on pig birth weight (Table 8.3). Similarly, there is no evidence that the stillbirth rate is reduced, whether expressed as number per litter or as percentage of total born.

Fat supplementation of an ad libitum-fed lactation diet consistently reduced the amount of feed consumed, but increased the amount of ME consumed (Table 8.3). Both effects seem somewhat related to percent supplemental fat, although linear and quadratic effects of percent fat account for less than one fourth of the variation in response. ME intake was increased slightly more by fat additions of ≥10% than by fat additions of <10% (Table 8.3). Feed intake was reduced more by ≥10% added fat than by lower levels. It appears that in the three tests showing increased feed intake with added fat (O'Grady and Lynch 1978; Shurson et al. 1986; Schoenherr et al. 1987), the sows may have been heat stressed. Schoenherr et al. (1987) found that added fat increased feed intake in heat-stressed sows, but decreased it in sows housed in thermoneutral environments. Presumably the increase in ME intake that results from fat supplementation is enhanced during heat stress because of the lower heat increment of the fat-supplemented diet, as described earlier. Perhaps many lactating sows are subjected to mild heat stress in an attempt to provide an appropriate environment for their pigs.

As noted above, one objective of adding fat to sow diets is to reduce the nutrient

Table 8.3 Summary of Responses to Supplemental Fat in Sow Diets

Category	No. of Responses		Responses	Total No. of Comparisons
	Positive	Negative		
Survival (%)				
Lower treatment mean survival <80%, >1 kg added fat before farrowing	14	6	2.7±1.7	369
Lower survival 70.1–80.0%	10	4	4.2±1.9[a]	226
Lower survival <70%	4	2	0.4±3.4	143
Pig birth wt (g)				
Added fat before farrowing	14	15	4±7	1505
Stillbirths/litter				
Added fat before farrowing	5	7	−0.015±0.043	932
Lactation feed intake (kg/d)				
Added fat during lactation, ad libitum	3	16	−0.189±0.048[b]	833
≥10% added fat	2	7	−0.267±0.097[c]	317
>10% added fat	1	9	−0.141±0.052[c]	517
ME intake (Mcal/d)				
Added fat during lactation, ad libitum	19	0	1.24±0.18[b]	834
≥10% added fat	9	0	1.55±0.40[d]	317
<10% added fat	10	0	1.05±0.16[b]	517

Lactation wt change (kg)				
Added fat during lactation, ad libitum	11	4	1.5 ± 0.7[c]	697
Added fat during lactation, ME intake increased by				
≥1 Mcal/d	5	2	2.2 ± 1.1[a]	239
<1 Mcal/d	7	3	1.3 ± 0.9	584
Lactation backfat change (mm)				
Added fat during lactation	2	1	0.36 ± 0.43	188
Wean to estrus interval (d)				
Added fat during lactation, ad libitum	2	4	-0.56 ± 0.57	427
Conception (%)				
Added fat during lactation, ad libitum	2	1	0.3 ± 1.9	208
Litter weaning wt (kg)				
Added fat during lactation, ad libitum	18	6	1.65 ± 0.52[d]	1150
ME intake increased by				
≥1 Mcal/d	7	2	2.74 ± 1.00[c]	364
<1 Mcal/d	7	2	1.18 ± 0.75	552
Pig weaning wt (kg)				
Added fat during lactation	35	16	118 ± 42	1368
No creep feed	19	8	114 ± 46	1179
Creep feed	16	8	147 ± 87	189

[a] $P < .10$.
[b] $P < .001$.
[c] $P < .05$.
[d] $P < .01$.

drain on lactating sows. The increase in ME intake noted above is encouraging. Data on weight loss in lactating sows allowed ad libitum consumption (Table 8.3) demonstrate that supplemental fat reduces weight loss ($P < .05$) but that this response is disappointingly small (1.5 kg). The reduction of weight loss was only slightly improved when daily ME intake was increased by more than 1 Mcal as compared with when the ME intake increase was smaller. The response was not increased by increasing the fat level, and it was not related to the overall level of weight loss.

The reduction in backfat thickness during lactation was moderated by supplemental dietary fat in two of three cases (Nelssen et al. 1985; Johnston et al. 1986; Rozeboom et al. 1987), as shown in Table 8.3. This response failed to occur in the study (Nelssen et al. 1985) in which all sows were fed the same amount of ME during lactation. This study also reported the largest overall loss of backfat thickness. These limited data are not adequate to judge whether supplemental dietary fat will reduce the loss of backfat.

The ultimate reason for reducing the nutrient drain on lactating sows is to improve their subsequent reproductive performance. There is at present insufficient information to determine whether or not supplemental dietary fat contributes to this objective. There is no strong indication that supplemental fat reduces the interval from weaning to first estrus or improves conception (Table 8.3).

Adding fat to sow diets increases the transfer of nutrients to the suckling pigs, as the litter weaning weight was increased by supplemental dietary fat. This response was positively related to the increase in ME intake caused by the added fat (Table 8.3). Individual pig weaning weight was increased in most cases. Both litter and pig weaning weight responses to added fat were greatest when 10% to 14.9% fat was added. There is no indication from the data that the weaning weight response to fat is moderated by provision of creep feed.

FAT IN NEONATAL PIGLET DIETS

The energetic fragility of neonatal pigs and the prospect of improving their chances of survival by increasing the amount of fat provided to them via colostrum and milk were described in the previous section. Perhaps the fat could be provided directly to the pigs rather than indirectly through the sow. This route would likely be more efficient, particularly because the fat could be targeted to those pigs most likely to benefit.

We have administered to pigs four oral doses of corn oil (8 ml each dose) during the first 2 days after birth and found no effect on preweaning survival (Pettigrew et al. 1986). Examination of the data from only the low-birth-weight pigs (1000 to 1250 g) revealed that in this group mortality was delayed by the corn oil, but the overall preweaning mortality was not affected. We see four possible reasons for the lack of response in this trial. First, the hypothesis that pigs need supplemental energy may be incorrect. Second, the acceptable survival (>85%) in this test may indicate that these pigs did not need supplemental energy. Third, the modest dose may have been insufficient to provide the desired response. Fourth, the pigs may not have the digestive, absorptive, and/or metabolic capacity to utilize the fat.

Recent research in our laboratory has shown that newborn piglets have ample capacity to digest and absorb a large oral dose of fish oil (Chiang et al. 1987). Furthermore, they are able to metabolize a considerable amount of trioctanoin (8:0, a medium-chain fat), but much less triolein (18:1, a long-chain fat; Pettigrew et al. 1988). In fact, it appears that pigs can obtain about one third of their maintenance energy needs from exogenous medium-chain fats, administered in a dose of about 6 g/kg body weight every 12 hours. Oral doses of medium-chain fats increased serum glucose and nonesterified fatty acid concentrations and decreased urinary nitrogen excretion, supporting the notion that the pig used these fats effectively (Lepine et al. 1986; Odle et al. 1987). The response to corn oil was smaller (Odle et al. 1987). Further studies will determine whether or not provision of medium-chain fats will improve pig survival and whether or not the practice will improve the profitability of pork production.

FAT SOURCES

A range of animal, vegetable, and blended fats are available commercially. Production of various fats and of blends has been described by Howard (1984). Selection of fats for use in swine feeds should be based primarily on price and digestibility, with adequate consideration for handling characteristics and for contaminants. Some quality control measures for commercial fats have been established for the chemical industry, but these are of limited importance in animal feeding.

Factors affecting digestibility have been reviewed by Stahly (1984). Perhaps the most important is the ratio of unsaturated to saturated fatty acids; digestibility declines as this ratio falls below 1.5:1. Shorter-chain fatty acids are more easily digested, but these contain less energy per gram. A high level of nonesterified fatty acids reduces digestibility (Stahly 1984).

A number of dry fat products, in which fat is mixed with a carrier, can be purchased. They are generally easier to handle than are other fat products. Of course, the nutritional value of the product is affected by the nutritional value of the carrier. Certain feedstuffs (such as unextracted soybeans) contain important quantities of fat. They can be used as fat sources in swine diets when consideration of cost and handling characteristics indicates an economic advantage.

REFERENCES

Aherne, F.X., V. Danielsen, and H.E. Nielsen. 1982. *Acta Agr. Scand.* 8:151.

Allee, G.L. 1976. Swine Day '76. *Progress Report 283.* p. 26. Manhattan, KS: Agricultural Experiment Station, Kansas State University.

Allee, G.L. 1985. *Proceedings of the Georgia Nutrition Conference for the Feed Industry.* p. 136. Athens: University of Georgia.

Allee, G.L., D.H. Baker, and G.A. Leveille. 1971. *J. Nutr.* 101:1415.

Allee, G.L., and R.H. Hines. 1971. Swine Industry Day. *Progress Report 171.* p. 13. Manhattan, KS: Agricultural Experiment Station, Kansas State University.

Atkinson, R.E. 1984. In: *Fats in Animal Nutrition.* Wiseman, J. (Ed.). pp. 495–503. London: Butterworths.
Atteh, J.D., and S. Leeson. 1983. *Can. J. Anim. Sci.* 63:699.
Brooks, C.C. 1972. *J. Anim. Sci.* 34:217.
Cermak, J.P., and P.A. Ross. 1978. *Farm Build. Prog.* 51:11.
Chiang, S.H., et al. 1987. *J. Anim. Sci.* 65(Suppl. 1):307.
Chiba, L.I., et al. 1985. *J. Anim. Sci.* 61:763.
Christensen, K. 1985. *Beretning fra Statens Husdyrbrugsforsog* (No. 577), p. 122.
Clawson, A.J., et al. 1962. *J. Anim. Sci.* 21:62.
Frobish, L.T., et al. 1970. *J. Anim. Sci.* 30:197.
Gore, A.M., E.T. Kornegay, and H.P. Veit. 1986. *J. Anim. Sci.* 63:1.
Greeley, M.G., et al. 1964. *J. Anim. Sci.* 23:816.
Hale, O.M., J.C. Johnson, Jr., and E.P. Warren. 1968. *J. Anim. Sci.* 27:1577.
Hanke, H.E., G. Castro, and R.J. Meade. *Minnesota Swine Research Reports.* p. 24. St. Paul: University of Minnesota.
Hanke, H.E., et al. 1978. *Minnesota Swine Research Reports.* p. 27. St. Paul: University of Minnesota.
Hanke, H.E., et al. 1980. *Minnesota Swine Research Reports.* p. 15. St. Paul: University of Minnesota.
Hillier, J.C. 1950. *Okla. Agri. Exp. Sta.* MP–17:84.
Howard, A.J. 1984. In: *Fats in Animal Nutrition.* Wiseman, J. (Ed.) London: Butterworths.
Johnston, L.J., et al. 1986. *J. Anim. Sci.* 63:804.
Just, A. 1982. *Livestock Prod. Sci.* 9:501.
Keaschall, K.E., et al. 1983. *J. Anim. Sci.* 56:286.
Lawrence, N.J., and C.V. Maxwell. 1983. *J. Anim. Sci.* 57:936.
Leibbrandt, V.D., et al. 1975. *J. Anim. Sci.* 40:1081.
Lepine, A.J., R.D. Boyd, and J.A. Welch. 1986. *J. Anim. Sci.* 63(Suppl.1):275.
Lewis, A.J., et al. 1980. *J. Anim. Sci.* 51:361.
Maynard, L.A., et al. 1979. *Animal Nutrition.* 7th ed. pp. 199–200. New York: MacGraw-Hill Book Co.
Miller, K.P., H.E. Hanke, and R.J. Meade. 1977. *Minnesota Swine Research Reports.* p. 42. St. Paul: University of Minnesota.
Moser, B.D. 1975. *Nebraska Swine Report.* p. 25. Lincoln, NE: Institute of Agriculture and Natural Resources, University of Nebraska-Lincoln.
Moser, B.D. 1977. *Feedstuffs* 49:20.
Moser, B.D., and L. Bitney. 1976. *Nebraska Swine Report.* p. 15. Lincoln, NE: Institute of Agriculture and Natural Resources, University of Nebraska-Lincoln.
Moser, B.D., and A.J. Lewis. 1981. *Pig News Inform.* 2:265.
Nelssen, J.L., et al. 1985. *J. Anim. Sci.* 60:171.
Odle, J., N.J. Benevenga, and T.D. Crenshaw. 1987. *J. Anim. Sci.* 65(Suppl. 1):307.
O'Grady, J.F., and P.B. Lynch. 1978. *Irish J. Agric. Res.* 17:1.
Peo, E.R. Jr., et al. 1957. *J. Anim. Sci.* 16:885.
Pettigrew, J.E. 1981. *J. Anim. Sci.* 53:107.
Pettigrew, J.E., et al. 1986. *J. Anim. Sci.* 62:601.
Pettigrew, J.E., et al. 1988. *Anim. Prod.* 46:518 (Abstr.).
Pollman, D.S., K.C. Behnke, and G.L. Allee. 1983. *Anim. Feed. Sci. Technol.* 8:99.
Rozeboom, D.W., et al. 1987. *Minnesota Swine Res. Rep.* p. 49. St. Paul: University of Minnesota.
Sauer, W.C., et al. 1980. *Acta Agric. Scand.* 30:499.
Schoenherr, W.D., T.S. Stahly, and G.L. Cromwell. 1987. *J. Anim. Sci.* 65(Suppl. 1):318.
Seerley, R.W. 1984. In: *Fats in Animal Nutrition.* Wiseman, J. (Ed.). pp. 333–352. London: Butterworths.
Seerley, R.W., J.P. Briscoe, and H.C. McCampbell. 1978. *J. Anim. Sci.* 46:1018.
Seerley, R.W., M.C. McDaniel, and H.C. McCampbell. 1978. *J. Anim. Sci.* 47:427.

Seerley, R.W., G.E. Poley, and R.C. Wahlstrom. 1964. *J. Anim. Sci.* 23:1016.
Seerley, R.W. et al 1974. *J. Anim. Sci.* 38:64.
Shurson, G.C., et al. 1986. *J. Anim. Sci.* 62:672.
Stahly, T.S. 1984. In: *Fats in Animal Nutrition.* Wiseman, J. (Ed.). pp. 313–331. London: Butterworths.
Stahly, T.S., and G.L. Cromwell. 1979. *J. Anim. Sci.* 49:1478.
Stahly, T.S., G.L. Cromwell, and J.R. Overfield. 1981. *J. Anim. Sci.* 53:1269.
Tribble, L.F., et al. 1979. *J. Anim. Sci.* 48:541.
Wagner, G.R., et al. 1963. *J. Anim. Sci.* 22:202.
Waterman, R. 1973. *Report of Swine Research.* p. 68. East Lansing, MI: Michigan State University Agricultural Experiment Station.

Chapter 9

Amino Acids in Swine Nutrition

A.J. Lewis

PROTEINS AND NONPROTEIN NITROGEN

Crude and True Protein

The protein content of swine diets is generally determined by a chemical procedure known as the Kjeldahl method (AOAC 1984). Actually, the Kjeldahl method does not determine protein, but nitrogen (N) content. Protein is calculated from N by multiplying by 100/16 (or 6.25). This multiplication factor is used because the average N content of proteins is 16 g N/100 g protein. The protein content determined in this manner is usually referred to as crude protein. The term crude is used because there are two assumptions inherent in the conversion from N to protein that are not always valid.

The first assumption is that all proteins contain 16% N. Although the assumption is not true, the use of a single conversion factor works quite well because normal diets contain mixtures of proteins and average N contents are usually close to 16%. Furthermore, the protein requirements of swine have been established using the same set of assumptions; thus the same basis has been used for establishing the composition of feedstuffs and the dietary requirements of swine. Other conversion factors are used for a few specialized products. For example, the conversion factor for wheat and its products is 5.70, and for milk and dairy products it is 6.38 (AOAC 1984).

A second assumption in the conversion from N to protein is that all of the N is present in proteins. In most feedstuffs given to swine, part of the N is from compounds other than proteins. For example, about 10% of the crude protein of corn and 13% of the crude protein from soybean meal is nonprotein nitrogen (NPN) (Van Soest and Sniffen 1984). NPN sources inflate the estimate of protein content. Except for a few feedstuffs such as silages and immature root crops, however, most of the NPN is in the form of amino acids, which are the components of proteins and related compounds. These substances are assumed to have the same nutritional value as proteins themselves. The amount of true protein that is present in a feedstuff can be determined by separating the actual protein by precipitation and then conducting a Kjeldahl analysis of the precipitate. Thus, the term crude protein comprises true protein and NPN. The usual crude protein value is accurate enough for most purposes in swine nutrition.

Use of Nonprotein Nitrogen

In addition to the forms of NPN found naturally in most feedstuffs, there are various simple forms of NPN, such as urea and ammonium salts, that are available for addition to livestock feeds. Many simple sources of NPN are considerably cheaper than protein sources, and therefore the nutritional value of simple NPN compounds is of economic importance. To be of value, NPN must be in a form that can be converted to protein within the pig. The utilization of simple forms of NPN by swine has been the subject of a considerable amount of research. Most experiments have examined the utilization of urea; others have tested ammonium salts.

In experiments where ^{15}N-labeled urea has been administered orally (Liu et al. 1955) or added to the feed (Grimson et al. 1971), N from urea has been found in various body proteins including the liver, kidney, muscle, blood, and intestinal wall, although the amounts incorporated have been rather small. An initial step in the utilization of N from urea seems to be the hydrolysis of urea by bacterial urease in the intestine. Deguchi et al. (1978) observed that whereas ^{15}N from dietary urea was incorporated into body proteins in pigs with a normal intestinal flora, there was no such incorporation in germ-free pigs.

Results of practical feeding experiments to examine the nutritional value of urea for swine have not been encouraging. In most experiments (Hanson and Ferrin 1955; Hays et al. 1957; Kornegay et al. 1965; Kornegay 1972), there has been little or no benefit from the addition of urea to practical swine diets, even when the dietary protein content was relatively low. Some experiments have provided evidence of utilization of urea when crystalline amino acids were also included in the diet, but generally the benefits have been small and variable (Grimson and Bowland 1971; Kornegay et al. 1970; Kornegay 1972). Generally from 1% to 3% urea has been included in diets.

The nutritional value for swine of a variety of ammonium salts has also been examined; compounds tested have included diammonium phosphate, ammonium polyphosphate, and ammonium acetate. An active intestinal flora is not necessary for the utilization of ammonium salts. Deguchi et al. (1980) reported that ^{15}N from diammonium citrate was incorporated into amino acids in germ-free pigs. In one germ-free pig, ^{15}N was detected in all the amino acids of proteins; in another, ^{15}N was found in all amino acids except histidine, lysine, and threonine.

Experiments in which ammonium salts have been tested in practical diets have not produced promising results. Wehrbein et al. (1970) reported that the replacement of increasing amounts of intact protein by a mixture of ammonium salts progressively decreased performance. Subsequent experiments (Platter et al. 1973; Sokol et al. 1979; Clawson and Armstrong 1981), some with additions of crystalline amino acids, also failed to demonstrate significant nutritional contributions from the NPN sources.

Recent research has demonstrated that in pigs fed normal diets (containing no simple forms of NPN), there is considerable recycling of urea of endogenous origin in the digestive tract (Thacker et al. 1982; Thacker et al. 1984; Mosenthin et al. 1986).

ESSENTIALITY OF AMINO ACIDS

It has been known for many years that when swine are fed diets that are deficient in protein they do not grow or reproduce normally (see reviews by Pond 1973; Baker and Speer 1983). Therefore, proteins were considered to be essential dietary constituents. It is now clearly recognized, however, that it is not proteins per se but their components, amino acids, that are the essential ingredients. Young pigs gain weight when fed diets containing no protein, but an appropriate mixture of amino acids (Shelton et al. 1950; Beeson et al. 1951; Mertz et al. 1952; Eggert et al. 1955). Furthermore, sows are able to maintain a normal pregnancy during the last 84 days of gestation when fed a diet that contains crystalline amino acids as the sole source of N (Easter and Baker 1976).

Essential and Nonessential Amino Acids

There are twenty different amino acids that commonly occur in proteins, but not all of them are essential dietary components. Swine are able to synthesize some amino acids and these do not need to be provided in the diet; they are referred to as nonessential (or dispensable) amino acids. Other amino acids cannot be synthesized by swine, or at least they cannot be synthesized at a rate sufficient to permit optimum growth or reproduction; they are referred to as essential (or indispensable). Experiments to determine which amino acids are essential, and which nonessential, were conducted in the 1940s and 1950s by researchers at Cornell and Purdue universities. A classification based on their results is presented in Table 9.1.

Conditionally Essential Amino Acids

Some amino acids are essential dietary components in certain situations, but not in others. Arginine is required for the growth of young pigs (Southern and Baker 1983), but sows are able to synthesize arginine at a rate sufficient to meet their needs for postpubertal growth and pregnancy (Easter et al. 1974; Easter and Baker 1976). Histidine is required during pregnancy (Easter and Baker 1977), but it does not seem to be a dietary requirement for maintenance of adult female swine (Baker et al. 1966). Proline is not a dietary requirement for swine for most stages of their life cycle, but very young pigs (1 to 5 kg) are unable to synthesize proline rapidly enough to meet their requirements (Ball et al. 1986).

The requirement for the two sulfur amino acids (methionine and cystine) is usually met by a mixture of these amino acids. Cystine can by synthesized from methionine (but not vice versa), and, therefore, methionine can meet the total need for sulfur amino acids. Cystine can satisfy at least 50% of the sulfur amino acid requirement (Shelton et al. 1951b; Becker et al. 1955; Mitchell et al. 1968; Baker et al. 1969b).

Phenylalanine can be converted to tyrosine, and thus it can meet the requirement for both of the two aromatic amino acids. Tyrosine cannot be converted to phenylala-

Table 9.1 Nutritional Classification of Amino Acids for Swine

Amino Acid	*References*
Essential	
Arginine	a,b
Histidine	c,d
Isoleucine	e
Leucine	a,b,c
Lysine	g,h,i
Methionine	j,k,l
Phenylalanine	a,b,m
Threonine	n,o
Tryptophan	p,q,r
Valine	a,b,s
Nonessential	
Alanine	
Asparagine	
Aspartic acid	
Cysteine	
Glutamic acid	
Glutamine	
Glycine	
Proline	
Serine	
Tyrosine	

References: a, Beeson et al. 1951; b, Mertz et al. 1952; c, Eggert et al. 1955; d, Rechcigl et al. 1956; e, Brinegar et al. 1950a; f, Eggert et al. 1954; g, Mertz et al. 1949; h, Brinegar et al. 1950b; i, Shelton et al. 1951a; j, Bell et al. 1950; k, Shelton et al. 1951b; l, Curtin et al. 1952; m, Mertz et al. 1954; n, Beeson et al. 1953; o, Sewell et al. 1953; p, Beeson et al. 1948; q, Beeson et al. 1949; r, Shelton et al. 1951c; s, Jackson et al. 1953.

nine, but it can satisfy at least 50% of the total aromatic amino acid requirement (Robbins and Baker 1977).

AMINO ACID BALANCE (PROTEIN QUALITY)

Ideal Protein

Proteins differ considerably in their nutritional value for swine, some, such as milk proteins, are high in nutritional value; others, such as sesame meal, are low. It has been established that the nutritional value (quality) of a protein is primarily dependent on its amino acid composition, especially the content of essential amino acids. In the past there was a large amount of work done to establish the best methods of assessing protein quality (Hegsted 1974). Today, however, with more knowledge about the amino acid composition of proteins and the amino acid requirements of swine, the emphasis has moved toward assessing how well proteins and mixtures of proteins meet amino acid requirements. A protein that contains a perfect balance of amino acids, both among the essential amino acids and between essential and nonessential amino acids, has been defined as an ideal protein (Cole 1979; ARC 1981).

Estimates of the proportions of amino acids in ideal protein for growing swine have been derived from an examination of various types of data, including the composition of pig tissue, the composition of sows' milk, and combinations of individual estimates of amino acid requirements. The validity of assuming that there is one set of ideal proportions among amino acids for all stages of growth has been questioned (Lewis et al. 1977). Nevertheless, the concept of an ideal protein has proved very useful, especially in explaining some of the variation in pig responses to different levels and sources of proteins (ARC 1981). A comparison of the ideal proportions among essential amino acids assumed by Agricultural Research Council (ARC) (1981), Institut National de la Recherche Agronomique (INRA) (1984), and National Research Council (NRC) (1988), expressed relative to tryptophan, is presented in Table 9.2.

Amino Acid Disproportions

In theory, any departure from the pattern of amino acids of ideal protein will lead to a reduction in swine performance, at least in terms of the efficiency with which dietary protein is utilized. In practice, however, swine seem to be relatively tolerant of quite wide variations in the pattern of amino acids, as long as all amino acid requirements are met. Nevertheless, if the dietary amino acid pattern deviates too far from the ideal, swine performance will be reduced. The negative effects caused by the ingestion of disproportionate amounts of amino acids have been classified into three main types: toxicity, imbalance, and antagonism (Harper et al. 1970).

Toxicities, characterized by the consumption of a large excess of an individual amino acid, are rare in practical swine nutrition. They would be caused only by misinformation or errors in mixing of a diet that included crystalline amino acids. Unfortunately, of the four amino acids that are currently available in a feed grain form

Table 9.2 Estimates of the Composition of Ideal Protein for Growing Swine[a]

Amino Acid	*ARC (1981)*	*INRA (1984)*	*NRC (1988)*
Arginine	—	1.6	3.0–1.0
Histidine	2.3	1.4	1.8
Isoleucine	3.8	3.3	3.7
Leucine	7.0	4.0	5.0
Lysine	7.0	5.6	7.0–6.0
Methionine + cystine	3.5	3.3	3.4
Phenylalanine + tyrosine	6.7	5.5	5.5
Threonine	4.2	3.3	4.0
Tryptophan	1.0	1.0	1.0
Valine	4.9	3.9	4.0

[a]Proportions of each amino acid relative to tryptophan.
(Data from ARC 1981; INRA 1984; NRC 1988.).

(lysine, methionine, tryptophan, and threonine), two (methionine and tryptophan) have the highest relative toxicity of the essential amino acids. In rats, the addition of 3% methionine to the diet is severely toxic (Benevenga and Harper 1967). The rat's requirement for sulfur amino acids is 0.60%, thus the margin of safety is rather small. Swine appear to be particularly sensitive to excess methionine (Baker 1977). In contrast, excesses of lysine (Edmonds and Baker 1986; Lewis et al. 1986) and especially threonine (Edmonds and Baker 1986) are well tolerated by young pigs.

Imbalances are also caused by excessive intake(s) of (an) amino acid(s), but usually the extent of the disproportion is less and there are no clear toxic features that are specific for the amino acid(s) involved. Imbalances are caused by the exacerbation of the deficiency of the most limiting amino acid, and they can be corrected by the appropriate addition of that amino acid. In an experiment by Wahlstrom and Libal (1974), as little as 0.2% added methionine reduced the performance of growing-finishing pigs, but this effect was alleviated by the addition of 0.2% lysine (the first limiting amino acid).

Antagonisms are specific relationships between amino acids in which an excessive amount of one amino acid increases the requirement of a structurally related amino acid. There are two groups of amino acids in this category: arginine and lysine; and leucine, isoleucine, and valine.

Although there are clear examples of arginine-lysine antagonism (primarily high levels of lysine antagonizing arginine) in poultry (Austic and Scott 1975), the situation is much less clear in swine. Corn-soybean meal diets typical of those fed throughout much of the United States contain considerable amounts of arginine, and it has been suggested (Harmon 1980) that the excess arginine may antagonize lysine, which is usually first limiting. However, experiments since that time in which the arginine content of diets has been reduced (by selecting ingredients low in arginine) have generally failed to show any improvement in swine performance (Miller et al. 1981a,b; Kelley et al. 1983; Anderson et al. 1984a). Furthermore, experiments that have examined the effects of crystalline arginine added to swine diets have also indicated that the amounts of excess arginine present in most practical diets probably cause little if any problem (Southern and Baker 1982; Hagemeier et al. 1983; Anderson et al. 1984b). However, excessive supplements of crystalline arginine can reduce feed intake and growth rate.

The potential leucine-isoleucine-valine antagonism also seems to be of minor importance in practical swine diets. Many diets (especially those based on corn) contain relatively high levels of leucine, but experiments with swine in which this antagonism between the branched-chain amino acids has been investigated indicate that it is unlikely to be a cause of reduced performance in most practical situations (Oestemer et al. 1973; Henry et al. 1976).

LIMITING AMINO ACIDS IN FEEDS

In most practical swine diets, the amino acid "disproportion" of greatest concern is simply a deficiency of one or more amino acids. Feedstuffs with a high protein content are usually relatively expensive and thus there is a tendency to limit their inclusion in diets. When the dietary protein content is inadequate to meet the requirements of all essential amino acids, swine performance will be restricted. The amino acid that is present in the least amount relative to its requirement is said to be the first-limiting amino acid, and the extent to which it is adequate will determine animal performance. If the deficiency of this amino acid is corrected, then the amino acid next lowest in relation to its requirement (second-limiting) will dictate animal performance. Information about which amino acids are most limiting in natural feedstuffs is important in formulating swine diets.

Cereal Grains

Cereal grains form the basis of most swine diets throughout the world and generally supply 40% to 50% of the protein in the diets of growing-finishing pigs. Thus the amino acid composition of cereals is of great importance. The most limiting amino acids of the common cereal grains are listed in Table 9.3.

It is evident that the primary amino acid limitations of all the cereals are very similar. With the exception of corn, lysine is invariably the first-limiting amino acid. The low concentration of lysine in all cereals, relative to the pig's requirement, makes it the most important amino acid in swine nutrition.

In corn, lysine and tryptophan are about equally limiting for growing pigs. Some experiments (Gallo and Pond 1968) have indicated that lysine is first-limiting, others (Baker et al. 1969a) have indicated tryptophan, whereas in yet others (Lewis et al. 1979) lysine and tryptophan have been co-limiting. In terms of supporting nitrogen retention in young gravid gilts, corn is first-limiting in lysine and second-limiting in tryptophan (Allee and Baker 1970).

After lysine, threonine is next in importance. Threonine is second-limiting in all cereals except corn, and is third-limiting in corn (Grosbach et al. 1985). There are less data about further amino acid limitations, but it seems that histidine is third-limiting in barley (Fuller et al. 1979), and tryptophan is third-limiting in sorghum (Cohen and Tanksley 1976; Purser and Tanksley 1976). What is very clear in terms of practical diet formulation throughout most of the world (where swine diets are generally based on corn, sorghum, barley, or wheat) is that three amino acids—lysine, tryptophan, and threonine—are of central importance.

Table 9.3 Limiting Amino Acids in Cereal Grains for Swine

	Limiting Amino Acids		
Cereal Grain	*First*	*Second*	*Third*
Barley	Lysine	Threonine	Histidine
Corn	Lysine and tryptophan		Threonine
Oats	Lysine		
Sorghum	Lysine	Threonine	Tryptophan
Triticale	Lysine	Threonine	
Wheat	Lysine	Threonine	

(Adapted, by permission, from Lewis 1985.)

Protein Supplements

Less is known about the amino acids that are limiting in protein supplements, because these ingredients are usually fed in combination with cereal grains and few have been examined as the sole source of protein. Nevertheless, there are certain common features that are important to consider.

Most plant protein sources are low in lysine and are probably first-limiting in this amino acid. Included in this category are corn gluten meal, cottonseed meal, linseed meal, peanut meal, safflower meal, sesame meal, and sunflower meal. Because of their low lysine content, it is difficult to obtain satisfactory swine performance if these protein sources provide the only source of supplemental amino acids in a cereal-based diet.

Two plant sources of protein, rapeseed meal (or canola meal) and soybean meal, have higher lysine contents. Although it is unclear which amino acid is first-limiting in rapeseed meal, it has been established that methionine is first-limiting in soybean meal (Berry et al. 1962, 1966). Because rapeseed meal and soybean meal have relatively high lysine and low sulfur amino acid contents, they combine well with (or complement) amino acid patterns of cereal grains, which are low in lysine and high in sulfur amino acids.

Animal protein sources contain relatively high amounts of lysine, and they are generally superior to plant sources as supplements to cereal-based diets. The amino acid patterns of milk products (dried skim milk and dried whey) and fish products (fish meal and fish protein concentrate) are particularly good. Meat products (meat meal, and meat and bone meal) are variable in composition, but they are low in tryptophan and also isoleucine. Tryptophan is usually the first-limiting amino acid in practical diets containing cereals and meat meals (Luce et al. 1964; Batterham 1970; Stockland et al. 1971; Stables and Carr 1976; Evans and Leibholz 1979a,b). Blood meal is very high in lysine but severely deficient in isoleucine (Becker et al. 1963).

Complete Diets

Because lysine is deficient in cereal grains and many protein supplements, it is usually the first-limiting amino acid in complete diets. The sequence of limiting amino acids in a corn-soybean meal diet has been evaluated in numerous experiments. The first three limiting amino acids are lysine, tryptophan, and threonine (Sharda et al. 1976; Corley and Easter 1980; Russell et al. 1983). The fourth-limiting amino acid seems to be either methionine (Russell et al. 1983, 1986) or valine (Kerr et al. 1985).

DIET FORMULATION ON THE BASIS OF AMINO ACIDS

For many years swine diets were formulated to satisfy crude protein requirements rather than to meet requirements for specific amino acids, and feed labeling regulations in the United States still require that the crude protein content of a feed be listed on the feed tag. With present knowledge of the amino acid requirements of swine and the amino acid composition of feedstuffs, the formulation of diets on the basis of amino acids rather than crude protein is a much more precise approach. This is especially true when a wide variety of different feedstuffs is available for consideration.

Diet formulation using computers makes it possible to consider all of the amino acids, but this is unnecessary. In theory, only the first-limiting amino acid needs to be considered; when the diet satisfies the requirement for it, the requirements for all of the other amino acids will be satisfied also. Thus, diets will almost always be formulated on a lysine basis. Levels of tryptophan and threonine, and possibly methionine and valine, should be checked to ensure that the requirements for these amino acids have been met.

Formulation on the basis of lysine rather than crude protein is crucial if two different cereal grains that have similar lysine contents but very different crude protein contents are being considered. If diets are formulated on a crude protein basis, the diet containing the cereal with the high protein content is liable to be lysine-deficient. An excellent example of this for corn-soybean meal versus wheat-soybean meal diets is the experiment of Cromwell et al. (1984).

AMINO ACID AVAILABILITY

The amino acid composition of a feedstuff or a diet can be determined by chemical procedures, commonly acid hydrolysis followed by ion exchange chromatography with colorimetric or fluorimetric detection of the amino acids. Chemical procedures do not, however, determine the amounts of amino acids that are available to a pig. To be "available," an amino acid must be absorbed and presented to the tissues in a form that can be used for normal metabolic functions. Until recently, little attention was paid to the differences in availability between different feedstuffs. Indeed, the 1979 edition of the *Nutrient Requirements of Swine* (NRC 1979) dismissed the topic with the statement "the availability of amino acids in the protein of common feed ingredients fed to swine has not been adequately determined." Since then, much effort has been devoted to determining availabilities, and there have been several excellent reviews of the subject (Tanksley and Knabe 1984; Sauer and Ozimek 1986; Sibbald 1987). This topic is discussed in detail in Chapter 19.

AMINO ACID—ENERGY REQUIREMENTS

The voluntary intake of pigs allowed ad libitum access to feed is influenced by the metabolizable energy (ME) concentration of the diet. When the dietary energy concentration is low, pigs increase feed intake, and vice versa (Clawson et al. 1962; Cole et al. 1967). As a consequence, changes in dietary ME concentration affect intakes of nutrients, including amino acids. Therefore, if a constant intake of an amino acid is to be maintained when diets of different ME concentration are fed, the amino acid concentration, expressed as a percentage of the diet, must be adjusted.

Many of the common feedstuffs fed to swine have a relatively uniform ME concentration, and the effects of energy density are minor. Some ingredients such as fats, however, have ME concentrations that are substantially greater than the majority of feedstuffs. Other ingredients such as those high in fiber contain relatively low ME concentrations. When energy concentrations differ considerably from those found in "standard" ingredients like corn and soybean meal, then amino acid requirements (in terms of dietary concentration) will be affected.

To obviate the difficulties inherent in expressing amino acid requirements in terms of dietary concentration, some organizations (ARC 1981; INRA 1984) list requirements as grams of amino acid per unit of energy (digestible or metabolizable). Although this may be an improvement, there are difficulties with this approach also. First, the ME concentration of the diet is not the only factor that affects the feed intake of pigs, and consequently pigs do not always adjust their feed intakes to maintain a constant ME intake. Amino acid concentrations themselves can influence feed intake, particularly when the levels of certain amino acids are marginal or deficient. Second, the ME values of ingredients may not be constant. For example, there is evidence in poultry that the ME value of fat is dependent on the amount added and also the age of the birds. Whether there are similar differences in swine is not certain.

Although there have been numerous investigations of protein-energy relationships in swine (e.g., Wagner et al. 1963; Greeley et al. 1964; Robinson and Lewis 1964; Seerley et al. 1964; Clawson 1967; Cooke et al. 1972a,b; Lodge et al. 1972a,b; Leibbrandt et al. 1975; Campbell and Dunkin 1983), no consensus about the optimum proportions between protein and energy has emerged. Some of the confusion has been caused by the variety of different protein and energy sources that have been investigated.

Attempts to define precise relationships between specific amino acids and dietary energy concentrations have also been rather discouraging. Experiments in which lysine:energy ratios have been varied (Abernathy et al. 1958; Mitchell et al. 1965; Anderson and Bowland 1967; Tribble et al. 1979; Lewis et al. 1980; Batterham et al. 1985) have not yielded consistent results.

Thus, although it is clear that there are important interrelationships between dietary energy and amino acids, and there is no doubt that amino acid concentrations should be adjusted when there are substantial differences in ME, it is not possible to make precise recommendations about these adjustments. Perhaps future research on this topic in which the availabilities of amino acids are taken into account will resolve some of the remaining questions.

USE OF CRYSTALLINE AMINO ACIDS

The amino acid requirements of swine can be met from intact proteins such as those contained in corn and soybean meal, or they can be provided by crystalline amino acids. Generally, it is much cheaper to use intact proteins to provide most of the amino acid needs, but crystalline sources of some amino acids are now available at prices that often merit their inclusion in swine diets.

D- and L-Isomers and Amino Acid Analogues

Amino acids have an asymmetric (or chiral) carbon atom in their structure, and thus can exist in two forms (as D- or L-isomers). Almost all amino acids that are produced in nature exist as the L-isomer, and this is therefore the form that is usually ingested and utilized by pigs. Chemical synthesis, however, yields a racemic mixture (50% D- and 50% L-isomers), and thus it becomes important to know to what extent (if any) the D-isomers of specific amino acids can be used by swine.

Lysine

As far as is known, there are no mammals that are able to utilize D-lysine. This is presumably because lysine does not participate in reversible transaminations, which are necessary for the inversion of D- to L-isomers. Consequently, it is assumed that relative to L-lysine, D-lysine has a potency of zero and DL-lysine a potency of 50%. Today, all of the major manufacturers of lysine use a fermentation process that yields lysine in the L-form, usually as the monohydrochloride (L-lysine.HCl). Feed grade lysine contains a minimum of 98% L-lysine.HCl. This is equivalent to 78% actual lysine. Use of feed grade lysine in the United States has increased substantially during the last 15 years (Dye 1984; Romoser 1984), much of it being used in swine feeds.

Tryptophan

Different species vary greatly in their ability to utilize D-tryptophan. Pigs can utilize D-tryptophan, although not as efficiently as the L-form. Feed grade tryptophan is available as both L-tryptophan and DL-tryptophan. The results of an experiment by Baker et al. (1971) with growing pigs indicated that D-tryptophan has a biological activity of 60% relative to L-tryptophan. Subsequent research by Arentson and Zimmerman (1985) revealed that there may be some variation in the efficiency with which the D-isomer is utilized. In their experiments, the average efficiency was about 70%. Based on these two reports, it seems that the potency of DL-tryptophan is 80% to 85% of that of L-tryptophan.

Threonine

There are four chemical isomers of threonine: D- and L-threonine and D- and L-allothreonine. In other species such as the rat (West and Carter 1938), only the natural form, L-threonine, is biologically available. This is because threonine, like lysine, does not participate in transamination reactions. It is assumed that the same is true for pigs, although this has never been tested. Feed grade threonine is in the L-form only.

Methionine

The D-form of methionine is well utilized by most species, and pigs seem to be no exception. Reifsnyder et al. (1984) reported that both DL-methionine and DL-methionine hydroxy analogue could directly replace the L-form in meeting the methionine requirement. There is evidence, however, that D-methionine may have less potency than L-methionine in very young pigs (Kim and Bayley 1983). Feed grade sources of methionine are available as DL-methionine and as methionine hydroxy analogue.

Frequency of Feeding

The efficiency with which crystalline lysine is utilized by swine is influenced by the number of daily meals that they receive. A considerable amount of research in Australia (reviewed by Batterham 1984) has demonstrated that pigs use crystalline lysine less efficiently when they are fed once per day than when they are fed six times per day (or, presumably, ad libitum). Subsequent research in the United States (Cooke et al. 1983, 1985) and the United Kingdom (Partridge et al. 1985) has confirmed that crystalline lysine is used less efficiently when pigs are fed infrequently than when they are allowed ad libitum access to feed. The reason for the lower efficiency is presumed to be related to the rapid absorption of crystalline lysine relative to other amino acids derived from intact proteins. The differential absorption rates would be expected to be deleterious when the number of daily feedings is limited, but of little consequence for a pig that consumes numerous small meals throughout the day.

Whether the frequency of feeding affects the utilization of other crystalline amino acids has not been examined, but if the effect is caused by rapid absorption, it would be expected to be a general phenomenon.

AMINO ACID REQUIREMENTS

Accurate estimates of the amino acid requirements of swine are of considerable economic importance, and their measurement has been an active area of research since the original determination of which amino acids are essential. Requirements are influenced by many factors, including dietary protein level, dietary energy density, dietary cation concentration, and environmental temperature. Many of these have been discussed, or alluded to, previously. Two other factors that influence the amino acid requirements of swine are the sex of the animal and the criterion that is used for assessment.

Effect of Sex

It is well known that there are differences in the body composition of boars, barrows, and gilts. At a given weight, boars are leaner than gilts, which in turn are leaner than barrows. One would expect that amino acid requirements would reflect these differences in body composition, and this has been confirmed by experimental observations. Several experiments have demonstrated that boars have higher protein and amino acid requirements than gilts, which have higher requirements than barrows (Speer et al. 1957; Baker et al. 1967; Blair et al. 1969; Henry et al. 1971; Tanksley and Escobosa

1971; Ross et al. 1978; Tyler et al. 1983; NCR-42 Committee 1984; Williams et al. 1984; Batterham et al. 1985).

Until recently, standard tables of requirements have not separated the amino acid requirements for the different sexes, but current tables (INRA 1984; NRC 1988) now reflect some of these differences, at least for some stages of the life cycle.

Criterion of Assessment

The requirement for almost any nutrient depends to some extent on the response criteria that are measured in its establishment. This is certainly true for amino acid requirements. Estimates of amino acid requirements for maximal carcass leanness are usually higher than estimates for maximal rates of weight gain (Cahilley et al. 1963; Baker et al. 1967; Smith et al. 1967; Brown et al. 1973a,b), although there have been some exceptions to this (Meade 1972). Furthermore, the requirements for maximal feed efficiency are generally somewhat higher than for weight gain. The criterion of assessment also affects the estimates of the amino acid requirements of sows during lactation (Lewis and Speer 1975).

Tables of requirements do not usually state clearly what criteria were used as the basis of their estimates of requirements. Most seem to use a mixture of criteria, with European estimates seemingly placing more emphasis on carcass composition than North American estimates. The ARC (1981) placed primary emphasis on "adjusted" feed conversion efficiency in its estimates of requirements of growing pigs.

Comparison of Published Amino Acid Requirements

Nutrient (including at least some amino acid) requirements of swine have been published by several organizations in various countries including Australia, France, Germany, and The Netherlands, but the most well established are those of the Agricultural Research Council (United Kingdom) and National Research Council (United States). A brief history and background to the development of requirements by the ARC and NRC has been presented by Lewis (1984). Summaries of current (ARC 1981; NRC 1988) estimates of requirements are presented in Tables 9.4 through 9.6.

There are clearly large differences in the estimates of the amino acid requirements of growing pigs from weaning to market weight. The estimates of the ARC are considerably higher at all stages. It is not reasonable to believe that there are really such large differences in the requirements of pigs in the United States and the United Kingdom. The differences in estimates reflect, primarily, different approaches and assumptions made in their estimation. There is clearly a need for further research in this area. The estimates of requirements of sows during gestation and lactation are quite similar. Although this is pleasing, it is more a reflection that both organizations have utilized the same few experiments in arriving at their estimates of requirements rather than that the requirements of sows are better known than those of growing pigs.

Table 9.4 Amino Acid Requirements of Starting Pigs: Percentage of Diet

Amino Acid	*ARC*[a]	*NRC*[b]	*NRC*[c]
Arginine	—	0.50	0.40
Histidine	0.46	0.31	0.25
Isoleucine	0.76	0.63	0.52
Leucine	1.41	0.85	0.70
Lysine	1.41	1.15	0.90
Methionine + cystine	0.70	0.58	0.48
Phenylalanine + tyrosine	1.35	0.94	0.77
Threonine	0.85	0.68	0.56
Tryptophan	0.20	0.17	0.14
Valine	0.99	0.68	0.56

[a]For pigs 3 to 8 weeks old.
[b]For pigs 5 to 10 kg.
[c]For pigs 10 to 20 kg.
(Data from ARC 1981; NRC 1988.)

Table 9.5 Amino Acid Requirements of Growing and Finishing Pigs: Percentage of Diet

	Growing		*Finishing*	
Amino Acid	*ARC*[a]	*NRC*[b]	*ARC*[c]	*NRC*[d]
Arginine	—	0.25	—	0.10
Histidine	0.40	0.22	0.28	0.18
Isoleucine	0.65	0.45	0.47	0.37
Leucine	1.19	0.60	0.85	0.50
Lysine	1.19	0.70	0.85	0.60
Methionine + cystine	0.59	0.41	0.43	0.34
Phenylalanine + tyrosine	1.13	0.66	0.82	0.55
Threonine	0.71	0.48	0.51	0.40
Tryptophan	0.17	0.12	0.13	0.10
Valine	0.84	0.48	0.60	0.40

[a]For pigs 15 to 50 kg.
[b]For pigs 20 to 50 kg.
[c]For pigs 50 to 90 kg.
[d]For pigs 50 to 110 kg.
(Data from ARC 1981; NRC 1988.)

Future Research

Further research is needed to resolve differences in estimates of amino acid requirements. The current estimates are satisfactory for those amino acids that are rarely limiting. They are unsatisfactory, however, for the economically critical amino acids (lysine, tryptophan, and threonine). Research using dose-response and response-surface methodologies will help to define the consequences of inadequacy to over-

Table 9.6 Amino Acid Requirements of Sows: Percentage of Diet

	Gestation		*Lactation*	
Amino Acid	*ARC*	*NRC*	*ARC*	*NRC*
Arginine	—	0	0.42	0.40
Histidine	0.13	0.15	0.25	0.25
Isoleucine	0.37	0.30	0.44	0.39
Leucine	0.32	0.30	0.72	0.48
Lysine	0.43	0.43	0.63	0.60
Methionine + cystine	0.29	0.23	0.34	0.36
Phenylalanine + tyrosine	0.33	0.45	0.72	0.70
Threonine	0.36	0.30	0.44	0.43
Tryptophan	0.07	0.09	0.12	0.12
Valine	0.46	0.32	0.44	0.60

(Data from ARC 1981; NRC 1988.)

abundant intakes of these amino acids. Additional research is also needed to further define the optimum proportions between amino acids and energy for growing-finishing pigs.

REFERENCES

Abernathy, R.P., R. F. Sewell, and R.L. Tarpley. 1958. *J. Anim. Sci.* 17:635.
Allee, G.L., and D.H. Baker. 1970. *J. Anim. Sci.* 30:748.
Anderson, G.H., and J.P. Bowland. 1967. *Can. J. Anim Sci.* 47:47.
Anderson, L.C., et al. 1984a. *J. Anim. Sci.* 58:362.
Anderson, L.C., et al. 1984b. *J. Anim. Sci.* 58:369.
AOAC. 1984. *Official Methods of Analysis.* 14th ed. Washington, DC: Association of Official Analytical Chemists.
ARC. 1981. *The Nutrient Requirements of Pigs.* 2d ed. Slough, England: Commonwealth Agricultural Bureaux.
Arentson, B.E., and D.R. Zimmerman. 1985. *J. Anim. Sci.* 60:474.
Austic, R.E., and R.L. Scott. 1975. *J. Nutr.* 105:1122.
Baker, D.H. 1977. *Sulfur in Nonruminant Nutrition.* West Des Moines, IA: National Feed Ingredients Association.
Baker, D.H., and V.C. Speer. 1983. *J. Anim. Sci.* 57(Suppl. 2):284.
Baker, D.H., et al. 1966. *J. Nutr.* 88:382.
Baker, D.H., et al. 1969a. *J. Anim. Sci.* 28:23.
Baker, D.H., et al. 1969b. *J. Anim. Sci.* 29:581.
Baker, D.H., et al. 1967. *J. Anim. Sci.* 26:1059.
Baker, D.H., et al. 1971. *J. Anim. Sci.* 33:42.
Ball, R.O., J.L. Atkinson, and H.S. Bayley. 1986. *J. Nutr.* 55:659.
Batterham, E.S. 1970. *Aust. J. Exp. Agric. Anim. Husb.* 10:534.
Batterham, E.S. 1984. *Pig News Inform.* 5:85.
Batterham, E.S., L.R. Giles, and E.B. Dettmann. 1985. *Anim. Prod.* 40:331.
Becker, D.E., et al. 1955. *J. Anim. Sci.* 14:1086.
Becker, D.E., et al. 1963. *J. Anim. Sci.* 22:1093.
Beeson, W.M., E.T. Mertz, and H.D. Jackson. 1951. *J. Anim. Sci.* 10:1037 (Abstr.).

Beeson, W.M., H.D. Jackson, and E.T. Mertz. 1953. *J. Anim. Sci.* 12:870.
Beeson, W.M., E.T. Mertz, and D.C. Shelton. 1948. *Science* 107:599.
Beeson, W.M., E.T. Mertz, and D.C. Shelton. 1949. *J. Anim. Sci.* 8:532.
Bell, J.M., et al. 1950. *J. Nutr.* 40:551.
Benevenga, N.J., and A.E. Harper. 1967. *J. Nutr.* 93:44.
Berry, T.H., et al. 1962. *J. Anim. Sci.* 21:558.
Berry, T.H., et al. 1966. *J. Anim. Sci.* 25:722.
Blair, R., et al. 1969. *J. Agric. Sci. Cambridge* 72:379.
Brinegar, M.J., et al. 1950a. *J. Nutr.* 42:619.
Brinegar, M.J., et al. 1950b. *J. Nutr.* 42:129.
Brown, H.D., B.G. Harmon, and A.H. Jensen. 1973a. *J. Anim. Sci.* 37:708.
Brown, H.D., B.G. Harmon, and A.H. Jensen. 1973b. *J. Anim. Sci.* 37:1159.
Cahilly, G.M., Jr., et al. 1963. *J. Anim. Sci.* 22:726.
Campbell, R.G., and A.C. Dunkin. 1983. *Br. J. Nutr.* 49:221.
Clawson, A.J. 1967. *J. Anim. Sci.* 26:328.
Clawson, A.J., and W.D. Armstrong. 1981. *J. Anim. Sci.* 52:1.
Clawson, A.J., et al. 1962. *J. Anim. Sci.* 21:62.
Cohen, R.S., and T.D. Tanksley, Jr. 1976. *J. Anim. Sci.* 43:1028.
Cole, D.J.A. 1979. "Amino acid nutrition of the pig." In: *Recent Advances in Animal Nutrition—1978.* Haresign, W., and D. Lewis (Eds.). pp. 59–72. London: Butterworths.
Cole, D.J.A., J.E. Duckworth, and W. Holmes. 1967. *Anim. Prod.* 9:141.
Cooke, H., D.W. Giesting, and R.A. Easter. 1985. *J. Anim. Sci.* 61(Suppl. 1):319.
Cooke, R., G.A. Lodge, and D. Lewis. 1972a. *Anim. Prod.* 14:35.
Cooke, R., G.A. Lodge, and D. Lewis. 1972b. *Anim. Prod.* 14:219.
Cooke, H., et al. 1983. *J. Anim. Sci.* 57(Suppl. 1):240.
Corley, J.R., and R.A. Easter. 1980. *J. Anim. Sci.* 51(Suppl. 1):191.
Cromwell, G.L., T.S. Stahly, and H.J. Monegue. 1984. *J. Anim. Sci.* 59(Suppl. 1):103.
Curtin, L.V., et al. 1952. *J. Nutr.* 48:499.
Deguchi, E., et al. 1978. *J. Nutr.* 108:1572.
Deguchi, E., et al. 1980. *Am. J. Vet. Res.* 41:212.
Dye, L.J. 1984. *Profile of the Amino Acid Industry: Review of Suppliers and Products.* Chicago, IL.: NFIA Nutrition Institute on Amino Acids.
Easter, R.A., and D.H. Baker. 1976. *J. Nutr.* 106:636.
Easter, R.A., and D.H. Baker. 1977. *J. Nutr.* 107:120.
Easter, R.A., R.S. Katz, and D.H. Baker. 1974. *J. Anim. Sci.* 39:1123.
Edmonds, M.S., and D.H. Baker. 1986. *J. Anim. Sci.* 63(Suppl. 1):271.
Eggert, R.G., et al. 1954. *J. Nutr.* 53:177.
Eggert, R.G., et al. 1955. *J. Anim. Sci.* 14:556.
Evans, D.F., and J. Leibholz. 1979a. *Anim. Feed Sci. Technol.* 4:33.
Evans, D.F., and J. Leibholz. 1979b. *Anim. Feed Sci. Technol.* 4:43.
Fuller, M.F., et al. 1979. *Br. J. Nutr.* 41:321.
Gallo, J.T., and W.G. Pond. 1968. *J. Anim. Sci.* 27:73.
Greeley, M.G., et al. 1964. *J. Anim. Sci.* 23:816.
Grimson, R.E., and J.P. Bowland. 1971. *J. Anim. Sci.* 33:58.
Grimson, R.E., J.P. Bowland, and L.P. Milligan. 1971. *Can. J. Anim. Sci.* 51:103.
Grosbach, D.A., A.J. Lewis, and E.R. Peo, Jr. 1985. *J. Anim. Sci.* 60:487.
Hagemeier, D.L., G.W. Libal, and R.C. Wahlstrom. 1983. *J. Anim. Sci.* 57:99.
Hanson, L.E., and E.F. Ferrin. 1955. *J. Anim. Sci.* 14:43.
Harmon, B.G. 1980. "The role of amino acid balance in practical swine rations." In: *Proceedings of the 41st Minnesota Nutrition Conference.* pp. 132–138. St. Paul: University of Minnesota.
Harper, A.E., N.J. Benevenga, and R.M. Wohlhueter. 1970. *Physiol. Rev.* 50:428.
Hays, V.W., et al. 1957. *J. Anim. Sci.* 16:44.

Hegsted, D.M. 1974. "Assessment of protein quality." In: *Improvement of Protein Nutriture.* pp. 64–88. Washington, DC: National Academy of Sciences.
Henry, Y., P.H. Duee, and A. Rerat. 1976. *J. Anim. Sci.* 42:357.
Henry, Y., A. Rerat, and R. Tomassone. 1971. *Ann. Zootechnie* 20:521.
INRA. 1984. *L'alimentation des Animaux Monogastriques: Porc, Lapin, Volailles.* Paris: Institut National de la Recherche Agronomique.
Jackson, H.D., E.T. Mertz, and W.M. Beeson. 1953. *J. Nutr.* 51:109.
Kelly, K.A., et al. 1983. *J. Anim. Sci.* 57(Suppl. 1):252.
Kerr, B.J., L.E. Russell, and R.A. Easter. 1985. *J. Anim. Sci.* 61(Suppl. 1):326.
Kim, K.I., and H.S. Bayley. 1983. *Br. J. Nutr.* 50:383.
Kornegay, E.T. 1972. *J. Anim. Sci.* 34:55.
Kornegay, E.T., V. Mosanghini, and R.D. Snee. 1970. *J. Nutr.* 100:330.
Kornegay, E.T., et al. 1965. *J. Anim. Sci.* 24:951.
Leibbrandt, V.D., et al. 1975. *J. Anim. Sci.* 40:1070.
Lewis, A.J. 1984. "Comparison of ARC and NRC recommended requirements for energy and protein in growing pigs." In: *Recent Advances in Animal Nutrition-1984.* Haresign, W., and D.J.A. Cole (Eds.). pp. 61–73. London: Butterworths.
Lewis, A.J. 1985. "Use of synthetic amino acids in practical rations." In: *Proceedings of the Carolina Swine Nutrition Conference.* pp. 32–45. Raleigh: North Carolina State University.
Lewis, A.J., and V.C. Speer. 1975. "A multiple parameter approach to the estimation of amino acid requirements of lactating sows." In: *Protein Nutritional Quality of Foods and Feeds. Part 1.* Friedman, M. (Ed.). pp. 51–66. New York: Marcel Dekker Inc.
Lewis, A.J., E.R. Peo, Jr., and J.D. Hancock. 1986. *J. Anim. Sci.* 63(Suppl. 1):271.
Lewis, A.J., et al. 1977. *J. Nutr.* 107:1369.
Lewis, A.J., et al. 1979. *Nutr. Rep. Int.* 19:533.
Lewis, A.J., et al. 1980. *J. Anim. Sci.* 51:361.
Liu, C.H., et al. 1955. *J. Nutr.* 57:241.
Lodge, G.A., et al. 1972a. *Anim. Prod.* 14:47.
Lodge, G.A., B. Hardy, and D. Lewis. 1972b. *Anim. Prod.* 14:229.
Luce, W.G., E.R. Peo, Jr., and D.B. Hudman. 1964. *J. Anim. Sci.* 23:521.
Meade, R.J. 1972. "Supplementing practical swine diets with amino acids." In: *Proceedings of the 33rd Minnesota Nutrition Conference.* pp. 9–20. St. Paul: University of Minnesota.
Mertz, E.T., W.M. Beeson, and H.D. Jackson. 1952. *Arch. Biochem. Biophys.* 38:121.
Mertz, E.T., J.N. Henson, and W.M. Beeson. 1954. *J. Anim. Sci.* 13:927.
Mertz, E.T., D.C. Shelton, and W.M. Beeson. 1949. *J. Anim. Sci.* 8:524.
Miller, E.R., et al. 1981a. *J. Anim. Sci.* 53(Suppl. 1):93.
Miller, E.R., et al. 1981b. *J. Anim. Sci.* 53(Suppl. 1):255.
Mitchell, J.R., Jr., et al. 1965. *J. Anim. Sci.* 24:977.
Mitchell, J.R., Jr., et al. 1968. *J. Anim. Sci.* 27:1322.
Mosenthin, R., et al. 1986. *J. Anim. Sci.* 63(Suppl. 1):281.
NRC-42 Committee on Swine Nutrition. 1984. *J. Anim. Sci.* 59(Suppl. 1):95.
NRC. 1979. *Nutrient Requirements of Domestic Animals.* No. 2, *Nutrient Requirements of Swine.* 8th ed. Washington, DC: National Academy of Sciences–National Research Council.
NRC. 1988. *Nutrient Requirements of Domestic Animals.* No. 2, *Nutrient Requirements of Swine.* 9th ed. Washington, DC: National Academy of Sciences–National Research Council.
Oestemer, G.A., L.E. Hanson, and R.J. Meade. 1973. *J. Anim. Sci.* 36:674.
Partridge, I.G., A.G. Low, and H.D. Keal. 1985. *Anim. Prod.* 40:375.
Platter, P.D., et al. 1973. *J. Anim. Sci.* 37:514.
Pond, W.G. 1973. *J. Anim. Sci.* 36:175.
Purser, K.W., and T.D. Tanksley, Jr. 1976. *J. Anim. Sci.* 43:257 (Abstr.).
Rechcigl, M., Jr., et al. 1956. *J. Nutr.* 60:619.

Reifsnyder, D.H., C.T. Young, and E.E. Jones. 1984. *J. Nutr.* 114:1705.
Robbins, K.R., and D.H. Baker. 1977. *J. Anim. Sci.* 45:113.
Robinson, D.W., and D. Lewis. 1964. *J. Agric. Sci. Cambridge* 63:185.
Romoser, G.L. 1984. *History of Protein and Amino Acid Concepts and a Look at the Future.* Chicago: NFIA Nutrition Institute on Amino Acids.
Ross, R.D., D.M. Thrasher, and T.D. Bidner. 1978. *J. Anim. Sci.* 47(Suppl. 1):319.
Russell, L.E., G.L. Cromwell, and T.S. Stahly. 1983. *J. Anim. Sci.* 56:1115.
Russell, L.E., et al. 1986. *Anim. Prod.* 42:291.
Sauer, W.C., and L. Ozimek. 1986. *Livestock Prod. Sci.* 15:367.
Seerley, R.W., G.E. Poley, and R.C. Wahlstrom. 1964. *J. Anim. Sci.* 23:1016.
Sewell, R.F., et al. 1953. *J. Nutr.* 49:435.
Sharda, D.P., D.C. Mahan, and R.F. Wilson. 1976. *J. Anim. Sci.* 42:1175.
Shelton, D.C., W.M. Beeson, and E.T. Mertz. 1950. *Arch. Biochem. Biophys.* 29:446.
Shelton, D.C., W.M. Beeson, and E.T. Mertz. 1951a. *Arch. Biochem. Biophys.* 30:1.
Shelton, D.C., W.M. Beeson, and E.T. Mertz. 1951b. *J. Anim. Sci.* 10:57.
Shelton, D.C., W.M. Beeson, and E.T. Mertz. 1951c. *J. Anim. Sci.* 10:73.
Sibbald, I.R. 1987. *Can. J. Anim. Sci.* 67:221.
Smith, J., Jr., A.J. Clawson, and E.R. Barrick. 1967. *J. Anim. Sci.* 26:752.
Sokol, L., R.L. Harrold, and C.H. Haugse. 1979. *J. Anim. Sci.* 49(Suppl. 1):95.
Southern, L.L., and D.H. Baker. 1982. *J. Anim. Sci.* 55:857.
Southern, L.L., and D.H. Baker. 1983. *J. Anim. Sci.* 57:402.
Speer, V.C., et al. 1957. *J. Anim. Sci.* 16:607.
Stables, N.H.J., and J.R. Carr. 1976. *NZ J. Agric. Res.* 19:311.
Stockland, W.L., R.J. Meade, and J.W. Nordstrom. 1971. *J. Anim. Sci.* 32:262.
Tanksley, T.D., Jr., and A. Escobosa. 1971. *J. Anim. Sci.* 33:239 (Abstr.).
Tanksley, T.D., Jr., and D.A. Knabe. 1984. "Ileal digestibilities of amino acids in pig feeds and their use in formulating diets." In: *Recent Advances in Animal Nutrition—1984.* Haresign, W., and D.J.A. Cole (Ed.). London: Butterworths.
Thacker, P.A., et al. 1982. *Can. J. Anim. Sci.* 62:1193.
Thacker, P.A., W.C. Sauer, and H. Jorgensen. 1984. *J. Anim. Sci.* 59:409.
Tribble, L.F., et al. 1979. *J. Anim. Sci.* 48:541.
Tyler, R.W., et al. 1983. *J. Anim. Sci.* 57:364.
Van Soest, P.J., and C.J. Sniffen. 1984. Nitrogen Fractions in NDF and ADF. *Proc. Distillers Feed Conf.*, Cincinnati, OH. 39:73.
Wagner, G.R., et al. 1963. *J. Anim. Sci.* 22:202.
Wahlstrom, R.C., and G.W. Libal. 1974. *J. Anim. Sci.* 38:1261.
Wehrbein, G.F., et al. 1970. *J. Anim. Sci.* 31:327.
West, H.D., and H.E. Carter. 1938. *J. Biol. Chem.* 122:611.
Williams, W.D., et al. 1984. *J. Anim. Sci.* 58:657.

Chapter 10

Calcium, Phosphorus, and Vitamin D in Swine Nutrition

E.R. Peo, Jr.

Since the domestication of the pig and its evolution as a major meat commodity, cereal grains have served as the major source of energy for swine diets. With the discovery and isolation of vitamin B_{12} (Rickes et al. 1948), the movement away from the old commonly used "trios" protein supplement was quickly accomplished and all-plant-based swine diets are now the rule rather than the exception. Although all-plant diets (basically, cereal grain and soybean meal fortified with minerals and vitamins) are excellent, they pose some serious formulation problems. For example, cereal grains are practically devoid of calcium (Ca) but are relatively high in total phosphorus (P), some of which is biologically unavailable to the pig (Hays 1976). In addition, much of the P in cereal grains and soybean meal is present as phytic acid, a natural chelator of several divalent mineral cations (Nelson et al. 1968). Driven by these known problems, researchers have investigated not only the Ca and P requirements of all classes of swine but also the complexity of the many interactions associated with these two mineral elements (for major reviews, see Hays 1976; Peo 1976; Kornegay 1985). From the research, it is apparent that adequate Ca and P nutrition for all classes of swine is dependent upon three major factors: (1) an adequate supply of each element in available form in the diet; (2) a suitable ratio of available Ca and P in the diet; and (3) the presence of vitamin D. The significance of each of the factors and the interactions among them are important considerations for swine nutritionists.

CALCIUM

The mature body of the pig contains about 2% total Ca, 99% of which is present in hard tissues such as bones and teeth. The remaining 1% is widely distributed in the blood, extracellular fluids, and extraosseous tissues of the body (Pike and Brown 1984). Thus, the development of the skeleton of the pig should receive primary consideration in determining Ca requirements because it has a support role and serves as a reservoir and source of Ca for maintaining homeostasis of serum Ca. Although body Ca originates from the diet, serum Ca is maintained primarily through the action of parathormone and other modulation hormones such as thyrocalcitonin, calmodulin, and, to some extent, vitamin D, in liberating Ca from bone reserves (Maynard et al. 1975; Pike and Brown 1984; DeLuca and Schones 1976; Hadley 1984; Fitzpatrick et al. 1987; Garel 1987).

Regardless of dietary source, Ca must be solubilized (ionized) in order to be absorbed. This is accomplished by the low pH of the stomach. However, the pH in the newborn pig's stomach is about 4.0 (Cunningham and Brisson 1957). However, lactose in milk favors the development of an acid environment and thus, may be one of the rationales as to why lactose evolved as the major carbohydrate found in the milk of most mammals. While lactose may promote Ca absorption in the young pig, it appears to be ineffective in this respect in growing-finishing swine (Moser et al. 1980).

Several physical-chemical forces work against maintenance of solubility. As the ingesta passes from the stomach into the small intestine where Ca absorption takes place, the pH rises. This has a negative influence on solubility by creating an environment for the formation of tri-calcium phosphate, an insoluble complex. Also, the ratio of dietary Ca to P comes into play at this point, with a wide ratio of Ca to P creating a solubility problem similar to one caused by a high pH. That is, if Ca is in higher concentration than P (or vice versa), the opportunity for tri-calcium phosphate to be formed becomes greater and thus reduces absorption opportunities. In addition, as shown in Figure 10.1, Ca absorption and utilization are also affected by magnesium and sulfur (primarily SO_4 salt), two elements relatively high in swine diets. Other elements found in natural ingredients also might interfere with Ca absorption (Tillman 1966).

Absorption of Ca occurs in the proximal duodenum by a vitamin D-induced Ca binding protein active transport system (Stanbury 1980) regulated to meet Ca needs of the body. It is most active during pregnancy and lactation. Ca is also absorbed directly into the blood stream by passive ionic diffusion, largely in the mid and distal small intestine (Avioli 1972).

Erythrocytes are almost devoid of Ca but blood serum contains 9 to 12 mg/dl (Ullrey et al. 1967). There are two recognized forms of serum Ca: diffusable (60% of total) and nondiffusable. The diffusable form exists mainly as salts of phosphate or bicarbonate and represents Ca that freely exchanges with tissues demanding Ca. Nondiffusable Ca occurs in association with protein or is ionically bound but ultrafiltrable (Crampton and Lloyd 1959; Kaneko 1980).

Serum Ca serves the body in the following ways (Peo 1976):

1. to meet structural demands
2. for maintenance of cell membrane integrity and normal permeability
3. for normal function of nerve cells
4. as a link between excitation and contraction of muscles
5. as a link between excitation and secretion of endocrine glands
6. as a regulator, activator, or inhibitor of key enzymes such as those involved in blood coagulation

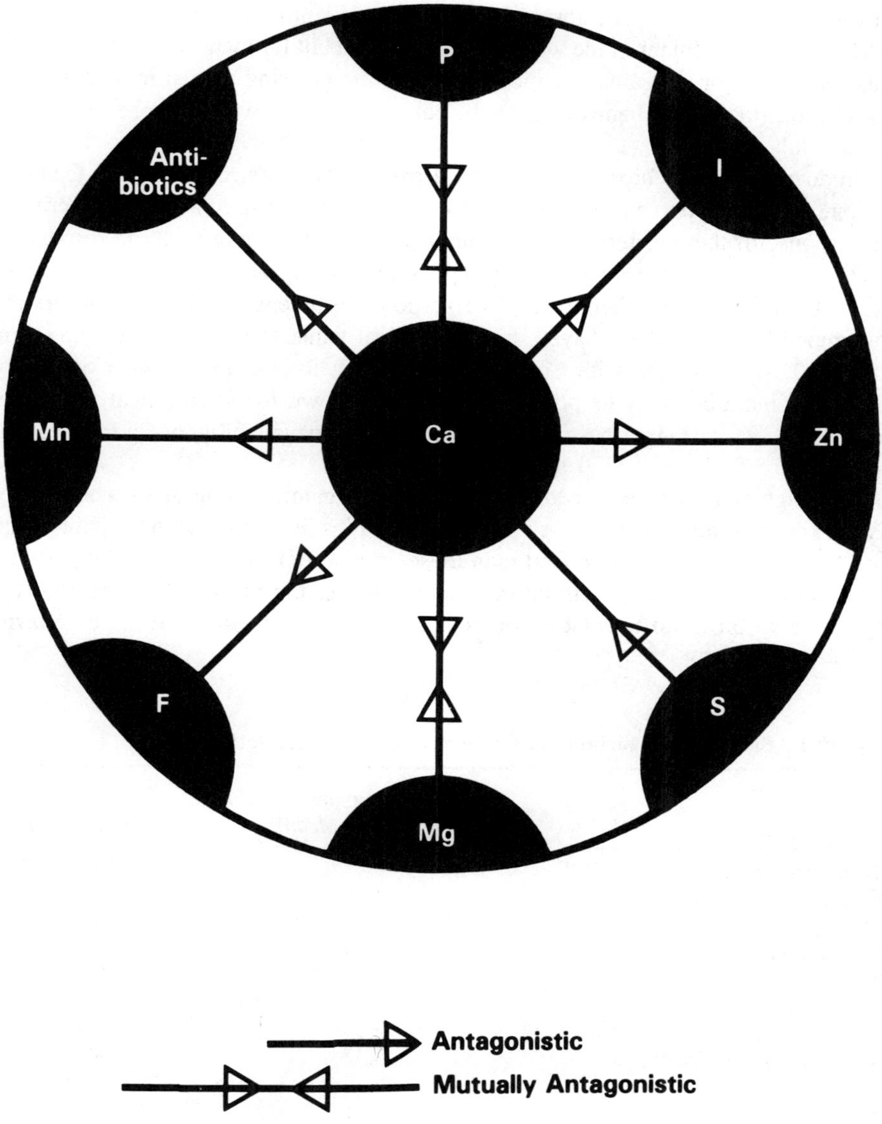

FIGURE 10.1 *Known interrelationships of calcium with other elements and certain antibiotics common to swine diets.*

After serving its role(s) in the body, Ca is excreted largely in the feces (Moore and Tyler 1955a, 1955b; Partridge 1980). Hence, determining the digestibility of Ca supplements ([Ca intake − fecal Ca ÷ Ca] intake) is of little value, since there is no practical way to determine whether fecal Ca originated from diet or body. Some estimates of true Ca (and P) absorption have been identified by Gueguen and Perez (1981). Thus, assessment of the value of a Ca supplement for swine must involve other traits. Net retention of Ca can be meaningful for the growing animal in a positive Ca balance, meeting the demands of growth, but net retention would not be as valuable for the adult.

In determining the bioavailability of Ca from various sources, growth, feed conversion, serum Ca, percent bone ash, and bone strength are used as response criteria. The response of these criteria to a test supplement, as compared with the response to a highly available reference standard, provides a much superior estimate of the usefulness of a Ca supplement than a simple digestion coefficient. To date, it appears that most mineral sources of Ca have a high biological value (Table 10.1), varying from 51% to 102% (compared with $CaCO_3$ as a standard; Ross et al. 1984). Conversely, Ca in plant materials may be poorly available, as shown for alfalfa meal (Cromwell et al. 1984a). Particle size does not seem to affect the bioavailability of Ca from various mineral sources (Pond et al. 1982; Ross et al. 1984).

Although poor gains and feed intake may be one manifestation of a Ca deficiency, it is not known if this is a direct or indirect effect. Pigs fed diets low in Ca gain weight more slowly and consume less feed than those on a sufficient diet (Peo 1976). But, is this because of the onset of structural failure causing the pig to not stand to eat as long as those on a sufficient diet or is it due to a failure of endogenous enzyme

Table 10.1 Biological Availability of Calcium in Certain Feedstuffs for Pigs

	Diameter (mm) (Geometric Mean)	*Availability (%)*[a]
Calcium carbonate		100
Fine grind	0.11	96
Medium grind	0.18	102
Coarse grind	0.40	102
Calcitic limestone	0.29	100
Dolomitic limestone (12% magnesium)	0.06	51
Dolomitic limestone (11% magnesium)	0.24	78
Gypsum (calcium sulfate)	0.32	99
Marble		
Fine grind	0.11	100
Medium grind	0.15	95
Oyster shell flour	0.10	98
Aragonite		100
Fine grind	0.17	93
Medium grind	0.54	100
Alfalfa meal[b]		22

[a] Determined by the slope-ratio (single point regression) procedure; criterion of response was bone breaking strength.

[b] Cromwell et al. 1984a, 1984b.

(Data from Ross et al. 1984; Cromwell et al. 1984a, 1984b).

systems? The former seems more plausible because of the known forces maintaining Ca homeostasis in the body (Hadley 1984).

Rickets (in the young) or osteomalacia (in the adult) are evident in pigs fed Ca-deficient diets. Some signs are stiffness of gait, enlarged and painful joints, deformities of the long bones (bent, bowed, broken), humped back or camel back syndrome, and posterior paralysis or the downer sow syndrome (Hart and Steenbock 1913; Maynard and Miller 1927; Maynard et al. 1975; Krider and Carrol 1971; White 1971; Nimmo et al. 1981a). Rickets and osteomalacia are easy to diagnose, but one should always remember that a deficiency of P or vitamin D will produce similar signs because all three (Ca, P, and vitamin D) are involved in normal bone metabolism.

Widely used reference bases for nutrient requirements of swine are the ones established by the National Academy of Sciences, National Research Council (NRC) on *Nutrient Requirement of Swine* (1988) and the Agricultural Research Council's (ARC) *Nutrient Requirements of Pigs* (1981). Their recommendations are shown in Table 10.2. Recommendations from universities, the feed industry, and consultants are usually higher than are those of the NRC and are identified as "allowances" rather than minimum requirements, as identified by the NRC. The stress of field production systems (Wahlstrom et al. 1975; Libal et al. 1977) and an allowance for variances in bioavailability may account for the disparity in requirements among the groups. A recent survey by Overfield et al. (1986), summarized in Table 10.2, shows how large the disparity can be.

In addition to its known involvement in rickets, Ca has an indirect effect on other diseases. Often, Ca carbonate is used as a diluent for other mineral nutrients or is pulled into the diet by least-cost computer formulations as a filler. This can elevate diet Ca to levels that interfere with zinc (Zn) utilization, leading to parakeratosis (Luecke et al. 1956; Lewis et al. 1956; Lewis et al. 1957; Stevenson and Earle 1956; Conrad and Beeson 1957; Newland et al. 1958; Whiting and Bezeau 1958; Wahlstrom 1957; Hoefer et al. 1960; Berry et al. 1961; Pond and Jones 1964). The disease can be alleviated by increasing the Zn content of the diet or by reducing Ca levels. The latter seems to be the more practical approach to the problems since Ca is also known to interfere with tetracycline absorption, which could reduce this important drug's effectiveness (Eggert et al. 1959; Costain and Lloyd 1962).

Ca has been implicated in the turbinate bone disease atrophic rhinitis (Brown et al. 1966). However, it appears that any possible relationship between Ca (or P) deficiency and atrophic rhinitis is coincidental to the causative agent (Peo et al. 1967; Libal et al. 1969; Baustad et al. 1967; Harmon et al. 1967; Lindley 1967; Krusemark et al. 1968; Washam et al. 1968; Wahlstrom and DeGoey 1968; Bunch et al. 1969; Logomarisino et al. 1969; Wahlstrom and Friedrikson 1969; Cromwell et al. 1970; Veum et al. 1970; Coalson et al. 1972; Cromwell et al. 1972; Stockland and Blaylock 1973; Logomarisino et al. 1974; Doige et al. 1975; Hays 1968).

While Ca is an important mineral nutrient, overuse can lead to serious consequences as a result of its antagonistic effects on other elements or drugs (Figure 10.1). Levels of fortification commensurate with those identified by the NRC (1988) should minimize any problems associated with deficient or excess levels of dietary Ca.

Table 10.2 Nutrient Requirements of Swine[a]

	Weight Class of Swine (kg)											
Nutrient	*1–5*[b]	*5*[c]	*5–10*[b]	*10–20*[b]	*25*[c]	*20–50*[b]	*45*[c]	*50–110*[b]	*90*[c]	*Bred Gilts, Sows*	*Boars*	*Lactating Sows*
NRC												
Calcium (%)	0.90		0.80	0.70		0.60		0.50		0.75	0.75	0.75
Phosphorus (%)	0.70		0.65	0.60		0.50		0.40		0.60	0.60	0.60
Vitamin D (IU)	220		220	200		150		150		200	200	200
ARC												
Calcium (%)		0.94			0.88		0.75		0.61	0.80	0.80	0.80
Phosphorus (%)		0.80			0.51		0.37		0.28	0.70	0.70	0.70
Vitamin D (IU)		104			104		104		104	—	—	—
University recommendations[d,e]												
Calcium (%)	0.80		0.77	0.66				0.59		0.82	0.83	0.79
Phosphorus (%)	0.67		0.64	0.55				0.49		0.66	0.66	0.63
Vitamin D_3 (IU)	206		206	135				142		235	255	214
Industry recommendations[d,f]												
Calcium (%)	0.86		0.82	0.74				0.63		0.95	0.86	0.93
Phosphorus (%)	0.73		0.69	0.60				0.52		0.77	0.72	0.76
Vitamin D_3 (IU)	600		535	450				340		710	505	705

[a]Nutrient requirements are % or amount/kg diet, on an as-fed basis.
[b]Weight class used by NRC (1988).
[c]Weight class used by ARC (1981).
[d]Overfield et al. (1986).
[e]Variability: calcium, 28; phosphorus, 42; vitamin D_3, 145.
[f]Variability: calcium, 29; phosphorus, 36; vitamin D_3, 190.
(Data from NRC 1988; ARC 1981; Overfield et al. 1986.)

PHOSPHORUS

Approximately 1% of the mature pig's body weight is P. Eighty percent is found primarily as salts of Ca and magnesium (Mg) in the hard tissues of the body. The remaining 20% is located in soft tissues where it exists as part of organic phosphates such as high energy adenosine triphosphate (ATP), a compound necessary for energy transductions essential for all cellular activity; as phospholipids, which are components of cell membranes and are involved in fat transport; as coenzyme forms of certain B vitamins; and as part of DNA and RNA, genetically coded compounds responsible for cell reproduction (Pike and Brown 1984; Anonymous 1978; Maynard et al. 1975; Hays 1976).

Biologically available P from feedstuffs is more completely absorbed (up to 90%) than Ca, with absorption taking place in the proximal end of the duodenum in the orthophosphate ($PO_4^{\equiv}$) form (Bartter 1964; Irving 1964). Whether or not P is absorbed by a passive or active system, or both, has not been elucidated. The phosphate ion may be a "tag along" to Ca. Although Ca and P share a mutual antagonism (Figures 10.1 and 10.2), normal dietary levels of Ca enhance P absorption (Fox et al. 1978).

The amount of P absorbed is dependent upon level of P, source, amount of Ca, Ca:P ratio, intestinal pH, and other mineral elements that are antagonistic to P absorption and utilization, as shown in Figure 10.2. There are many more mutual antagonisms between other elements and P than with Ca.

The P concentration of whole blood ranges from 35 to 45 mg/dl, while inorganic P concentrations are about 8 to 10 mg/dl in plasma (Ullrey et al. 1967; also Table 10.3), reflecting the need for P in the metabolic activities of erythrocytes. Plasma P is used to meet body needs for bone formation and cellular metabolism. Maintenance of plasma P is not as critical to life as is Ca, but low plasma P will result in impairment of all metabolic functions and, hence, lowered pig performance (Hays 1976).

P has more physiological functions than any other element. In addition to combining to form the hydroxyapatite mineral crystal of bones and teeth, P is found in every cell in the body, where it is involved in many metabolic processes including acid-base balance; muscle metabolism; and intermediary metabolism of carbohydrates, fats, protein, and nucleotides (Hays 1976).

P is excreted from the body via the feces and urine (Moore and Tyler 1955a, 1955b; Pike and Brown 1984). Thus, as with Ca, digestibility determinations are almost meaningless for estimating the biological value of a P supplement. Other criteria must be used. Because P is an expensive element, biological value is important. Of the methods available to estimate biological value, most are similar to the assay established by Gillis et al. (1954), with the exception that different traits serve as response criteria and statistics are used to compare the slopes of the regression lines achieved from animal response to a P source of known high biological value as compared with that of an unknown. Response criteria can be gain and feed conversion (good sensitivity), serum Ca and P (low sensitivity), percent bone ash (high sensitivity for the young, growing animal; low sensitivity for adults), serum alkaline phosphatase (good sensitivity), percent composition of bone ash (very low sensitivity), and physical traits of bone (high sensitivity) (Crenshaw et al. 1981a; Crenshaw et al. 1981b; Cromwell et.

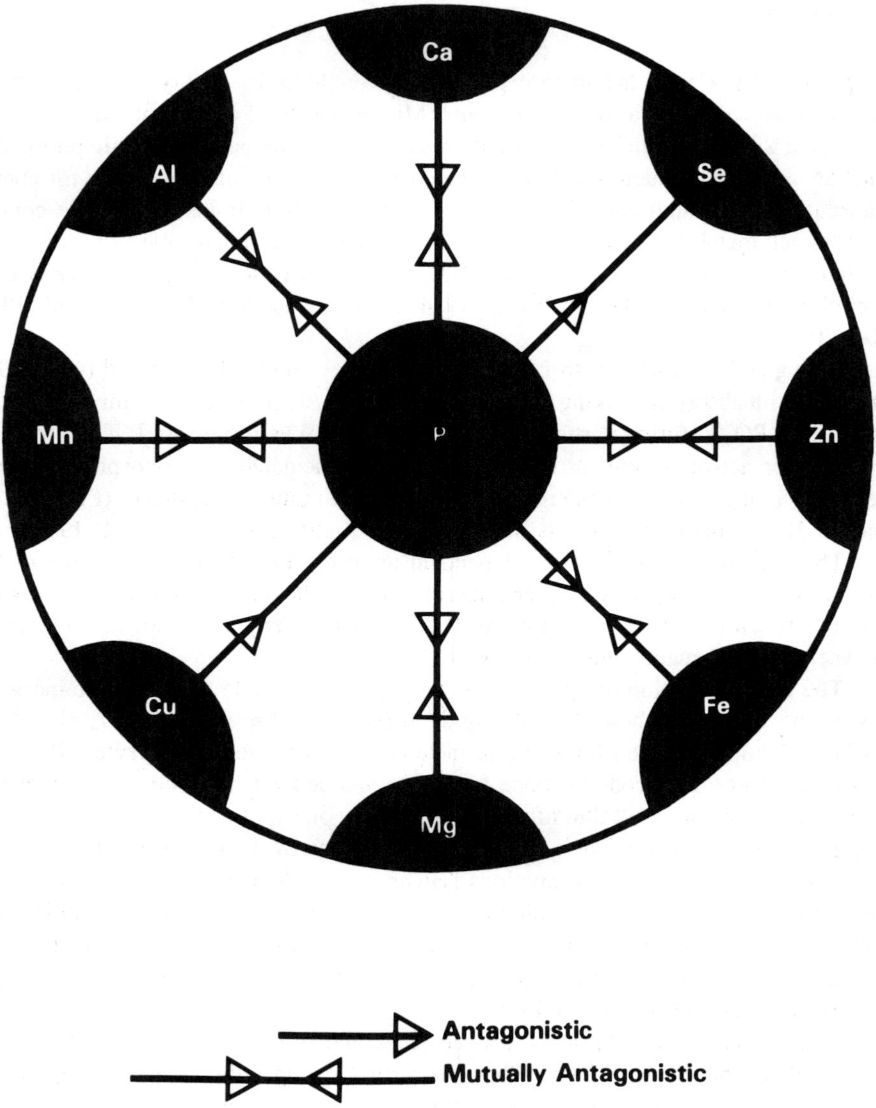

FIGURE 10.2 *Known interrelationships of phosphorus with other elements common to swine diets.*

al. 1972; Cromwell et al. 1970; Miller et al. 1966; Maxson et al. 1983; Reinhard et al. 1976; Reinhart and Mahan 1986; Koch et al. 1984; Koch and Mahan 1985; Koch and Mahan 1986; Combs 1962a; Boyd et al. 1983). The relative bioavailability of several P sources is shown in Table 10.4.

Table 10.3 Effect of Dietary Levels of Vitamin D_3 on Gains, Feed Intake, Feed Conversion, and Blood Serum Levels of Calcium, Phosphorus, and Alkaline Phosphatase of Nursery-Age Pigs

	Vitamin D_3 (IU/kg Diet)										
Criterion[a]	*550*	*5500*	*11,000*	*16,500*	*22,000*	*27,500*	*44,000*	*88,000*	*176,000*	*220,000*	*440,000*[b]
Avg. daily gain (g)	420	416	408	407	413	406	375	390	335	30	—
Avg. daily feed intake (g)	801	792	763	744	771	776	741	766	701	633	—
Feed/gain ratio	1.91	1.92	1.89	1.83	1.89	1.93	1.97	1.94	2.04	10.36	—
Serum											
Calcium (mg/dl)	11.7	11.2	11.8	11.5	11.6	11.6	12.0	12.0	14.4	16.7	—
Phosphorus (mg/dl)	9.8	10.3	10.1	9.7	9.9	9.9	9.8	9.8	8.1	7.8	—
Alkaline phosphatase IU/L	117.7	128.3	112.0	120.8	117.2	124.3	105.1	96.2	105.7	82.4	—

[a]Pooled data for three experiments adjusted to the mean response of the control within each experiment. The control level was 550 IU/kg for all three experiments. Initial weight of the pigs varied from 6.4 to 16 kg for 21- to 28-day trials, depending on the experiment.

[b]Five of the eight pigs died on this treatment during the first 7 days on test. Treatment terminated.

(Data from Hancock et al. 1986.)

Table 10.4 Biological Availability of Phosphorus in Certain Feedstuffs for Pigs

Ingredient	*Average*[a]	*Range*
Corn	15	9–29
Corn, high moisture	49	42–58
Grain sorghum	22	19–25
Grain sorghum, high moisture	43	42–43
Oats	30	23–36
Barley	31	—
Wheat	50	40–56
Wheat bran	35	—
Wheat middlings	45	34–55
Rice bran	25	—
Soybean meal, dehulled	25	18–35
Soybean meal	38	36–39
Peanut meal	12	—
Cottonseed meal	21	0–42
Alfalfa meal	100	—
Fish meal	100	—
Meat and bone meal	93	—
Dicalcium phosphate	100	—

[a]Values derived from pigs weighing 15 to 35 kg.
(Data from NRC 1988.)

Rickets in the young and osteomalacia in the adult are manifestations of abnormal P nutrition (deficiency or metabolism). In the resultant rachitic bone, there is an overproduction of preosseous tissue that fails to calcify for lack of P. This overproduction of preosseous tissue is also found at the site of broken bones in P-deficient (as well as in Ca- and vitamin D-deficient) animals and results in the so-called ''beaded rib syndrome,'' which is somewhat observable in swine by manual palpation of the rib cage but is more evident by visual inspection at slaughter or upon necropsy (Hays 1976; Peo 1976).

Another associated condition, osteoporosis, probably occurs only in extremely acute situations in pigs. Osteoporosis by classical definition means ''too little bone.'' The bone that is present is normal (Kaneko 1980). Others have defined osteoporosis as a pathological decrease in the volume of bone tissue per unit of volume organ (Fourman et al. 1968). In animals it is primarily of nutritional origin. Differentiation between osteomalacia and osteoporosis is difficult at best. In humans, osteoporosis has become a highly visible disease and is the most common cause of skeletal rarefraction in the elderly. Because pigs rarely reach the same physiological age as elderly humans, osteomalacia is more apt to be a problem than is osteoporosis. The exact cause of osteoporosis is unknown, but some factors associated with the onset of the condition are aging, accelerated bone loss from excess glucocorticoids, immobilization, vitamin C deficiency, iron overload, hypogonadism, malabsorption, hyperparathyroidism, and hyperthyroidism (Albanese 1977; Kaneko 1980; Paige 1983).

A proper Ca:P ratio is one of the major problems related to dietary adequacy of the two elements for swine. P is a rather expensive mineral element to add to swine diets; Ca is inexpensive. Thus, quite often swine diets approach or exceed the upper limits for Ca but barely meet the minimum requirements for P. The consequences of feeding excess Ca with a minimum level of P, thereby creating a wide ratio between the two, are poor weight gain and feed conversion and structural unsoundness (Peo 1976). Swine can perform reasonably well on high levels of dietary Ca as long as a desirable ratio exists between Ca and P (Libal et al. 1969). The optimum ratio appears to lie between 1 and 1.3:1, with outside limits of 0.9 and 1.6:1 (Combs et al. 1962b; Zimmerman et al. 1963; Peo 1976; Hays 1976; Henika 1978).

During the early part of this century, rickets commonly occurred in swine. Analysis of bone (Table 10.5) showed that it contained Ca and P in about a 2:1 ratio. Because cereal grains contain little Ca, the general recommendation at that time was to feed diets or mineral mixes with a Ca:P ratio similar to that found in bone. Reviews by Peo (1976), Hays (1976), and Kornegay (1985) on the role of Ca and P in swine nutrition certainly point out the fallacy of thinking that the ratio of Ca and P in bone is the ratio that should be in the feed. A more appropriate indicator is probably the composition of sows' milk (Table 10.5). The Ca:P ratio in sows' milk varies from 0.6 to 1.2:1. "You can't fool mother nature" is a rather true statement when one thinks about the purpose of sows' milk—to provide those nutrients needed for development of a young growing animal. If Ca and P were needed in a 2:1 ratio to optimize bone mineralization, it is logical to assume that the two elements would have been present in that ratio in milk.

Pigs fed varying levels of Ca and P respond in terms of gain, bone weight, and bone breaking strength according to the ratio of Ca and P fed. The data presented in Table 10.6 show how different traits respond to changes in ratio between the two elements. Varying Ca level seems to exert a greater influence (positive or negative) on the traits evaluated than does varying the level of P. However, the Ca:P ratio for swine is important (Henika 1978).

Table 10.5 Calcium and Phosphorus in Bone Ash and Sow's Milk

		Sow's Milk, Day of Lactation[a]			
Nutrient	*Bone Ash*[b]	*1*	*14*	*28*	*35*
Calcium (%)	36	0.05	0.25	0.15	0.18
Phosphorus (%)	17	0.09	0.22	0.14	0.15
Calcium:phosphorus ratio	2.1:1	0.6:1	1.14:1	1.07:1	1.2:1

[a] Data from Fahmy and Bernard (1971).

[b] Data from Maynard et al. (1975).

Table 10.6 Effect of Calcium:Phosphorus Ratio on Certain Traits of Swine

	Ca Levels (%)			
P (%)	*0.35*	*0.65*	*0.90*	*Average for P*[a]
		Average Daily Gain (g)		
0.30	690	663	534	631
0.50	754	754	708	735
0.70	690	745	772	740
Avg. for Ca[b]	713	722	672	
		Bone Weight (g)[c]		*Average for P*[d]
0.30	11.5	12.8	11.3	11.8
0.50	13.4	14.1	15.4	14.3
0.70	12.1	14.2	14.9	13.7
Avg. for Ca[e]	12.3	13.7	13.8	
		Bone Strength (kg)[f]		*Average for P*[g]
0.30	201	237	209	216
0.50	193	307	368	289
0.70	152	283	349	261
Avg. for Ca[h]	182	276	309	

[a] Linear and quadratic effect of P level ($P<.005$).
[b] Linear effect of Ca level ($P<.05$); Ca × P interaction ($P<.005$).
[c] Weight of dry, fat-free fourth metatarsal.
[d] Linear and quadratic effect of P level ($P<.025$).
[e] Linear effect of Ca level ($P<.05$).
[f] Breaking strength, kilogram of force, of dry, fat-free fourth metatarsal.
[g] Quadratic effect of P level ($P<.05$).
[h] Linear effect of Ca level ($P<.005$).
(Data from Peo 1967.)

VITAMIN D

Shortly after its discovery in 1922 (McCollum et al.), researchers found that vitamin D is a companion nutrient to Ca and P. Signs of vitamin D deficiency are similar to those manifested with Ca and P deficiency, making it difficult to distinguish the cause of the observed rickets or osteomalacia. Vitamin D exists in nature in two major forms: ergocalciferol, the plant source identified as vitamin D_2, and cholecalciferol, the animal source known as vitamin D_3. Both appear to be effective as a source of supplemental vitamin D for swine (Bethke et al. 1946) but recent evidence suggests that pigs discriminate in their metabolism of the two forms of vitamin D (Horst et al. 1982). Vitamins D_2 or D_3 arise from their previtamin forms by photoisomerization, an ultraviolet light-energy-dependent reaction (Lawson 1980).

Vitamin D administered in the diet is absorbed largely in the distal small intestine. The absorbed vitamin D is transported via the lymph-blood systems to the liver where it is converted to 25-OH-D_3 and probably secreted back into the blood stream. Evidence suggests that vitamin D is not stored to any large extent in the liver, since the blood of pigs contains 2.4 to 14.3 times the amount of vitamin D found in the liver (Quarterman et al. 1964). Unmetabolized calciferol is found in adipose tissue and voluntary muscle. The release of vitamin D from storage is probably accomplished by the partition characteristics of calciferol between the adipose tissue lipid phase and a specific binding protein in plasma (Mawer 1980).

Synthesis of 25-OH-D_3 occurs almost entirely in the liver. The hydroxylation reaction is carried out by a microsomal enzyme and involves the insertion of molecular oxygen by the use of reduced nicotinamide adenine dinucleotide phosphate (NADPH) as a cofactor (Lawson 1980). Plasma 25-OH-D_3 is an acceptable criterion of the vitamin D status of the animal. Although 25-OH-D_3 has all of the biological effects of D_3 (Lawson 1980), 1,25-$(OH)_2$-D_3 appears to be the active form. This form of D_3 is classified as a steroid hormone because it is produced in a single tissue (only the kidney) and has target tissues (intestines and bone). The conversion of 25-OH-D_3 to 1,25-$(OH)_2$-D_3 is accomplished through the action of 1,25-OH-D_3-1 hydroxylase in concert with the cofactors NADPH, ferredoxin, and a flavoprotein, the latter being an integral part of the hydroxylase enzyme. It appears that cytochrome P_{450} is not involved in the hydroxylation (Lawson 1980). Active D_3 stimulates Ca absorption and Ca mobilization from bone (see Figure 10.3). Low dietary Ca has been shown to markedly

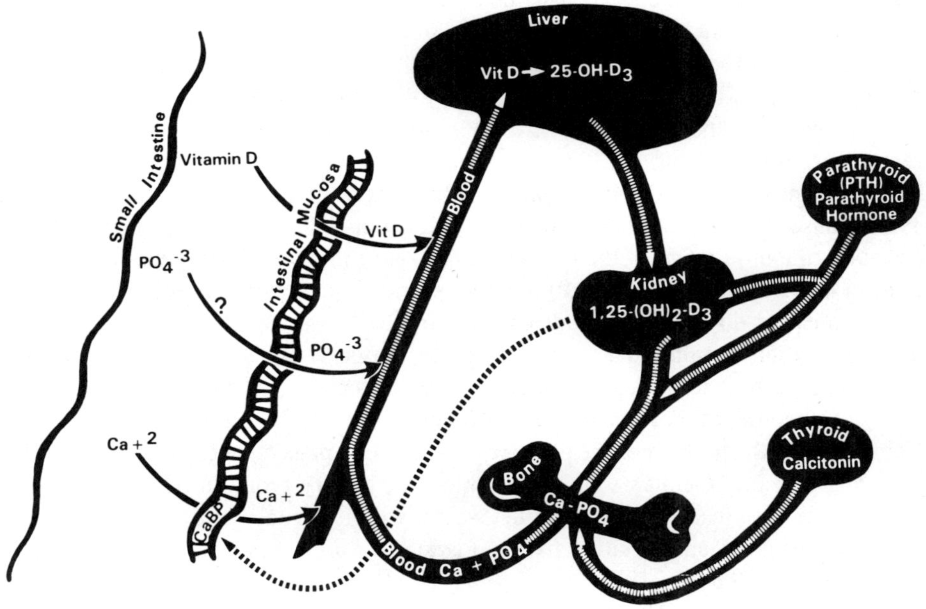

(Adapted, by permission of the authors, from Church and Pond. 1975. *Basic Animal Nutrition and Feeding.* p. 156. Corvallis, OR: O&B Books, as modified by J.D. Hancock. 1986. Nebraska Agricultural Research Division, University of Nebraska, Lincoln.)

FIGURE 10.3 *Known interrelationships among calcium, phosphorus, vitamin D_3, activated vitamin D_3, thyroid and parathyroid hormones, and body tissues.*

stimulate 1-hydroxylase activity, but the effect of dietary P levels on the enzyme remains controversial (Henry 1980). Similarly, the effect of parathyroid hormone on the metabolism of 25-(OH)-D_3 has not been thoroughly documented (Henry 1980; Arnaud 1983).

The interactions among Ca, P, vitamin D, and the thyroid-parathyroid hormones that have been elucidated and generally accepted are the pathways identified in Figure 10.3. As for vitamin D, calcium homeostasis is the only parameter for which there is unequivocal evidence for its essential role in the body (Toverud et al. 1987).

PRACTICAL CONSIDERATIONS IN CALCIUM, PHOSPHORUS, AND VITAMIN D NUTRITION

The NRC (1988) and ARC (1981) requirements for Ca, P, and vitamin D shown in Table 10.2 represent the best analytical summation of research findings concerning the requirements for these three nutrients. Also listed in Table 10.2, for comparison, are the results of a large survey on recommendations of requirements for these three nutrients by university and feed industry nutritionists (Overfield et al. 1986). Surprisingly, the requirements for Ca and P are reasonably close among the three groups except perhaps for breeding stock, particularly gestating sows. NRC and ARC requirements are expressed as minimum requirements. Regarding expensive nutrients, the NRC and ARC requirements are also the industry standard. With relatively inexpensive nutrients, overfortification is often the rule. Since P is an expensive nutrient, minimal fortification of brood sow diets was previously the general practice. Today, industry nutritionists are adding 25% more P to diets of gestating and lactating swine than is recommended by the NRC (1988); 15% more than is recommended by university researchers (Overfield et al. 1986).

The dam stores Ca during gestation to help meet the needs of lactation (Hansard 1965; Hansard et al. 1966; Itoh et al. 1967). If the mineral reserves are not filled during gestation, the physiology of the lactating sow is such that the skeleton will be depleted to meet the demand for Ca (and P) for milk production. A rarified skeleton can result in the so-called downer sow syndrome (Figure 10.4), which occurs in late lactation or shortly after weaning and is manifested by vertebral and femoral fractures commonly caused by excessive fighting as groups of females are mixed together or by riding one another as they come into heat (Nimmo et al. 1981b; Kornegay et al. 1985). Compounding the problem is the practice of selecting replacement females from market hogs and breeding them as soon as possible. The dietary requirements for Ca and P necessary to sustain an animal to market weight will not sustain a growing gilt through her first pregnancy and lactation (Nimmo et al. 1981a,b), although the issue remains controversial (Kornegay 1985).

The sows shown in Figure 10.4 had been fed the levels of Ca and P recommended by the NRC (1979) for growing-finishing swine from weaning through lactation. It is obvious that these levels of Ca and P (0.65% and 0.50% of the total diet) are not adequate for reproducing swine when limited in total feed intake (1.82 kg/day) through pregestation and gestation. Therefore, it is recommended that gilts selected from

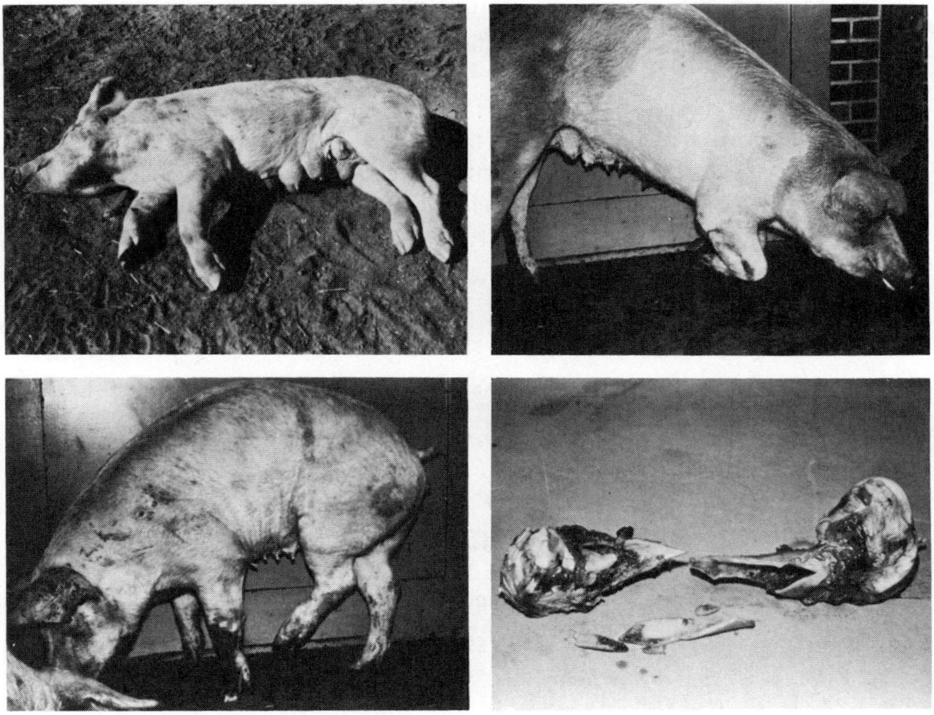

FIGURE 10.4 *Different manifestations of the downer-sow syndrome.* Clockwise from upper left: *prostration; buckled knees; spontaneous fracture of femur identified on necropsy; and failure to stand on one or more of the hind limbs. (Nebr. Agr. Res. Div. IANR, Univ. of Nebraska, Lincoln.)*

market stock be fed levels of Ca and P recommended for breeding stock for at least 60 days before breeding (Levis et al. 1985). Similarly, boars should be fed higher levels of Ca and P during their growth and development than are market hogs. The 1988 NRC recommendations for boars are, again, minimum requirements. From a practical standpoint, the requirements for Ca and P could be inflated by 30% without affecting animal performance and would be good insurance for strong skeletal development (Nimmo et al. 1981b).

The NRC and ARC requirements for vitamin D for all classes of swine along with the variances in requirements used by different university and industry nutritionists are shown in Table 10.2. Industry and university recommendations for vitamin D supplementation of swine diets exceed the NRC requirements by 320% and 17.5%, respectively (Overfield et al. 1986). Overfortification poses no particular problem unless formulation or mixing errors result in superlevels. Vitamin D is toxic at high levels (Table 10.3). The consequences of toxic doses of vitamin D are slow growth, poor feed conversion, bone abnormalities, calcification of the soft tissue, and death (Chineme et al. 1976; Long 1984; Hancock et al. 1986). Although the 5- to 50-kg pig can tolerate up to 44,000 IU D_3/kg diet, the practical maximum safe level is about 22,000 IU/kg diet, well above any intentional fortification levels (Hancock et al. 1986; Peo et al. 1986).

Calcium, phosphorus, and vitamin D are critical nutrients for growth and maintenance of the hard and soft tissues by the pig's body. They cannot be considered separately because of the known interacting forces that exist among them (Figures 10.1, 10.2, and 10.3). Recognizing this mutual relationship is essential for successful swine nutrition.

REFERENCES

Agricultural Research Council. 1981. *The Nutrient Requirements of Pigs.* Slough, England: Commonwealth Agricultural Bureaux.

Albanese, A.A. 1977. *Bone Loss, Causes, Detection and Therapy.* New York: Alan R. Liss, Inc.

Arnaud, C.D. 1983. In: *Assay of Calcium Regulating Hormones.* Bikle, D.D., (Ed.). pp. 1–19. New York: Springer-Verlag.

Avioli, L.V. 1972. *Arch. Intern. Med.* 129:345.

Bartter, F.C. 1964. In: *Mineral Metabolism.* Vol. 2, Part A. Comar, C.L., and F. Bronner (Eds.). pp. 315–339. New York: Academic Press.

Baustad, B., J. Teige, Jr., and S. Tollersrud. 1967. *Acta Vet. Scand.* 8:369.

Berry, R.K., et al. 1961. *J. Anim. Sci.* 20:433.

Bethke, R.M., et al. 1946. *Ohio Agric. Exp. Sta. Bul.* No. 667.

Boyd, R.D., D. Hall, and J.F. Wu. 1983. *J. Anim. Sci.* 57:396.

Brown, W.R., L. Krook, and W.G. Pond. 1966. *Cornell Vet.* 56:(Suppl. 1):1.

Bunch, R.J., M.J. Brinegar, and L.H. Neagle. 1969. *J. Anim. Sci.* 29:130.

Chineme, C.N., L. Krook, and W.G. Pond. 1976. *Cornell Vet.* 66:387.

Coalson, J.A., et al. 1972. *J. Anim. Sci.* 35:1194.

Combs, G.E. 1962a. *Feedstuffs.* 34:46.

Combs, G.E., et al. 1962b. *J. Anim. Sci.* 21:3.

Conrad, J.H., and W.M. Beeson. 1957. *J. Anim. Sci.* 16:589.

Costain, R.A., and L.E. Lloyd. 1962. *J. Anim. Sci.* 21:751.

Crampton, E.W., and L.E. Lloyd. 1959. *Fundamentals of Nutrition.* San Francisco: W.H. Freeman and Co.

Crenshaw, T.D., et al. 1981a. *J. Anim. Sci.* 52:1319.

Crenshaw, T.D., et al. 1981b. *J. Anim. Sci.* 53:827.

Cromwell, G.L., et al. 1970. *J. Anim. Sci.* 30:519.

Cromwell, G.L., et al. 1972. *J. Anim. Sci.* 34:746.

Cromwell, G.L., T.S. Stahly, and H.J. Moneque. 1984a. *Kentucky Agric. Exp. Sta. Prog. Rpt.* 174:17.

Cromwell, G.L., R.D. Ross, and T.S. Stahly. 1984b. *Feed Management* 35:23.

Cunningham, H.M., and G.J. Brisson. 1957. *J. Anim. Sci.* 16:573.

DeLuca, H.F., and H.K. Schnoes. 1976. *Ann. Rev. Biochem.* 45:631.

Doige, C.E., B.D. Owen, and J.H.L. Mills. 1975. *Can. J. Anim. Sci.* 55:147.

Eggert, R.C., W.T. Akers, and C.N. Huhtanen. 1959. *J. Anim. Sci.* 18:1505.

Fahmy, M.H., and C. Bernard. 1971. *Can. J. Anim. Sci.* 51:351.

Fitzpatrick, L.A., M.L. Brandi, and G.A. Aurbach. 1987. In: *Current Research on Calcium Regulating Hormones.* Cooper, C.W. (Ed.). pp. 21–30. Austin, TX: University of Texas Press.

Fourman, P., et al. 1968. *Calcium Metabolism and the Bone.* 2d ed. Oxford, England: Blackwell.

Fox, J., A.D. Care, and R. Swaminathan. 1978. *Br. J. Nutr.* 39:431.
Garel, J.M. 1987. In: *Current Research on Calcium Regulating Hormones.* Cooper, C.W. (Ed). pp. 67–78. Austin, TX: University of Texas Press.
Gillis, M.B., L.C. Norris, and G.F. Heuser. 1954. *J. Nutr.* 52:115.
Gueguen, L., and J.M. Perez. 1981. *Proc. Nutr. Soc.* 40:273.
Hadley, Mac E. 1984. *Endocrinology.* Englewood Cliffs, NJ: Prentice-Hall.
Hancock, J.D., et al. 1986. *J. Anim. Sci.* 63(Suppl. 1):268.
Hansard, S.L. 1965. In: *Proceedings of Symposium, Swine in Biomedical Research.* Bustad, L.K., and R.O. McClellan (Eds.). pp. 78–96. Seattle, WA: Frayn Printing Co.
Hansard, S.L., et al. 1966. *J. Nutr.* 89:335.
Harmon, B.G., et al. 1967. *J. Anim. Sci.* 26:1476.
Hart, E.B., and H. Steenbock. 1913. *J. Biol. Chem.* 14:75.
Hays, V.W. 1968. *Proc. Distillers Feed Res. Council* 23:48.
Hays, V.W. 1976. *Literature Review on Phosphorus in Swine Nutrition.* pp. 1–60. West Des Moines, IA: National Feed Ingredients Association.
Henika, R.G. 1978. *Nutr. News* 41:9.
Henry, H.L. 1980. In: *Vitamin D, Molecular Biology and Clinical Nutrition.* Norman, A.W. (Ed.). pp. 127–148. New York: Marcel Dekker.
Hoefer, J.A., et al. 1960. *J. Anim. Sci.* 19:249.
Horst, R.L., et al. 1982. *Biochem. J.* 204:185.
Irving, J.T. 1964. In: *Mineral Metabolism.* Vol. 2, Part A. pp. 249–313. New York: Academic Press.
Itoh, H., et al. 1967. *J. Anim. Sci.* 26:335.
Kaneko, J.J. 1980. *Clinical Biochemistry of Domestic Animals.* 3rd ed. New York: Academic Press.
Koch, M.E., and D.C. Mahan. 1985. *J. Anim. Sci.* 60:699.
Koch, M.E., and D.C. Mahan. 1986. *J. Anim. Sci.* 62:163.
Koch, M.E., D.C. Mahan, and J.E. Corley. 1984. *J. Anim. Sci.* 59:1546.
Kornegay, E.T. 1985. *Calcium and Phosphorus in Animal Nutrition.* West Des Moines, IA: National Feed Ingredients Association.
Krider, J.L., and W.E. Carroll. 1971. *Swine Production.* 4th ed. New York: McGraw Book Co.
Krusemark, L.L., et al. 1968. *J. Anim. Sci.* 27:1153.
Lawson, D.E.M. 1980. In: *Vitamin D, Molecular Biology and Clinical Nutrition.* Norman, A.W. (Ed.). pp. 93–126. New York: Marcel Dekker.
Levis, D.G., et al. 1985. *Neb. Agric. Ext. Cir.* EC84:212.
Lewis, P.K., Jr., W.G. Hoekstra, and R.H. Grummer. 1957. *J. Anim. Sci.* 16:578.
Lewis, P.K., Jr., et al. 1956. *J. Anim. Sci.* 15:741.
Libal, G.W., et al. 1969. *J. Anim. Sci.* 28:331.
Libal, G.W., et al. 1977. *S. Dakota Agric. Exp. Sta. AS Series* 77–37.
Lindley, C.E. 1967. *Hog Farm Mgmt.* 4:22.
Logomarisino, J.V., et al. 1969. *J. Anim. Sci.* 29:139.
Logomarisino, J.V., et al. 1974. *J. Anim. Sci.* 39:544.
Long, G.G. 1984. *J. Am. Vet. Med. Assoc.* 184:164.
Luecke, R.W., et al. 1956. *J. Anim. Sci.* 15:347.
Mawer, E.B. 1980. In: *Vitamin D, Molecular Biology and Clinical Nutrition.* Norman, A.W. (Ed.). pp. 149–196. New York: Marcel Dekker.
Maxson, P.F., and D.C. Mahan. 1983. *J. Anim. Sci.* 56:1124.
Maynard, L.A., and R.C. Miller. 1927. *Proc. Soc. Anim. Prod.* 27:68.
Maynard, L.A., et al. 1975. *Animal Nutrition.* 7th ed. New York: McGraw-Hill Book Co.
McCollum, E.V., et al. 1922. *J. Biol. Chem.* 54:249.
Miller, E.R., D.E. Ullrey, and R.W. Luecke. 1966. *Proceedings of the 7th International Congress of Nutrition.* Vols. 1–5. Braunsweig, West Germany: Friedr. Vieweg and Sohn Verlag.
Moore, J.H., and C. Tyler. 1955a. *Br. J. Nutr.* 9:63.

Moore, J.H., and C. Tyler. 1955b. *Br. J. Nutr.* 9:81.
Morrison, F.B. 1959. *Feeds and Feeding.* 22d ed. Clinton, IA: Morrison Publishing Co.
Moser, R.L., et al. 1980. *J. Anim. Sci.* 51:89.
National Research Council. 1979. *Nutrient Requirements of Swine.* 8th ed. Washington, DC: National Academy of Sciences.
National Research Council. 1988. *Nutrient Requirements of Swine.* 9th ed. Washington, DC: National Academy of Sciences.
Nelson, T.S., L.W. Ferrara, and N.L. Storer. 1968. *Poult. Sci.* 47:1372.
Newland, H.W., et al. 1958. *J. Anim. Sci.* 17:886.
Nimmo, R.D., et al. 1981a. *J. Anim. Sci.* 52:1330.
Nimmo, R.D., et al. 1981b. *J. Anim. Sci.* 52:1343.
Overfield, J., et al. 1986. *Proceedings Nutrition Symposium, November 12–13.* pp. 1–29. St. Louis, MO: National Feed Ingredients Association.
Paige, D.M. 1983. *Manual of Clinical Nutrition.* Pleasantville, NJ: Nutrition Publications, Inc.
Partridge, I.G. 1980. *Proc. Nutr. Soc.* 39:185.
Peo, E.R., Jr. 1976. *Literature Review on Calcium in Swine Nutrition.* pp. 1–65. West Des Moines, IA: National Feed Ingredients Association.
Peo, E.R., Jr., et al. 1967. *J. Anim. Sci.* 26:910.
Peo, E.R., Jr., et al. 1986. *Neb. Swine Rep.* EC-86-219:14.
Pike, R.L., and M.L. Brown. 1984. *Nutrition, An Integrated Approach.* New York: J. Wiley and Sons, Inc.
Pond, W.G., and J.R. Jones. 1964. *J. Anim. Sci.* 23:1057.
Pond, W.G., et al. 1982. *Nutr. Rep. Int.* 26:1027.
Quarterman, J., A.C. Dalgarno, and A. Adam. 1964. *Br. J. Nutr.* 18:79.
Reinhard, M.K., et al. 1976. *J. Anim. Sci.* 43:770.
Reinhart, G.A., and D.C. Mahan. 1986. *J. Anim. Sci.* 63:457.
Rickes, E.L., et al. 1948. *Science* 107:396.
Ross, R.D., G.L. Cromwell, and T.S. Stahly. 1984. *J. Anim. Sci.* 59:125.
Stanbury, S.W. 1980. In: *Vitamin D, Molecular Biology and Clinical Nutrition.* Norman, A.W. (Ed.). pp. 251–308. New York: Marcel Dekker, Inc.
Stevenson, J.W., and I.P. Earle. 1956. *J. Anim. Sci.* 15:1036.
Stockland, W.L., and L.G. Blaylock. 1973. *J. Anim. Sci.* 37:906.
Tillman, A.D. 1966. *Proceedings of the 14th Annual Pfizer Research Conference.* Recent developments in beef cattle feeding. p. 7. Terre Haute, IN: Pfizer & Co., Inc.
Toverud, S.U., A. Boass, and S.A. Clark. 1987. In: *Current Research on Calcium Regulating Hormones.* Cooper, C.W. (Ed.). pp. 233–240. Austin, TX: University of Texas Press.
Ullrey, D.E., et al. 1967. *J. Anim. Sci.* 26:1024.
Veum, T.L., L.D. Kinter, and M.K. Schmidt. 1970. *J. Anim. Sci.* 31:1029.
Wahlstrom, R.C. 1957. *S. Dakota Agric. Exp. Sta. Cir.* 137.
Wahlstrom, R.C., and L. DeGoey. 1968. *S. Dakota Agric. Exp. Sta. AS Series* 68–32.
Wahlstrom, R.C., and J.F. Fredrikson. 1969. *S. Dakota Agric. Exp. Sta. AS Series* 69:37.
Wahlstrom, R.C., G.W. Libal, and S.L. Robbins. 1975. *S. Dakota Agric. Exp. Sta. AS Series* 75:52.
Wahlstrom, R.C., et al. 1982. *Nutr. Rep. Int.* 26:873.
Washam, R.D., et al. 1968. *J. Anim. Sci.* 27:1159.
White, R.G. 1971. The Relationship of Dietary Calcium and Phosphorus to Atrophic Rhinitis in Growing-Finishing Swine. M.S. thesis. University of Nebraska, Lincoln.
Whiting, F., and L.M. Bezeau. 1958. *Can. J. Anim. Sci.* 38:109.
Zimmerman, D.R., et al. 1963. *J. Anim. Sci.* 22:658.

Chapter 11

Sodium, Potassium, Magnesium, and Chloride in Swine Nutrition

T.D. Crenshaw

The inorganic elements required in macronutrient quantities (> 100 mg/kg of the diet) include calcium (Ca), phosphorus (P), sodium (Na), potassium (K), chloride (Cl), and magnesium (Mg). The Ca and P requirements are two- to eightfold greater than Na, K, and Cl requirements, and fifteenfold greater than Mg requirements (Table 11.1). Yet, the body regulates fluid concentrations such that Na, K, and Cl concentrations are considerably higher than Ca concentrations and in some compartments higher than P concentrations. Because of these differences in dietary requirements and the abundance of K and Mg in commonly utilized feed ingredients, scant attention is usually paid to Na, K, Cl, and Mg in swine nutrition. These nutrients are often ignored, but they are essential for life. Within 3 days after consuming a diet essentially devoid of any one of these elements, reductions in feed intake are observed.

This chapter describes the physiological roles of Na, K, Cl, and Mg and factors that affect their requirements. Although Ca and P have been discussed in Chapter 10, these elements will be mentioned again as they interrelate with Na, K, Cl, and Mg.

CHEMICAL PROPERTIES AND PHYSIOLOGICAL FUNCTIONS

Physiological roles of Na, K, Cl, and Mg can be grouped into functions that involve osmotic balance, acid-base balance, membrane potential, substrate transport, and enzymatic cofactors. The functions of each element are uniquely related to its chemical properties and the homeostatic regulation of compartments within the body.

Chemical Properties

Chemical properties of Na, K, Cl, and Mg are listed in Table 11.2. Unless specified otherwise in this chapter, the elements are considered to be in the ionic state because

Table 11.1 Requirements and Consumption of Macro Minerals by Ten-Kilogram Pigs

	Minimum Requirement[a]		*Daily Intake*[b]	
Element	*g*	*%*	*g*	*mmol*
Ca	6.6	0.70	4.63	116
P	5.7	0.60	3.97	41
Na	1.0	0.10	1.99	87
Cl	0.8	0.08	2.32	65
K	2.5	0.26	4.97	127
Mg	0.4	0.04	1.10	45

[a] Values are expressed as either g/d or as a percent of a corn-soybean meal diet (90% dry matter) recommended for 10- to 20-kg pigs (NRC 1988).

[b] Assumes a typical corn-soybean meal diet with a feed intake of 662 g/d (NRC 1986) for a 10-kg pig. Feed intake was predicted from the digestible energy intake (DE) where DE = 462 BW (body weight in kilograms) − 9.72 BW^2 − 1529 (NRC 1986).

Table 11.2 Chemical Properties of Macronutrient Elements

				Weight Equivalents[b]	
Element	*Atomic Weight*[a]	*Valence*	*Ionic Radius*	*mmol*	*mEq*
Na	22.99	+1	0.95	43.50	43.50
Mg	24.31	+2	0.65	41.14	82.27
K	39.10	+1	1.33	25.58	25.58
Ca	40.08	+2	0.99	24.95	49.90
Cl	35.45	−1	1.81	28.20	28.20
P	30.97	—[c]	—	10.40[d]	18.71

[a] The phosphorus present in biological systems exists as a phosphate in either dibasic (molecular weight = 95.97) or monobasic (molecular weight = 96.97) ion complexes.

[b] Equivalent to 1 g of each element.

[c] At physiological pH (7.4) the ratio of dibasic ($HPO_4^{=}$) to monobasic ($H_2PO_4^{-}$) phosphate ions yields a net valence of 1.8.

[d] One gram equivalent of phosphate at a pH of 7.4.

this is the state in which they participate in biological reactions. Certainly the covalently bound forms of Ca and P in bone mineral and the high-energy phosphate bonds are important, but the predominant state of Na, K, Cl, and Mg in the body is ionic.

Because of the biological importance of the ionic state, concentrations of Na, K, Cl, and Mg are best expressed as equivalents rather than weight. An equivalent is the molecular weight times the valence. Na, K, and Cl are monovalent, so the number of equivalents equals the number of moles. Divalent ions such as Ca, Mg, and dibasic phosphate provide two equivalents for each mole. Table 11.2 lists the equivalents for 1 g of each element.

Atomic weight comparisons of the macroelements suggest a pairing of Na and Mg, K and Ca, and Cl and P. The difference within each pair can be attributed to one or two protons and the number of associated electrons. For example, Na and Mg have similar atomic weights (these differ by approximately 1 g atom) but Mg has one additional electron in the M orbital. In physiological systems, phosphate ions exist in a ratio of dibasic ($HPO_4^{=}$) to monobasic ($H_2PO_4^{-}$) phosphate. The ratio of the two phosphate ions can be calculated using the Henderson-Hasselbalch equation:

$$[pH = pKa + \log (HPO_4^{=}/H_2PO_4^{-})]$$

The negative log of the dissociation constant (pKa) for an inorganic phosphate solution is 7.12, but with corrections for ionic strength and temperature a pKa of 6.8 is generally accepted for phosphate in physiological fluids. Using a pKa of 6.8 and a pH of 7.4, the concentration of dibasic phosphate would be approximately four times greater than the concentration of monobasic phosphate. Most phosphate ions are located intracellularly where the pH may range from 7.4 to 7.8. The dibasic to monobasic phosphate ratio would be greater than 6:1. Typically, a valence of 1.8 is used for calculating phosphate equivalents in physiological fluids.

Among the biologically important cations (Table 11.2), Mg has the smallest ionic radius and readily forms complexes with other ions and dipolar molecules (Aikawa 1981). The more predominant Mg complexes involve phosphate and carboxylate anions. The divalent strength and small size of Mg contribute to its role in biological phosphorylation reactions. While Ca has the same valence and forms complexes, the Ca complexes are stronger than Mg complexes and not easily dissociated. Contrary to Mg, compounds of Na, K, and Cl readily dissociate in aqueous solutions and rarely form complexes in biological systems. The strong dissociation constants of these ions contribute to their role as electrolytes in the regulation of osmotic and acid-base balance.

Body Composition and Compartments

Based on chemical analysis, the pig is composed of three to five times more Ca and P than Na, K, or Cl and greater than ten times more Ca and P than Mg (Table 11.3).

Table 11.3 Distribution of Macro Minerals in a Ten-Kilogram Pig

	Total[a]		*Exchangeable*[b]	
Element	*g*	*mmol*	*%*	*mmol*
Ca	85.0	2121	1	21
P	53.1	1715	20	343
Na	12.0	522	70	339
Cl	13.4	378	85	321
K	19.8	506	98	496
Mg	3.2	132	50	66

[a] Total amounts of each element were calculated from regression equations (Mudd et al. 1969).
[b] Estimates of the percent exchangeable macro minerals are based on the amount of each mineral in soft tissue.

Relative to daily amounts (g) consumed (Table 11.1), a pig contains 13 to 18 times more Ca and P, but only three to six times the amounts of Na, K, Cl, or Mg consumed per day. The proportions of body element content to daily consumption reflect the selective retention and storage of Ca and P in the skeleton, and also indicate that pigs cannot adapt to a diet deficient in Na, K, Cl, and Mg as easily as they can to a diet deficient in Ca and P. The body accumulation of Na, K, Cl, and Mg is under rigid endocrine control with little storage, but Ca and P can be accumulated in bone, which can serve as a reservoir to supply Ca and P when dietary intakes are insufficient.

The mineral elements are distributed among three pools within the body: extracellular fluid, intracellular fluid, and the bone. Minerals within the fluid pools and a small fraction of the bone pool are readily exchangeable with ingested elements. In the bone pool, minerals that are covalently bound in hydroxyapatite-like crystals are not rapidly exchanged. The proportions of each element within the bone pool are estimated in Table 11.3. Based on estimates of the elements present in the readily exchangeable pools (i.e., soft tissue), K is the most abundant and Ca the least abundant. Almost all the K is in the intracellular fluid, and it accumulates in the body in proportion to protein accretion and water. Ninety-nine percent of the body Ca is located in bone and is not readily exchangeable.

There are major differences in the ionic composition of the extracellular and intracellular fluid pools (Table 11.4). Na^+ comprises $>90\%$ of the cations in extracellular fluid and Cl^- comprises approximately 70% of the anions. In the intracellular fluid, the distribution shifts such that Na^+ contributes $<5\%$ of the cations. K^+ contributes $>75\%$ of the intracellular cations. Phosphate is the major intracellular anion. Ca^{++} and Mg^{++} are of minor importance in the total balance of electrolytes, although fluid levels of these cations are rigidly regulated.

Regulation and Function

The large differences in the ionic composition of the fluid compartments imply deliberate regulation by the body. Simple diffusion of molecules across the semipermeable cell membranes that separate these compartments would result in an equilibrium of ions between the extracellular and intracellular fluids. Active transport mechanisms exist in the membranes to maintain the concentration gradients and the unequal distributions of ions within each compartment. Maintenance of these pools is essential for regulation of osmotic balance, cation-anion balance, and the membrane potentials required for substrate transport.

One of the major active transport complexes in cell membranes is Na-K ATPase. This protein complex transports Na from within the cell into the extracellular fluid in exchange for K. Energy expenditure for ion transport has been estimated at 30% to 40% of basal energy (Baldwin et al. 1980). Adjustments in dietary cation-anion balance would probably not alter the amount of energy expenditure for ion transport. Most of the energy consumed by ion transport can be attributed to that required to counteract passive diffusion and maintain concentration gradients.

Table 11.4 Average Cation and Anion Concentration of Physiological Fluids

	Body Fluid Compartments[a]		
	Extracellular	*Interstitial*	*Intracellular*
Cations			
Na^+	142	145	10
K^+	4	4	159
Ca^{++}	5	3	1
Mg^{++}	2	2	40
Total	153	154	210
Anions			
Cl^-	103	117	3
HCO_3^-	28	31	10
$HPO_4^=$, $H_2PO_4^-$	4	4	75
$SO_4^=$	1	1	2
Protein	17	—	45
Others	—	1	75
Total	153	154	210

[a] Concentration expressed as mEq/L.

(Adapted, by permission, from Berliner and Giebisch 1979, and Guyton 1981.)

The kidneys function to regulate the body content of Na, K, and Cl by changes in glomerular filtration rate and the fractional reabsorption of ions. The kidneys also contain transporters that, under certain circumstances, actively secrete ions into the collecting ducts. The body does not seem to control the levels of Na, K, or Cl absorbed. Thus, the body depends on the kidneys for homeostatic maintenance of Na, K, and Cl. The regulation of body Mg levels is not well understood. Some evidence indicates that Mg is influenced by the same factors that influence Ca and P homeostasis (Pointillart and Gueguen 1978).

Two preeminent physiological roles of the macrominerals involve osmolarity and cation-anion (acid-base) balance. The numerous other physiological functions, while important, will not be compromised unless severe deficiencies or toxicities occur. The homeostatic regulation of osmolarity and cation-anion balance ensures adequate concentrations of ions for most physiological processes. The major endocrine control systems affecting osmolarity and cation-anion balance include the antidiuretic hormone system, the renin-angiotensin system, and the aldosterone system.

Cellular osmolarity is simply the concentration of molecules, regardless of charge, within a semipermeable membrane. Na and Cl contribute $>80\%$ of the extracellular fluid osmotic load while K contributes 50% of the intracellular osmotic load. Regulation of cation and anion concentrations to maintain osmotic fluid balance predominates over mechanisms involved in the regulation of acid-base balance (Schwartz et al. 1968). Serum Na levels play the major role in maintenance of osmotic pressure. The osmoreceptors located in the hypothalamus respond only to plasma Na, with no response to changes in plasma K and only slight response to changes in plasma urea or glucose concentrations (Guyton 1981).

Secondary to effects on osmolarity, the fluid balance of Na, K, and Cl affects acid-base homeostasis. These elements are considered to be strong ions, since they are essentially 100% dissociated in physiological fluids. Acid-base balance is affected by the strong ion difference (SID). The SID (Steward 1980) is the sum of all the strong base (cation) concentrations minus the sum of all the strong acid (anion) concentrations. In mammalian fluids, the SID is always positive and provides an excess of about 50 mEq/L. The excess cations are balanced by organic anions (not strong anions) so that electroneutrality is maintained. Additional effects of cation-anion balance on acid-base homeostasis may be attributed to compensation via changes in renal amino acid metabolism and bone accretion.

The nutritional application of cation-anion balance via manipulation of dietary mineral balance must consider the influence of cation-anion balance on homeostasis, particularly renal compensation. Typical diets consumed by swine are acidogenic (Crenshaw and Golz 1986) even though the diets contain approximately 200 mEq excess cations per kilogram based on the summation of dietary Na + K − Cl. The kidneys of pigs fed a typical corn-soybean meal diet compensate for excess acid so that blood pH and partial pressure of carbon dioxide are maintained within normal ranges. Thus, a chronic rather than acute acid load is imposed on the animal, and the kidneys compensate to maintain homeostasis. Evidence for renal compensation to a chronic acid load includes a urine pH <7.2 with a normal blood pH. Under conditions of a chronic acid load the bicarbonate buffer system does not contribute to the long-term disposal of H^+. The carbon dioxide and water excreted by a respiratory response to an acid load are offset by renal bicarbonate (and an associated H^+) production to replenish circulating bicarbonate levels (Guyton 1981). The kidneys are responsible for the long-term regulation of acid excretion, but the kidneys cannot concentrate H^+ below a urine pH of 4.5 (Ganong 1973). Hydrogen ions are eliminated via renal ammoniagenesis from glutamine and monobasic phosphate excretion (Halperin and Jungas 1983; Brosnan and Brosnan 1982). Under an acid load Na is reabsorbed with bicarbonate to maintain blood base levels, but urinary K, and possibly Cl excretion, are increased.

NUTRIENT ALLOWANCES

The amounts of supplemental Na, K, Cl, and Mg required for swine diets composed of natural ingredients depend on the concentration and availability of these ions within the feed ingredients, the requirements of the animal, and the interactions of other nutrients with these ions. Because of the chemical properties of Na, K, and Cl, there is little reason to suspect that these elements would not be readily available to the animal for absorption (Peeler 1972; Miller and Kornegay 1983; Crenshaw 1983). Indeed, Combs and Miller (1985) reported that the availabilities of K in corn and soybean meal were 90% to 95% and 97%, respectively, as available as the K of potassium acetate. The amounts of these minerals absorbed will depend on the nature of the diet and resulting water flux along the intestinal tract. Net secretion of endogenous Na, K, and Cl occurred in the proximal intestine of 20-kg pigs, and different amounts were absorbed from purified versus natural ingredient diets (Partridge 1978).

Most plant ingredients included in swine diets accumulate K and Mg in sufficient quantities to meet minimal requirements (NRC 1988), but the same plants are deficient in Na and Cl. The K content in plants is generally proportional to the plant protein content. Protein feedstuffs contain three to six times more K than most cereal grains but even the cereal grains exceed K and Mg concentrations required for swine growth. Thus, there is little likelihood of a K or Mg deficiency when natural feed ingredients are provided. Most experiments designed to evaluate minimum requirements of K and Mg have used purified diets.

Using purified or semipurified diets, minimum requirements of K have been found to range from 0.15% to 0.35% of the diet (Hughes and Ittner 1942; Meyer et al. 1950; Jensen et al. 1961; Combs et al. 1985). Minimum Mg requirements are approximately 0.03% to 0.04% of the diet (Bartley et al. 1961; Miller et al. 1965a,b,c). Supplementing natural ingredient diets with inorganic sources of K or Mg has not improved growth performance in swine (Mayo et al. 1959; Svajgr et al. 1969; Krider et al. 1975; Patience et al. 1987a; Jesse et al. 1988; Brumm and Schricker 1989).

Improvements in growth performance have been observed when diets consisting of natural ingredients were supplemented with Na and Cl (Hagsten and Perry 1976; Hagsten et al. 1976; Alcantara et al. 1980). The minimum Na requirements for growing pigs range from 0.08% to 0.10% of the diet (Meyer et al. 1950; Alcantara et al. 1980; Honeyfield and Froseth 1985; Honeyfield et al. 1985). The minimum Cl requirement is probably 0.08% (Honeyfield and Froseth 1985), but very few experiments with pigs have been designed to determine Cl requirements specifically. Conclusions from most of the earlier research indicated that Cl requirements were met if salt (NaCl) was supplemented at a level (0.20%) to meet the Na requirement. More recently, Honeyfield et al. (1985) suggested that Na and Cl should be considered separately in diet formulations rather than assuming that Cl levels are met with NaCl additions. The investigators concluded that Na and Cl should be provided in a 1:1 molar ratio in the total diet. Since NaCl provides a 1:1 ratio and is the major source of Na and Cl in natural ingredient diets, attention to the ratio would only be required if ingredients with excessive levels of either Na or Cl were intentionally included in the diet.

Limited research has been directed toward establishing requirements for gestating or lactating swine. Recommended (NRC 1988) levels of Na, K, Cl, and Mg are based largely on extrapolation of work with growing animals. Cromwell et al. (1989) reported a depression in birth weights and weaning weights of offspring from sows when dietary NaCl levels were decreased from 0.50% to 0.25%. In a second experiment, however, there were no differences in performance when NaCl levels were decreased from 0.25% to 0.125%. The workers concluded that sows should be fed diets with 0.50% NaCl.

Perhaps more important than establishing minimum requirements for Na, K, Cl, and Mg is an understanding of the interactions among these elements and with other nutrients. Interactions between Na and Cl (Honeyfield et al. 1985) and between K and

Cl (Crenshaw and Golz 1986) have been reported in experiments conducted with pigs. Based on work with poultry and limited research with pigs, Austic and Calvert (1981) suggested that swine diets should be formulated to provide 250 mEq excess cations/kg of diet based on the summation of Na + K − Cl. Patience et al. (1987a) observed a depression in the growth rate of swine fed diets with excess anions (−85 mEq/kg) but no difference in the performance of animals fed diets that ranged from 0 to 341 mEq excess cations. Variation in the magnitude of response to altered dietary Na, K, and Cl levels may be due to variation in the quality of protein and the relative rates of tissue accretion in the animals. Growth performance was improved in pigs fed diets with deficient protein or lysine levels when the deficient diets were supplemented with Na or K (Leibholz et al. 1966; Austic and Calvert 1981). The beneficial response is apparently not due to improvements in nitrogen, energy, or amino acid digestibility (Moughan and Smith 1984; Patience et al. 1986) or to apparent shifts in the digestibility of other macrominerals (Patience et al. 1987b). Based on the physiological functions of Na, K, and Cl and the major role of the kidneys in the regulation of these ions, the beneficial responses are most likely mediated through changes in renal metabolism.

Toxic dietary levels of Na, K, Cl, and Mg have not been defined for swine (NRC 1980). The maximum tolerable levels for swine suggested by the National Research Council (1980) include 8% NaCl, 3% K, and 0.3% Mg. The previous dietary level to which the animal was adapted will influence the short-term response to excessive levels. Both the quality and quantity of water available to the pig will influence the animals' response to excessive mineral levels. Water restriction will create a salt toxicity at dietary sodium chloride levels that do not alter animal performance if ample water is available to the animal (Bohstedt and Grummer 1954). Australian recommendations for pigs (CSIRO 1987) indicate that water should not contain more than 6000 mg/L total dissolved salts but also acknowledge that pigs can consume larger quantities of minerals if previously adjusted to high mineral intakes. Apparently the pig can excrete large quantities of minerals if ample water is provided and the minerals are balanced with a fixed counter ion.

REFERENCES

Aikawa, J.K. 1981. *Magnesium: Its Biological Significance.* Boca Raton, FL: CRC Press, Inc.
Alcantara, P.F., et al. 1980. *J. Anim. Sci.* 50:1092.
Arnauld, J., and P.A. LaChance. 1980. *J. Nutr.* 110:2480.
Austic, R.E., and C.C. Calvert. 1981. *Fed. Proc.* 40:63.
Baldwin, R.L., et al. 1980. *J. Anim. Sci.* 51:1416.
Bartley, J.C., et al. 1961. *J. Anim. Sci.* 20:137.
Berliner, R.W., and G. Giebisch. 1979. "Body fluids and the excretion of urine." In: *Best and Taylor's Physiological Basis of Medical Practice.* 10th ed. Brodeck, J.R. (Ed). Baltimore: Williams and Wilkins Co.
Bohstedt, G., and R.H. Grummer. 1954. *J. Anim. Sci.* 13:933.
Brosnan, J.T., and M.E. Brosnan. 1982. *Adv. Nutr. Res.* 4:77.
Brumm, M.C., and B.R. Schricker. 1989. *J. Anim. Sci.* 67:1411.
Combs, N.R., and E.R. Miller. 1985. *J. Anim. Sci.* 60:715.
Combs, N.R., et al. 1985. *J. Anim. Sci.* 60:709.

Crenshaw, T.D. 1983. *Potassium in Nonruminant Nutrition.* West Des Moines, IA: National Feed Ingredients Association.
Crenshaw, T.D., and D.I. Golz. 1986. *Proceedings of the 9th Annual International Mineral Nutrition Conference.* Rexadale, Canada.
Cromwell, G.L., et al. 1989. *J. Anim. Sci.* 67:374.
CSIRO. 1987. *Feeding Standards for Australian Livestock. Pigs.* East Melbourne, Australia: CSIRO.
Ganong, W.F. 1973. *Review of Medical Physiology.* 6th ed. Los Altos, CA: Lange Medical Publications.
Guyton, A.C. 1981. *Textbook of Medical Physiology.* 6th ed. Philadelphia: W.B. Saunders, Co.
Hagsten, I., and T.W. Perry. 1976. *J. Anim. Sci.* 42:1191.
Hagsten, I., et al. 1976. *J. Anim. Sci.* 42:12.
Halperin, M.L., and R.L. Jungas. 1983. *Kidney Int.* 24:709.
Honeyfield, D.C., and J.A. Froseth. 1985. *J. Nutr.* 115:1366.
Honeyfield, D.C., et al. 1985. *J. Anim. Sci.* 60:691.
Hughes, E.H., and N.R. Ittner. 1942. *J. Agric. Res.* 64:189.
Jensen, A.H., et al. 1961. *J. Anim. Sci.* 20:464.
Jesse, G.W., et al. 1988. *J. Anim. Sci.* 66:1325.
Krider, J.L., et al. 1975. *J. Anim. Sci.* 40:1027.
Leibholz, J.M., et al. 1966. *J. Anim. Sci.* 25:37.
Mayo, R.H., et al. 1959. *J. Anim. Sci.* 18:264.
Meyer, J.H., et al. 1950. *J. Anim. Sci.* 9:300.
Miller, E.R., et al. 1965a. *J. Nutr.* 85:13.
Miller, E.R., et al. 1965b. *J. Nutr.* 85:347.
Miller, E.R., et al. 1965c. *J. Nutr.* 85:209.
Miller, E.R., and E.T. Kornegay. 1983. *J. Anim. Sci.* 57(Suppl. 2):315.
Moughan, P.J., and W.C. Smith. 1984. *J. Sci. Food Agric.* 35:1183.
Mudd, A.J., et al. 1969. *J. Agric. Sci.* 73:181.
NRC. 1980. *Mineral Tolerance of Domestic Animals.* Washington, DC: National Academy Press.
NRC. 1986. *Predicting Feed Intake of Food Producing Animals.* Washington, DC: National Academy Press.
NRC. 1988. *Nutrient Requirements of Swine.* 9th ed. Washington, DC: National Academy of Sciences.
Partridge, I.G. 1978. *Br. J. Nutr.* 39:527.
Patience, J.F., et al. 1986. *Nutr. Res.* 6:263.
Patience, J.F., et al. 1987a. *Nutr. Res.* 64:457.
Patience, J.F., et al. 1987b. *Nutr. Res.* 64:1079.
Peeler, H.T. 1972. *J. Anim. Sci.* 35:695.
Pointillart, A., and L. Gueguen. 1978. *Ann. Biol. Anim. Biochem. Biophys.* 18:1247.
Schwartz, W.B., et al. 1968. *N. Engl. J. Med.* 279:630.
Steward, P.A. 1980. *How to Understand Acid-Base.* New York: Elsevier.
Svajgr, A.J., et al. 1969. *J. Anim. Sci.* 29:439.

Chapter 12

Vitamin E and Selenium in Swine Nutrition

D.C. Mahan

HISTORICAL PERSPECTIVE

Selenium (Se) and vitamin E are recognized as important dietary constituents for swine, but our understanding of their biochemical roles has changed dramatically over the past three decades. In 1922, Evans and Bishop identified a fat-soluble compound categorized as an antisterility vitamin that today is generically termed vitamin E. Selenium was, however, initially characterized as a toxic element, causing lameness and death of livestock that consumed certain range plants in the North Central plains of the United States (Franke 1934).

It was not until 1957 (Schwarz and Foltz) that Se was established as a dietary essential. It was with the subsequent discovery of glutathione peroxidase (GSH-Px) by Mills (1957) and the later discovery of Se as an integral component of this enzyme (Rotruck et al. 1973) that research escalated in both laboratory and domesticated animals.

It is now recognized that both nutrients are metabolic and dietary essentials, that an interrelationship exists between them, that other factors can influence their availability and metabolism, and that they are essential for the health and well-being of livestock.

SOURCES

Soil Factors Affecting Selenium Availability

Vast amounts of information have been collected on Se concentration in feedstuffs throughout the world. The central region of the United States, extending into central

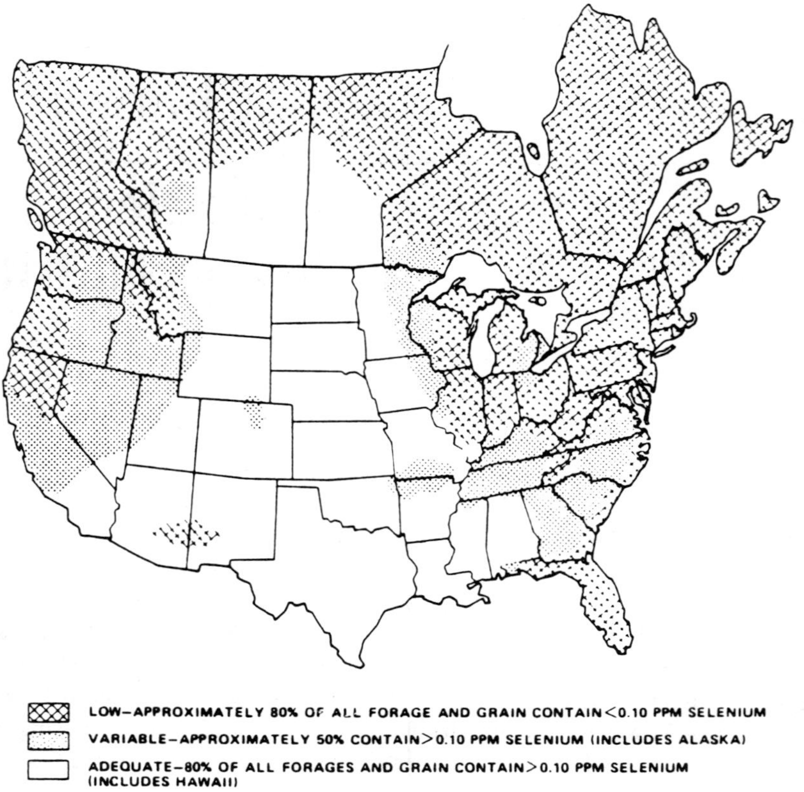

(Reprinted, by permission, from NRC 1983.)

FIGURE 12.1 *Regional distribution of forages and grain containing low, variable, or adequate levels of selenium in the United States and Canada.*

Canada, can produce crops with adequate, and in some cases, high, Se concentrations, whereas feedstuffs raised in other areas may precipitate an Se deficiency (Figure 12.1).

In well-aerated, alkaline soils, inorganic Se exists in the oxidized state (i.e., selenate and selenite), the form more readily available to plants; whereas in acid, poorly aerated soils subject to excessive rain, irrigation, or leaching, soil Se complexes with iron (Fe) hydrous oxide or is converted to the unavailable selenide state (Swaine 1955). Soil minerals, such as sulfate, can interfere with selenate and may compete with absorption sites at the root membrane (Mayland 1985).

Certain soil microorganisms oxidize Se from the reduced to the oxidized state, subsequently increasing its availability to plant tissue (Sarathchandra and Watkinson 1981). The liming of soils and the application of fertilizer sources rich in Se can elevate plant Se (Cary et al. 1967). The application of selenite to soil can increase the grain's Se content (Pond et al. 1971; Nielsen et al. 1979), but because of possible misapplication, differing soil factors that affect the availability of Se, and the possibility of its leaching into the potable water table, this approach may not be desirable. Fly ash from the coal burning process produces a product high in Se that is readily absorbed by plant tissue and retained by animal tissue (Mandisodza et al. 1979).

The Se content of some soils is high (>80 ppm), termed seleniferous, but the majority of soils range from 0.1 to 2 ppm, most not exceeding 0.5 ppm Se (Swaine 1955; Cary et al. 1967; Levesque 1974). "Indicator" plants grown on seleniferous soils accumulate Se in high concentrations (>1000 ppm) while other plants do not exceed 50 ppm when raised on the same soil. As with other minerals, the concentration of Se in soil might show little relationship to its concentration in plant tissue. Although the concentration of Se in grain is governed largely by soil availability factors and plant species, most cereal grains available for swine diets are below the pig's Se requirement (Table 12.1).

Cereal Grains

Upon absorption in plant tissue, Se often replaces the sulfur (S) component of organic metabolites, but it also is found in water-soluble form. The largest proportion of Se is incorporated into the grain protein component, notably as seleno-amino acids (selenomethionine, Se-methylselenomethionine, selenocystine, selenocysteine). Allaway et al. (1981) and Olson et al. (1970) reported that most Se in wheat is selenomethionine. Although excessive heat can vaporize Se, the normal pelleting, drying, and heating processes used in feed manufacturing does not effect Se losses.

Plant vitamin E occurs in eight isomeric forms (tocopherols and tocotrienols) but is found largely in the free-alcohol form in green forages and grain seeds. The isomeric forms of highest biological importance are the tocopherols. Alpha-tocopherol has

Table 12.1 Tocopherol and Selenium Concentrations in Selected Feedstuffs[a]

	Tocopherol Isomer				
Feedstuff	α	β[b]	γ	δ[b]	*Se*
Animal fat	6	Tr	8	Tr	
Barley	4	3	0.5		0.10
Corn	6		38	Tr	0.04
Corn oil	112	50	602	18	
Cottonseed meal	8		10		0.90
Cottonseed oil	389		387		
Milo	5		15		0.10
Oats	7	2	3		0.30
Soybean meal	2		14	Tr	0.10
Soybean oil	101		593	264	
Wheat	10	9		0.08	0.04
Wheat germ oil	1330	710	260	271	

[a]All values are in milligrams per kilogram.

[b]Trace (Tr) amounts detected in some samples.

(Adapted, by permission, from the data of Cort et al. 1983; Machlin 1984; and NRC 1988.)

the highest relative biopotency (i.e., 100%); the beta form ranges from 15% to 40%; the gamma form, 3% to 19%, while the delta form has <1% activity (Ullrey 1981). The concentration and isomeric form of these tocopherols vary with plant species and stage of plant maturity. Because many feedstuffs commonly used in swine diets generally contain more of the gamma than the alpha isomer (Table 12.1), a total vitamin E analysis tends to overestimate cereal grain vitamin E potency.

The waxy covering of grain seeds prevents oxygen and moisture penetration. Consequently, any harvesting or feed processing method that disrupts this protective barrier exposes the free-alcohol tocopherol form to oxidative destruction. The germ portion of the grain is rich in the tocopherols. Lightweight corn and corn grain affected by disease contain less vitamin E than does normal corn (Adams et al. 1975). Corn storage results in a lower tocopherol concentration with the rate of destruction exacerbated by moisture (Young et al. 1975). Excessive heat, grinding, pelleting, feed storage, moisture, and mold can lower the natural dietary tocopherol levels of grains (Adams et al. 1975).

Animal Products

Most Se incorporated into animal tissue has a lower (<25%) biological availability than that from plants (>60%). Great variations in Se availability occur in animal tissues. For instance, its biological value in bovine milk is equivalent to selenite (Mathias et al. 1967), whereas that in meat and bone meal or poultry by-products has a biological activity less than 20% (Cantor et al. 1975). Fish meal products have a lower availability due to tissue binding of Se and mercury (Hg).

Animal tissue contains largely alpha-tocopherol and would be expected to have a higher vitamin E potency as compared with plant tocopherol, which contains a high proportion of the gamma-isomer.

Investigators have demonstrated that feeding supplemental vitamin E to swine will improve the shelf life of pork (Tagwerker 1981). Because swine can deposit unsaturated fats, pork is more susceptible to fatty acid oxidation than are other meats. Dammers et al. (1958) suggested that 40 mg vitamin E/kg diet was the minimum quantity required to give pork a satisfactory shelf life.

Commercial Sources

The Food and Drug Administration (FDA) (1987) currently permits manufactured premixes to contain no more than 200 mg Se/kg (90.8 mg/lb) with a maximum supplemental level of 0.3 ppm inorganic Se in the complete swine diet. Sodium selenite is currently used in feed premixes, but other forms are equally effective. Selenate and selenite retain their bioavailability under normal feed and premix storage conditions (Olson et al. 1973) unless reduced to the selenide form (Groce et al. 1973a).

Commercial forms of vitamin E usually are the acetate ester (i.e., tocopheryl acetate) with the succinate ester having a lower bioavailability (Machlin 1984). Alpha-tocopheryl acetate is commercially available in a meal carrier or as an injectable product in an oil base. The product is stable under normal handling procedures or diet mixtures (Dove and Ewan 1987).

Dietary Factors Affecting Selenium and Vitamin E Availability

The oxidative state of several minerals can affect the biological utilization of Se. Because of the strong electronegative characteristic of Se and other metals in its class, Se is able to attract electrons from other metals, effectively chelating them. It is this binding force that allows Se to reduce the availability and toxicity of other metals, but these elements in turn may reduce the availability of Se (Hill 1975).

Early research conducted with Se involved alleviating its toxicity effects. Wahlstrom et al. (1955, 1956) reported that organic arsenicals provided effective protection against toxic levels of Se. Arsenic blocks the biosynthesis of dimethylselenide, the product formed and exhaled when excess Se is administered; it can also chelate and divert Se to the biliary system (Olson et al. 1963; Levander and Baumann 1966). Whanger (1981) and Frost (1981) documented the involvement of Se in detoxifying several heavy metals (Hg, cadmium [Cd], lead [Pb], silver [Ag], thallium [Tl], arsenic [As]), and noted that vitamin E enhances the detoxifying effects of Se. Van Vleet et al. (1977) presented evidence that Se and vitamin E therapy prevented cobalt (Co) toxicity. Van Vleet et al. (1977, 1982) demonstrated that the independent feeding of several elements (Ag, zinc [Zn], Cd, tellurium [Te], Co, copper [Cu], Hg, tin [Sn], Pb, As, Fe, and S) at relatively high dietary levels could induce the Se-vitamin E deficiency in ducklings. Although some of these minerals and organic arsenicals are routinely added to swine diets, no Se deficiencies have been reported when normal dietary levels of these trace minerals are fed (Hitchcock et al. 1978; Thulin et al. 1985). Lowry et al. (1985a,b) presented evidence that the retention of Se was reduced by high dietary P but not by elevated dietary Ca levels.

Tocopherols in free form are easily oxidized in the presence of unsaturated or rancid fats (Obel 1953) and certain trace minerals (i.e., Fe, Cu) but not the stabilized commercial alpha-tocopheryl acetate (Dove and Ewan 1987).

SELENIUM AND VITAMIN E METABOLIC ROLE

Metabolism

Absorption and Vascular Transport

Organic Se is absorbed effectively but at a slower rate than the inorganic form (Groce et al. 1973a), dependent on the rate of hydrolysis of the dietary protein sources and the competitive absorption site between selenomethionine and methionine. The absorption of other organic seleno-compounds does not appear to be inhibited by their respective S analogues (NRC 1983).

Inorganic dietary Se as selenite or selenate is absorbed throughout the small intestine but largely from the ileum in the nonruminant. Upon absorption, Se is rapidly incorporated within the erythrocyte, but then a large portion appears to be released (Jenkins and Hidiroglou 1972). Other Se appears to be bound to plasma proteins.

The absorption of natural tocopherols and/or their esters is considered to be relatively low (e.g., <40%) and dependent on factors affecting fat absorption and excretion. Vitamin E appears to be absorbed mainly in the upper two thirds of the small intestine. The micelle and factors involving its formation (i.e., fat, bile, pancreatic lipase) appear necessary for optimum vitamin E absorption. The type of fat fed can influence tocopherol absorption; unsaturated fatty acids have an inhibitory effect, while medium-chain fatty acids have a stimulating effect. The acetate or succinate ester is hydrolyzed from the tocopherol component for effective absorption.

Tocopherols are absorbed through the enterocyte into the lacteals, circulated in the lymph, and bound to lipoprotein fractions in the blood. A high correlation exists between serum triglyceride and tocopherol concentrations. Although gamma-tocopherol is frequently the most abundant tocopherol isomer in cereal grains and their oils (Table 12.1), the alpha-isomer is at a higher concentration in swine tissue, suggesting selective retention of the isomers.

Metabolic Conversion

When seleno-amino acids are absorbed, they can be incorporated into tissue protein or metabolized with the Se reduced to the selenide form. Selenates and selenites are reduced to the biologically active selenide form. Diplock et al. (1971) demonstrated that vitamin E was effective in maintaining a greater tissue pool of selenide, probably serving as an antioxidant protector. Although Se can be tightly bound to various proteins, much of the selenide is metabolized to selenocysteine. Selenocysteine is the active catalytic form of Se that appears necessary for the formation of GSH-Px, but the metabolic mechanism is yet unclear. Other chemical Se forms associated with protein tissue are not clear. Riboflavin is involved in the activity of glutathione reductase, an enzyme essential for the production of reduced glutathione. A deficiency of riboflavin can reduce GSH-Px activity (Brady et al. 1979; Parsons et al. 1985).

Vitamin E is a vital component of biological membranes. A proposed mechanism model suggests that cellular membranes are composed of globular proteins with a viscous coating of various phospholipids and cholesterol as integral constituents of the membrane. Vitamin E bound to plasma protein becomes coupled with the membrane phospholipid, serving in an antioxidative role by preventing damage to membrane surfaces. Dietary fats or membrane phospholipids containing a high unsaturated fatty acid content result in oxidative damage, thus elevating the dietary requirement for vitamin E (Drochner 1976).

Tissue Distribution

Selenium retained in swine tissue reflects both the quantity and source of dietary Se provided (Ku et al. 1972, 1973; Young et al. 1976, 1977b; Mahan and Moxon 1978b,

1980; Kurkela and Kaantee 1984). Organic Se, largely selenomethionine, is incorporated into muscle tissue at higher concentrations than Se from selenite. Although the pig cannot synthesize methionine, inorganic Se is increased in animal tissue, particularly in nonmuscular tissue, as the dietary level increases (Mahan et al. 1975, 1978a,b). Tissues vary in their Se concentration, with kidney, liver, testes, and glandular (e.g., pancreas, spleen) tissue having the highest levels and muscle tissue the lowest values (Groce et al. 1973b; Mahan and Moxon 1978a,b, 1980). The liver perhaps best reflects the animal's Se status; in a deficiency condition, there is a more rapid decline of Se in that organ (Mahan et al. 1977; Peplowski et al. 1981) while upon toxicosis there is a marked increase relative to other tissue.

Blood Se may also reflect the animal's Se status, with normal serum concentrations ranging from 0.08 to 0.15 ppm (Mahan and Moxon 1978a; Meyer et al. 1981). Hair Se can reflect Se retention on a long-term basis (Mahan et al. 1974; Goehring et al. 1984a,b), with dark hair having a higher Se content than white hair (Wahlstrom et al. 1984). Genetic and litter differences in Se retention have been reported (Jensen et al. 1979, 1984; Stowe and Miller 1985).

Selenium is transferred through the placenta; higher concentrations occur in piglet tissue when sows are fed higher dietary Se levels (Mahan et al. 1977). Colostrum has a higher Se content than mature sow milk. Because the milk of later parities has a lower Se concentration than from earlier parities, the progeny of mature sows are more likely to encounter the deficiency condition earlier postweaning (Mahan et al. 1977).

Tissues vary in their concentration of vitamin E, with the major reservoir in the liver, which accumulates tocopherol in a linear logarithmic fashion relative to intake. Plasma tocopherol levels in swine appear to be below those of other species (Lindberg 1973). Because there is a relatively high correlation between plasma and liver tocopherol, plasma tocopherol has been used in establishing vitamin E status (Ullrey 1981).

Vitamin E appears to be largely concentrated in the cellular membrane fraction and intracellular structures; its bioavailability is limited once incorporated (Machlin 1984). Adipose tissue contains substantial amounts of tocopherol, but most is unavailable for other biological purposes (Machlin et al. 1979).

Alpha-tocopherol is the major isomer in porcine tissue, and gamma-tocopherol is second highest in tissue concentration. The presence of the additional methyl group on the chromonal ring may have an effect on alpha-tocopherol tissue retention (Machlin 1984).

Colostrum has a higher tocopherol content than mature sow milk (Nielsen et al. 1973; Mahan et al. 1975; Loudenslager et al. 1986), and both milks exhibit a decline with sow reproductive age. Mammary transfer of tocopherol results in higher tissue and plasma tocopherol concentrations in pigs of early versus later parities. Nursing pigs receive relatively high levels of alpha-tocopherol from sow's colostrum and milk, but their plasma tocopherol concentrations decline rapidly following weaning (Mahan and Moxon 1980; Meyer et al. 1981).

Excretion

The biologically active selenide form may be bound with heavy metals; stored in tissue; converted to selenocysteine, GSH-Px, or other chemical forms; or excreted. Normal

Se excretion patterns in swine, as in other nonruminants, are through the urine and feces. Urinary Se is in the form of trimethylselenide, a reduced form of the element (Palmer et al. 1970). As dietary or injected amounts of Se increase, excretion through the kidney increases (Mahan 1985).

Elemental Se and metal selenides are excreted in the feces. The biliary system diverts a large proportion of the reduced Se to the intestinal lumen. Intestinal bacteria can convert dietary selenite into insoluble selenide or microbial seleno-proteins. The proportion of microbial Se produced is higher in ruminants, but it constitutes approximately 45% of total fecal Se in the nonruminant (Levander and Baumann 1966). Animal feces thus return inert Se to the soil, where it is unavailable for plant absorption unless microbiological or soil chemical oxidative processes convert it to a more usable form.

High levels of injected or fed Se result in the volatile methylated Se metabolite dimethylselenide being exhaled through the lungs.

Functional Role

Since it was discovered that Se is a component of factor 3 (Schwarz and Foltz 1957), it has become clear that this element complements other nutrients.

Antioxidant

Oxygen is used in energy-yielding metabolic processes in the body, but there are metabolic by-products that can result in extensive damage to cellular tissue. Hydrogen peroxide, hydroperoxides, superoxides, various radicals including the hydroxyl radical, and possibly singlet oxygen can be formed as products of reactions in body cells.

Cellular tissue contains various protective systems that ultimately destroy the reactive peroxide products. The major cellular mechanisms providing protection are vitamin E, GSH-Px, catalase, and superoxide dismutase. These systems are compartmentalized within the cell and complement one another. Although difficult to demonstrate in vivo, vitamin E serves as an antioxidant that scavenges free radicals before they can attack cellular and intracellular membranes. Glutathione peroxidase destroys H_2O_2 and hydroperoxides in the cytosol and mitochrondrial matrix space. Catalase degrades H_2O_2 to form the hydroxyl radical (Chance et al. 1979; NRC 1983).

Hydrogen extraction from unsaturated fatty acids is thought to result in the formation of peroxide radicals. The hydrophobic nature of cellular and intracellular membranes attract the aliphatic hydrocarbon side chain of vitamin E, allowing tocopherol rather than the lipoprotein component of the membrane to become oxidized (Drochner 1976). This prevents disorientation of the membrane structure and thus maintains cellular integrity. Disruption of the mitochondrial membrane, which normally contains high levels of tocopherol, is an early pathological finding in vitamin E-deficient animals (Machlin 1984). Selenium as a component of the enzyme GSH-Px, along with catalase and superoxide dismutase, serves compartmentally in the cytosol as a reducing agent that attacks the peroxides of cellular metabolism.

There is a Se-dependent and a Se-independent form of GSH-Px (Lawrence and Burk 1978). Meyer et al. (1981) demonstrated that the Se-dependent form in pig liver was responsive to dietary selenite, whereas the independent form was not. Although liver tissue increases in Se content at a declining rate as the dietary concentration of the element increases, GSH-Px remains stable. Consequently, the activity of this enzyme is perhaps the best criterion of the Se status of the pig (Hakkarainen et al. 1978a,b; Chavez 1979). Workers have reported high correlations between tissue Se and GSH-Px activities in deficient swine (Adkins and Ewan 1984), but the correlation coefficient declines as the dietary Se level increases above the animal's requirement (Meyer et al. 1981). Consequently, during deficient conditions, the incorporation of Se into GSH-Px appears to be of high biological priority, but as more Se becomes available to body tissue, it is bound to protein tissue in a nonselective way or is used in the formation of other tissue seleno-compounds.

Arachidonic Acid and Prostaglandin Metabolism

Arachidonic acid found in the phospholipid of membranes is involved in the synthesis of different prostaglandins. Vitamin E stimulates the incorporation of linoleic acid into arachidonic acid, a reaction that involves free-radical metabolism (Diplock 1981). Prostaglandin synthesis is reduced in the testis and muscle of vitamin E-deficient animals (Chan et al. 1980) and appears to be involved in smooth muscle contraction. Platelet aggregation is increased and prostaglandin E is inhibited under vitamin E deficiency (Mustard and Packham 1970; Lake et al. 1977). The role of vitamin E in the synthesis of the prostaglandins may help to explain many clinical deficiency signs encountered with both growing and reproducing swine.

Immunity

Both linoleic and arachidonic acid have been shown to influence immunoregulatory mechanisms in vivo. The effect may be direct, since plasma membrane fluidity of lymphoid cells increases the probability of affecting cell-antigen interactions by polyunsaturated fatty acids (Sheffy and Schultz 1979). Larsen and Tollersrud (1981) demonstrated enhanced T cell proliferation when Se or vitamin E were administered. Nockels (1979) demonstrated an increase in plaque-forming cells and demonstrated that vitamin E fed to nonimmunized hens increased the primary immune response of their immunized progeny.

Evidence also suggests that Se and vitamin E may be involved in the immune response in swine. Ellis and Vorhies (1976) demonstrated improved humoral response to an *Escherichia coli* bacterin when young pigs were fed high levels (110 IU/kg) of supplemental vitamin E. Subsequent research by others (Teige 1977; Teige et al. 1977, 1978; Nockels 1979; Peplowski et al. 1981) demonstrated that dietary Se and vitamin E were effective in enhancing the immune response in pigs. Peplowski et al. (1981) presented evidence that the humoral responses to sheep red blood cell injections were additive for both vitamin E and Se with similarly enhanced immunocompetent humoral responses whether the nutrients were injected or provided in the feed. The results of Teige et al. (1977, 1978) and Saxegaard and Teige (1977) suggest that swine deficient in Se and vitamin E are more susceptible to swine dysentery. However, the effects of various stress conditions (e.g., cold, crowding) have not resulted in beneficial immunogenic responses to supplemental vitamin E (Kornegay et al. 1986; Yen et al. 1986).

Sperm Maturation

Male rats born from females fed an Se-deficient diet had fewer spermatozoa in the caudal epididymes, poorer sperm motility, and more spermatids with tail breakage (Wu et al. 1973). Selenium was found localized in the spermatid tail midpiece, that portion that contains the mitochondria (Wu et al. 1979). In Se-deficient mouse spermatids, the mitochondria were found to be disoriented, to have excessive cytoplasmic content, and to have a loose apposition of the plasma membrane with an irregularity in the structure of the center core (Calvin et al. 1981). Later rat work demonstrated a selenocysteine-rich polypeptide component surrounding the mitochrondria that provided a linking function that could stabilize the mitochondrial helix during spermatid development (Calvin et al. 1981). Research with the boar has demonstrated reduced sperm motility and higher sperm morphological abnormalities with Se deficiencies (Marin-Guzman et al. 1988).

Other Functions

Labored breathing resulting from stress conditions is reported in Se- and vitamin E-deficient swine, implying the involvement of these nutrients in red blood cell development or maturation. Baustad and Nafstad (1972) reported morphological abnormalities of blood and bone marrow cells.

Sweeney and Brown (1972) demonstrated progressive vascular damage in connective tissue components, suggesting the involvement of Se and vitamin E in collagen and connective tissue synthesis. Lake et al. (1977) reported the involvement of vitamin E in collagen-induced platelet aggregation. The spraddle leg condition in neonatal pigs implies not only weakened muscles in young neonates but the possible impairment of connective tissue development.

SELENIUM AND VITAMIN E DEFICIENCY IN SWINE

Contributing Factors

Semipurified diets containing unsaturated or rancid fats readily produce deficiencies of Se and vitamin E in young swine (Obel 1953; Eggert et al. 1957; Grant 1961a,b; Lannek et al. 1961; Ewan et al. 1969). Analagous responses when cereal grain-oilseed diets are fed are fewer and were unheard of during the early 1960s, but field incidences escalated from that period (Michel et al. 1969; Trapp et al. 1970; Van Vleet et al. 1970) until Se was approved as a dietary supplement. There have been several swine industry changes over the past three decades that have contributed to the onset of this problem.

1. Swine confinement has eliminated soil as an Se source from the pig's natural diet.
2. Swine confinement has resulted in reduced green forage consumption, a source of vitamin E.
3. Swine confinement has resulted in increased growth rates with higher daily requirements for all nutrients.
4. Increased crop yields can deplete the soil of Se for incorporation into plant tissue.
5. Continuous cropping of corn, less crop rotation, and irrigation has resulted in a lower soil pH, thus reducing soil Se available for plant absorption.
6. Increased usage of simplified cereal grain-soybean meal swine diets has resulted in the dietary deletion of several products that originally contributed Se and tocopherol.
7. The use of high-moisture grains results in feedstuffs with a lower vitamin E content.
8. The incorporation of unsaturated fats into swine diets can exacerbate the tissue requirement for vitamin E.
9. Higher levels of some dietary trace minerals (i.e., Cu, Fe) destroy the alpha-tocopherol content of feed.
10. Finer grinding, pelleting, and long storage periods of feedstuffs and prepared feeds reduce the natural vitamin E potency.
11. Earlier weaning can result in lower quantities of Se and vitamin E stored in the body tissue of young swine at weaning.
12. High sow productivity, early weaning, early rebreeding, and longer retention of sows in the herd can deplete maternal tissue reserves of both Se and vitamin E.
13. Genetic differences in swine's ability to retain and/or utilize Se (and possibly vitamin E) are only now becoming apparent.
14. Storage of grains and feedstuffs for extended periods and the possible contamination with toxin-producing molds could destroy natural tocopherol.

Growing Swine

Tissues with the highest rate of development that use Se and vitamin E for metabolic purposes are those in which the deficiency is likely to be encountered. In growing swine, these are the intestine, liver, muscle, vascular, and adipose tissues. Extreme deficiencies will interfere with normal growth processes and feed utilization because both GSH-Px and vitamin E are associated with the mitochrondrion, the cellular organelle where oxidative phosphorylation occurs. Independent deficiency signs cannot be clearly delineated for each nutrient and will be considered associated unless evidence indicates otherwise.

Swine Performance

Swine fed semipurified diets fortified with Se or vitamin E will generally have improved growth rates and feed conversions (Forbes and Draper 1957; Ewan et al.

1969; Glienke and Ewan 1977; Adkins and Ewan 1984); whereas when cereal grains serve as the basal feedstuff, animal performance is generally not improved by the addition of Se or vitamin E (Mahan and Moxon 1978a,b; Nielsen et al. 1979; Meyer et al. 1981; Goehring et al. 1984a). Cereal grains may contain low Se and vitamin E but appear to be adequate to prevent reductions in animal performance. However, it has been noted that the largest, fastest growing weanling pigs are more prone to sudden death, implying that labile tissue Se and vitamin E reserves have been depleted by daily nutrient needs that are higher than those of slower growing animals. This combination of factors may be the cause of death in the larger pigs, which generally occurs 1 to 2 weeks following weaning (Mahan and Moxon 1980).

Tissue Signs

Swine fed semipurified diets deficient in Se, vitamin E, or both nutrients exhibit more marked deficiency signs than those fed practical diets. Feeding unsaturated or rancid fats and factors resulting in low dietary levels of these nutrients can, however, exacerbate the deficiency with both types of diets.

Clinical observations encountered under experimental and field conditions include liver deterioration and hemorrhages (hepatosis dietetica); heart tissue abnormalities (weakened, thin walled, enlarged, pale striations); light-colored, pale striated muscle tissue (nutritional muscular dystrophy); and cecal and colonic hemorrhages (Grant and Thafvelin 1958; Grant 1961b; Ewan et al. 1969; Nafstad and Tollersrud 1970; Bengtssen et al. 1978). These workers report that Se and vitamin E supplementation can prevent the deficiencies, with tocopherol reportedly delaying the onset of Se deficiency (Bengtssen et al. 1978). Gastric ulcers appear to be associated with vitamin E and Se deficiency, and some evidence suggests that Se deficiency may be more responsible than vitamin E deficiency (Mahan et al. 1975).

Increased fluid accumulation in the pericardial sac, edema in the intestinal membranes, and steatitis or yellow discoloration of body fat are signs that appear to be associated more with vitamin E than with Se deficiency (Eggert et al. 1957).

Blood Profiles

The leakage of cellular fluids (exudative diathesis) can elevate various enzymes (generally amino acid transferases) in the circulating fluids (Wretlind et al. 1959; Ewan et al. 1969; Tollersrud 1973) under deficient conditions. These enzymes are generally not organ specific, but some enzymes may reflect muscle rather than liver necrosis. Exercise and dietary protein have been shown to result in moderate increases in plasma concentrations of some enzymes (Tollersrud 1973), but not of the magnitude encountered in the Se- and vitamin E-deficient condition. Low blood concentrations of Se and vitamin E generally occur prior to the elevation of these blood enzymes.

Reduced prothrombin time, increased red blood cell hemolysis, and morphological abnormalities of bone marrow cells have all been demonstrated to reflect a vitamin E-deficient condition (Baustad and Nafstad 1972; Jensen et al. 1979, 1983). Although anemia has also been reported with vitamin E deficiencies (Obel 1953; Grant 1961b;

Nafstad 1965; Nafstad and Nafstad 1968; Baustad and Nafstad 1972), the effect is not always encountered (Ewan et al. 1969; Michel et al. 1969; Fontaine et al. 1977a,b, c; Niyo et al. 1980).

Iron Toxicity

British and Scandinavian workers (Lannek et al. 1962; Tollerz and Lannek 1964; Patterson et al. 1967, 1969, 1971) demonstrated that neonatal pigs deficient in Se and vitamin E were sensitive to iron-dextran injections and died from an apparent Fe toxicity within a few hours of injection. Iron can induce myodegeneration, resulting in peroxidative damage to muscle cells, possibly because of an increased affinity of skeletal muscle for Fe. The injection of vitamin E, not Se, 1 day prior to Fe injection provides protection from Fe toxicity (Tollerz and Lannek 1964; Tollerz 1973). However, Miller et al. (1973) were unable to repeat the Fe toxicity response in piglets born of sows fed corn-soybean meal diets without supplemental Se or vitamin E. Other work reported by Ullrey (1981) produced death when 8-day-old piglets from dams fed 5% lipid were injected with 750 mg Fe and were orally fed 5 to 10 ml of aerated cod-liver oil daily. Loudenslager et al. (1986) suggested that the consumption of colostrum provided protection. These workers demonstrated a decline in serum tocopherol and an increase in GSH-Px activity after Fe was administered. These results suggest that Fe toxicity may be a problem when Se and vitamin E deficiencies are extreme, but when the neonatal pig is adequate or borderline in its status of these nutrients and consumes colostrum prior to Fe injections, it is able to tolerate normal quantities of injected Fe without detrimental effects.

Disease and Stress Conditions

Various disease or disease-related problems are frequently associated with the Se-vitamin E deficiency. Thomlinson and Buxton (1963) presented evidence that young swine deficient in Se and vitamin E can be hypersensitive to *E. coli,* resulting in an anaphylactic reaction with signs resembling gut edema. A response termed *generalized Shwartzman reaction* (GSR), an anaphylactic reaction, occurred when injections of *E. coli* endotoxins were administered to vitamin E-deficient pigs with supplemental vitamin E protective against GSR (Teige et al. 1973; Teige 1977).

Gut edema and postweaning diarrhea are diseases frequently observed in conjunction with Se-vitamin E deficiency in weanling pigs. A proposed model may relate these clinical observations to the functional role of these nutrients. Under conditions of Se-vitamin E deficiency, cellular membrane integrity is reduced, allowing the leakage of cellular fluids and providing an entry site for infectious agents. Under deficient conditions coupled with stress (e.g., weaning, parturition), pathogenic organisms may enter the cellular environment. Unless these pathogens are destroyed by the oxygen burst mechanism of the phagocytic leucocytes or by the immune system, a disease condition may occur.

Reproducing Swine

Reproductive Performance

Adamstone et al. (1949) first reported vitamin E deficiency in adult swine. Their study demonstrated that a vitamin E-deficient diet resulted in lowered litter size, attributable to embryonic death rather than interference in ovulation or implantation mechanisms. The progeny born from deficient sows exhibited muscular incoordination and necrosis of muscle fibers. Piatkowski et al. (1979), however, did not demonstrate fetal atrophy in first-litter gilts fed a semipurified diet deficient in Se and vitamin E, nor did Chavez (1985) demonstrate a lower number of pigs born from gilt litters.

When practical diets were fed, Mahan et al. (1974) demonstrated that sows fed corn-soybean meal diets with 0.1 ppm Se had a larger litter size in parity 2 than a group without added Se, but no effect was observed in parity 1. The feeding of high-moisture corn resulted in a lower number of pigs born (Whitehair and Miller 1985) or poor reproductive performance (Young et al. 1977a, 1978). Nielsen et al. (1979) did not observe an increased litter size when Se and vitamin E were supplemented to a low-Se barley diet.

The progeny from older versus younger sows have lower tissue reservoirs of Se at weaning, suggesting maternal depletion of these nutrients with age (Mahan et al. 1977). Confined sows are more prone to exhibit the reproductive deficiency (Mahan et al. 1974) than those housed on pasture (Wilkinson et al. 1977a).

The results of the above studies suggest that Se and vitamin E deficiency can affect litter size, notably via embryonic losses. Lowered reproductive performance will generally not occur when gilt litters are fed practical diets; but the deficiency is more likely to occur in both the mature sow and her progeny, particularly under conditions exacerbating the deficiency onset.

Tissue Signs

Maternal tissue in gilts or sows develops at a slower rate than that of growing swine. Although Se- and vitamin E-deficient tissues (e.g., pale striated muscle, gastric ulcers) occur in adult animals fed a vitamin E- and Se-deficient semipurified diet, the time necessary to develop these myopathies is longer than in younger animals (Mahan et al. 1974; Piatkowski et al. 1979). Tissue myopathies in sows fed corn-soybean meal diets without supplemental Se or vitamin E did not occur after two reproductive cycles (Mahan et al. 1974).

Blood and Milk Profile

Because maternal tissue degeneration does not occur rapidly in adult swine, cellular enzyme leakage does not occur readily. Mahan et al. (1974) demonstrated that serum glutamic oxalo-acetic transaminase (GOT) and glutamic pyruvic transaminase (GPT) enzymes were elevated after 60 days postcoitum when gilts were fed a semipurified diet devoid of supplemental Se or vitamin E, whereas no elevation of these enzymes occurred when corn-soybean meal diets were provided.

Serum Se concentrations are higher during pregnancy than during lactation (Mahan et al. 1975), implying that lactation has a larger nutritional drain on tissue Se reservoirs than does pregnancy. Vrzgula et al. (1980) demonstrated a low blood vitamin E concentration over two reproductive phases when the diet was devoid of vitamin E.

Parturition Problems

Although retained placenta is a reported sign of the Se-vitamin E deficiency in dairy cattle (Julien et al. 1976), it has not been demonstrated in swine. However, extended parturition times and inadequate expression of milk from mammary tissue have been observed in both species, implying inadequate smooth muscle contractions. These responses imply inadequate prostaglandin production.

Progeny from Se- and vitamin E-deficient sows are weak at birth with a reduced desire to nurse the dam. The poor release of milk from mammary tissue of deficient sows and the declining glycogen reserves of neonatal swine compounds the problem. Spraddle-legged pigs have been reported born to sows deficient in Se and vitamin E (Adams 1975).

Sperm Production

Rat sperm, particularly the tail midpiece, is morphologically affected under Se-deficient conditions (Wu et al. 1973). Although Segerson et al. (1981) reported no impairment of boar sperm motility or morphology when a low-Se semipurified diet was fed from 77 to 250 days of age, recent evidence from Marin-Guzman et al. (1988) demonstrated lower sperm production and motility when Se-deficient boar sperm was collected over extended periods.

Disease Conditions

Disease conditions are associated with the Se-vitamin E deficiency during the reproductive period (Trapp et al. 1970). Whitehair and Miller (1985) reported a high incidence of mastitis, metritis, and agalactia (MMA) in sows fed a dried high-moisture corn diet; however, when a similar diet fortified with Se and vitamin E was provided, MMA was not evident. Their results are consistent with the observations of Ringarp (1960), who reported a high MMA incidence when poor-quality feed was fed to reproducing sows. Although MMA is a complex disease that occurs during a stressful period, these results suggest that vitamin E and/or Se may be effective in reducing its incidence.

SELENIUM AND VITAMIN E TOXICOSIS

Selenium

The minimum lethal dose of Se depends on the chemical form of the element, animal age, and other physiological and dietary factors. Responses to high dietary Se levels are categorized as acute (the quantity that induces toxicosis in a relatively short time) or chronic (the effects of which are seen over extended time periods).

Elemental Se is relatively nontoxic and has a median lethal dose (LD_{50}) of 6700 ppm in rats (Cummins and Kirmura 1971). Dimethylselenide, the principal metabolite exhaled through the lung under toxicosis conditions, has an LD_{50} of 1600 ppm; while the urinary metabolite, trimethylselenide, has an LD_{50} of 49.4 ppm (McConnel and Portsman 1952; Obermeyer et al. 1971). Selenite will produce toxicosis signs in weanling swine at dietary levels of 5 to 9 ppm (Mahan et al. 1984; Goehring et al. 1984a,b). When selenite is injected at 1.65 mg Se/kg body weight (Diehl et al. 1975) or is administered orally at 2.7 to 3.6 mg/kg body weight (Miller 1938; Miller and Williams 1940), selenosis will result.

Younger animals are more prone to toxicosis at lower Se levels than are older animals (Halverson et al. 1966), with Se- and vitamin E-deficient animals being more susceptible to Se toxicity at lower dietary concentrations (Jaffe and Mondragen 1975; Van Vleet and Ruth 1977; Van Vleet et al. 1977). Protein diets lower in both quality and quantity (Gortner 1940) are conducive to Se toxicosis. Feeding a semipurified diet as compared with one containing natural grain (Harr et al. 1967) produces selenosis more readily.

Acute Se toxicosis results from the ingestion of large quantities of seleniferous feedstuffs, a diet with extremely high levels of inorganic Se, or a large quantity of injected Se. Acute selenosis is generally not a problem under most swine feeding programs, but it may occur under conditions of poor feed mixing techniques, inadequate weighing of Se premixes, or misapplication of injectable Se. Immediate signs of selenosis include labored breathing, pulmonary edema, vomiting, prostration, frothing at the mouth, and abnormal staggering movement. Death occurs within hours or a few days of injection (Orstadius 1960; Herigstad et al. 1973; Diehl et al. 1975). The effects of ingesting a large quantity of Se ($>$20 ppm) include feed refusal, loss of weight, respiratory distress, spinal paralysis, incoordination, loss of hair, and death (Miller 1938, 1940; Herigstad et al. 1973; Harrison et al. 1983; Mahan and Moxon 1984).

Chronic Se toxicosis occurs when diets or feedstuffs contain 5 to 9 ppm Se. Symptoms are characterized in growing swine by reduced growth and feed intakes, loss of hair, and separation of the hoof from the foot at the coronary band site (Goehring et al. 1984; Mahan and Moxon 1984). Chronic selenosis in reproducing sows results in lower conception rates; small, weak piglets, and a high percentage of stillbirths (Wahlstrom and Olson 1959).

Elevated serum Se and enzyme (GOT) levels, with high Se concentrations in all tissues, particularly the liver, result as quantities injected or ingested increase (Diehl et al. 1975; Mahan and Moxon 1984).

The toxic effects of Se from feeding seleniferous grains may be counteracted by administering sodium arsenite (Moxon 1937, 1941). The organic arsenicals, arsanilic acid at 0.01% and 3-nitro-4 hydroxyphenylarsonic acid at 0.005% of the diet, are less dangerous than inorganic arsenic (Wahlstrom et al. 1955). Linseed meal provides protection against selenosis (Moxon 1937; Wahlstrom et al. 1956), largely because of its cyanogenic glucoside (linustatin, neolinustatin) properties (Palmer et al. 1974, 1980).

Vitamin E

Although the biological need for vitamin E may be elevated under conditions of low Se or when various dietary factors exacerbate the vitamin E requirement, the feeding of vitamin E at 220 mg/kg diet has not resulted in detrimental performance responses (Peplowski et al. 1981).

SELENIUM AND VITAMIN E REQUIREMENTS

Because both Se and vitamin E are incorporated into tissue components and are involved in metabolism, the dietary requirement will vary by period of production. Factors that influence feed intake, stress conditions, and body reservoirs of Se and vitamin E complicate the issue of clearly defining dietary requirements. From existing evidence, the young growing pig and the adult lactating female have the greatest biological requirements.

The dietary requirements for Se may frequently vary from the 0.3 ppm supplemental limit approved by the FDA (1987). Because of tissue storage capacity for Se, the approved dietary limit should meet the pig's needs if it is consistently provided throughout the animal's life cycle. Vitamin E, on the other hand, is more subject to variable dietary and tissue factors and is not as labile as tissue Se. Therefore, different allowances for vitamin E will be needed in the various production phases.

Growing Swine

The neonatal pig has a low vitamin E reservoir while Se is stored in tissue, reflecting the level fed the sow (Mahan et al. 1977; Vrzgula et al. 1982; Chavez 1985). Consequently, the neonate is dependent on an exogenous source of both nutrients, particularly vitamin E. Colostrum and mature milk contain substantial quantities of both nutrients. Therefore, unless the sow is depleted of these nutrients by extended lactations or reproductive cycles in which she is fed a diet low in Se or vitamin E, the young pig should receive adequate quantities while nursing the sow. Although the deficiency has been reported in the neonatal pig, Se or vitamin E injections in the neonate and pretreatment of the sow have been effective in reducing baby pig mortality (Van Vleet et al. 1973).

Weaning appears to exacerbate the deficiency in young swine. Pigs with lower body weights at weaning have lower body reservoirs of Se and are dependent on a higher dietary level postweaning than are heavier pigs (Mahan 1987). Selenite in drinking water quickly and effectively increases tissue Se (Mahan and Moxon 1978a).

The stresses of weaning, infection, and the effects of various dietary components that chelate Se or oxidize natural tocopherol have all been shown to increase the dietary requirements of Se and vitamin E. Under conditions where deficiency problems exist, the injection of 0.05 mg Se and 20 mg vitamin E/kg body weight has provided effective therapy in reducing pig mortality (Mahan et al. 1973; Niyo et al. 1977; Mahan and Moxon 1980).

Evidence suggests that the 21-day-old weanling pig fed a practical diet requires 0.5 ppm supplemental Se for approximately 14 days postweaning. The Se requirement declines to 0.35 ppm by 5 weeks postweaning (Meyer et al. 1981; Mahan 1987). Although the vitamin E requirement for swine has not been clearly determined, and factors concerning its absorption and utilization are as yet unclear, it would appear that 20 IU/kg diet should meet the needs of the weanling pig. Under conditions where dietary fat is fed, supplemental levels of 30 to 40 IU/kg may be necessary.

The requirement for both Se and vitamin E during the later growth and finishing period is lower than for weanling swine (Mahan et al. 1977; Wilkinson et al. 1977b). The requirement for Se declines to approximately 0.1 ppm and the vitamin E requirement to 10 to 20 IU/kg diet by market weight.

Reproduction

Selenium and vitamin E for gestating swine are needed for maintenance, maternal, and fetal tissue development. Piatkowski et al. (1979) determined that each fetus accumulates approximately 0.05 mg Se, suggesting that the dam's gestation requirement for Se is relatively low. The injection of selenite (0.05 mg/kg body weight) 3 to 6 weeks prior to farrowing has in some but not all cases improved reproductive performance.

Colostrum has a relatively high concentration of Se and vitamin E, and mature milk contains both nutrients at lower concentrations. Lactation imposes a higher dietary requirement on the sow for both nutrients; a still greater need exists under conditions of high milk production, larger litter size, and longer lactations. The lower milk concentrations of these nutrients occur with advancing reproduction cycles (Mahan et al. 1974, 1977), suggesting that aged sows may become depleted.

Sow gestation and lactation research establishing the dietary requirements for Se and vitamin E is lacking, but 0.3 ppm supplemental Se and 20 to 30 IU vitamin E/kg diet should meet sows' needs. When deficiency problems are present, elevated therapeutic dietary levels of vitamin E (60 to 80 IU/kg) have resulted in improved reproductive performance and higher colostrum tocopherol concentrations.

The growing boar's dietary need for Se and vitamin E is considered similar to that of the young gilt and barrow, even though the testis accumulates large quantities of Se. Because it is difficult to produce Se or vitamin E deficiency in breeding boars (Segerson et al. 1981), 0.3 ppm Se and 22 IU vitamin E/kg diet should be adequate.

REFERENCES

Adams, C.R., H.F. Eoff, and Z.R. Zimmerman. 1975. *Roche Agreport* 401.

Adamstone, F.B., J.L. Krider, and M.F. James. 1949. *Ann. N.Y. Acad. Sci.* 52:260.

Adkins, R.S., and R.C. Ewan. 1984. *J. Anim. Sci.* 58:346.

Allaway, W.H., E.E. Cary, and C.F. Ehlig. 1981. In: *Selenium in Biology and Medicine.* Muth, O.H. (Ed.). pp. 273–296. Westport, CT: AVI Publishing Co.

Baustad, B., and I. Nafstad. 1972. *Br. J. Nutr.* 28:183.
Bengtssen, G., et al. 1978. *J. Anim. Sci.* 46:143.
Brady, P.S., et al. 1979. *J. Nutr.* 109:1615.
Calvin, H.I., E. Wallace, and G.W. Cooper. 1981. In: *Selenium in Biology and Medicine.* Muth, O.H. (Ed.). p. 319. Westport, CT: AVI Publishing Co.
Cantor, A.H., M.L. Scott, and T. Noguchi. 1975. *J. Nutr.* 105:96.
Cary, E.E., G.A. Wieczorek, and W.H. Allaway. 1967. *Soil Sci. Soc. Am. Prod.* 31:21.
Chan, A.C., C.E. Allen, and P.V.J. Hegarty. 1980. *J. Nutr.* 110:66.
Chance, B., H. Sies, and A. Boveris. 1979. *Physiol. Rev.* 59:527.
Chavez, E.R. 1979. *Can. J. Anim. Sci.* 59:67.
Chavez, E.R. 1985. *Can. J. Anim. Sci.* 65:497.
Cort, W.M., et al. 1983. *J. Agric. Food Chem.* 31:1330.
Cummins, L.M., and E.T. Kimura. 1971. *Toxicol. Appl. Pharmacol.* 20:89.
Dammers, J., K. Stolk, and G. Van Wieringen. 1958. *Vesl. Landbouwkund* 64:5.
Diehl, J.S., D.C. Mahan, and A.L. Moxon. 1975. *J. Anim. Sci.* 40:844.
Diplock, A.T. 1981. In: *Selenium in Biology and Medicine.* Muth, O.H. (Ed.). p. 303. Westport, CT: AVI Publishing Co.
Diplock, A.T., H. Baum, and J.A. Lucy. 1971. *Biochem. J.* 123:721.
Dove, C.R., and R.C. Ewan. 1987. *J. Anim. Sci.* 65(Suppl. l):302.
Drochner, W. 1976. *Ubers. Tierernahrung* 4:93.
Eggert, R.O., et al. 1957. *J. Anim. Sci.* 16:1037 (Abstr.).
Ellis, R.P., and M.W. Vorhies. 1976. *J. Am. Vet. Med. Assoc.* 68:231.
Evans, H.M., and K.S. Bishop. 1922a. *Science* 56:650.
Evans, H.M., and K.S. Bishop. 1922b. *J. Metab. Res.* 1:335.
Ewan, R.C., et al. 1969. *J. Anim. Sci.* 9:912.
Fontaine, M., V.E.O. Valli, and L.G. Young. 1977a. *Can. J. Comp. Med.* 41:57.
Fontaine, M., V.E.O. Valli, and L.G. Young. 1977b. *Can. J. Comp. Med.* 41:64.
Fontaine, M., et al. 1977c. *Can. J. Comp. Med.* 41:41.
Food and Drug Administration. U.S. Department of Health and Human Services. 1987. Fed. Reg. 52:21001.
Forbes, R.M., and H.H. Draper. 1957. *J. Anim. Sci.* 16:1037 (Abstr.).
Franke, K.W. 1934. *J. Nutr.* 8:597.
Frost, D.V. 1981. In: *Selenium in Biology and Medicine.* p. 490. Westport, CT: AVI Publishing Co.
Glienke, L.R., and R.C. Ewan. 1977. *J. Anim. Sci.* 45:1334.
Goehring, T.B., et al. 1984a. *J. Anim. Sci.* 59:725.
Goehring, T.B., et al. 1984b. *J. Anim. Sci.* 59:733.
Gortner, R.A. 1940. *J. Nutr.* 19:105.
Grant, C.A., and B. Thafvelin. 1958. *Nord. Vet. Med.* 10:657.
Grant, C.A., B. Thafvelin, and R. Christell. 1961a. *Acta Pharmacol. Toxicol.* 18:285.
Grant, C.A. 1961b. *Acta Vet. Scand.* 2(Suppl. 3):1.
Groce, A.W., et al. 1973a. *J. Anim. Sci.* 37:942.
Groce, A.W., et al. 1973b. *J. Anim. Sci.* 37:948.
Hakkarainen, J., et al. 1978a. *Acta Vet. Scand.* 19:269.
Hakkarainen, J., et al. 1978b. *J. Anim. Sci.* 46:1001.
Halverson, A.W., I.S. Palmer, and P.L. Guss. 1966. *Toxicol. Appl. Pharmacol.* 9:477.
Harr, J.R., et al. 1967. In: *Selenium in Biology and Medicine.* Muth, O.H. (Ed.). p. 153. Westport, CT: AVI Publishing Co.
Harrison, L.H., et al. 1983. *Vet. Pathol.* 20:265.
Herigstad, R.R., C.K. Whitehair, and O.E. Olson. 1973. *Am. J. Vet. Res.* 34:1227.
Hill, C.H. 1975. *Fed. Proc.* 34:2096.
Hitchcock, J.P., et al. 1978. *J. Anim. Sci.* 46:425.
Jaffe, W.G., and C. Mondragon. 1975. *Br. J. Nutr.* 33:387.
Jenkins, K.J., and M. Hidiroglou. 1972. *Can. J. Physiol. Pharmacol.* 50:927.
Jensen, P.T., V. Danielsen, and H.E. Nielsen. 1979. *Acta Vet. Scand.* 20:92.

Jensen, P.T., et al. 1983. *Acta Vet. Scand.* 24:135.
Jensen, A.M., et al. 1984. *Acta Vet. Scand.* 25:436.
Julien, W.E., et al. 1976. *J. Dairy Sci.* 59:1960.
Kornegay, E.T., et al. 1986. *J. Anim. Sci.* 63:484.
Ku, P.K., et al. 1972. *J. Anim. Sci.* 34:208.
Ku, P.K., et al. 1973. *J. Anim. Sci.* 37:501.
Kurkela, P., and E. Kaantee. 1984. *J. Agric. Sci. Finland* 56:61.
Lake, A.M., M.J. Stuart, and F.A. Oski. 1977. *J. Pediatr.* 90:722.
Lannek, N., et al. 1961. *Res. Vet. Sci.* 2:67.
Lannek, N., P. Lindberg, and G. Tollerz. 1962. *Nature (London)* 195:1006.
Larsen, H.J., and S. Tollersrud. 1981. *Res. Vet. Sci.* 31:301.
Lawrence, R.A., and R.F. Burk. 1978. *J. Nutr.* 108:211.
Levander, O.A., and C.A. Baumann. 1966. *Toxicol. Appl. Pharmacol.* 9:106.
Levesque, M. 1974. *Can. J. Soil Sci.* 54:63.
Lindberg, P. 1973. *Acta Vet. Scand.* 19(Suppl.):39.
Loudenslager, M.J., et al. 1986. *J. Anim. Sci.* 63:1905.
Lowry, K.R., D.C. Mahan, and J.R. Corley. 1985a. *J. Anim. Sci.* 60:1438.
Lowry, K.R., D.C. Mahan, and J.R. Corley. 1985b. *J. Anim. Sci.* 60:1429.
Machlin, L.J. 1984. In: *Handbook of Vitamins. Nutritional, Biochemical and Clinical Aspects.* Machlin, L.J. (Ed.). pp. 99–146. New York: Marcel Dekker.
Machlin, L.J., J. Keating, J. Nelson, et al. 1979. *J. Nutr.* 109:105.
Mahan, D.C. 1985. *J. Anim. Sci.* 61:173.
Mahan, D.C. 1987. *J. Anim. Sci.* 65(Suppl. 1):132.
Mahan, D.C., and A.L. Moxon. 1978a. *J. Anim. Sci.* 46:384.
Mahan, D.C., and A.L. Moxon. 1978b. *J. Anim. Sci.* 47:456.
Mahan, D.C., and A.L. Moxon. 1980. *Nutr. Rep. Int.* 21:829.
Mahan, D.C., and A.L. Moxon. 1984. *J. Anim. Sci.* 58:1216.
Mahan, D.C., A.L. Moxon, and J.H. Cline. 1975. *J. Anim. Sci.* 40:624.
Mahan, D.C., A.L. Moxon, and M. Hubbard. 1977. *J. Anim. Sci.* 45:738.
Mahan, D.C., et al. 1973. *J. Anim. Sci.* 36:1104.
Mahan, D.C., et al. 1974. *J. Anim. Sci.* 39:536.
Mandisodza, K.T., et al. 1979. *J. Anim. Sci.* 49:535.
Marin-Guzman, J., D.C. Mahan, and R.E. Whitmoyer. 1988. *J. Anim. Sci.* 66(Suppl. 1):327.
Mathias, M.M., D.E. Hogue, and J.K. Loosli. 1967. *J. Nutr.* 93:14.
Mayland, H.F. 1985. In: "Selenium Responsive Diseases in Food Animals." Las Vegas, February 18. Western States Vet. Conf. p. 5.
McConnel, K.P., and O.W. Portsman. 1952. *J. Biol. Chem.* 195:277.
Meyer, W.R., D.C. Mahan, and A.L. Moxon. 1981. *J. Anim. Sci.* 52:302.
Michel, R.L., C.K. Whitehair, and K.K. Keahey. 1969. *J. Am. Vet. Med. Assoc.* 155:50.
Miller, E.R., et al. 1973. *Rep. Swine Res.* 232. MI State Univ. p. 43.
Miller, W.T. 1938. *J. Agric. Res.* 56:831.
Miller, W.T., and K.T. Williams. 1940. *J. Agric. Res.* 60:163.
Mills, G.C. 1957. *J. Biol. Chem.* 229:189.
Moxon, A.L. 1937. *S. Dakota Agric. Exp. Sta. Bull. No. 311.*
Moxon, A.L. 1941. *Proc. S. Dakota Acad. Sci.* 21:34.
Mustard, J.F., and M.A. Packham. 1970. *Pharmacol. Rev.* 22:97.
Nafstad, I. 1965. *Pathol. Vet.* 2:277.
Nafstad, I., and H.J. Nafstad. 1968. *Pathol. Vet.* 5:520.
Nafstad, I., and S. Tollersrud. 1970. *Acta Vet. Scand.* 11:452.
Nielsen, H.E., et al. *Acta Agric. Scand. Suppl.* 19:35.
Nielsen, H.E., et al. *Acta Vet. Scand.* 20:276.
Niyo, Y., et al. 1977. *Am. J. Vet. Res.* 38:1479.
Niyo, Y., et al. 1980. *Am. J. Vet. Res.* 41:474.
Nockels, C.F. 1979. *Fed. Proc.* 38:2134.

NRC. 1983. *Selenium in Nutrition.* Revised Edition. pp. 22–27.
NRC. 1988. *Nutrient Requirements of Swine.* 9th Revised Edition. Washington, DC: National Academy Press.
Obel, A.L. 1953. *Acta Pathol. Microbiol. Scand.* 94(Suppl.):1.
Obermeyer, B.D., et al. 1971. *Toxicol. Appl. Pharmacol.* 20:135.
Olson, O.E., C.E. Holmquist, and C.W. Carlson. 1973. *Poult. Sci.* 52:403.
Olson, O.E., et al. 1963. *J. Agric. Food Chem.* 11:531.
Olson, O.E., et al. 1970. *Phytochemistry* 9:1181.
Orstadius, K. 1960. *Nature* 188:1117.
Palmer, I.S., and O.E. Olson. 1974. *J. Nutr.* 104:306.
Palmer, I.S., et al. 1980. *J. Nutr.* 110:145.
Palmer, I.S., et al. 1970. *Biochim. Biophys. Acta* 208:260.
Parsons, M.J., et al. 1985. *J. Anim. Sci.* 60:451.
Patterson, D.S.P., et al. 1967. *Biochem. J.* 104:2.
Patterson, D.S.P., et al. 1969. *Zentralbl. Vet. Med. A.* 16:199.
Patterson, D.S.P. et al. 1971. *Zentralbl. Vet. Med. A.* 18:453.
Peplowski, M.A. et al. 1981. *J. Anim. Sci.* 51:344.
Piatkowski, T.C., et al. 1979. *J. Anim. Sci.* 48:1357.
Pond, W.G., et al. 1971. *J. Anim. Sci.* 33:996.
Ringarp, N. 1960. *Acta Agric. Scand.* 7(Suppl.):140.
Rotruck, J.T., et al. 1973. *Science* 179:588.
Sarathchandra, S.U., and J.H. Watkinson. 1981. *Science* 211:600.
Saxegaard, F., and J. Teige, Jr. 1977. *Acta Vet. Scand.* 18:563.
Schwarz, K., and C.M. Foltz. 1957. *J. Am. Chem. Soc.* 79:3292.
Segerson, E.C., W.R. Getz, and B.H. Johnson. 1981. *J. Anim. Sci.* 53:1360.
Sheffy, B.E., and R.D. Schultz. 1979. *Fed. Proc.* 38:2139.
Stowe, H.D., and E.R. Miller. 1985. *J. Anim. Sci.* 60:200.
Swaine, D.J. 1955. *Common. Bur. Soil. Sci. Tech. Commun.* 48:91.
Sweeney, P.R., and R.G. Brown. 1972. *Am. J. Pathol.* 68:479.
Tagwerker, F.J. 1981. "Vitamins and Quality of Food Products of Animal Origin." Roche Seminar, Osaka and Tokyo, Japan.
Teige, J., Jr. 1977. *Acta Vet. Scand.* 18:140.
Teige, J., Jr., K. Nordstoga, and J. Aursjo. 1977. *Acta Vet. Scan.* 18:384.
Teige, J., Jr., F. Saxegaard, and A. Froslie. 1978. *Acta Vet. Scand.* 19:133.
Teige, J., Jr., et al. 1973. *Acta Vet. Scand.* 14:92.
Thomlinson, J.R., and A. Buxton. 1963. *Immunology* 6:126.
Thulin, A.J., et al. 1985. *J. Anim. Sci.* 61(Suppl 1):74.
Tollersrud, S. 1973. *Acta Agric. Scand.* 19(Suppl.):124.
Tollerz, G. 1973. *Acta Agric. Scand.* 19(Suppl.):184.
Tollerz, G., and N. Lannek. 1964. *Nature* 201:846.
Trapp, A.L., et al. 1970. *J. Am. Vet. Med. Assoc.* 157:289.
Ullrey, D.E. 1981. *J. Anim. Sci.* 53:1039.
Van Vleet, J.F. 1982. *Am. J. Vet. Res.* 43:851.
Van Vleet, J.F., and G.R. Ruth. 1977. *Am. J. Vet. Res.* 38:1299.
Van Vleet, J.F., W. Carlton, and H.J. Olander. 1970. *J. Am. Vet. Med. Assoc.* 157:1208.
Van Vleet, J.F., K.B. Meyer, and H.J. Olander. 1973. *J. Am. Vet. Med. Assoc.* 163:452.
Van Vleet, J.F., A.H. Rebar, and V.J. Ferrans. 1977. *Am. J. Vet. Res.* 38:991.
Vrzgula, L., et al. 1980. *Arch. Exper. Vet. Med. Leipzig* 36:775.
Wahlstrom, R.C., and O.E. Olson. 1959. *J. Anim. Sci.* 18:141.
Wahlstrom, R.C., L.D. Kamstra, and O.E. Olson. 1955. *J. Anim. Sci.* 14:105.
Wahlstrom, R.C., L.D. Kamstra, and O.E. Olson. 1956. *J. Anim. Sci.* 15:794.
Wahlstrom, R.C., et al. 1984. *Nutr. Rep. Int.* 29:143.
Whanger, P.D. 1981. In: *Selenium in Biology and Medicine.* Spallholz, M.G. (Ed.). Westport, CT: AVI Publishing Co.

Whitehair, C.K., and E.R. Miller. 1985. In: *Selenium Responsive Diseases in Food Animals.* West States Vet. Conf. p. 11. Las Vegas, February 18.
Wilkinson, J.E., et al. 1977a. *J. Anim. Sci.* 44:224.
Wilkinson, J.E., et al. 1977b. *J. Anim. Sci.* 44:229.
Wretlind, B., K. Orstadius, and P. Lindberg. 1959. *Zentralbl. Vet. Med. A.* 6:963.
Wu, A.S.H., et al. 1973. *Biol. Reprod.* 8:625.
Wu, A.S.H., et al. 1979. *Biol. Reprod.* 20:793.
Yen, J.T., et al. 1986. *Nutr. Rep. Int.* 31:877.
Young, L.G., et al. 1975. *J. Anim. Sci.* 40:495.
Young, L.G., et al. 1976. *Can. J. Comp. Med.* 40:92.
Young, L.G., et al. 1977a. *J. Anim. Sci.* 45:1051.
Young, L.G., et al. 1977b. *J. Anim. Sci.* 44:590.
Young, L.G., et al. 1978. *J. Anim. Sci.* 47:639.

Chapter 13

Vitamins A and K in Swine Nutrition

D.E. Ullrey

VITAMIN A

Chemical Structure and Nomenclature

Vitamin A is a generic term for derivatives of beta-ionone that have, to some degree, the biological activity of all-*trans* retinol (Anonymous 1982). Esters of all-*trans* retinol are known as retinyl esters. A palmitic acid ester of retinol is named retinyl palmitate. If the terminal group of retinol is a carboxyl, it is known as retinoic acid. An aldehyde form of retinol, active in vision, is 11-*cis* retinal. Another naturally occurring compound, once known as vitamin A_2, is 3-dehydroretinol. Structures of these compounds are shown in Figure 13.1.

The international standard for vitamin A is all-*trans* retinyl acetate, 0.344 μg of which has 1 IU of biological activity for the rat. All-*trans* retinol and all-*trans* retinyl palmitate have 1 IU biological activity per 0.300 μg and 0.549 μg, respectively.

Over 400 carotenoids have been isolated from nature, with about 50 possessing biological activity. The most active of these provitamins is all-*trans* beta-carotene, although cryptoxanthin, and alpha- and gamma-carotene also are found in significant concentrations in feedstuffs and have appreciable provitamin A activity. Their structures are shown in Figure 13.2.

All-*trans* beta-carotene is the international standard for provitamins A, and 0.6 μg has 1 IU of provitamin A activity for the rat.

Concentrations in Feedstuffs

Preformed vitamin A is found only in animal products, and concentrations are extremely variable because of differences in levels in the animals from which the products

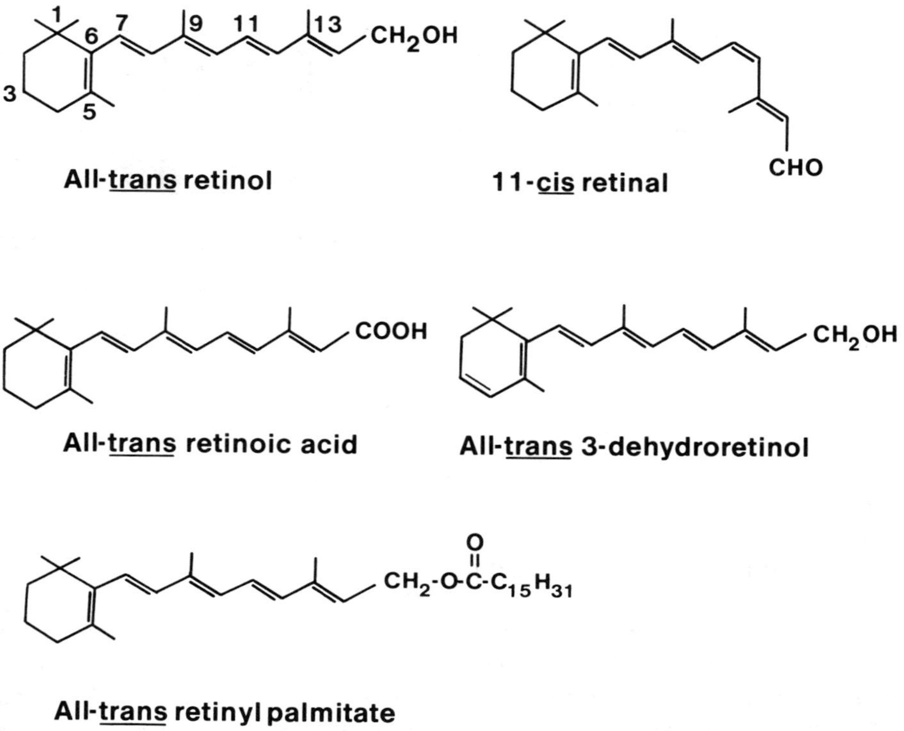

FIGURE 13.1 *Chemical structure of all-*trans *retinol and several major derivatives.*

were derived and because of losses during processing and storage. Vitamin A concentrations found in dried whole milk and dried whey have been reported to be 11,600 and 500 IU/kg dry matter, respectively (NRC 1986). Fish meal made from alewives was reported to contain 4300 IU vitamin A/kg dry matter. Vitamin A concentrations in other animal products commonly used in swine feeds are unknown or are presumed to be low due to low fat content or vitamin A destruction.

Provitamin A compounds (carotenes and carotenoids) may be found in small quantities in certain animal products but are most concentrated in yellow and green plant feedstuffs. Yellow corn and yellow corn by-products, such as corn gluten meal, have considerable provitamin A activity. White corn, barley, oats, rye, sorghum grains, and wheat essentially have none. Growing green plants, such as alfalfa, have very high provitamin A concentrations. When these plants are cut and dried to produce dehydrated alfalfa meal, much of that provitamin A activity is retained. However, just as for vitamin A, provitamin A activity declines with processing and storage, and levels found in feedstuffs are extremely variable. Carotene concentrations found in certain plant products used in swine diets are shown in Table 13.1.

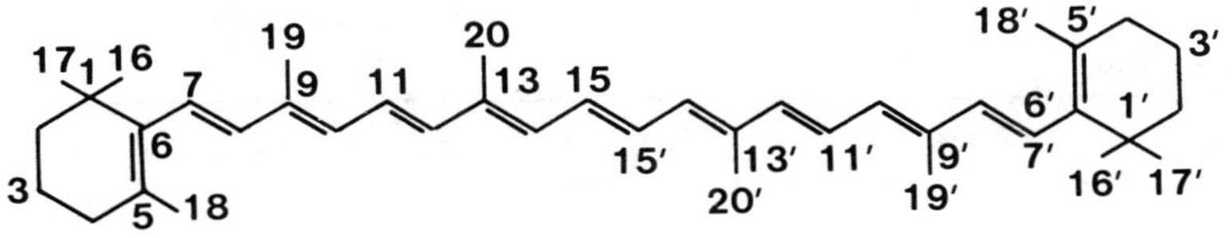

All-trans β-carotene

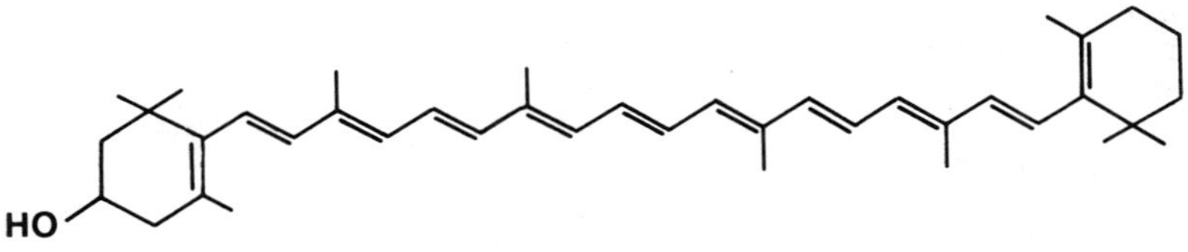

Cryptoxanthin

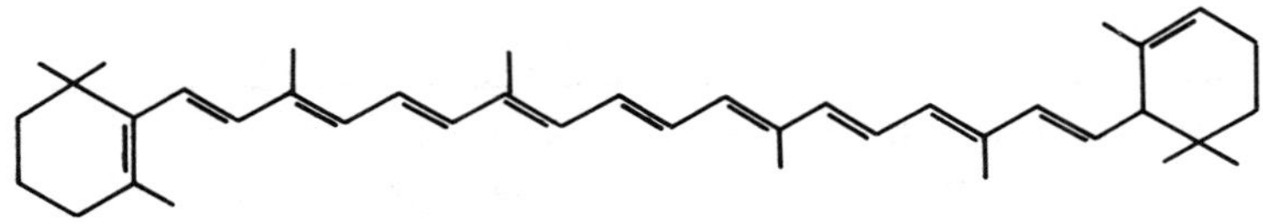

α-carotene

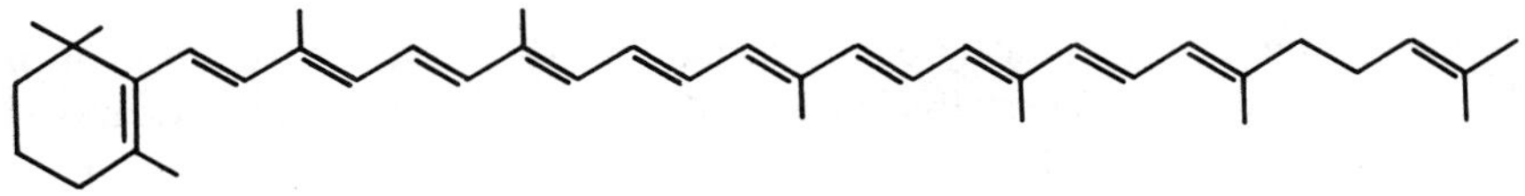

γ-carotene

FIGURE 13.2 *Chemical structure of all-*trans *beta-carotene and several important derivates.*

Commercial Sources

Several stabilized forms of vitamin A are available commercially. Retinyl palmitate is one of the most common, but retinyl acetate and retinyl propionate are manufactured, also. These products are imbedded, along with antioxidants, in a gelatin-carbohydrate matrix to create beadlets that retain 90% or more of their initial activity for at least 6 months when mixed in feeds and stored under good conditions. When temperatures and humidity are high, loss may be considerably greater (Olson 1984).

All-*trans* beta-carotene can be produced by a fermentative process (Ciegler et al. 1963). One milligram of this carotene has about 190 IU of provitamin A activity for swine (Ullrey et al. 1965; Hendricks et al. 1967), but its primary intended use was as a coloring agent in human foods.

Table 13.1 Carotene Concentrations (Dry Basis) Found in Plant Products Used in Swine Diets[a]

Plant Product	*Dry Matter (%)*	*Beta-Carotene (mg/kg)*
Alfalfa, fresh, early bloom	23	174
Alfalfa meal, dehydrated (17% CP)	92	131
Barley grain	88	2
Brewers' grain, dried	92	1
Corn distillers' solubles, dried	93	1
Corn gluten meal (60% CP)	90	34
Corn grain, yellow	89	3
Cottonseed meal, solv. (41% CP)	91	—[b]
Oats grain	89	0
Peanut meal, solv.	92	—[b]
Rye grain	88	0
Sorghum grain	89	0
Soybean meal, solv. (44% CP)	90	0
Wheat grain	89	0
Wheat middlings	89	—[b]

[a]Values for fresh alfalfa are from NRC 1984. Other values are from NRC 1985.
[b]Presumed to be zero based on carotene concentrations in related products.

Stability and Bioavailability

Retinol in pure form is easily oxidized, particularly when exposed to light in a hot, humid environment. When dissolved in seed oils with natural antioxidants, such as alpha-tocopherol and beta-carotene, retinol is quite resistant to destruction.

Carotenes and carotenoids are very unstable in pure form but in feeds behave similarly to retinol. They can be oxidized to inactive forms during storage by enzymatic action or by exposure to light and oxygen. The loss of provitamin A activity during storage of sun-cured hay is about 7% per month (Waite and Sastry 1949).

The bioavailability of dietary retinol or retinyl esters for the pig appears to be equivalent on a molar basis. Thus, 1 IU of vitamin A activity can be derived from 0.300 μg of all-*trans* retinol, 0.344 μg of all-*trans* retinyl acetate, or 0.549 μg of all-*trans* retinyl palmitate.

The bioavailability of carotenes and carotenoids in feedstuffs is dependent on the isomers present and the amounts consumed per day, smaller amounts being used more efficiently. Yellow corn contains three compounds with provitamin A activity: beta-carotene, beta-zeacarotene, and cryptoxanthin. These are present in approximate proportions of 25:25:50. When fed in concentrations comparable to those found in typical corn-soybean meal diets used for pigs, 1 mg of this carotene/carotenoid mixture has about 260 IU of vitamin A activity for support of liver vitamin A storage, as compared with all-*trans* retinyl palmitate (Wellenreiter et al. 1969). Schöne et al. (1988) found that 1 mg of synthetic beta-carotene added in concentrations of 2, 4, 8, 50, and 100 mg/kg to a vitamin A-free and beta-carotene–free grain-soybean meal diet for growing pigs was equivalent to 360, 320, 290, 130, and 80 μg of retinol, respectively.

Metabolism

Absorption

After food is consumed, preformed vitamin A compounds and provitamin A carotenes and carotenoids are released from proteins by gastric pepsin and duodenal proteases (Olson 1984). These lipid-soluble materials become a part of fat globules that are acted on by pancreatic lipase and retinyl ester hydrolase in the presence of bile salts to form mixed micelles containing retinol, carotenes and carotenoids, sterols, phospholipids, monoglycerides and diglycerides, and fatty acids. These micelles diffuse into the glycoprotein layer surrounding the microvillus and contact the cell membranes, allowing transfer of provitamin A and vitamin A compounds into the mucosal cells. A mucosal beta-carotene dioxygenase splits provitamin A compounds at the 15,15′ position, releasing retinal, which is converted to retinol (Fidge et al. 1969). Much of the retinol, derived either from preformed vitamin A in the diet or from carotenoid cleavage, is esterified in the mucosal cell with palmitic acid or with smaller quantities of other fatty acids, such as oleic or stearic. These retinyl esters plus triglyceride, phospholipid, and protein become part of chylomicra that are released into the lymph and, thus, are transported via the portal circulation to the liver. In the liver, a specific retinol-binding protein is synthesized and binds to all-*trans* retinol for transport in the plasma (Huang et al. 1972). Chew et al. (1983) found that retinol makes up over 85% of total plasma vitamin A in swine, while the remainder is retinyl esters. Beta-carotene was not found in swine plasma.

Tissue Deposition

A number of tissues (retina, intestine, skin) have cell surface receptors that recognize retinol-binding protein. Retinol is released, is transferred across the cell membrane, and is bound by cellular retinol-binding proteins in the cytosol. Normally, over 90% of vitamin A stores are found in the liver, with a much smaller, but significant, store in the kidneys. The storage form is probably a lipoglycoprotein complex with over 95% of vitamin A as retinyl esters and the remainder as unesterified retinol (Chew et al. 1983; Olson 1984).

Swine ovarian follicular fluid was found to contain 37 μg retinol/dl but no beta-carotene. Porcine corpora lutea contained neither beta-carotene nor retinol (Chew et al. 1983). Testicular tissue of boars of breeding age contained 48 to 107 IU of vitamin A/100 g, isolated as retinol after alkaline hydrolysis (Booth 1974).

Intermediary Metabolism

A variety of vitamin A metabolites have been identified in several tissues. In the liver, retinol may be phosphorylated by adenosine triphosphate (ATP) to retinyl phosphate, and then interact with guanosine diphosphate (GDP) mannose to form retinyl phosphomannose. Retinol also may be transformed into its beta-glucuronide. Retinol may be oxidized to retinoic acid, and retinoic acid may be transformed to a beta-glucuronide or a 5,6-epoxy derivative, or oxidized to a 4-hydroxide and, finally, to a 4-ketoretinoic acid. This latter compound may form a beta-glucoronide, be oxidatively chain-shortened, or be demethylated (Olson 1984).

Excretion

The proportion of dietary carotenoids that is excreted in the feces appears to be directly related to level of intake. In other words, the efficiency of absorption declines with increasing dietary carotenoid concentration. Since swine normally do not circulate carotenoids in their plasma, carotenoid derivatives, other than derivatives of retinol, are not found in bile or urine (Olson 1984).

Absorbed vitamin A may be stored, conjugated, or oxidized and then excreted. Derivatives, such as glucuronide conjugates of retinol, retinoic acid, and 4-ketoretinoic acid, generally are excreted in the feces via the bile. Oxidatively chain-shortened and demethylated derivatives generally are excreted in the urine (Olson 1984).

Biochemical Functions

Vision

While the biochemical details of the visual process are still controversial, it has been known for years (Wald 1968) that a photon striking the dark-adapted retina will activate the visual pigment rhodopsin, producing a transient conformational change and generating an electrical signal that travels via the optic nerves to the visual center of the brain. Vital to normal function is 11-*cis* retinal, a component of rhodopsin. Retinol in the plasma is transferred into the rod cell and is oxidized to all-*trans* retinal by retinol reductase, requiring nicotinamide-adenine-dinucleotide phosphate (NADP). All-*trans* retinal is then isomerized to 11-*cis* retinal.

Growth

The weight gain of baby pigs that are born to depleted mothers is affected very little by low vitamin A intakes after birth (Heaney et al. 1963). Skeletal growth appears to be restricted, but soft tissue growth continues. The primary effect of vitamin A deficiency on growth of bone seems to involve faulty bone remodeling. In the absence of adequate vitamin A, bones do not increase in dimension normally, and foramena through which nerves and blood vessels pass do not properly enlarge. It has been demonstrated in rats that, while only dietary retinol will support vision, either retinol or retinoic acid will support growth. Both compounds also will support growth in pigs (Nelson et al. 1964).

Tissue Differentiation

It has been known for a long time that mucus-secreting epithelial cells become keratinized when vitamin A deficiency occurs in the rat, and in vitro studies with chick mesenchymal cells established that differentiation into columnar or squamous epithelium could be influenced by adequate or limited supplies of vitamin A in the culture medium. A current hypothesis indicates that retinyl phosphate serves as a carrier of sugars in the synthesis of specific glycoproteins, which may act as cell surface receptors or as regulators of cellular differentiation (Wolf et al. 1979; DeLuca et al. 1979).

Deficiency Signs

More than 70 years ago, signs of vitamin A deficiency were described in swine (Hart et al. 1916). Incoordination, emaciation, blindness, and posterior paralysis were seen. Others (Hale 1935; Hostetler et al. 1935; Guilbert et al. 1937, 1940; Braude et al. 1941, 1951; Hentges et al. 1952a, 1952b; Sorensen et al. 1954; Goodwin and Jennings 1958; Frape et al. 1959; Hjarde et al. 1959; Nelson et al. 1962; Heaney et al. 1963; Wellenreiter et al. 1969; Booth 1974; Brief and Chew 1983) have confirmed and extended these observations and have reported reduced growth rate, ataxia, night blindness, elevated cerebrospinal fluid pressure, abnormal skeletal remodeling, squamous metaplasia of epithelial tissue, reduced spermatogenesis, developmental abnormalities including microphthalmia and anophthalmia, increased embryonic mortality, and weakness in newborn pigs. Dvorak (1973) found no differences in adrenocortical activity between vitamin A-supplemented and mildly hypovitaminotic pigs despite the observation of Wolf et al. (1958) that vitamin A deficiency in rats resulted in decreased glucocorticoid production or secretion and presumably an impaired response to stress.

Assessment of Vitamin A Status

Clinical

Growth rate appears to be relatively insensitive to vitamin A deficiency (Frape et al. 1959; Nelson et al. 1952). A detailed report by Hostetler et al. (1935) indicated that the first clinical sign of vitamin A deficiency in young pigs (15 kg initial weight) was depressed appetite, appearing after 93 to 122 days. Locomotor incoordination appeared 10 to 20 days later. The pigs squealed when approached, were restless, and walked in circles. A profuse watery discharge from the eye, with some purulence, developed, followed by corneal ulceration and opacity. Exophthalmos was seen, and there was a partial or total loss of vision. These workers did not report evidence of night blindness, which has been proposed as one of the earliest signs of vitamin A deficiency. However, tests for night blindness are very difficult to conduct with swine. Clonic spasms and loss of the ability to stand were seen at about 240 days. Abscesses were common at necropsy.

Biochemical

When vitamin A concentrations in swine plasma or serum are expressed as total retinol, mean values on adequate practical diets appear to fall in the range of 20 to 40 μg/dl

(Grummer et al. 1948; Heaney et al. 1963; Eaton et al. 1964; Ullrey et al. 1965; Wellenreiter et al. 1969). If weaned pigs are fed a diet containing no supplemental vitamin A nor any measurable beta-carotene for up to 10 weeks, serum retinol concentrations decline about 0.3 to 0.7 μg/dl/day. When 1000 IU vitamin A (as retinyl palmitate)/kg diet are fed to depleted pigs, serum vitamin A concentrations are restored to normal within 2 weeks (Ullrey et al. 1965). However, liver vitamin A concentration (expressed as retinol) is proportional to dietary vitamin A concentration over a broad range. After 9 weeks of repletion, pigs fed diets containing 0, 250, 500, 1000, or 2000 IU vitamin A/kg had mean liver retinol concentrations of 1, 3, 9, 27, or 76 μg/g (dry basis), respectively. Significant linear correlations between concentrations of vitamin A in the diet and in the liver were found by Hennig et al. (1985), but plasma vitamin A concentrations were not different between 1000 and 4000 IU vitamin A/kg diet. These workers estimated that the threshold of liver vitamin A concentration was 35 IU/g liver, below which plasma vitamin A concentrations would fall from a plateau of about 45 IU/dl. However, the correlation was only 0.52, and application of the relationship to individual animals must be made with caution. Free-living adult wild boars were found to have 2000 and 1400 IU/g liver in females and males, respectively (Drescher-Kaden and Hoppe 1972). Piglets had 400 IU and juveniles between 13 and 24 months of age had 700 IU/g liver. It should be noted that, while the concentrations of vitamin A in different locations within the pig liver seem to be similar, samples taken next to a previous liver biopsy may have a lower vitamin A concentration than at other locations, presumably because of tissue scarring and interference with normal blood flow (Jones et al. 1956).

Plasma vitamin A (as retinol) concentrations and cerebrospinal fluid pressure were inversely related after 75 days of a vitamin A intake from retinyl palmitate equivalent to 0, 2.2, 22, or 220 μg retinol/kg body weight (Nelson et al. 1964). Comparable effects on cerebrospinal fluid pressure were seen when like amounts of retinoic acid were fed. However, no level of supplemental retinoic acid sustained normal plasma or liver vitamin A concentrations.

Grummer et al. (1948) found that newborn pigs before nursing had a mean plasma vitamin A (as retinol) concentration of 10 μg/dl. The ingestion of colostrum resulted in an immediate increase, reaching a peak of 34 μg/dl plasma during the first week. After weaning, these values declined to 20 μg/dl or less. Bowland et al. (1949) analyzed colostrum and milk from ten sows on pasture and ten sows in dry lot. No carotene was present, and mean vitamin A concentrations (as retinol) tended to be higher in colostrum and milk from sows on pasture. The colostrum and milk retinol concentrations in relation to stage of lactation found by Bowland et al. (1949) are shown in Table 13.2. Dvorak (1986) also found that newborn pigs had very low plasma vitamin A concentrations before ingestion of colostrum. Afterward, plasma vitamin A concentrations rose abruptly to several times their initial values. Liver vitamin A concentrations in newborn pigs have been reported to be about 60 μmol retinol/kg, with a large standard deviation (Steinhardt et al. 1985).

Table 13.2 Vitamin A Concentration in Sows' Colostrum and Milk Throughout Lactation[a]

	Stage of Lactation									
Sow Location	*1 d*	*3 d*	*1 wk*	*2 wk*	*3 wk*	*4 wk*	*5 wk*	*6 wk*	*7 wk*	*8 wk*
Pasture										
Mean	145	153	79	51	53	51	51	52	53	57
Low	65	61	33	29	27	38	38	40	38	40
High	254	331	155	78	78	67	61	71	78	86
Dry lot										
Mean	129	137	64	35	39	38	31	32	33	36
Low	83	68	19	18	20	18	11	18	20	19
High	166	301	151	72	63	64	52	48	70	71

[a] All values are in micrograms retinol per deciliter.

(Adapted, by permission, from Bowland et al. 1949.)

Requirement

The vitamin A requirements of swine can be met either by preformed vitamin A or by various provitamin A-active carotenes and carotenoids. Of the provitamin A compounds, beta-carotene has the greatest biological activity for swine, although pigs appear less efficient than rats in converting beta-carotene to vitamin A (Ullrey 1972). Based on liver storage of vitamin A, 1 mg of the carotenes and carotenoids in corn has about 260 IU of provitamin A activity for growing-finishing pigs (Wellenreiter et al. 1969).

Because liver vitamin A stores may be substantial, they can be used during periods of low vitamin A intake. Thus, estimates of dietary vitamin A requirement depend on the degree of vitamin A depletion or repletion. In addition, estimates of requirement depend on the criterion chosen. Weight gain is less sensitive to dietary vitamin A supply than are cerebrospinal fluid pressure, plasma vitamin A concentration, or liver vitamin A stores. Using various criteria, Sheffy et al. (1954) and Frape et al. (1959) concluded that pigs, during the first 8 weeks of life, required 220 to 1760 IU of vitamin A/kg of diet.

Growing-finishing pigs require 100 to 380 IU/kg diet for maximum daily gain and 1000 to 2700 IU/kg diet for normal cerebrospinal fluid pressure or moderate liver storage (Guilbert et al. 1937; Braude et al. 1941; Hentges et al. 1952a; Myers et al. 1959; Hjarde et al. 1961; Nelson et al. 1963; Ullrey et al. 1965). Schöne and Lüdke (1984) found that as long as liver vitamin A concentrations were >50 IU/g at weaning and >100 IU/g at the start of finishing, dietary vitamin A concentrations of 250 IU/kg produced the same weight gains from weaning to market as did 2000 IU vitamin A/kg diet. Likewise in these pigs, based on serum protein profile and the development of antibodies to human gamma globulin or to a lipopolysaccharide from *Salmonella dublin,* Lüdke et al. (1985) were unable to demonstrate a dietary vitamin A requirement higher than 250 IU/kg. Dietary vitamin A requirements may be increased by elevated intakes of nitrite or nitrate (Koch et al. 1963; Seerley et al. 1965; Wood et al 1967; Hutagalung et al. 1968), although there may be some adaptation over time to elevated nitrite intakes (Schöne and Lüdke 1984).

Estimates of vitamin A requirements for reproduction are affected to a major degree by liver stores. Only in the fourth pregnancy of sows fed diets without supplemental vitamin A did Braude et al. (1941) see evidence of deficiency. When gilts received adequate vitamin A until 9 months of age, no signs of deficiency were seen during two reproductive cycles (Hjarde et al. 1961; Selke et al. 1967). Heaney et al. (1963) fed a low vitamin A diet to gilts from 4 months of age through two reproductive cycles and found no effects on litter size, birth weights, survival rates, or gains after birth. Parrish et al. (1951) proposed that 7000 IU of vitamin A/day during gestation and lactation would support normal serum and liver vitamin A concentrations.

The National Research Council (1988a) has proposed vitamin A requirements of 2200, 1750, and 1300 IU/kg diet (90% dry matter) for pigs that weigh 1 to 10, 10 to 20, and 20 to 110 kg, respectively. The proposed vitamin A requirement for bred gilts and sows and adult boars was 4000 IU/kg diet and for lactating gilts and sows was 2000 IU/kg diet.

Toxicity

Signs

Hypervitaminosis A in swine results in rough hair coat, scaly skin, hyperirritability, hyperesthesia, bleeding from cracks in the skin above the hooves, blood in urine and feces, ataxia, inability to rise, periodic tremors, and death (Anderson et al. 1966).

Toxic Levels

When young pigs (5 to 10 kg) were fed diets containing 880,000, 660,000, or 440,000 IU of added vitamin A/kg, toxicity signs appeared in 18, 32, or 43 days, respectively (Anderson et al. 1966). No toxicity signs were seen within 8 weeks when 220,000 IU of vitamin A were added/kg diet. Wolke et al. (1968) observed lesions in endochondral and intramembranous bone within 5 weeks when diets providing 6614 or 19,842 μg of retinyl acetate/kg of body weight/day were fed to weaned pigs.

The National Research Council (1988b) has proposed a maximum dietary vitamin A tolerance level of 20,000 IU/kg for growing swine and 40,000 IU/kg for breeding swine.

VITAMIN K

Chemical Structure and Nomenclature

Vitamin K is a generic descriptor for menadione (menaquinone; 2-methyl-1,4-naphthoquinone) and all derivatives that exhibit antihemorrhagic activity in animals fed a vitamin K-deficient diet. In the past, menadione has been known as vitamin K_3. This compound does not occur as such in natural feed ingredients. A naturally occurring derivative found in green plants and to a lesser extent in animal tissues is 2-methyl-3-phytyl-1,4-naphthoquinone (phylloquinone; phytylmenaquinone; vitamin K_1). A series of vitamin K compounds with unsaturated side chains has been found in bacteria and animal tissues. These have the class name 2-methyl-3-multiprenyl-1,4-naphthoquinone (menaquinone-n; prenylmenaquinone-n; vitamin $K_{2(n)}$). Structures are shown in Figure 13.3.

Concentrations in Feedstuffs

While both chemical and bioassays have been used for vitamin K analyses, a reliable data base for animal feed ingredients does not exist. In general, green leafy plant tissues are good sources of phylloquinone. The National Research Council (1974, 1981) has reported about 10 mg of vitamin K (presumably phylloquinone)/kg of dehydrated alfalfa meal. Herring fish meal has been reported to have about 2 mg of vitamin K (probably mostly prenylmenaquinones)/kg (NRC 1981). Corn, oats, and wheat have been reported to have about 0.2 to 0.3 mg of vitamin K (presumably phylloquinone)/kg

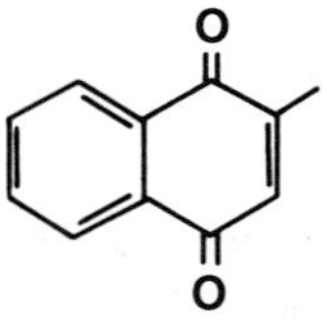

Menadione

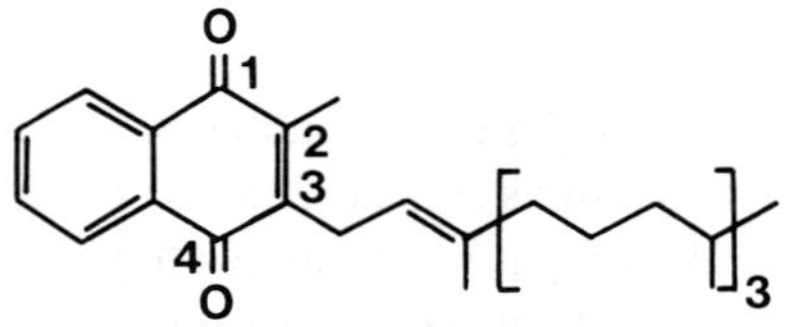

Phytylmenaquinone (vitamin K$_1$)

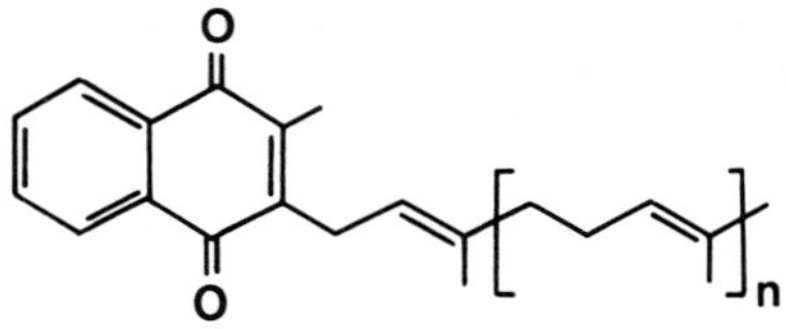

Prenylmenaquinone-n (vitamin K$_2$)

FIGURE 13.3 *Chemical structure of menadione, phytylmenaquinone (vitamin K_1), and prenylmenaquinone-n (vitamin K_2).*

(Olson 1973). Vitamin K-active compounds found in animal tissues probably have their origin both from the diet and from bacterial synthesis in the gastrointestinal tract. Intestinally synthesized prenylmenaquinones may be absorbed from the gut near or below the site of synthesis or as a consequence of coprophagy (Berdanier and Griminger 1968; Schulze and Haenel 1969).

Commercial Sources

Menadione was synthesized over 40 years ago (Fieser et al. 1941) and, when fed, was thought to have direct vitamin K activity. However, it is now usually assumed that menadione is alkylated to a biologically active menaquinone by intestinal microorganisms or by tissue alkylating enzymes (Suttie 1984). In any case, orally administered menadione has high biological antihemorrhagic activity. However, lipids must be present in the diet to promote absorption, and the stability of menadione in feeds is uncertain.

Thus, water-soluble derivatives of menadione have been developed. Menadione sodium bisulfite has been used commercially, but stability can be improved by crystallization in the presence of an excess of sodium bisulfite, forming menadione sodium bisulfite complex. This compound has been widely used in poultry and swine feeds. A third water-soluble derivative has been produced by the addition of dimethylpyrimidinol to menadione sodium bisulfite, resulting in a product called menadione pyrimidinol bisulfite. This product is equal to or somewhat superior to menadione sodium bisulfite complex for poultry (Griminger 1965; Dua and Day 1966; Charles et al. 1968) and swine (Seerley et al. 1976). The formulas of these commercial forms are presented in Figure 13.4.

Parenteral vitamin K preparations include water-soluble menadiol sodium diphosphate and water-miscible formulations of phylloquinone. The latter is relatively safe when administered intramuscularly. However, menadione and its water-soluble derivatives react with free tissue sulfhydryl groups, causing hemolytic anemia, hyperbilirubinemia, kernicterus, and brain damage in the neonate. Thus, parenteral use of menadiol sodium diphosphate is not recommended.

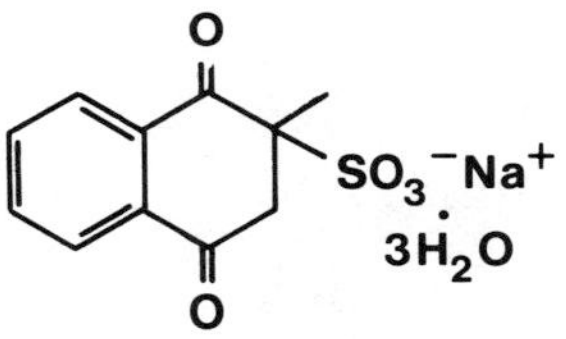

Menadione sodium bisulfite

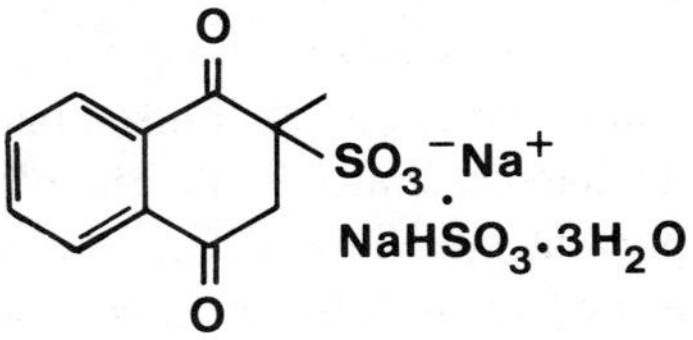

Menadione sodium bisulfite complex

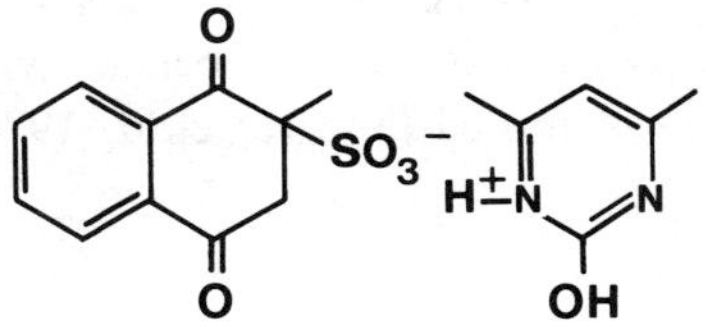

Menadione pyrimidinol bisulfite

FIGURE 13.4 *Chemical structures of commercial vitamin K forms.*

Antagonists

Coumin derivatives were the first antagonists of vitamin K to be discovered. Spoiled sweet clover, which caused a hemorrhagic disease of cattle, was found to contain 3,3′-methyl-bis-(4-hydroxycoumarin), or dicumarol. Several substituted hydroxycoumarins have been found to have significant anticoagulant activity, as do certain substituted indandiones, alkylated naphthoquinones, pyridinols, and pyrimidines (Suttie 1984).

Reports of a hemorrhagic syndrome in swine, in which blood-clotting Factors VII and X were deficient, suggested the presence of a vitamin K antagonist in moldy corn (Osweiler et al. 1970). The mold *Fusarium tricinctum* has been found to produce the toxin diacetoxyscirpenol, which produces edema and hemorrhage in the rat (Gilgan et al. 1966; Bamburg et al. 1968). Since Clardy et al. (1970) identified scirpenol-like compounds in feeds producing hemorrhage in swine, and since vitamin K improved prothrombin and blood clotting times (Muhrer et al. 1970), it has been suggested that scirpenols may be antagonostic to vitamin K in swine (Speer 1971).

While not structural antagonists, certain sulfa drugs and antibiotics can decrease intestinal synthesis of vitamin K by altering the intestinal flora.

Metabolism

Absorption

The polar vitamin K compounds are incorporated into mixed lipid micelles under the influence of bile and pancreatic lipase. During contact of the micelles with the microvillar membranes, the vitamin K compounds are transferred to the intestinal mucosal cells and then to the lymphatic system. Phylloquinone appears to be well absorbed in the proximal intestine of the rat by an energy-dependent process. Phylloquinone absorption in the distal gut is relatively poorer (Hollander 1973). Menaquinone absorption can occur in either the proximal or distal intestine by a passive process without carrier mediation (Hollander et al. 1976). The efficiency of this process generally appears sufficient to prevent vitamin K deficiency in mammals (Hollander et al. 1977). Menadione is absorbed from both the small intestine and colon by a passive process (Hollander and Truscott 1974a, 1974b).

Transport

Absorbed phylloquinone is associated with chylomicrons in the lymph (Blomstrand and Forsgren 1968). In the plasma, phylloquinone is associated with lipoproteins, but no specific carrier protein has been identified (Shearer et al. 1970).

Tissue Deposition

Phylloquinone, injected into the rat, rapidly concentrates in the liver but has a half-life of only about 17 hours (Thierry et al. 1970). Injected menadione is poorly concentrated in the liver, is widely distributed in all tissues, and is very rapidly excreted. Menadione is stored mainly as menaquinone-4. Menaquinones-6 to 13, found in liver and other tissues, presumably are of bacterial origin (Matschiner 1970).

Intermediary Metabolism

Menadione can be converted to a biologically active form, menaquinone-4, by alkylation in the liver. Some phylloquinone is converted to phylloquinone 2,3-epoxide. There is no evidence, however, that phylloquinone and the menaquinones must be metabolically transformed before they can serve as cofactors for the vitamin-K–dependent carboxylases (Suttie 1984).

Excretion

Glucuronides and sulfates of menadione have been found both in bile and urine. Several urinary glucuronides of phylloquinone have been identified. The degradative metabolism and excretion of phylloquinone and the menaquinones is much slower than that of menadione.

Biochemical Functions

Blood coagulation has been described as a cascade in which fibrinogen is ultimately converted to fibrin. The process is triggered by a series of events, initiated by intrinsic factors in the blood or by tissue factors released from a site of tissue injury. Subsequent to initiation, a proteinase, in conjunction with accessory components of an activation complex, converts an inactive precursor to an active proteolytic enzyme that becomes the proteinase in the next stage of the cascade. Four inactive precursors that require vitamin K for activation to the next stage are Factors VII, IX, and X, and prothrombin. The ultimate activation of prothrombin to thrombin promotes the fibrinogen to fibrin conversion and formation of a stable clot.

The vitamin-K–dependent step has been shown to be the formation of gamma-carboxyglutamic acid residues. Thus, synthesis of prothrombin requires a vitamin-K–dependent carboxylase, an endogenous precursor protein, oxygen, carbon dioxide, and vitamin K. The resultant gamma-carboxyglutamic acid residues provide binding sites for calcium ions that are needed for further activation (Suttie 1984).

Other vitamin-K–dependent proteins also have been identified, including osteocalcin that is found in association with the skeleton. The functions of these proteins are still under investigation (Suttie 1980).

Deficiency

Signs

Blood in the urine, subcutaneous hemorrhage, prolonged bleeding from the umbilicus or as a consequence of mild trauma, and extended blood clotting time have been seen in swine (Schendel and Johnson 1962; Fritschen et al. 1971; Brooks et al. 1973; Seerley et al. 1976; Sasaki et al. 1982).

Clinical Assessment

Vitamin K status can be assessed by commercially available, modified one-stage assays of prothrombin. Serum is used to supply Factors VII and X, and Russell's viper venom is used to activate Factor X. Under these conditions, prothrombin concentration is limiting, and the rate of clot formation is related to the amount of prothrombin in the test plasma (Suttie 1984).

Requirement

When 1- and 2-day-old pigs were fed a purified, liquid diet containing sulfathiazole and oxytetracycline to limit intestinal microbial synthesis of vitamin K, 5 μg of menadione sodium phosphate/kg of body weight was required in the diet (Schendel and Johnson 1962). Coprophagy was minimized by use of wire-bottomed cages and careful cleaning. Seerley et al. (1976) found that 1.1 mg of menadione pyrimidinol bisulfite/kg of diet prevented the hemorrhage induced in weanling pigs by the anticoagulant pivalyl. Hall et al. (1986) proposed that 2 mg of menadione as menadione pyrimidinol bisulfite/kg of diet was needed to prevent the effects of pivalyl in pigs weighing 72 kg.

Neufville et al. (1973) reported that a dietary vitamin K supplement of 4 mg/kg improved ($P < .10$) gains of 4-kg weaned pigs as compared with pigs fed the basal diet. The same supplemental level fed to sows for 3 days prior to farrowing and during 2 weeks of lactation resulted in no advantage in the number of pigs weaned, weight at weaning, or percent survival (Wallace et al. 1974).

Hemorrhage has been reported under field conditions, and mycotoxin-contaminated feed ingredients were thought to be the cause (Muhrer et al. 1970; Osweiler 1970; Fritschen et al. 1971). Vitamin K supplements equivalent to 2.0 mg of menadione/kg of diet prevented the syndrome.

When a hemostatic disorder, resulting in subcutaneous hemorrhage and excessive bleeding after castration, was noted in farm pigs, single intramuscular injections of 3 mg of vitamins K_1 or K_2 per kilogram of body weight produced an equal therapeutic response (Sasaki et al. 1985).

The National Research Council (1988a) has proposed a vitamin K requirement for pigs of 0.5 mg of menadione/kg of diet. However, it is difficult to demonstrate a requirement when coprophagy is permitted and when the diet contains neither anticoagulants nor antimicrobial agents that limit intestinal vitamin K synthesis.

Toxicity

Seerley et al. (1976) reported no toxic signs when 110 mg of menadione pyrimidinol bisulfite/kg of diet were fed for 16 weeks to weanling pigs. The National Research Council (1988b) has proposed that the toxic level of menadione or its derivatives is at least 1000 times the dietary requirement.

REFERENCES

Anderson, M.D., et al. 1966. *J. Anim. Sci.* 25:1123.
Anonymous. 1982. *J. Nutr.* 112:7.
Bamburg, J.R., et al. 1968. *Tetrahedron* 24:3329.
Berdanier, C.D., and P. Griminger. 1968. *Int. J. Vitam. Res.* 38:376.
Blomstrand, R., and L. Forsgren. 1968. *Int. Z. Vitam. Forsch.* 38:46.
Booth, W.D. 1974. *J. Reprod. Fertil.* 40:219.
Bowland, J.P., et al. 1949. *J. Anim. Sci.* 8:98.
Braude, R., et al. 1941. *Biochem. J.* 35:693.
Braude, R., et al. 1951. *Vet. Record* 63:671.
Brief, S., and B.P. Chew. 1983. *J. Anim. Sci.* 57(Suppl. 1):237.
Brooks, C.C., et al. 1973. *J. Anim. Sci.* 37:1344.
Charles, O.W., et al. 1968. *Poultry Sci.* 47:754.
Chew, B.P., et al. 1983. *J. Anim. Sci.* 57(Suppl. 1):324.
Ciegler, A., et al. 1963. *Biotech. Bioeng. J.* 5:109.
Clardy, D.O., et al. 1970. *Proceedings of the Research Workers Animal Disease Conference.* Chicago.
DeLuca, L.M., et al. 1979. *Fed. Proc.* 38:2535.
Drescher-Kaden, U., and P. Hoppe. 1972. *Z. Tierphysiol. Tiernahr. Futtermittelkd.* 29:276.
Dua, P.N., and E.J. Day. 1966. *Poultry Sci.* 45:94.
Dvorak, M. 1973. *Acta Vet. Brno* 42:3.
Dvorak, M., et al. 1986. *Acta Vet. Brno* 55:263.
Eaton, H.D., et al. 1964. *J. Nutr.* 82:343.
Fidge, N.H., et al. 1969. *Biochem. J.* 114:689.
Fieser, L.F., et al. 1941. *J. Biol. Chem.* 137:659.
Frape, D.L., et al. 1959. *J. Nutr.* 68:173.
Fritschen, R.D., et al. 1971. *Nebr. Swine Rep. EC71* 219:22.
Gilgan, M.W., et al. 1966. *Arch. Biochem. Biophys.* 114:1.
Goodwin, R.F.W., and A.R. Jennings. 1958. *J. Comp. Pathol.* 68:82.
Griminger, P. 1965. *Poultry Sci.* 44:211.
Grummer, R.H., et al. 1948. *J. Anim. Sci.* 7:222.
Guilbert, H.R., et al. 1937. *J. Nutr.* 13:543.
Guilbert, H.R., et al. 1940. *J. Nutr.* 19:91.
Hale, F. 1935. *Am. J. Ophthalmol.* 18:1087.
Hall, D.D., et al. 1986. *J. Anim. Sci.* 63(Suppl. 1):268.
Hart, E.B., et al. 1916. *J. Biol. Chem.* 25:239.
Heaney, D.P., et al. 1963. *J. Anim. Sci.* 22:925.
Hendricks, D.G., et al. 1967. *J. Nutr.* 93:37.
Hennig, A., et al. 1985. *Arch. Tierernahr.* 35:19.
Hentges, J.F., Jr., et al. 1952a. *J. Anim. Sci.* 11:266.
Hentges, J.F., Jr., et al. 1952b. *J. Am. Vet. Med. Assoc.* 120:213.
Hjarde, W., et al. 1959. *Second Annual Report.* p. 144. Copenhagen: Royal Veterinary Agricultural College, Sterility Research Institute.
Hjarde, W., et al. 1961. *Acta Agric. Scand.* 11:13.
Hollander, D. 1973. *Am. J. Physiol.* 225:360.
Hollander, D., and T.C. Truscott. 1974a. *J. Lab. Clin. Med.* 83:648.
Hollander, D., and T.C. Truscott. 1974b. *Am. J. Physiol.* 226:1516.
Hollander, D., et al. 1976. *Am. J. Physiol.* 230:251.
Hollander, D., et al. 1977. *Am. J. Physiol.* 233:E124.
Hostetler, E.H., et al. 1935. *Technical Bulletin No. 52.* Raleigh, NC: North Carolina Agricultural Experiment Station.
Huang, C.C., et al. 1972. *Comp. Biochem. Physiol.* 42B:57.
Hutagalung, R.I., et al. 1968. *J. Anim. Sci.* 27:79.

Jones, E.W., et al. 1956. *Cornell Vet.* 46:360.
Koch, B.A., et al. 1963. *J. Anim. Sci.* 22:840 (Abstr.).
Lüdke, H., et al. 1985. *Arch. Tierernahr.* 35:97.
Matschiner, J.T. 1970. "Vitamin K." In *The Fat-Soluble Vitamins.* DeLuca, H.F., and J.W. Suttie (Eds.). p. 377. Oxford, England: Pergamon Press.
Muhrer, M.E., et al. 1970. *J. Anim. Sci.* 31:1025 (Abstr.).
Myers, G.S., Jr., et al. 1959. *J. Anim. Sci.* 18:288.
National Research Council. 1974. *Nutrient Requirements of Dogs.* Washington, DC: National Academy Press.
National Research Council. 1981. *Nutrient Requirements of Coldwater Fishes.* Washington, DC: National Academy Press.
National Research Council. 1984. *Nutrient Requirements of Beef Cattle.* Washington, DC: National Academy Press.
National Research Council. 1985. *Nutrient Requirements of Dogs, Revised.* Washington, DC: National Academy Press.
National Research Council. 1986. *Nutrient Requirements of Cats.* Washington, DC: National Academy Press.
National Research Council. 1988a. *Nutrient Requirements of Swine.* Washington, DC: National Academy Press.
National Research Council. 1988b. *Vitamin Tolerance of Animals.* Washington, DC: National Academy Press.
Nelson, E.C., et al. 1962. *J. Nutr.* 76:325.
Nelson, E.C., et al. 1964. *J. Nutr.* 82:263.
Neufville, M.H. 1973. *J. Anim. Sci.* 37(Suppl. 1):288.
Olson, J.A. 1984. "Vitamin A." In: *Handbook of Vitamins.* Machlin, L.J. (Ed.). pp. 1–43. New York: Marcel Dekker, Inc.
Olson, R.E. 1973. "Vitamin K." In *Modern Nutrition in Health and Disease.* Goodhart, R.S., and M.E. Shils (Eds.). pp. 166–174. Philadelphia: Lea and Febiger.
Osweiler, G.D. 1970. "Porcine hemorrhage disease." In: *Proceedings of Pork Producers Day.* Report AS3531. Ames, IA: Iowa State University.
Osweiler, G.D., et al. 1970. *Modern Vet. Pract.* 51:35.
Parrish, D.B., et al. 1951. *J. Anim. Sci.* 10:551.
Sasaki, Y. 1982. *Jpn. J. Vet. Sci.* 44:933.
Sasaki, Y. 1985. *Jpn. J. Vet. Sci.* 47:435.
Schendel, H.E., and B.C. Johnson. 1962. *J. Nutr.* 76:124.
Schöne, F., and H. Lüdke. 1984. *Arch. Tierernahr.* 34:205.
Schöne, F., et al. 1988. *Arch. Tierernahr.* 38:193.
Schulze, J., and H. Haenel. 1969. *Z. Versuchstierkd.* 11:190.
Seerley, R.W., et al. 1965. *J. Anim. Sci.* 24:1014.
Seerley, R.W., et al. 1976. *J. Anim. Sci.* 42:599.
Selke, M.R., et al. 1967. *J. Anim. Sci.* 26:759.
Shearer, M.J., et al. 1970. *Br. J. Haematol.* 18:297.
Sheffy, B.E., et al. 1954. *J. Anim. Sci.* 13:999 (Abstr.).
Sorenson, D.K., et al. 1954. *Am. J. Vet. Res.* 15:258.
Speer, V.C. 1971. *Proc. Dist. Feed Res. Council* 26:39.
Steinhardt, M. 1985. *Arch Exp. Vet. Med. Leipzig* 39:183.
Suttie, J.W. 1984. "Vitamin K." In: *Handbook of Vitamins.* Machlin, L.J. (Ed.). pp. 147–198. New York: Marcel Dekker, Inc.
Suttie, J.W. (Ed.). 1980. *Vitamin K Metabolism and Vitamin K-Dependent Proteins.* Baltimore: University Press.
Thierry, M.J., et al. 1970. *Am. J. Physiol.* 219:854.
Ullrey, D.E. 1972. *J. Anim. Sci.* 35:648.
Ullrey, D.E., et al. 1965. *J. Nutr.* 85:375.
Waite, R., and K.N.S. Sastry. 1949. *J. Agric. Sci.* 39:174.

Wald, G. 1968. *Science* 162:230.
Wallace, H.D. 1974. *Florida Agricultural Experiment Station Research Report AL-1974-9.* Gainesville: University of Florida.
Wellenreiter, R.H., et al. 1969. *J. Nutr.* 99:129.
Wolf, G., et al. 1958. *J. Biol. Chem.* 230:979.
Wolf, G., et al. 1979. *Fed. Proc.* 38:2540.
Wolke, R.E., et al. 1968. *Am. J. Vet. Res.* 29:1009.
Wood, R.D., et al. 1967. *J. Anim. Sci.* 26:510.

Chapter 14

The Water-Soluble Vitamins in Swine Nutrition

D.A. Cook and R.A. Easter

Using chemically defined diets, it can be shown that the pig has a dietary requirement for all of the water-soluble vitamins with the exception of ascorbic acid. In general, however, feed ingredients and microbial synthesis in the gastrointestinal tract provide sufficient quantities of vitamin B_6, thiamin, folic acid, and possibly biotin to meet the pig's requirement. There is clear evidence of improved reproductive performance when choline and pantothenic acid are added to a corn-soybean meal diet. However, choline is clearly not required in similar diets for growing-finishing swine, while the data for pantothenic acid are inconclusive. Vitamin B_{12}, riboflavin, and niacin, on the other hand, must be added to the diet to prevent the development of frank deficiencies.

Much research was conducted during the "vitamin era" between 1930 and 1955 to establish the qualitative vitamin needs of pigs. Since that time, most experiments have been directed at verification of quantitative requirements and solution of problems related to human medicine. The careful reader will no doubt conclude that there is a need for additional vitamin research. The following review provides a summary of current knowledge. Other than the vitamins discussed in this chapter and elsewhere in this text, there is no evidence that compounds having a "vitamin" function in metabolism remain to be discovered.

THIAMIN

History

The discovery of thiamin stems from early studies of the cause of beriberi, a disease once prevalent in many countries where the staple food was polished rice. K. Takaki, M.D., is credited with the first real breakthrough in the prevention of beriberi (Gubler 1984). In 1885, as the surgeon general of the Japanese Navy, Takaki suggested decreasing the carbon:nitrogen ratio of the diet of crews by increasing the protein intake. This virtually eliminated beriberi among ships' crews. However, this suggestion was not widely accepted at the time as it was contrary to the current view of the medical profession on the causes of the disease. Due to the recent acceptance of Pasteur's work on the microbial cause of disease, it was felt that the disease was the result of a microorganism or toxin. Shortly thereafter, it was shown that rice bran, extracts of rice bran, or whole rice could alleviate the symptoms of the disease. Thiamin was subsequently identified as the active factor in rice bran that prevented beriberi (Jansen and Donath 1926). In later studies, Kinnersley and Peters (1928) isolated the vitamin, and in 1936 a synthetic process was developed for the production of thiamin (Robinson 1966).

Many of the events leading to the discovery of thiamin are also considered key to the development of the present vitamin concept. Early work by Christian Eijkman and his successor, Gerrit Grijns, investigating a polyneuritis in chickens resembling beriberi, is credited as being the first adventure in the experimental characterization of a nutritional deficiency. Additionally, it provided an animal model in which to study a human disorder (Gubler 1984). In fact, the word *vitamin* was first coined in reference to thiamin when a young chemist, Casimir Funk, convinced he had isolated the active antiberiberi factor that appeared to possess an amine function, coined the name *vitamine* to refer to thiamin as an amine essential for life (Funk 1911).

Nomenclature

"The compound 3-(4-amino-2-methylpyrimidin-5-ylmethyl)-5-(2-hydroxyethyl)-4-methylthiazolium, formerly known as vitamin B_1, vitamin F, aneurin(e), or thiamine, should be designated thiamin" (Anonymous 1987).

Metabolic Functions

The only known biologically active form of thiamin is the coenzyme thiamin pyrophosphate (TPP) (Lohmann and Schuster 1937). Thiamin is converted to TPP by means of the enzyme thiamin pyrophosphokinase and adenosine triphosphate (Sauberlich 1967). Thiamin, in the form of TPP, is essential for the metabolism of carbohydrates and proteins. Thiamin pyrophosphate functions as a coenzyme in the oxidative decarboxylation of alpha-ketoacids. Specifically, TPP is a coenzyme in the pyruvate dehydrogenase complex, the alpha-ketoglutarate complex, and the decarboxylation of the branched-chain alpha-ketoacids derived from the deamination of leucine, isoleucine, and valine (Gubler 1984). In addition, TPP functions in the transketolase reaction of the pentose phosphate shunt (Kochetov 1982). It is also believed that thiamin, in the form of thiamin triphosphate, might play a role in nerve conduction (Gubler et al. 1976).

Deficiency and Toxicity Signs

Hughes (1940b) noted anorexia and an associated reduction in weight gain in thiamin-deficient pigs. Similar signs were noted by VanEtten and co-workers (1940), who also noted a depression in body temperature, occasional vomiting, and a flabby heart. Other signs include bradycardia, hypertrophy of the heart, myocardial degeneration, and sudden death associated with heart failure (Wintrobe et al. 1943a; Ellis and Madsen 1944; Heineman et al. 1946; Miller et al. 1955). Electrocardiograms of thiamin-deficient pigs were shown to consistently exhibit sinus arrhythmia (Miller et al. 1957b). Transketolase activity has also been noted to be decreased in response to a thiamin deficiency (Peng and Heitman 1973).

No clinical signs of thiamin toxicity have been reported for swine. Levels as high as 100 mg/kg of body weight have been fed to young pigs with no ill effects noted (Ellis and Madsen 1944). In studies on acute toxicity in laboratory animals, excess thiamin appears to block nerve transmission and results in the development of clinical signs such as restlessness, epileptiform convulsions, cyanosis, and labored breathing (NRC 1987). It has been suggested that levels as high as 1000 times the requirement might be safe for most species.

Nutritional Requirements

Hughes (1939) demonstrated thiamin to be essential for normal growth and well-being of swine. Miller et al. (1955) estimated the thiamin requirement of baby pigs (2 to 10 kg) to be 1.5 mg/kg for a diet containing 10% fat. A requirement of 1.0 mg of thiamin/kg of diet was determined for pigs weaned at 3 weeks of age and fed to 40 kg of weight (VanEtten et al. 1940; Ellis and Madsen 1944). It has also been reported that the requirement for thiamin decreases as dietary energy from fat increases (Ellis and Madsen 1944). Peng and Heitman (1974) reported a requirement of 1.1 mg/kg of diet to maximize weight gain and 0.85 mg/kg of diet to maximize feed intake for pigs weighing from 30 to 90 kg.

The use of erythrocyte transketolase activity as an indicator of thiamin status has also been investigated. Estimates of thiamin requirements based on this method are as great as four times the level required to maximize weight gain (Peng and Heitman 1973). In addition, it was shown that increasing the environmental temperature from 20 °C to 35 °C resulted in an increase in the thiamin requirement as determined by this method (Peng and Heitman 1974). However, it has been suggested that this change may be the result of a reduction in feed intake coinciding with the elevation in environmental temperature (NRC 1988).

Sulfur dioxide treatment of feed ingredients has been shown to destroy thiamin activity (Gray 1980). Early studies investigating the thiamin requirement of pigs utilized this treatment to develop thiamin-deficient diets (VanEtten et al. 1940; Ellis and Madsen 1944). The antimicrobial activity of sulfur dioxide has been well established (Schroeter 1966), and thus recently the possibility of feeding sulfur dioxide-treated, high-moisture grains to pigs has gained interest. Gibson et al. (1987) demonstrated that 61% of the dietary thiamin in a diet containing sulfur dioxide-treated, high-moisture barley is destroyed within 7 days of mixing. Thus the workers concluded that its value in preserving swine diets based on high-moisture grains may be limited due to the rapid rate at which dietary thiamin is destroyed.

There was early interest in the use of swine to clear bracken-infested pastures due to their ability to "root" up the rhizomes (Evans et al. 1963). It was not known at the time if pigs would develop "bracken poisoning" due to the thiaminase enzyme contained in the plant. However, Evans and co-workers (1963) reported that the rhizomes alone, when included in a complete ration, would produce a thiamin deficiency. Another antithiamin factor, thiaminase I, has been identified in a number of fresh water fish (Tanphaichitr and Wood 1984). Signs of a thiamin deficiency have developed in association with the feeding of moderate levels of unprocessed fish known to contain thiaminase I (Green et al. 1941; Krampitz and Woolley 1944).

There is a general lack of information on the thiamin requirement for gestating and lactating sows. The only work that has been reported on this subject was confounded by a deficiency of other factors that were as yet not recognized as essential (Ensminger et al. 1947).

Determination of Status

Deficiency signs have been used in the past to determine the thiamin status of an animal. However, deficiency signs can be confused with other diseases. Furthermore, it is evident that subclinical or borderline inadequacies may affect the individual's performance and well-being. Thus, various biochemical procedures have been developed to detect preclinical thiamin deficiencies. Urinary thiamin excretion and blood pyruvate and lactate levels have been used in the past but have many limitations. Baker et al. (1964) developed a microbiological assay as a diagnostic tool for any body fluid or tissue that has been shown to be highly sensitive, accurate, and reproducible. However, erythrocyte transketolase activity is considered the most reliable index of the functional state of thiamin. Brin and co-workers (1960) demonstrated that this method is a reliable index of the availability of the coenzyme, thiamin diphosphate, and is well correlated with the degree of deficiency.

RIBOFLAVIN

History

Riboflavin does not have the dramatic background associated with some other vitamins; rather, its discovery was the result of patient, deliberate investigation. Originally known as vitamin B_2 and also as ovoflavin, it was isolated from egg white and was shown to be effective in promoting growth in rats in Kuhn's laboratory at the Kaiser Wilhelm Institute for Medical Research in 1932. Shortly thereafter, it was also extracted from milk. The structure was determined and the compound synthesized in 1934 by Kuhn and by Karrer and co-workers (Cooperman and Lopez 1984). Early riboflavin research with the pig was conducted by Hughes (1939, 1940a) and Krider and co-workers (1949).

Nomenclature

"The compound with the formula . . . 7,8-dimethyl-10-(1′-D-ribityl)isoalloxazine, formerly known as vitamin B_2, vitamin G, lactoflavin(e), or riboflavine, is designated riboflavin" (Anonymous 1987).

Metabolic Functions

Riboflavin participates in metabolism as a component of either flavin adenine dinucleotide (FAD) or flavin mononucleotide (FMN). Both FAD and FMN are the prosthetic groups for a number of flavin-linked dehydrogenases. Examples of these enzymes are nicotinamide adenine dinucleotide (NADH) dehydrogenase, succinate dehydrogenase, xanthine oxidase, and glutathione reductase. Involved is the transfer of hydrogens in an oxidation-reduction reaction, which involves the isoalloxazine ring of riboflavin. Given the role of FAD and FMN in hydrogen transfer reactions, it should be apparent that the flavoprotein enzymes are critical in the metabolism of carbohydrates, proteins, and fats. For a more detailed discussion of the biochemical functions of riboflavin, see Cooperman and Lopez (1984).

Deficiency and Toxicity Signs

Signs typical of riboflavin deficiency have been described previously (NRC 1988) and include a reduction in growth rate, stiffness of gait, alopecia, seborrhea, vomiting, and cataracts. Examination of pigs with severe riboflavin deficiency reveals increased blood neutrophil granulocytes, reduced immune response, discolored kidney and liver tissue, fatty liver, and degeneration of the myelin of the sciatic and brachial nerves. Females with severe deficiency have also been shown to have collapsed follicles and degenerating ova.

There is insufficient data available to estimate a maximum tolerable level of riboflavin for pigs. Seymour and co-workers (1968) found no detrimental effect when diets containing 8.8 mg of riboflavin/kg of body weight were fed to 5-week-old pigs. Furthermore, riboflavin does not appear to be well absorbed from the gut; therefore, high levels included in the diet should not pose a hazard to the pig (NRC 1987).

Nutritional Requirements

The necessity of riboflavin in the pig's diet was first established by Hughes (1939). Subsequent work has estimated the riboflavin requirement for baby pigs (2 to 20 kg) to be between 2.0 and 3.0 mg/kg in a synthetic diet (Forbes and Haines 1952; Miller et al. 1954). Estimates of the riboflavin requirement in a synthetic diet for growing pigs have ranged from 1.1 to 2.9 mg/kg of diet (Hughes 1940a; Krider et al. 1949; Mitchell et al. 1950; Terrill et al. 1955). Krider and co-workers (1949) and Miller and Ellis (1951) reported estimates of 1.8 to 3.1 mg of riboflavin/kg for growing pigs fed a practical diet. Mitchell et al. (1950) reported that the riboflavin requirement was dependent on environmental temperature. The investigators reported that the riboflavin requirement of the growing pig was approximately 1.2 mg/kg of diet at 28 °C, whereas the requirement was 2.3 mg/kg at 4 °C. However, Seymour and co-workers (1968) reported no consistent interaction between riboflavin and environmental temperature.

Miller and co-workers (1953) reported that an inadequacy in riboflavin (1.1 mg/kg of diet) for reproducing swine resulted in reproductive failure. This was later confirmed by Frank et al. (1984), in that of six gilts fed 0.77 mg of riboflavin/kg of diet, four gilts farrowed approximately 7 days prematurely, two had stillborn litters, and the remaining two failed to farrow by day 121 of gestation. Esch and co-workers (1981) reported that a riboflavin deficiency can lead to anestrus. The riboflavin requirement for gestating swine has been estimated to be between 6.4 and 6.6 mg/day, based on farrowing performance and erythrocyte glutathione reductase activity (Frank et al. 1984). Subsequent work by this group (Frank et al. 1985) utilizing similar criteria has estimated the riboflavin requirement for lactation to be 15.5 to 16.5 mg/day under an ad libitum feeding regimen. Recent work has indicated a response to the addition of 100 mg riboflavin/day to a corn-soybean meal diet from day 4 to 10 following onset of estrus (Bazer and Zavy 1988). The supplemental riboflavin resulted in an increase in litter size, embryonic survival, and allantoic fluid volume at day 30 of gestation, as well as an increase in conception rate and more piglets at birth, day 21, and day 42 of lactation.

Determination of Status

Early work utilized deficiency signs, riboflavin excretion in the urine, and growth and reproductive performance as indicators of riboflavin status. However, recently, the measurement of erythrocyte glutathione reductase (EGR), a flavin-dependent enzyme, has been widely accepted as an indicator of riboflavin status (Bamji and Sharada 1972; Nichoalds 1974; Prentice and Bates 1981). EGR activity is determined in the presence and absence of exogenous FAD and is expressed as a ratio, the EGR activity coefficient. This assay was validated as an indicator of riboflavin status in swine by Esch et al. (1981).

NIACIN

History

The first biochemical function of nicotinic acid was demonstrated by Warburg and co-workers (1935) when they isolated the compound from coenzyme II (NADP) and later found that it functioned as part of a hydrogen transport system (Warburg and Christian 1936). Shortly thereafter, Elvehjem et al. (1938) demonstrated that the active component of liver extracts that was successful in treating black tongue in dogs was niacinamide. It was also shown at this time that nicotinic acid cured pellagra in humans, the parallel of black tongue in dogs (Fouts et al. 1937; Smith et al. 1937; Spies et al. 1938). Krehl et al. (1945) established the link between tryptophan and niacin when they demonstrated that tryptophan was as active as nicotinic acid in the treatment of nicotinic acid deficiency. Heidelberger et al. (1949) provided the first proof of the conversion of tryptophan to nicotinic acid. Cho-Chung and Pitot (1968) later demonstrated the important mechanism of the feedback of NADPH on the tryptophan pyrolase enzyme in the regulation of the conversion of tryptophan to niacin.

Nomenclature

"The term *niacin* should be used as a generic descriptor for pyridine 3-carboxylic acid and derivatives exhibiting qualitatively the biological activity of nicotinamide" (Anonymous 1987). The compound pyridine 3-carboxylic acid, also known as niacin or vitamin PP, should be referred to as nicotinic acid. Nicotinamide is the preferred term for the compound also known as niacinamide or nicotinic acid amide (Anonymous 1987).

Metabolic Functions

Nicotinamide and nicotinic acid act as precursors for the coenzymes nicotinamide adenine dinucleotide (NAD) and nicotinamide adenine dinucleotide phosphate (NADP), in which nicotinic acid serves as a more efficient substrate (Ijichi et al. 1966). NAD is the coenzyme for a number of dehydrogenases participating in the metabolism of fat, carbohydrate, and amino acids (Rao and Goplan 1984). NADP also participates in dehydrogenation reactions, particularly in the hexose monophosphate shunt.

The coenzymes of nicotinamide have also been implicated in other biological reactions such as the synthesis and repair of DNA (Olivera and Lehman 1967; Zimmerman et al. 1967) and synthesis of protein (Honjo et al. 1971). Nicotinic acid has been reported to be a component of the glucose tolerance factor, but its function is as yet not known (Mertz 1975).

Deficiency and Toxicity Signs

Niacin deficiency signs in swine have been described previously (NRC 1988) and include anorexia, reduced weight gain, vomiting, diarrhea, dry skin, dermatitis, rough hair coat, hair loss, ulcerative gastritis, buccal mucosa ulcerations, inflammation and necrosis of the cecum and colon, and normocytic anemia.

No signs of a niacin toxicity in swine have been reported. Toxicity signs such as vasodilation, nausea, vomiting, and occasional skin lesions have been reported in other animals (Robie 1967). A level of 350 mg of nicotinamide/kg of body weight is presumed safe under cases of chronic exposure (NRC 1987).

Nutritional Requirements

The requirement for niacin is complicated by the presence of excess tryptophan in the diet and by its limited availability in certain feed ingredients. With the exception of the newborn, all classes of pigs have been shown to have the ability to convert excess tryptophan to niacin (Luecke et al. 1948; Powick et al. 1948; Cartwright et al. 1948). In addition, Firth and Johnson (1956) have estimated that 1 mg of niacin can be obtained from each 50 mg of tryptophan in excess of the requirement. The niacin in yellow corn, oats, wheat, and grain sorghum has been shown to be in a bound form and to be largely unavailable to the young pig (Kodicek et al. 1956; Luce et al. 1966; Harmon et al. 1969, 1970).

The dietary niacin requirement of the baby pig (1 to 8 kg) was estimated to be not >20 mg/kg of available niacin in the diet that was determined to contain the minimum amount of tryptophan necessary for normal growth (Firth and Johnson 1956). The workers also concluded that the 2- to 3-day-old pig is unable to convert tryptophan to nicotinic acid. For growing pigs (10 to 50 kg), the niacin requirement has been estimated to be approximately 10 to 15 mg/kg of available niacin in diets containing tryptophan levels near the requirement (Braude et al. 1946; Kodicek et al. 1959; Harmon et al. 1969). Although niacin is typically added to growing-finishing diets (NRC 1988), recent studies have demonstrated no improvement in performance when corn-soybean meal diets, supplemented with niacin, were fed to growing-finishing pigs (average weight, 41 to 45 kg) (Yen et al. 1978; Copelin et al. 1980). However, it has been suggested that the diets used contained calculated tryptophan in excess of the requirement (NRC 1988). No information is available for the niacin requirement of the gestating or lactating sow. However, recent evidence has shown no benefit of niacin supplementation to a corn-soybean meal-oat diet (14% crude protein) to sow and litter performance (Ivers et al. 1989).

Determination of Status

Urinary excretion of N′-methyl-nicotinamide and N′-methyl-2-pyridone-5-carboxamide have been shown to decrease during niacin deficiency (Luce et al. 1966, 1967). Recent work has suggested the determination of the activity of erythrocyte nicotinic acid mononucleotide pyrophosribosyl transferase as a possible method to assess niacin nutritional status in swine (Arienti et al. 1982).

PANTOTHENIC ACID

History

Work by Norris and Ringrose (1930) and Ringrose et al. (1931) is generally recognized as having led to the eventual identification of pantothenic acid. These researchers observed the development of a deficiency syndrome, first called chick pellagra, after feeding a diet composed largely of casein, middlings, and yellow corn. Pantothenic acid was, however, first identified as a growth factor for yeast by Williams and co-workers (1933), and subsequently was isolated in 1939 (Williams 1939; Williams et al. 1939) and synthesized in 1940 (Williams and Major 1940). The term *pantothenic acid* was derived from the Greek word "pantos," meaning everywhere, as tissue extracts from a variety of biological materials provided the growth factor for yeast (Fox 1984).

Nomenclature

"The compound N-(2,4-dihydroxy-3,3-dimethyl-1-oxobutyl)-beta-alanine, formerly known as pantoyl-beta-alanine, should be designated pantothenic acid" (Anonymous 1987).

Metabolic Functions

Pantothenic acid, in the form of pantotheine, is the functional group of the biologically active coenzyme A (CoA), acyl carrier protein, and guanosine 5′-triphosphate (GTP)-dependent acyl CoA synthetase (Olson 1984). CoA functions as a carrier of acyl groups in enzymatic reactions involved in biological acetylations (including choline, sulfonamides, para-aminobenzoate) and in the synthesis of fatty acids, cholesterol, sphingosine, citrate, acetoacetate, porphyrins, and sterols, as well as in the oxidation of fatty acids, pyruvate, and alpha-ketoglutarate (Fox 1984; Olson 1984). Pantothenic acid, in the form of 4′-phosphopantotheine, is incorporated into acyl carrier protein, which acts as an acyl carrier in fatty acid synthesis and is also the prosthetic group of GTP-dependent acyl CoA synthetase, which converts succinyl CoA to GTP plus CoA (Olson 1984).

Deficiency and Toxicity Signs

The primary sign noted in pantothenic acid deficiency in growing swine is that of an abnormal gait in the hind legs referred to as "goose stepping." This abnormal gait was first described by Wintrobe et al. (1940) and later confirmed by Hughes and Ittner (1942) as being the result of pantothenic acid deficiency. Other deficiency signs that have been observed include reduced growth, anorexia, diarrhea, dry skin, rough hair coat, alopecia, and reduced immune response (Hughes and Ittner 1942; Wintrobe et al. 1943b; Luecke et al. 1948, 1950, 1952; Wiese et al. 1951; Stothers et al. 1955). Gestating and lactating gilts fed a low pantothenic acid diet were observed to develop fatty livers, enlarged adrenal glands, intramuscular hemorrhage, eccentric dilatation of the heart, rectal congestion, atrophic ovaries, and infantile uteri (Ullrey et al. 1955). Pigs born to the gilts that did farrow exhibited locomotor incoordination and diarrhea and had a low rate of survival.

Pantothenic acid is generally considered to be nontoxic as no adverse response to the ingestion of elevated levels of pantothenic acid has been reported in any species (Omaye 1984).

Nutritional Requirements

The content of pantothenic acid has been shown to be highly available in barley, wheat, and soybean meal, but low in corn and grain sorghum (Southern and Baker 1981). For this reason, synthetic pantothenic acid is typically added to all swine diets in the form of calcium pantothenate. As only the d-isomer of pantothenic acid is biologically available, the d-form of calcium pantothenate has 92% activity, whereas the racemic mixture (*dl*) contains only 46% activity (NRC 1988).

Stothers and co-workers (1955) determined the pantothenic acid requirement of baby pigs (2 to 10 kg) to be approximately 15.0 mg/kg of diet. The requirement for pigs from 5 to 50 kg has been estimated to range from approximately 4.0 to 9.0 mg/kg of diet (Luecke et al. 1953; Barnhart et al. 1957; Sewell et al. 1962; Palm et al. 1968). Estimates of the pantothenic acid requirement of growing-finishing swine (approximately 20 to 90 kg) range from approximately 6.0 to 10.5 mg/kg of diet (Catron et al. 1953; Pond et al. 1960; Davey and Stevenson 1963; Palm et al. 1968; Meade et al. 1969; Roth-Maier and Kirchgessner 1977).

Ullrey et al. (1955) reported that pantothenic acid at a level below 5.9 mg/kg of diet resulted in poor reproductive performance. This finding has been confirmed by Davey and Stevenson (1963) and Teague et al. (1970). In addition, Bowland and Owen (1952) reported normal reproductive performance when a barley-based diet was supplemented with 6.6 mg pantothenic acid/kg. For optimal reproductive performance the requirement for pantothenic acid has been estimated to be 12.0 to 12.5 mg/kg of diet (Ullrey et al. 1955; Davey and Stevenson 1963).

Determination of Status

Clinical signs typically have been used to determine the pantothenic acid status of swine. Requirement studies have consistently used growth as the response criterion for lack of a better determinant. Luecke et al. (1950) found that blood levels of pantothenic acid seemed to be related to the levels consumed, and Owen and Bowland (1952) demonstrated that both blood and milk levels of lactating sows increased as the intake of pantothenic acid increased. However, in the latter study, the pantothenic acid level was also dependent on the day of lactation in which the sampling occurred. The CoA activity in blood as determined by the sulfanilimide acetylation test has been suggested as a possible method of assessing nutritional status (Ellestad et al. 1970).

VITAMIN B_6

History

Goldberger and Lillie (1926) fed rats a diet deficient in what was considered to be the rat pellagra-preventative factor, and the animals developed what was referred to as "rat pellagra." György (1934) later observed that this factor cured skin lesions in rats and suggested that it be called vitamin B_6. It was then demonstrated that vitamin B_6 did not cure human pellagra but did cure "rat pellagra" (Birch et al. 1935). Vitamin B_6 was subsequently isolated in 1938 by three groups working independently (Lepkovsky 1938; Keresztesy et al. 1938; György 1938) and synthesized by Harris and Folkers (1939). Snell (1945) identified two additional natural forms of the vitamin, pyridoxal and pyridoxamine.

Nomenclature

"The term vitamin B_6 should be used as a generic descriptor for all 3-hydroxy-2-methylpyridine derivatives exhibiting qualitatively the biological activity of pyridoxine in rats" (Anonymous 1987). The compound, 3-hydroxy-4,5-bis(hydroxymethyl)-2-methylpyridine, formerly known as vitamin B_6, adermin, or pyridoxal, should be designated pyridoxine. It should be noted that the term *pyridoxine* is not synonymous with the generic term *vitamin B_6*. The compound, also known as pyridoxaldehyde, should be designated pyridoxal. The compound, 3-hydroxy-4-methylamino-5-hydroxymethyl-2-methylpyridine, should be designated pyridoxamine (Anonymous 1987).

Metabolic Functions

The main active form of vitamin B_6 is pyridoxal phosphate (PLP), which serves as a coenzyme in many metabolic reactions. PLP has a functional role, particularly in amino acid metabolism, but also in carbohydrate and lipid metabolism. PLP is involved in transaminations, nonoxidative deamination, decarboxylation, and desulfhydration of amino acids. It also appears to affect the conformation of glycogen phosphorylase, as phosphorylase a (active form) contains 4 moles PLP, whereas phosphorylase b (inactive form) contains only 2 moles (Yunis et al. 1960). The role of PLP in lipid metabolism is as yet unclear, but it has been shown that carcasses of deficient animals contain less lipid than do those of controls (Sauberlich 1968). A more detailed discussion of the metabolic functions of vitamin B_6 is offered by Driskell (1984).

Deficiency and Toxicity Signs

As with many other vitamins, a deficiency of vitamin B_6 results in a reduction in feed intake and growth rate. Other signs that have been observed include the development of a brown exudate around the eyes, impaired vision, vomiting, ataxia, epileptiform seizures, coma, and death (Hughes and Squibb 1942; Wintrobe et al. 1942, 1943c; Lehrer et al. 1951; Miller et al. 1957a). Examination of blood samples taken from deficient animals has revealed microcytic hypochromic anemia; a reduction in albumin, hematocrit, hemoglobin, red blood cells, and lymphocytes; and an increase in gamma globulin (Hughes and Squibb 1942; Miller et al. 1957a; Harmon et al. 1963). Other signs characteristic of vitamin B_6 deficiency determined at necropsy include degeneration of sensory neurons and fat infiltration of the liver (Wintrobe et al. 1942). A reduction in antibody production as a result of vitamin B_6 deficiency has also been reported (Harmon et al. 1963).

Levels of vitamin B_6 as high as 9.2 mg/kg of diet have been fed to early weaned pigs with no detrimental effects (Adams et al. 1967). However, toxicity signs, such as ataxia, muscle weakness, and loss of balance, have been reported in other animals (Phillips et al. 1978). It is suggested that dietary levels of at least 50 times the requirement are safe for most species (NRC 1987).

Nutritional Requirements

The vitamin B_6 content of a grain-soybean meal diet for swine is generally adequate to meet the animal's requirement, and thus it is considered unnecessary to supplement the diet (NRC 1988). Easter et al. (1983) demonstrated no benefit from the addition of supplemental vitamin B_6 in nursery, grower, or finisher diets composed of corn and soybean meal. Yen et al. (1976) have reported availability values of vitamin B_6 for the chick to be approximately 40% in corn and approximately 60% in soybean meal. Estimates of the absolute requirement for vitamin B_6 range from 1.0 to 2.0 mg/kg of diet in the baby pig (2 to 10 kg) (Miller et al. 1957a; Kösters and Kirchgessner 1976a,b) and from 1.2 to 1.8 mg/kg of diet for the nursery pig (10 to 20 kg) (Sewell et al. 1964; Kösters and Kirchgessner 1976a,b). No estimates for the growing-finishing pig are available.

Studies conducted with gestating-lactating females have met with mixed results. Draper and co-workers (1958) found no benefit from the addition of pyridoxine to a corn-soybean meal-based diet for gestating females as measured by the excretion of xanthurenic acid. Ritchie et al. (1960) reported no improvement in reproductive or lactation performance when the diet was supplemented with 10 mg vitamin B_6/kg of diet. However, Easter and co-workers (1983) reported an improvement in litter size at birth and weaning when a corn-soybean meal diet was supplemented with 1 ppm of pyridoxine. Russell and co-workers (1985a) fed purified diets providing 0.45, 1.5, 2.1 or 83 mg of vitamin B_6/day to postpubertal gilts and utilized the erythrocyte glutamic-oxaloacetic transaminase coefficient as an indicator of the vitamin B_6 status of the gilts. They demonstrated that the minimum requirement for vitamin B_6 was >2.1 mg/day. This finding was further supported by examining whole muscle glutamic-oxaloacetic transaminase activity, which was greatly reduced in deficient gilts (Russell et al. 1985b).

Determination of Status

Clinical signs of a vitamin B_6 deficiency in young growing animals appear within 2 to 3 weeks following the removal of the vitamin from the diet (Miller et al. 1957a). Thus, a more sensitive measurement of vitamin B_6 status is required. One of the earliest methods utilized was the tryptophan loading test (Greenburg et al. 1949), which measures the excretion of xanthurenic acid following a test dose of tryptophan. Other methods that have been used include measurement of urinary 4-pyridoxic acid (Baysal et al. 1966), plasma pyridoxal phosphate (Lumeng et al. 1978) and serum transaminases (Linkswiler 1967). However, due to its simplicity and ease of measurement, the assay for erythrocyte glutamic-oxaloacetic transaminase activity has been suggested as the method of choice in assessing vitamin B_6 status (Russell et al. 1985a).

BIOTIN

History

The series of studies that led to the eventual discovery and isolation of biotin span nearly half a century. At the turn of the century, Wildiers (1901) discovered that a factor present in yeast and wort was required for the growth of certain strains of yeast. He named this factor "bios." Bios was later fractionated (Lucas 1924; Lash Miller 1924), and still later, Kögl (1935) isolated "biotin" from one of the fractions of bios.

Meanwhile, Boas (1927) reported that rats fed dried egg white developed characteristic pathological signs. It was observed that these signs could be alleviated by a factor present in liver and other sources. Boas named this factor "protective factor X." Other researchers, working independently, also discovered this factor in liver and called it "vitamin H" (György 1931) and "protective factor against egg white injury" (Lease and Parson 1934).

Kögl and Tonnis (1936) subsequently isolated biotin as its crystalline methyl ester from egg yolk, and vitamin H concentrates were isolated from liver (György et al. 1937). From comparison of the physical, chemical, and biological properties, it was later shown that biotin and vitamin H were one and the same (György et al. 1940; du Vigneaud et al. 1940). Du Vigneaud and co-workers (1942) established the structure of biotin, and subsequently Harris et al. (1945) were the first to synthesize biotin chemically.

Nomenclature

"The compound with the formula hexahydro-2-oxo-1H-thieno[3,4-d]imidazole-4-pentanoic acid, formerly referred to as vitamin H or coenzyme R, should be designated biotin" (Anonymous 1987).

Metabolic Functions

Biotin serves as the prosthetic group on enzymes involved in carboxylation reactions. All biotin enzymes present in animal tissues are dependent on adenosine triphosphate (ATP) and Mg^{2+} ions, which are required for enzyme activation via the attachment of the biotinyl moiety to the apoenzyme (Bonjour 1984). The active site of biotin enzyme consists of a carboxylase subsite that catalyzes the carboxylation of the biotinyl moiety, a transferase subsite that catalyzes the transfer of the carboxyl group from biotin to the substrate and the biotinyl-carrying site. The biotin prosthetic group functions as a mobile carboxyl carrier, as it is bound to the enzyme by a flexible arm that allows it to oscillate back and forth between the carboxylase and transferase subunits (Wood and Barden 1977).

Of the biotin enzymes known to exist, only four are found in animal tissues. These include pyruvate, acetyl-CoA, propionyl-CoA, and 3-methylcrotonyl-CoA carboxylases. An extensive review of the relevant aspects of these enzymes regarding biochemical nutrition, their metabolic functions, and their regulation is offered by Achuta Murthy and Mistry (1977).

Pyruvate carboxylase, a mitochondrial enzyme, is involved in both gluconeogenesis and lipogenesis. The reaction that it catalyzes yields oxaloacetate from pyruvate and has an absolute requirement for acetyl-CoA. In combination with phosphoenolpyruvate carboxykinase, pyruvate carboxylase can achieve the formation of phosphoenolpyruvate, which is a key reaction in the production of glucose from three carbon precursors, such as pyruvate, lactate, and gluconeogenic amino acids. In addition, pyruvate carboxylase is important in lipogenesis, as oxaloacetate is necessary for the translocation of acetyl-CoA from the mitochondria to the cytosol, the site of fatty acid synthesis.

Acetyl-CoA carboxylase is a key enzyme in de novo synthesis of fatty acids. This enzyme catalyzes the carboxylation of acetyl-CoA to malonyl CoA, which is the first committed step in fatty acid synthesis.

Propionyl-CoA carboxylase catalyzes the carboxylation of propionyl-CoA to methyl-malonyl-CoA, which through a series of reactions can result in the synthesis of oxaloacetate. Thus, propionate, produced as the result of oxidation of odd-numbered fatty acids; degradation of branched-chain amino acids, methionine, and threonine; and fermentation in hindgut, can enter into the tricarboxylic acid cycle or gluconeogenesis.

3-Methylcrotonyl-CoA carboxylase catalyzes the carboxylation of 3-methylcrotonyl CoA, an intermediate in the catabolism of leucine, to 3-methylglutaconyl-CoA, which following a series of reactions results in the production of acetyl-CoA and acetoacetate.

Deficiency and Toxicity Signs

A biotin deficiency in swine has been produced by the inclusion of large amounts of desiccated egg white in the diet (Cunha et al. 1946; Hamilton et al. 1983). This is due to the presence of avidin in the raw egg white, which forms a complex with biotin in the intestinal tract, making it unavailable to the pig. A biotin deficiency has also been produced by the addition of specific sulfa drugs to a synthetic diet (Lindley and Cunha 1946; Cunha et al. 1948; Lehrer et al. 1952), which is presumably the result of a reduction in bacterial synthesis of the vitamin in the intestinal tract. Deficiency signs that have been reported include alopecia, spasticity of the hind legs, dermatitis, skin ulcerations, a brown exudate on the skin and about the eyes, transverse cracking of the hooves, cracking and bleeding of the foot pads, diarrhea, and an inflammation of the mucous membranes of the mouth (Cunha et al. 1946, 1948; Lindley and Cunha 1946; Lehrer et al. 1952).

Studies with swine indicate that pigs can safely tolerate levels of biotin as high as ten times the nutritional requirement, and considering that the vitamin is not well retained, the maximum tolerable level may be considerably higher (NRC 1987).

Nutritional Requirements

The supply of biotin to the pig is affected by the biotin content of the diet, as well as the digestibility and availability of the biotin in the feed ingredients and the level of synthesis by the intestinal microflora. Recently, Sauer and co-workers (1988) determined the apparent digestibility of biotin in a number of protein supplements and cereal grains for the growing pig. Apparent digestibilities determined at the distal ileum were 55.4%, 2.7%, and 3.9% in soybean meal, meat and bone meal, and canola meal, respectively, and 4.8%, 4.0%, and 21.6% in barley, corn, and wheat, respectively. Bioavailabilities determined in the chick had previously been used to estimate the availability of biotin for the pig (Kornegay 1986). However, in view of the findings of Sauer and co-workers, these may not be applicable as bioavailability values determined in the chick are, generally, higher than digestibility values determined in the pig.

Typically, supplementation of diets with biotin has produced no improvement in performance of growing pigs. Newport (1981) reported no improvement in growth rate or feed efficiency of 2- to 28-day-old pigs when a filtered skim milk diet containing approximately 10 μg of biotin/kg of dry matter was supplemented with 50 μg of biotin/kg of diet. Moreover, the addition of 55 to 880 μg of biotin/kg of diet has been shown to have no beneficial effect on performance of nursery pigs (Peo et al. 1970; Hanke and Meade 1971; Washam et al. 1975; Hamilton and Veum 1986) and growing-finishing pigs (Meade 1971; Simmins and Brooks 1980; Easter et al. 1983; Bryant et al. 1985b; Hamilton and Veum 1986). In contrast to these findings, Adams et al. (1967) reported an improvement in performance of nursery pigs when 110 μg of biotin/kg of diet was added to a corn-milo-soybean meal diet. Peo et al. (1970) also reported a response to supplemental biotin in one trial when 440 μg/kg of diet were added.

Biotin supplementation of sow diets has been reported to reduce hoof cracks and foot pad lesions and, in general, to improve the integrity of the foot as well as to improve skin and hair coat condition (Halama 1979; Grandhi and Strain 1980; Misir and Blair 1984; Webb et al. 1984; Bryant et al. 1985a,b; Simmins and Brooks 1985). However, no improvement was observed by Bane et al. (1980), Hamilton and Veum (1984), Tribble et al. (1984), and Lewis et al. (1989). Penny and co-workers (1981) reported biotin supplementation to be ineffective in alleviating established foot lesions, but suggested that supplementation during growth and development may be helpful.

Biotin supplements of 100 to 550 μg/kg of diet have been reported to improve reproductive performance as measured by number of pigs farrowed and weaned, litter weaning weight, and weaning to estrus interval (Brooks et al. 1977; Halama 1979; Penny et al. 1981; Easter et al. 1983; Simmins and Brooks 1983; Hamilton and Veum 1984; Misir and Blair 1984; Tribble et al. 1984; Bryant et al. 1985c; Lewis et al. 1989). However, the responses in these studies were inconsistent for the reproductive criteria measured, and in addition, Grandhi and Strain (1980) reported no improvement in reproductive performance. Thus, due to the many confounding factors, it is difficult to estimate the biotin requirement for reproduction.

Determination of Status

Determination of biotin in whole blood, serum, and urine have been employed as indicators of biotin status (Bonjour 1984). However, these values can be variable depending on the assay used as well as on the level of biotin intake. Misir and co-workers (1986) have determined serum biotin levels indicative of various nutritional states for sows.

FOLIC ACID

History

Wills and Mehta (1930) discussed a macrocytic anemia associated with pregnancy, which was often fatal among women of Bombay. The disease was subsequently produced in monkeys and shown to be cured by extracts from liver and yeast. In the decade following, a bacterial growth factor was found to be present in spinach leaves (Mitchell et al. 1941) and in liver (Stokstad 1943) that had properties similar to a factor in liver and yeast that was shown to prevent anemia in chicks (Hogan and Parrott 1940) and in monkeys (Day et al. 1945). The factor was subsequently isolated (Stokstad et al. 1948), its structure was determined (Mowat et al. 1948), and it was synthesized (Waller et al. 1948). Mitchell and co-workers (1941) named the factor *folic acid,* as the word *folic* is derived from the Latin word folium, meaning foliage or leaf. The chemists who determined its structure named the factor pteroylglutamic acid (Waller et al. 1948).

Nomenclature

"The term *folate* should be used as a generic descriptor for folic acid and related compounds exhibiting qualitatively the biological activity of folic acid" (Anonymous 1987). The compound, pteroylmonoglutamic acid, formerly known as vitamin B_c, should be referred to as folic acid. Folic acids and folates (plural) should be used as general terms in reference to a group of compounds based on the N-[(6-pteridinyl) methyl]-p-aminobenzoic acid skeleton conjugated with one or more L-glutamic acid residues. Related compounds exhibiting folic acid activity should be named and abbreviated in accordance with the International Union of Pure and Applied Chemistry-

International Union of Biochemistry (IUPAC-IUB) Commission on Biochemical Nomenclature (1966) (Anonymous 1987).

Metabolic Functions

The metabolic role of folic acid coenzymes in mammalian tissues is in the transfer of single carbon moieties, such as methyl, formyl, formate, or hydroxymethyl. The coenzymatically active forms of the vitamin are the tetrahydro derivatives. Some of the specific reactions and the enzymes in which these coenzymes are involved are methylation of homocysteine to methionine (methionine synthetase), the interconversion of serine and glycine (serine hydroxymethyltransferase), the synthesis of purines (glycinamide ribonucleotide and 5-amino-4-imidazole-carboxamide ribonucleotide transformylases) and pyrimidines (thymidylate synthetase), and the oxidation of histidine (10-formyltetrahydrofolate dehydrogenase) and threonine (serine hydroxymethyltransferase). For a more detailed discussion of enzymatic reactions in which folic acid is involved, see Brody et al. (1984).

Deficiency and Toxicity Signs

Signs of a folic acid deficiency have been previously described (NRC 1988) and include a reduction in growth rate, fading hair color, macrocytic and normocytic anemia, leukopenia, thrombopenia, reduced hematocrit, and bone marrow hyperplasia. It should be noted, however, that, in general, a synthetic diet containing 1 to 2% of a sulfa drug or a folic acid antagonist was necessary to produce a folic acid deficiency (Cunha et al. 1948; Heinle et al. 1948; Cartwright et al. 1949, 1950; Johnson et al. 1950).

Folic acid is generally considered to be nontoxic as no adverse effects have been reported following the ingestion of high levels of the vitamin in any of several species (NRC 1987).

Nutritional Requirements

It is generally accepted that the growing pig can obtain sufficient folic acid from that which is contained in common feed ingredients and from bacterial synthesis in the intestine. Johnson et al. (1948) found no response to folic acid supplementation when a synthetic milk diet, which contained 2% sulfathaladine, was fed to 4-day-old pigs, and Cunha et al. (1947) reported similar findings in 8-week-old pigs fed a synthetic diet. Moreover, Newcomb and Allee (1986) found no beneficial effect in pigs weaned at 17 to 27 days fed a corn-soybean meal-whey diet supplemented with 1.1 mg of folic acid/kg. However, Lindemann and Kornegay (1986) reported an improvement in average daily gain in pigs weaned at 28 days when 0.5 mg of folic acid/kg was added to the diet. The investigators noted, however, that the response was mediated through an increase in feed intake as efficiency of feed utilization was not affected. The supplementation of a corn-soybean meal diet with 200 μg of folic acid/kg was shown to have no effect on growth or feed efficiency when fed during the starter, grower, or finisher phases (Easter et al. 1983).

Matte et al. (1984a) demonstrated that serum folates decrease by 50% from weaning to day 60 of gestation and suggested that this could indicate a possible deficiency of folic acid during mid gestation. These researchers reported an increase in litter size farrowed with the administration of 15 mg of folic acid intramuscularly ten times from weaning to day 60 of gestation (Matte et al. 1984b). Tremblay et al. (1986) demonstrated that the addition of 4.3 mg of supplemental folic acid/kg of diet maintained serum folates similar to those obtained with ten injections of 15 mg of folic acid administered from weaning to day 56 of gestation. It recently has been reported that the addition of 1 mg of folic acid/kg to a corn-soybean meal diet resulted in an improvement in the total number of pigs born and born live over three parities (Lindemann and Kornegay 1989). In addition, Thaler and co-workers (1989) found an increase in the number of pigs born, born live, and alive on days 14 and 21 of lactation during a two-parity study of the addition of 1.65 mg of folic acid/kg of diet. However, Easter et al. (1983) reported no improvement in number of pigs born or weaned when 200 μg of folic acid/kg was added to a corn-soybean meal diet. Tremblay et al. (1989) showed a reduction in embryonic mortality at day 30 of gestation with the addition of 5 mg/kg of diet. Pharazyn and Aherne (1987) showed no beneficial effect of folic acid supplementation of a wheat-barley–based diet fed during lactation. In addition, Matte and Girard (1989) reported that piglets from sows injected with 15 mg of folic acid per week from day 2 of lactation to weaning had significantly higher serum folate levels, but no response in growth rate of the piglets was observed.

Determination of Status

The most commonly used assay for folic acid status is the direct estimation of serum and red cell folate (Longo and Herbert 1976). However, the whole blood deoxyuridine (dU) suppression test can be used both to determine folic acid status and to distinguish between a folic acid and a vitamin B_{12} deficiency (Das et al. 1980).

VITAMIN B_{12}

History

Vitamin B_{12}, cyanocobalamin, was the last vitamin to be discovered. However, the history behind its discovery began in the early 1800s. Vitamin B_{12} is best known for its association with Addisonian pernicious anemia. Combe (1824) was the first to attribute a case of pernicious anemia to a disorder of the digestive system. Addison (1855) gave a detailed description of the symptoms associated with pernicious anemia. However, it was not until the early 1900s that the feeding of liver as a successful treatment was demonstrated (Minot and Murphy 1926). Shortly thereafter, Castle (1929) demonstrated that the antipernicious anemia principle in liver required prior binding to an "intrinsic factor" secreted by the stomach for proper intestinal absorption.

Vitamin B_{12}, cyanocobalamin, was subsequently isolated by two groups working independently in 1948 (Rickes et al. 1948; Smith 1948). West (1948), using the vitamin isolated by Rickes and co-workers, definitively demonstrated the association between vitamin B_{12} and pernicious anemia. A subsequent isolation of vitamin B_{12} resulted in the discovery of another form of the vitamin, which had an absorption spectrum different from that which was reported for cyanocobalamin (Pierce et al. 1949). This preparation, first termed vitamin B_{12b}, was later found not to contain cyanide and was, therefore, named hydroxocobalamin (Jukes and Stokstad 1951). Hydroxocobalamin was shown to have the same biological acitivity as cyanocobalamin (Lichtman et al. 1949), and it was thus determined that the cyanide was apparently an artifact of the original isolation procedure. It is presently recognized that animals contain three main cobalamins: hydroxocobalamin, adenosylcobalamin, and methylcobalamin (Linnel et al. 1974).

Nomenclature

"The term vitamin B_{12} should be used as a generic descriptor for all corrinoids exhibiting qualitatively the biological activity of cyanocobalamin" (Anonymous 1987). The compound formerly referred to as vitamin B_{12}, or cyanocobalamine, should be designated cyanocobalamin. The compound formerly referred to as vitamin B_{12b} should be designated hydroxocobalamin. Related compounds with vitamin B_{12} activity should be named in accordance with the IUPAC-IUB-CBN, The Nomenclature of Corrinoids, 1973 Recommendations (IUPAC-IUB Commission on Biochemical Nomenclature 1974).

Metabolic Functions

Two coenzyme forms of vitamin B_{12} are known to exist in animals. These include methylcobalamin, which functions as a methyl carrier, and adenosylcobalamin, which serves as a hydrogen carrier (Stadtman 1971). The function of methylcobalamin as a methyl carrier is the basis for the interrelationship between vitamin B_{12} and folate. In one such reaction, an enzyme-bound methylcobalamin is formed as an intermediate in the transfer of the methyl moiety of N^5-methyltetrahydrofolate to homocysteine in the resynthesis of methionine (Ellenbogen 1984). In another reaction, a cobalamin-dependent enzyme removes the methyl group from methylfolate, thereby generating tetrahydrofolate, from which is made the 5,10-methylenetetrahydrofolate required for thymidylate synthesis (Herbert 1984). In the form of adenosylcobalamin, vitamin B_{12} is a coenzyme for methylmalonyl-CoA mutase, which catalyzes the conversion of methyl-malonyl-CoA to succinyl-CoA (Ellenbogen 1984). This reaction is a step in the catabolism of propionyl-CoA, which is derived from the breakdown of valine and isoleucine.

Deficiency and Toxicity Signs

A vitamin B_{12} deficiency in pigs is evidenced by a reduction in growth rate and feed intake, rough hair coat, dermatitis, enlarged liver, extreme irritability and sensitivity to touch, posterior incoordination, and unsteadiness of gait (Anderson and Hogan 1950b; Neumann and Johnson 1950; Neumann et al. 1950; Richardson et al. 1951; Catron et al. 1952). Examination of blood samples from deficient pigs has indicated normocytic anemia and high neutrophil with concomitantly low lymphocyte counts (Neumann and Johnson 1950, Cartwright et al. 1951). Similar to pernicious anemia in humans, a double deficiency of vitamin B_{12} and folic acid has been reported to result in the development of macrocytic anemia and bone marrow hyperplasia (Johnson et al. 1950; Cartwright et al. 1952).

No data are available to suggest an upper safe level of vitamin B_{12} for pigs. Data with chicks suggest an upper safe level at three times the requirement, whereas data regarding mice indicate that dietary levels of at least several hundred times the requirement are safe (NRC 1987).

Nutritional Requirements

In early work, a synthetic milk ration was determined to be deficient in an unknown growth factor contained in purified casein (Neumann et al. 1948). It was subsequently discovered that this deficiency could be alleviated by adding the antipernicious anemia liver extract (Johnson and Neumann 1948). The factor contained in this extract was shortly thereafter identified as vitamin B_{12}. Thus, it is obvious that the pig requires a source of vitamin B_{12} in the diet. However, studies investigating the response to supplemental vitamin B_{12} have met with variable results. This may be partially explained by the fact that ingredients from plant sources are devoid of vitamin B_{12}, whereas animal by-products contain the vitamin (NRC 1988). However, it has been suggested that microbial synthesis of vitamin B_{12} in the intestinal tract, as well as that supplied via coprophagy, may satisfy the pig's requirement for the vitamin (Bauriedel et al. 1954; Hendrickx et al. 1964). Nonetheless, due to the commercial availability of vitamin B_{12} supplements, it is routinely added to grain-soybean meal diets.

Estimates of the vitamin B_{12} requirement of young pigs (1.5 to 20 kg) have ranged from 15 to 20 μg/kg of dry matter in the diet (Anderson and Hogan 1950b; Nesheim et al. 1950; Frederick and Brisson 1961). However, Neumann and co-workers (1950) reported suboptimal performance over a similar weight range in pigs receiving 34 μg of vitamin B_{12}/kg of diet dry matter. This diet, however, contained sulfasuxidine to inhibit intestinal synthesis of vitamin B_{12}. These studies utilized a synthetic milk diet, and the pigs were housed in wire-floored cages to avoid coprophagy. For pigs ranging in weight from 10 to 45 kg and housed in wire-floored cages, the requirement ranges from 8.8 to 11.0 μg/kg of diet (Richardson et al. 1951; Catron et al. 1952).

The addition of 11 to 1100 μg of vitamin B_{12}/kg of diet has been shown to improve reproductive performance of sows (Anderson and Hogan 1950a; Frederick and Brisson 1961; Teague and Grifo 1966). However, Teague and Grifo (1966) found no improvements in the number of pigs farrowed and weaned or in their weights at birth or weaning until the third and fourth parities of the sows, when 110 to 1100 μg of vitamin B_{12}/kg of diet were added to a corn-soybean meal diet. Due to the limited information available and wide range of levels of supplementation used, it is difficult to determine an exact requirement of vitamin B_{12} for gestation and lactation, but a level of 15 μg/kg of diet has been suggested (NRC 1988).

Determination of Status

Early studies utilized gross observations and performance, as well as red and white blood cell counts, as indicators of status. However, more recently, a number of diagnostic tests have been investigated in the area of human nutrition. One of the most commonly used tests is that of serum vitamin B_{12} levels (Herbert 1979). Newer tests for vitamin B_{12} status include the peripheral blood lymphocyte vitamin B_{12} level (Herbert 1984) and the whole blood dU suppression test (Das et al. 1980).

CHOLINE

History

The name choline arises from the word *chole,* which is German for bile, as it was originally isolated from hog bile by Strecker (1862). Strecker (1868) subsequently demonstrated choline is a constituent of lecithin. It has been said that the early studies of choline follow closely the discovery of insulin by Banting and Best in 1922 (Chan 1984). It was noted that the administration of insulin to depancreatized dogs helped mobilize excess lipid from the liver. Subsequent studies demonstrated that choline is the active constituent of dietary lecithin that provides the lipotropic activity (Allan et al. 1924; Hershey 1930; Best and Hershey 1932). Best and Huntsman (1932) were the first to demonstrate the nutritional importance of choline, as they reported the development of fatty livers in rats fed a low-choline, high-fat diet, which could be prevented by choline supplementation.

Nomenclature

"The compound with formula $(CH_3)_3N^+CH_2CH_2OH$ should be designated choline" (Anonymous 1987).

Metabolic Functions

Choline is considered part of a labile methyl pool capable of contributing methyl groups for the biosynthesis of methionine and other methylated compounds, including purines and pyrimidines (Kuksis and Mookerjea 1984). It is believed, however, that choline must first be oxidized to betaine before it can donate its methyl groups. Choline is also a precursor for acetylcholine, which is formed by reaction with acetyl-CoA by enzymatic action of choline acetylase (Freeman and Jenden 1976). Choline is also a precursor for the de novo synthesis of phosphatidylcholine (Kennedy and Weiss 1956) and sphingomyelin (Stoffel and Melzner 1980). Thus, as a constituent of phospholipids, choline plays a role in the structure of biological membranes.

Deficiency Signs

The clinical signs of a choline deficiency have been previously described (NRC 1988). Gross observation reveals a reduction in weight gain, rough hair coats, and an unsteady and staggering gait. Examination of blood samples from deficient animals indicates a reduction in red cell number and a decrease in hematocrit and hemoglobin concentrations. Upon necropsy, fat infiltration of the liver and kidney has been observed. As a result of severe choline deficiency, kidney glomeruli can become occluded due to massive fat infiltration.

No clinical signs of a choline toxicity have been observed in swine (NRC 1987). However, Southern et al. (1986) reported a reduction in growth when diets containing 2000 mg choline/kg were fed to nursery, growing, and finishing pigs.

Nutritional Requirements

Molitoris and Baker (1976) determined the bioavailability of choline in soybean meal to be approximately 65% for the chick. No estimate is available for the bioavailability of choline in feed ingredients for the pig. However, studies investigating the addition of choline to corn-soybean meal and corn-isolated soybean protein diets fed to nursery, growing, and finishing pigs have shown no response in weight gain to supplemental choline (Bryant et al. 1977; Russet et al. 1979b; NCR-42 Committee on Swine Nutrition 1980; Southern et al. 1986).

Johnson and James (1948) reported that the addition of 260 mg of choline/kg to a synthetic milk diet (13% solids) that contained 0.8% methionine prevented development of a choline deficiency in 1- to 4-day-old pigs. Neumann and co-workers (1949), using the same diet and pigs of similar weight and age, determined that 1000 mg of choline/kg of dry matter were required to maximize weight gain and feed efficiency and to prevent fat infiltration of the liver and kidneys. Nesheim and Johnson (1950) later demonstrated that the addition of 0.8% methionine to this diet (1.6% total methionine) alleviated the need for supplemental choline. The investigators thus concluded that even at this early age, the pig can utilize excess methionine as a methyl donor for choline synthesis. Kroenig and Pond (1967) further supported this finding when they demonstrated in 3-week-old pigs that only when methionine became limiting did choline elicit a growth response. Russet and co-workers (1979a,b) have determined the choline requirement of pigs 3 to 8 weeks of age to be approximately 330 mg/kg of a semipurified diet (23% crude protein) in the presence of 0.31% methionine and 0.33% cystine.

Choline supplementation of sow diets during gestation and lactation has proved effective in improving reproductive performance. Kornegay and Meacham (1973) reported an increase in the number of live pigs farrowed during the fifth and sixth parity when 880 mg of choline/kg was added to a corn-soybean meal diet. Stockland and Blaylock (1974) fed a corn-soybean meal diet supplemented with 412 mg of choline/kg to gestating and lactating sows over three parities and found an increase in pigs farrowed, farrowed alive, and weaned, as well as an improvement in conception rate. The NCR-42 Committee on Swine Nutrition (1976) reported an increase in total pigs per litter, an increase in live pigs per litter, and more pigs at 2 weeks of age, as well as a reduction in spraddle-legged pigs, upon supplementation of a corn-soybean meal diet with 770 mg of choline/kg. Luce et al. (1985) reported that gilts fed a choline-supplemented diet during gestation farrowed heavier pigs, but no reduction in spraddle-legged pigs was observed. A more recent report has indicated similar results when a sorghum-soybean meal diet was supplemented with 882 mg of choline/kg and fed during gestation and lactation (Maxwell et al. 1987). An increase in pig weight at day 42 and in litter weight at days 21 and 42 were observed. Choline supplementation of diets containing 8% to 10% vegetable or animal fat fed during lactation has been reported to have no effect on lactational performance in sows (Seerley et al. 1981; Boyd et al. 1982).

Determination of Status

A number of blood and plasma parameters have been used as indicators of choline status (Russet et al. 1979a,b), but none has been shown to be consistent, as many of the parameters can be confounded by the status of other nutrients such as methionine, folic acid, and vitamin B_{12}. Plasma choline level has been used in humans but has been shown to be more highly reflective of dietary consumption (Hirsch et al. 1978).

ASCORBIC ACID

History

Ascorbic acid may have influenced the course of history by spontaneously ending many military campaigns and long ocean voyages due to fatal outbreaks of scurvy when rations became depleted of ascorbic acid (Jaffe 1984). Scurvy was originally believed to be a venereal disease and was treated accordingly with disastrous results. Ascorbic acid, or vitamin C, was recognized as the antiscorbutic factor in fresh fruits and vegetables as early as 1734 (Chick 1953). However, it was not until 1932 that two different research groups isolated and identified this compound (Svirbely and Szent-György 1932; King and Waugh 1932). The pig, however, does not require a dietary source of ascorbic acid for growth and development because, unlike the human, the pig has the ability to synthesize ascorbic acid (Braude et al. 1950).

Nomenclature

"The term *vitamin C* should be used as a generic descriptor for all compounds exhibiting qualitatively the biological activity of ascorbic acid" (Anonymous 1987). L-ascorbic acid or simply ascorbic acid, formerly known as vitamin C, cevitamic acid, or hexuronic acid, should be used to designate the compound 2,3-didehydro-L-threo-hexano-1,4-lactone. "The compound L-threo-hexano-1,4-lactone should be designated L-dehydroascorbic acid or dehydroascorbic acid" (Anonymous 1987).

Metabolic Functions

Although ascorbic acid has long been known to prevent the occurrence of scurvy, the biochemical function of ascorbic acid is uncertain. An ascorbic acid deficiency may induce various liver lysosomal enzyme activities (Hoehn and Kanfer 1978) and impair the biosynthesis of collagen (Barnes and Kodicek 1972). The impairment in collagen synthesis appears to be due to decreased ability to hydroxylate lysine and proline. The hydroxylation of these amino acid residues is required for formation of cross links in the collagen matrix, which give strength to the collagen. Collagen is essential for normal growth of bone and cartilage. Ascorbic acid also enhances the formation of intracellular material, the formation of bone matrix, and the formation of tooth dentin (NRC 1988). Ascorbic acid is also involved in the hydroxylation of trimethyllysine and gamma-butyrobetaine in carnitine biosynthesis (Broquist 1982). Ascorbic acid, due to its reducing and chelating properties, also enhances the absorption of some metal ions from the diet and their mobilization and distribution throughout the body (Calabrese 1980). The vitamin has also been implicated in the metabolism of cholesterol (Turley et al. 1976), the synthesis of epinephrine and antiinflammatory steroids (Broquist 1982), wound healing (Irwin and Hutchins 1976), and leukocyte functions (Shilotri 1977).

Deficiency Signs

Ascorbic acid is not a dietary essential for the pig as it can be synthesized from carbohydrates such as glucose and galactose. Other species, such as primates and the guinea pig, lack the enzyme L-gulonolactone oxidase, which is required for ascorbic acid biosynthesis (Nishikimi and Udenfriend 1976). Thus, no deficiency signs have been observed in the pig. However, under certain environmental conditions, a reduction in plasma, serum, and liver ascorbic acid concentration has been reported (Riker et al. 1967; Brown et al. 1970, 1975; Dvorak 1974).

No signs of ascorbic acid toxicity have been reported in swine. Levels as high as 10 g/kg of diet have been fed to young pigs with no adverse effects noted (Chavez 1983). However, excess ascorbic acid has been reported to result in development of toxicity signs in humans and laboratory animals. These signs include allergic responses, oxaluria, uricosuria, and interference with mixed function oxidase systems (NRC 1987).

Nutritional Requirements

It is generally accepted that the pig does not require a dietary source of ascorbic acid (NRC 1988). Some research has suggested that under certain environmental conditions the pig may not be able to synthesize enough ascorbic acid for maximum growth. Riker et al. (1967) reported that plasma ascorbic acid levels were lower for pigs in a hot environment. Kornegay et al. (1986) found no benefit to supplemental ascorbic acid for weaning pigs exposed to cold. There is also a high correlation between energy intake and serum ascorbic acid concentrations (Brown et al. 1970). Ascorbic acid supplementation has been shown to significantly improve growth rate of 3-week-old pigs, especially at a low energy intake (Brown et al. 1975). Dvorak (1974) reported a reduction in liver ascorbic acid levels in 1- and 40-day-old pigs in response to fasting. Studies investigating the effect of ascorbic acid supplementation when no specific stress had been imposed have met with mixed results. Jewel et al. (1981) reported an increase in weight gain in pigs weaned at 1 day of age in one trial but were unable to show a response to supplemental ascorbic acid in a second trial. In pigs weaned at 3 to 4 weeks of age, a significant improvement in weight gain has been shown with supplemental ascorbic acid (Brown et al. 1975; Yen and Pond 1981). Parenteral dosing and feed supplementation with ascorbic acid has been reported to improve weight gain in pigs initially weighing 24 kg (Mahan et al. 1966). Cromwell and coworkers (1970) were only able to show an improvement in growth rate in two of three trials when supplemental ascorbic acid was added to the diet of growing pigs. No response to supplemental ascorbic acid has been reported in suckling pigs (Leibbrandt 1977), pigs weaned at 3 to 4 weeks of age (Mahan and Saif 1983; Nakano et al. 1983; Yen and Pond 1983, 1984, 1987; Chiang et al. 1985; Yen et al. 1985), or growing-finishing pigs (Hutagalung et al. 1969; Strittmatter et al. 1978). Housing system (Mahan and Saif 1983), crowding (Brown and Partridge 1971; Yen and Pond 1983, 1987), space allowance (NCR-89 Committee on Confinement Management of Swine 1989), carbadox (Mahan and Saif 1983; Yen and Pond 1984), and copper (Mahan and Saif 1983) have also been reported to have no interactive effect with supplemental ascorbic acid.

It has also been postulated that ascorbic acid supplementation may be effective in the prevention or alleviation of osteochondrosis in swine. It was thought that osteochondrosis might be related to insufficient collagen cross-linking due to a reduction in hydroxylation of lysine and proline. However, dietary supplementation with ascorbic acid has been shown to be ineffective in preventing this condition (Strittmatter et al. 1978; Cleveland et al. 1983; Nakano et al. 1983).

Navel bleeding in piglets was reported to be prevented by the addition of 1.0 g of ascorbic acid/day to the feed of pregnant sows beginning 6 days prior to farrowing (Sandholm et al. 1979). In addition, it was noted that the administration of a water-soluble vitamin K in the drinking water failed to prevent navel bleeding in newborn piglets. The investigators postulated that the defect in coagulation was due to immature collagen, which did not efficiently induce platelet plug formation, and that the piglets depend on their dam for their supply of ascorbic acid. However, in subsequent studies where navel bleeding was not considered to be a problem, there was no improvement found in piglet survival or growth rate when 1.0 to 10.0 g of ascorbic acid/day was added to sows' diets beginning in late pregnancy (Lynch and O'Grady 1981; Chavez 1983; Yen and Pond 1983).

Determination of Status

Due to the limited knowledge concerning the metabolic functions of ascorbic acid, no completely satisfactory or reliable biochemical procedures to identify a deficiency state or to assess nutritional status have been developed (Jaffe 1984). However, measurements of ascorbic acid content in serum, plasma, whole blood, leukocytes, and urine have been used to determine inadequacies (Sauberlich et al. 1974). Various fluorometric and colorimetric procedures are available for the measurement of ascorbic acid levels in biological samples (Sauberlich et al. 1974).

REFERENCES

Achuta Murthy, P.N., and S.P. Mistry. 1977. *Prog. Food Nutr. Sci.* 2:405.
Adams, C.R., et al. 1967. *J. Anim. Sci.* 26:903 (Abstr.).
Addison, T. 1855. *On the Constitutional and Local Effects of Disease of the Suprarenal Capsules.* London: Samuel Highely.
Allan, F.N., et al. 1924. *Br. J. Exp. Pathol.* 5:75.
Anderson, G.C., and A.G. Hogan. 1950a. *J. Nutr.* 40:243.
Anderson, G.C., and A.G. Hogan. 1950b. *Proc. Soc. Exp. Biol. Med.* 75:288.
Anonymous. 1987. *J. Nutr.* 117:7.
Arienti, G., et al. 1982. *Int. J. Vitam. Nutr. Res.* 52:142.
Baker, H., et al. 1964. *Am. J. Clin. Nutr.* 14:197.
Bamji, M.S., and D. Sharada. 1972. *J. Nutr.* 102:443.
Bane, D.P., et al. 1980. *Proc. Int. Pig. Vet. Soc.* 6:334.
Barnes, M.J., and E. Kodicek. 1972. *Vitam. Horm.* 30:1.
Barnhart, C.E., et al. 1957. *J. Anim. Sci.* 16:396.
Bauriedel, W.R., et al. 1954. *J. Agric. Food Chem.* 2:468.
Baysal, A., et al. 1966. *J. Nutr.* 89:19.
Bazer, F.W., and T.T. Zavy. 1988. *J. Anim. Sci.* 66(Suppl. 1):324.
Best, C.H., and J.M. Hershey. 1932. *J. Physiol. (Lond.)* 75:49.
Best, C.H., and M.E. Huntsman. 1932. *J. Physiol. (Lond.)* 75:405.
Birch, T.W., et al. 1935. *Biochem. J.* 29:2830.
Boas, M.A. 1927. *Biochem. J.* 21:712.
Bonjour, J.P. 1984. In: *Handbook of Vitamins.* Machlin, L.J. (Ed.). pp. 403–435. New York: Marcel Dekker, Inc.
Bowland, J.P., and B.D. Owen. 1952. *J. Anim. Sci.* 11:757 (Abstr.).
Boyd, R.D., et al. 1982. *J. Anim. Sci.* 54:1.
Braude, R., et al. 1946. *Biochem. J.* 40:843.
Braude, R., et al. 1950. *Br. J. Nutr.* 4:186.
Brin, M., et al. 1960. *J. Nutr.* 71:273.
Brody, T., et al. 1984. In: *Handbook of Vitamins.* Machlin, L.J. (Ed.). pp. 459–496. New York: Marcel Dekker, Inc.
Brooks, P.H., et al. 1977. *Vet. Rec.* 101:46.
Broquist, H.P. 1982. *Fed. Proc.* 41:2840.
Brown, R.G., and I.G. Partridge. 1971. *Can. J. Anim. Sci.* 51:824.

Brown, R.G., et al. 1975. *Can. J. Anim. Sci.* 55:353.
Brown, R.G., et al. 1970. *Can. J. Anim. Sci.* 50:605.
Bryant, K.L., et al. 1977. *Research Report AL-1977-1.* Gainesville, FL: Florida Agricultural Experiment Station.
Bryant, K.L., et al. 1985a. *J. Anim. Sci.* 60:154.
Bryant, K.L., et al. 1985b. *J. Anim. Sci.* 60:136.
Bryant, K.L., et al. 1985c. *J. Anim. Sci.* 60:145.
Calabrese, E.J. 1980. *Nutrition and Environmental Health—The Influence of Nutritional Status on Pollutant Toxicity and Carcinogenicity.* Vol. 1 of *The Vitamins.* New York: Wiley and Sons.
Cartwright, G.E., et al. 1948. *Arch Biochem.* 19:109.
Cartwright, G.E., et al. 1949. *Blood* 4:301.
Cartwright, G.E., et al. 1950. *J. Lab. Clin. Med.* 36:675.
Cartwright, G.E., et al. 1951. *Blood* 6:867.
Cartwright, G.E., et al. 1952. *Blood* 7:992.
Castle, W.B. 1929. *Am. J. Med. Sci.* 178:748.
Catron, D.V., et al. 1952. *J. Nutr.* 47:461.
Catron, D.V., et al. 1953. *J. Anim. Sci.* 12:51.
Chan, M.M. 1984. In: *Handbook of Vitamins.* Machlin, L.J. (Ed.). pp. 549–570. New York: Marcel Dekker, Inc.
Chavez, E.R. 1983. *Can. J. Anim. Sci.* 63:683.
Chiang, S.H., et al. 1985. *Nutr. Rep. Int.* 31:573.
Chick, H. 1953. *Proc. Nutr. Soc.* 12:210.
Cho-Chung, Y.S., and H.C. Pitot. 1968. *Eur. J. Biochem.* 3:401.
Cleveland, E.R., et al. 1983. *J. Anim. Sci.* 57(Suppl. 1):387.
Combe, J.S. 1824. *Trans. Med.-Chirurg. Soc.* (Edinburg). 1:194.
Cooperman, J.M., and R. Lopez. 1984. In: *Handbook of Vitamins.* Machlin, L.J. (Ed.). pp. 299–327. New York: Marcel Dekker, Inc.
Copelin, J.L., et al. 1980. *J. Anim. Sci.* 51(Suppl. 1):190.
Cromwell, G.L., et al. 1970. *J. Anim. Sci.* 31:63.
Cunha, T.J., et al. 1946. *J. Anim. Sci.* 5:219.
Cunha, T.J., et al. 1947. *J. Nutr.* 34:173.
Cunha, T.J., et al. 1948. *J. Nutr.* 36:215.
Das, K.C., et al. 1980. *Clin. Chem.* 26:72.
Davey, R.J., and J.W. Stevenson. 1963. *J. Anim. Sci.* 22:9.
Day, P.L., et al. 1945. *J. Biol. Chem.* 157:423.
Draper, H.H., et al. 1958. *J. Anim. Sci.* 17:68.
Driskell, J.A. 1984. In: *Handbook of Vitamins.* Machlin, L.J. (Ed.). pp. 379–401. New York: Marcel Dekker, Inc.
du Vigneaud, V., et al. 1940. *Science* 92:62.
du Vigneaud, V., et al. 1942. *J. Am. Chem. Soc.* 64:188.
Dvorak, M. 1974. *Nutr. Metab.* 16:215.
Easter, R.A., et al. 1983. *Nutr. Rep. Intl.* 28:945.
Ellenbogen, L. 1984. In: *Handbook of Vitamins.* Machlin, L.J. (Ed.). pp. 497–547. New York: Marcel Dekker, Inc.
Ellestad, J.J., et al. 1970. *Fed. Proc.* 29:820.
Ellis, N.R., and L.L. Madsen. 1944. *J. Nutr.* 27:253.
Elvehjem, C.A., et al. 1938. *J. Biol. Chem.* 123:137.
Ensminger, M.E., et al. 1947. *J. Anim. Sci.* 6:409.
Esch, N.W., et al. 1981. *Biol. Reprod.* 25:659.
Evans, I.A., et al. 1963. *J. Comp. Pathol.* 73:229.
Firth, J., and B.C. Johnson. 1956. *J. Nutr.* 59:223.
Forbes, R.M., and W.T. Haines. 1952. *J. Nutr.* 47:411.
Fouts, P.J., et al. *Proc. Soc. Ex. Biol. Med.* 37:405.

Fox, H.M. 1984. In: *Handbook of Vitamins.* Machlin, L.J. (Ed.). pp. 437–457. New York: Marcel Dekker, Inc.
Frank, G.R., et al. 1984. *J. Anim. Sci.* 59:1567.
Frank, G.R., et al. 1985. *J. Anim. Sci.* 61(Suppl. 1):315.
Frederick, G.L., and G.J. Brisson. 1961. *Can. J. Anim. Sci.* 41:212.
Freeman, J.J., and D.J. Jenden. 1976. *Life Sci.* 19:949.
Funk, C. 1911. *J. Physiol. (Lond.)* 43:395.
Gibson, D.M., et al. 1987. *Can. J. Anim. Sci.* 67:841.
Goldberger, J., and R.D. Lillie. 1926. *Public Health Rep.* 41:1025.
Grandhi, R.R., and J.H. Strain. 1980. *Can. J. Anim. Sci.* 60:961.
Gray, T.J.B. 1980. In: *Toxicology.* Tilbury, R.H. (Ed.). London: Applied Science Publishers Ltd.
Green, R.G., et al. 1941. *J. Nutr.* 21:243.
Greenburg, L.D., et al. 1949. *Arch. Biochem.* 21:237.
Gubler, C.J. 1984. In: *Handbook of Vitamins.* Machlin, L.J. (Ed.). pp. 245–297. New York: Marcel Dekker, Inc.
Gubler, C.J., et al. 1976. *Thiamin.* New York: Wiley & Sons.
György, P. 1931. *Z. Arztl. Fortbild.* 28:377.
György, P. 1934. *Nature* 133:498.
György, P. 1938. *J. Am. Chem. Soc.* 60:983.
György, P., et al. 1937. *Proc. Soc. Exp. Biol. Med.* 37:313.
György, P., et al. 1940. *Science* 91:243.
Halama, A.K. 1979. *Wien. Tierärztliche Monatsschrift.* 66:370.
Hamilton, C.R., and T.L. Veum. 1984. *J. Anim. Sci.* 59:151.
Hamilton, C.R., and T.L. Veum. 1986. *J. Anim. Sci.* 62:155.
Hamilton, C.R., et al. 1983. *Int. J. Vitam. Nutr. Res.* 53:44.
Hanke, H.G., and R.J. Meade. 1971. 1970-71 Minnesota Swine Research Report H-120. St. Paul, MN: University of Minnesota Press.
Harmon, B.G., et al. 1963. *J. Nutr.* 79:269.
Harmon, B.G., et al. 1969. *J. Anim. Sci.* 28:848.
Harmon, B.G., et al. 1970. *J. Anim. Sci.* 31:339.
Harris, S.A., and K. Folkers. 1939. *Science* 89:347.
Harris, S.A., et al. 1945. *J. Am. Chem. Soc.* 67:2096.
Heidelberger, C., et al. 1949. *J. Biol. Chem.* 179:151.
Heinemann, W.W., et al. 1946. *J. Nutr.* 31:107.
Heinle, R.W., et al. 1948. *J. Lab. Clin.Med.* 33:1647.
Henderickx, H.K., et al. 1964. *J. Anim. Sci.* 23:1036.
Herbert, V. 1979. In: *Textbook of Medicine.* 15th ed. Beeson, P.B., W. McDermott, and J.B. Wyngaarden (Eds.). p. 1709. Philadelphia: W.B. Saunders.
Herbert, V. 1984. In: *Nutrition Reviews Present Knowledge in Nutrition.* 5th ed. pp. 347–364. Washington, DC: The Nutrition Foundation, Inc.
Hershey, J.M. 1930. *Am. J. Physiol.* 93:657.
Hirsch, M.J., et al. 1978. *Metabolism* 27:953.
Hoehn, S.K., and J.N. Kanfer. 1978. *Can. J. Biochem.* 56:353.
Hogan, A.G., and E.M. Parrot. 1940. *J. Biol. Chem.* 132:507.
Honjo, T., et al. 1971. *J. Biol. Chem.* 246:4251.
Hughes, E.H. 1939. *J. Nutr.* 17:527.
Hughes, E.H. 1940a. *J. Nutr.* 20:223.
Hughes, E.H. 1940b. *J. Nutr.* 20:239.
Hughes, E.H., and N.R. Ittner. 1942. *J. Anim. Sci.* 1:116.
Hughes, E.H., and R.L. Squibb. 1942. *J. Anim. Sci.* 1:320.
Hutagalung, R.I., et al. 1969. *J. Anim. Sci.* 29:700.
Ijichi, H., et al. 1966. *J. Biol. Chem.* 241:3701.
Irwin, M.I., and B.K. Hutchins. 1976. *J. Nutr.* 106:823.
IUPAC-IUB Commission on Biochemical Nomenclature. 1966. *J. Biol. Chem.* 241:2991.

IUPAC-IUB Commission on Biochemical Nomenclature. 1974. *Biochemistry.* 13:1555.
Ivers, D.J., et al. 1989. *J. Anim. Sci.* 67(Suppl. 2):120.
Jaffe, G.M. 1984. In: *Handbook of Vitamins.* Machlin, L.J. (Ed.). pp. 199–244. New York: Marcel Dekker, Inc.
Jansen, B.C.P., and W.F. Donath. 1926. *Proc. Kon. Ned. Akad. Wetensch. (Amsterdam) 29:* 1390.
Jewell, D.E., et al. 1981. *J. Anim. Sci.* 53(Suppl. 1):98.
Johnson, B.C., and M.F. James. 1948. *J. Nutr.* 36:339.
Johnson, B.C., and A.L. Neumann. 1948. *J. Anim. Sci.* 7:528.
Johnson, B.C., et al. 1948. *J. Anim. Sci.* 7:486.
Johnson, B.C., et al. 1950. *J. Lab. Clin. Med.* 36:537.
Jukes, T.H., and E.L.R. Stokstad. 1951. *Vitam. Horm.* 9:1.
Kennedy, E.P., and S.B. Weiss. 1956. *J. Biol. Chem.* 222:193.
Keresztesy, J.C., and J.R. Stevens. 1938. *Proc. Soc. Exp. Biol. Med.* 38:64.
King, C.G., and W.A. Waugh. 1932. *Science* 75:357.
Kinnersly, H.W., and R.A. Peters. 1928. *Biochem. J.* 22:419.
Kochetov, G.A. 1982. *Ann. N.Y. Acad. Sci.* 378:382.
Kodicek, G., et al. 1956. *Br. J. Nutr.* 10:51.
Kodicek, G., et al. 1959. *Br. J. Nutr.* 13:363.
Kögl, F. 1935. *Chem. Ber.* 68:16.
Kögl, F., and B. Tonnis. 1936. *Hoppe Seylers Z. Physiol. Chem.* 242:43.
Kornegay, E.T. 1986. *Livest. Prod. Sci.* 14:65.
Kornegay, E.T., and T.N. Meacham. 1973. *J. Anim. Sci.* 37:506.
Kornegay, E.T., et al. 1986. *J. Anim. Sci.* 63:484.
Kösters, W.W., and M. Kirchgessner. 1976a. *Z. Tierphysiol. Tiernahr. Futtermittelkd.* 37:235.
Kösters, W.W., and M. Kirchgessner. 1976b. *Z. Tierphysiol. Tiernahr. Futtermittelkd.* 37:247.
Krampitz, L.O., and D.W. Wooley. 1944. *J. Biol. Chem.* 152:9.
Krehl, W.A., et al. 1945. *Science* 101:487.
Krider, J.L., et al. 1949. *J. Anim. Sci.* 8:121.
Kroenig, G.H., and W.G. Pond. 1967. *J. Anim. Sci.* 26:352.
Kuksis, A., and S. Mookerjea. 1984. In: *Nutrition Reviews Present Knowledge in Nutrition.* 5th ed. pp. 383–399. Washington, DC: The Nutrition Foundation, Inc.
Lash Miller, W. 1924. *Science* 59:197.
Lease, J.J., and H.T. Parsons. 1934. *Biochem. J.* 288:2109.
Lehrer, W.P., Jr., et al. 1951. *J. Anim. Sci.* 10:65.
Lehrer, W.P., Jr., et al. 1952. *J. Nutr.* 47:203.
Leibbrandt, V.D. 1977. *J. Anim. Sci.* 45(Suppl. 1):98.
Lepkovsky, S. 1938. *Science* 87:169.
Lewis, A.J., et al. 1989. *J. Anim. Sci.* 67(Suppl. 1):114.
Lichtman, H., et al. 1949. *Proc. Soc. Exp. Biol. Med.* 72:643.
Lindemann, M.D., and E.T. Kornegay. 1986. *J. Anim. Sci.* 63(Suppl. 1):98.
Lindemann, M.D., and E.T. Kornegay. 1989. *J. Anim. Sci.* 67:459.
Lindley, O.C., and T.J. Cunha. 1946. *J. Nutr.* 32:47.
Linkswiler, H. 1967. *Am. J. Clin. Nutr.* 20:547.
Linnel, J.C., et al. 1974. *Clin. Sci. Mol. Med.* 46:163.
Lohmann, K., and P. Schuster. 1937. *Biochem. Z.* 294:188.
Longo, D.L., and V. Herbert. 1976. *J. Lab. Clin. Med.* 87:138.
Lucas, G.H.W. 1924. *J. Phys. Chem.* 28:1180.
Luce, W.G., et al. 1966. *J. Nutr.* 88:39.
Luce, W.G., et al. 1967. *J. Anim. Sci.* 26:76.
Luce, W.G., et al. 1985. *Nutr. Rep. Int.* 32:245.
Luecke, R.W., et al. 1948. *J. Nutr.* 36:417.
Luecke, R.W., et al. 1950. *J. Anim. Sci.* 9:78.
Luecke, R.W., et al. 1952. *J. Anim. Sci.* 11:238.

Luecke, R.W., et al. 1953. *J. Anim. Sci.* 12:605.
Lumeng, L., et al. 1978. *J. Nutr.* 108:545.
Lynch, P.B., and J.F. O'Grady. 1981. *Irish J. Agric. Res.* 20:217.
Mahan, D.C., and L.J. Saif. 1983. *J. Anim. Sci.* 56:631.
Mahan, D.C., et al. 1966. *J. Anim. Sci.* 25:1019.
Matte, J.J., and C.L. Girard. 1989. *J. Anim. Sci.* 67:426.
Matte, J.J., et al. 1984a. *J. Anim. Sci.* 59:158.
Matte, J.J., et al. 1984b. *J. Anim. Sci.* 59:1020.
Maxwell, C.V., et al. 1987. *J. Anim. Sci.* 64:1044.
Meade, R.J. 1971. *1970-71 Minnesota Swine Research Report H-218.* St. Paul, MN: University of Minnesota Press.
Meade, R.J., et al. 1969. *Minnesota Agricultural Experiment Station Technical Bulletin 263.* St. Paul, MN: University of Minnesota Press.
Mertz, W. 1975. *Nutr. Rev.* 33:129.
Miller, C.O., and N.R. Ellis. 1951. *J. Anim. Sci.* 10:807.
Miller, C.O., et al. 1953. *J. Nutr.* 51:163.
Miller, E.R., et al. 1954. *J. Nutr.* 52:405.
Miller, E.R., et al. 1955. *J. Nutr.* 56:423.
Miller, E.R., et al. 1957a. *J. Nutr.* 62:407.
Miller, E.R., et al. 1957b. *Proc. Soc. Bio. Med.* 94:209.
Minot, G.R., and W.P. Murphey. 1926. *JAMA* 91:923.
Misir, R., and R. Blair. 1984. *J. Anim. Sci.* 59(Suppl. 1):254.
Misir, R., and R. Blair. 1986. *Res. Vet. Sci.* 40:212.
Mitchell, H.K., et al. 1941. *J. Am. Chem. Soc.* 63:2284.
Mitchell, H.H., et al. 1950. *J. Nutr.* 41:317.
Molitoris, B.A., and D.H. Baker. 1976. *J. Anim. Sci.* 42:481.
Mowatt, J.H., et al. 1948. *J. Am. Chem. Soc.* 70:14.
Nakano, T., et al. 1983. *Can. J. Anim. Sci.* 63:421.
National Research Council. 1987. *Vitamin Tolerance of Animals.* Washington, DC: National Academy Press.
National Research Council. 1988. *Nutrient Requirements of Swine.* Washington, DC: National Academy Press.
Nesheim, R.O., and B.C. Johnson. 1950. *J. Nutr.* 41:149.
Nesheim. R.O., et al. 1950. *Arch. Biochem.* 27:240.
Neumann, A.L., and B.C. Johnson. 1950. *J. Nutr.* 40:403.
Neumann, A.L., et al. 1948. *Proc. Soc. Exp. Biol. Med.* 69:513.
Neumann, A.L., et al. 1949. *J. Nutr.* 38:195.
Neumann, A.L., et al. 1950. *J. Anim. Sci.* 9:83.
Newcomb, M.D., and G.L. Allee. 1986. *J. Anim. Sci.* 63(Suppl. 1):108.
Newport, M.J. 1981. *Anim. Prod.* 33:333.
Nichoalds, G.E. 1974. *Clin. Chem.* 20:624.
Nishikimi, N., and S. Udenfriend. 1976. *Proc. Natl. Acad. Sci. USA* 73:2066.
Norris, L.C., and A.T. Ringrose. 1930. *Science* 71:643.
North Central Region-42 Committee on Swine Nutrition. 1976. *J. Anim. Sci.* 42:1211.
North Central Region-42 Committee on Swine Nutrition. 1980. *J. Anim. Sci.* 50:99.
North Central Region-89 Committee on Confinement Management of Swine. 1989. *J. Anim. Sci.* 67:624.
Olivera, B.M., and I.R. Lehman. 1967. *Proc. Natl. Acad. Sci. USA* 57:1700.
Olson, R.E., 1984. In: *Nutrition Reviews Present Knowledge in Nutrition.* Washington, DC: The Nutrition Foundation, Inc.
Omaye, S.T. 1984. *Adv. Exp. Med. Biol.* 177:169.
Owen, B.D., and J.P. Bowland. 1952. *J. Nutr.* 48:317.
Palm, B.W., et al. 1968. *J. Anim. Sci.* 27:1596.
Peng, C.L., and H. Heitman, Jr. 1973. *Br. J. Nutr.* 30:391.

Peng, C.L., and H. Heitman, Jr. 1974. *Br. J. Nutr.* 32:1.
Penny, R.H.C., et al. 1981. *Vet. Rec.* 109:80.
Peo, E.R., Jr., et al. 1970. *J. Anim. Sci.* 31:209 (Abstr.).
Pharazyn, A., and F.X. Aherne. 1987. *66th Annual Feeder's Day Report.* Edmonton, Alberta: University of Alberta.
Phillips, W.E., et al. 1978. *Toxicol. Appl. Pharmacol.* 44:323.
Pierce, J.V., et al. 1949. *J. Am. Chem. Soc.* 71:2952.
Pond, W.G., et al. 1960. *J. Anim. Sci.* 19:1115.
Powick, W.C., et al. 1948. *J. Anim. Sci.* 7:228.
Prentice, A.M., and C.J. Bates. 1981. *Br. J. Nutr.* 45:53.
Rao, B.S.N., and C. Gopalan. 1984. In: *Nutrition Reviews Present Knowledge in Nutrition.* 5th ed. pp. 318–331. Washington, DC: The Nutrition Foundation, Inc.
Richardson, D., et al. 1951. *J. Nutr.* 44:371.
Rickes, E.L., et al. 1948. *Science* 107:396.
Riker, J.T., III, et al. 1967. *J. Nutr.* 92:99.
Ringrose, A.T., et al. 1931. *Poult. Sci.* 10:166.
Ritchie, H.D., et al. 1960. *J. Nutr.* 70:491.
Robie, T.R. 1967. *J. Schiz.* 1:133.
Robinson, F.A. 1966. *Vitamin Co-Factors of Enzyme Systems.* Toronto: Pergamon Press.
Roth-Maier, D.A., and M. Kirchgessner. 1977. *Z. Tierphysiol. Tiernahr. Futtermiytelkd.* 38: 121.
Russell, L.E., et al. 1985a. *J. Nutr.* 115:1124.
Russell, L.E., et al. 1985b. *J. Nutr.* 115:1117.
Russet, J.C., et al. 1979a. *J. Anim. Sci.* 49:708.
Russet, J.C., et al. 1979b. *J. Anim. Sci.* 48:1366.
Sandholm, M., et al. 1979. *Vet. Rec.* 104:337.
Sauberlich, H.E. 1967. *Am. J. Clin. Nutr.* 20:528.
Sauberlich, H.E. 1968. In: *The Vitamins: Chemistry, Physiology, Pathology, Assay.* Vol. 2. 2d ed. Sebrell, W.H., Jr., and R.S. Harris (Eds.). pp. 39–80. New York: Academic Press.
Sauberlich, H.E., et al. 1974. *Laboratory Tests for the Assessment of Nutritional Status.* Boca Raton, FL: CRC Press.
Sauer, W.C., et al. 1988. *J. Anim. Sci.* 66:2583.
Schroeter, L.C. 1966. *Sulfur Dioxide.* 1st ed. Toronto: Pergamon Press.
Seerley, R.W., et al. 1981. *J. Anim. Sci.* 52:542.
Sewell, R.F., et al. 1962. *Fed. Proc.* 21:468.
Sewell, R.F., et al. 1964. *J. Anim. Sci.* 23:694.
Seymour, E.W., et al. 1968. *J. Anim. Sci.* 27:389.
Shilotri, P.G. 1977. *J. Nutr.* 107:1513.
Simmins, P.H., and P.H. Brooks. 1980. *Anim. Prod.* 30:469 (Abstr.).
Simmins, P.H., and P.H. Brooks. 1983. *Vet. Rec.* 112:425.
Simmins, P.H., and P.H. Brooks. 1985. *Anim. Prod.* 40:544.
Smith, D.T., et al. 1937. *JAMA* 109:2054.
Smith, E.L. 1948. *Nature (Lond.)* 161:638.
Snell, E.E. 1945. *J. Biol. Chem.* 157:491.
Southern, L.L., and D.H. Baker. 1981. *J. Anim. Sci.* 53:403.
Southern, L.L., et al. 1986. *J. Anim. Sci.* 62:992.
Spies, T.D., et al. 1938. *J. Am. Med. Assoc.* 110:622.
Stadman, T.C. 1971. *Science* 171:859.
Stockland, W.L., and L.G. Blaylock. 1974. *J. Anim. Sci.* 39:1113.
Stoffel, W., and I. Melzner. 1980. *Z. Physiol. Chem.* 361:755.
Stokstad, E.L.R. 1943. *J. Biol. Chem.* 149:573.
Stokstad, E.L.R., et al. 1948. *J. Am. Chem. Soc.* 70:3.
Stothers, S.C., et al. 1955. *J. Nutr.* 57:47.
Strecker, A. 1862. *Ann Chemie Pharmacie* 123:353.

Strecker, A. 1868. *Ann Chemie Pharmacie* 148:77.
Strittmatter, J.E., et al. 1978. *J. Anim. Sci.* 47(Suppl. 1):16.
Svirbely, J.L., and A. Szent-György. 1932. *Biochem. J.* 26:865.
Tanphaichitr, V., and B. Wood. 1984. In: *Nutrition Reviews Present Knowledge in Nutrition.* pp. 273–284. Washington, DC: The Nutrition Foundation.
Teague, H.S., and A.P. Grifo, Jr. 1966. *J. Anim. Sci.* 25:895 (Abstr.).
Teague, H.S., et al. 1970. *Ohio Agricultural Research Development Center Animal Science Mimeograph 200.* Wooster, OH: Ohio State University Press.
Terrill, S.W., et al. 1955. *J. Anim. Sci.* 14:593.
Thaler, R.C., et al. 1989. *J. Anim. Sci.* 66(Suppl. 1):114.
Tremblay, G.F., et al. 1986. *J. Anim. Sci.* 63:1173.
Tremblay, G.F., et al. 1989. *J. Anim. Sci.* 67:724.
Tribble, L.R., et al. 1984. *J. Anim. Sci.* 59(Suppl. 1):245.
Turley, S.D., et al. 1976. *Atherosclerosis* 24:1.
Ullrey, D.E., et al. 1955. *J. Nutr.* 57:401.
VanEtten, C., et al. 1940. *J. Nutr.* 20:607.
Waller, C.W., et al. 1948. *J. Am. Chem. Soc.* 70:19.
Warburg, O., and W. Christian. 1936. *Biochem. Z.* 287:291.
Warburg, O., et al. 1935. *Biochem. Z.* 282:157.
Washam, R.D., et al. 1975. *J. Anim. Sci.* 40:179.
Webb, N.G., et al. 1984. *Vet. Rec.* 114:185.
West, R. 1948. *Science* 107:398.
Wiese, A.C., et al. 1951. *J. Anim. Sci.* 10:80.
Wildiers, E. 1901. *Le Cellule* 18:313.
Williams, R.J. 1939. *Science* 89:486.
Williams, R.J., and R.T. Major. 1940. *Science* 91:246.
Williams, R.J., et al. 1933. *J. Am. Chem. Soc.* 55:2912.
Williams, R.J., et al. 1939. *J. Am. Chem. Soc.* 61:454.
Wills, L., and M.M. Mehta. 1930. *Indian J. Med. Res.* 17:777.
Wintrobe, M.M., et al. 1940. *Bull. Johns Hopkins Hosp.* 67:377.
Wintrobe, M.M., et al. 1942. *J. Nutr.* 24:345.
Wintrobe, M.M., et al. 1943a. *Bull. Johns Hopkins Hosp.* 73:169.
Wintrobe, M.M., et al. 1943b. *Bull. Johns Hopkins Hosp.* 73:313.
Wintrobe, M.M., et al. 1943c. *Bull. Johns Hopkins Hosp.* 72:1.
Wood, H.G., and R.E. Barden. 1977. *Annu. Rev. Biochem.* 46:385.
Yen, J.T., and W.G. Pond. 1981. *J. Anim. Sci.* 53:1292.
Yen, J.T., and W.G. Pond. 1983. *J. Anim. Sci.* 56:621.
Yen, J.T., and W.G. Pond. 1984. *J. Anim. Sci.* 58:132.
Yen, J.T., and W.G. Pond. 1987. *J. Anim. Sci.* 64:1672.
Yen, J.T., et al. 1976. *J. Anim. Sci.* 42:866.
Yen, J.T., et al. 1977. *J. Anim. Sci.* 45:269.
Yen, J.T., et al. 1978. *J. Anim. Sci.* 47(Suppl. 1):325.
Yen, J.T., et al. 1985. *Nutr. Rep. Int.* 31:877.
Yunis, A.A., et al. 1960. *J. Biol. Chem.* 235:3163.
Zimmerman, S.B., et al. 1967. *Proc. Natl. Acad. Sci. USA* 57:1841.

Chapter 15

Iron, Copper, Zinc, Manganese, and Iodine in Swine Nutrition

E.R. Miller

The essential trace elements are now recognized as important nutrients for swine (NRC 1988; ARC 1981). However, it was not until 1955 that their practical importance was generally recognized. In that year Tucker and Salmon (1955) reported that zinc (Zn) in the diet of growing pigs prevented or cured parakeratosis (Kernkamp and Ferrin 1953), which had been widely observed in the United States in growing pigs fed diets that were primarily composed of corn and plant proteins. Also in that year, Barber et al. (1955a,b,c) reported growth promotion of pigs by the addition of 250 ppm of copper (Cu) as $CuSO_4 \cdot 5H_2O$ to the diet. In that year as well, Barber et al. (1955d), Brownlie (1955), and McDonald et al. (1955) reported the efficacy of a single intramuscular injection of iron-dextran as an effective hematinic to prevent baby pig anemia, which had been long recognized (McGowan and Crichton 1923) as a problem in confinement rearing of swine.

Also in 1955, it became apparent that the Zn requirement of swine was dependent on several dietary factors that influenced Zn absorption and utilization (Luecke et al. 1956). Much of the research in trace element nutrition of swine in recent years has dealt with the interactions among the trace elements and with other components of the diet.

The trace elements for which there has been a demonstrated nutritional requirement by swine include iron (Fe), Cu, Zn, manganese (Mn), iodine (I), selenium (Se), and cobalt (Co). Selenium, because it is an integral part of glutathione peroxidase functioning with reduced glutathione as an important biological antioxidant system, is discussed with vitamin E in Chapter 12. The only demonstrated requirement of the pig for cobalt is as a component of vitamin B_{12}, which is discussed in Chapter 14. Other trace elements, including chromium, tin, nickel, molybdenum, vanadium, silicon, and fluorine, are considered to be dietary essentials for some animals and probably are for swine as well. However, these trace elements have not been demonstrated unequivocally to be dietary essentials for swine and are not covered in this chapter. This chapter is concerned with functions, signs of deficiency and toxicity, requirements, availability of feed forms, and interactions of Fe, Cu, Zn, Mn, and I in swine nutrition.

IRON

Iron Functions

Iron functions in the body as a component of hemoglobin of erythrocytes and myoglobin of muscle for O_2 and CO_2 transport and in the enzymes catalase, peroxidase, cytochrome oxidase, succinic dehydrogenase, aconitase, and xanthine oxidase in cellular metabolism. Thus, Fe is vital to cellular and whole body energetics. The presence of Fe in the body in ferritin and hemosiderin for Fe storage, in transferrin for plasma Fe transport, in uteroferrin for placental Fe transport, and in transferrin and lactoferrin in milk for Fe transfer to the suckling pig is also important (Furugouri 1981).

Iron Deficiency

Iron deficiency anemia is a universal concern for the nursing pig reared in modern confinement facilities (Miller 1981). The reasons for rapid development of anemia in nursing pigs are as follows:

1. The nursing pig reared in confinement is denied access to a natural source of iron from the soil.
2. The pig is born with a low total body Fe, amounting to <50 mg, about 80% of which is in hemoglobin (Venn et al. 1947), and efforts to increase placental transfer through high levels of Fe in the gestation diet (Brady et al. 1978) have been ineffective. Uteroferrin is an Fe-containing glycoprotein involved in maternal to fetal Fe transport in swine (Ducsay et al. 1982). While this may provide a means of increasing fetal Fe stores, Fe-dextran injections of the sow during gestation do not result in enough increase in fetal Fe storage to prevent the rapid development of anemia in the nursing pig (Ducsay et al. 1984).
3. Sow's colostrum and milk are low in Fe (about 2 ppm in colostrum and 1 ppm in milk), and attempts to increase mammary transfer of Fe by feeding high Fe concentrations in the lactation diet (Brady et al. 1978) or by Fe-dextran injections (Pond et al. 1961) have not been successful.
4. Absorption of colostral constituents (immunoglobulins, nutrients, and fluids) by the newborn pig results in a 50% increase in plasma volume during the first day of life (Ramirez et al. 1963), and this hemodilution triggers the iron deficiency anemia (Furugouri 1981).
5. Rapid growth rate of the nursing pig (doubling birth weight by 1 week and redoubling by 3 weeks of age; Cunha 1977) places a heavy demand on the erythropoietic system. Since the erythrocyte is 30% to 34% hemoglobin and hemoglobin contains 0.35% Fe, there is a constant demand for Fe to support erythropoiesis of the rapidly growing nursing pig (Miller et al. 1961).

Iron deficiency anemia in the nursing pig may vary from a borderline chronic anemia to acute anemia. Signs of chronic anemia are poor growth, listlessness, rough hair coat, wrinkled skin, and a paleness of the snout, ears, and mucous membranes.

This may be readily observed in white pigs. Blood hemoglobin concentration of chronically anemic pigs may range from 5 to 8 g/dL. Signs of acute anemia are labored breathing or a spasmodic movement of the diaphragm muscles following exercise. This is referred to as "thumps." In the most acute state, fast-growing pigs may die suddenly. Blood hemoglobin of acutely anemic pigs may range from 3 to 5 g/dL. Iron deficiency may lower the resistance of the pig to disease (Miller 1985), and respiratory problems and enteritis may appear more frequently in chronically anemic pigs.

Iron Requirement

The Fe requirement of the baby pig may be met orally or parenterally. The oral Fe requirement of baby pigs reared on artificial diets or condensed cow's milk is 60 to 150 mg/kg of milk solids (Matrone et al. 1960; Ullrey et al. 1960; Manners and McCrea 1963; Miller et al. 1982). Venn et al. (1947) calculated that nursing pigs need to retain at least 7 mg Fe daily to maintain body Fe concentration. If this retained Fe went totally for erythropoiesis, it would be adequate for synthesis of 2 g of hemoglobin (0.35% Fe) daily in about 100 billion new erythrocytes (mean corpuscular hemoglobin of 20×10^{-9} mg; Miller et al. 1961). Expected values of blood volume, total circulating erythrocytes, and total blood hemoglobin at birth and 3 weeks of nursing pigs receiving adequate iron are given in Table 15.1.

The Fe requirement of the nursing pig may be met orally by weekly dosing with pills, paste, or solutions containing Fe or by providing a constant supply of liquid or dry iron preparations in the creep area of the farrowing stall (Miller et al. 1969b). The Fe requirement of the nursing pig is met typically, however, with a single intramuscular injection of 100 to 200 mg of Fe as Fe-dextran or gleptoferron (Parsons et al. 1979a; Pollman et al. 1983). Iron-dextran may also be administered orally within the first few hours of life, before gut closure, and be effectively utilized (Thoren-Tolling 1975). Beyond weaning, the Fe requirement is largely met by ingredients in natural diets, especially the usual phosphorus sources, which typically provide 80 to 100 ppm of Fe to the diet (Kornegay 1972).

Table 15.1 Birth and 21-Day Blood Values of Nursing Pigs Receiving an Adequate Amount of Iron Either Orally or Parenterally

	Age of Nursing Pigs	
	Birth	*21 d*
Body weight (g)	1300	6000
Total blood volume (ml)[a]	120	500
Total blood erythrocytes (10^{10})[b]	60	250
Total blood hemoglobin (g)[c]	12	50

[a] Calculated from Ramirez et al. 1963.

[b] To maintain erythrocyte count of $5 \times 10^6/mm^3$ (Miller et al. 1961).

[c] To maintain hemoglobin concentration of 10 g/dl (Venn et al. 1947).

Table 15.2 Bioavailability of Iron from Various Sources

Iron Source	*RBV*[a]	*Reference*
$FeSO_4 \cdot 7H_2O$	100	
$FeSO_4 \cdot 2H_2O$	100	Miller et al. (1978)
$FeSO_4 \cdot H_2O$	92	Miller et al. (1978)
Ferric ammonium citrate	100	Harmon et al. (1967)
Ferric choline citrate	140	Miller et al. (1981)
Disodium Fe EDTA	90	Anderson et al. (1974)
Ferric polyphosphate	97	Anderson et al. (1974)
Reduced Fe	33–70	Anderson et al. (1974)
Sodium Fe pyrophosphate	33	Anderson et al. (1974)
Ferrous carbonate	0–74	Ammerman et al. (1974)
Ferric citrate	100	Ullrey et al. (1973)
Ferrous fumarate	100	Towlerton (1968)
Ferric oxide	0	Pickett et al. (1961)
Blood meal (flash-dried)	55	Parsons et al. (1979b)
Defluorinated phosphate	35–85	Kornegay (1972)

[a] Relative biological value (RBV) using $FeSO_4 \cdot 7H_2O$ as standard (100).

Iron Availability

Procedures for determining the bioavailability of the mineral elements are covered in Chapter 20. With Fe compounds, the slope-ratio technique using hemoglobin response in mildly deficient pigs from the test Fe source as compared with a standard Fe source ($FeSO_4 \cdot 7H_2O$) is appropriate. Relative biological values of several Fe sources as compared with $FeSO_4 \cdot 7H_2O$ (100) for pigs have been determined and are presented in Table 15.2.

Iron Toxicity

Campbell (1961) determined that administering orally 600 mg of Fe from ferrous sulfate per kilogram of body weight to 3- to 10-day-old pigs resulted in clinical signs of Fe toxicity including incoordination, shivering, hyperpnea, and tetanic convulsions. These signs were observed 1 to 3 hours after Fe dosing. All pigs had profuse diarrhea. Histopathologically, there was edema of the stomach wall, hyperemia, and extensive mucosal necrosis.

Oral or parenteral Fe administration to baby pigs for prevention of anemia has resulted in mortality in some litters (Behrens 1957; Bray 1958; Nilson 1960; Blandford and Lodge 1961; Ullrey et al. 1961; Lannek et al. 1962; Arpi and Tollerz 1965; Oksannen 1967). Mortality usually occurred within 3 to 12 hours. Clinical signs included drowsiness, dyspnea, and coma. Gross necropsy findings were edema at injection site, pallor of skeletal muscles, swollen kidneys, epicardial hemorrhage, hydropericardium, hydrothorax, and necrosis of the liver. Microscopically, there was severe degeneration of muscle and nephrosis. Studies by Patterson et al. (1967, 1969,

1971) indicate that peroxidation of muscle lipids is the initial step in muscle degeneration and that susceptibility to Fe toxicity is related to the vitamin E-selenium status of the pigs.

Continuous feeding of diets of growing pigs containing 5000 ppm of Fe from ferrous sulfate produced rickets (O'Donovan et al. 1963; Furugouri 1972). This was from formation of Fe phosphate in the digestive tract resulting in lowered phosphorus absorption. Rickets was prevented by elevating the dietary P level. At the 5000-ppm level of dietary Fe, transferrin saturation and liver Fe storage were well below capacity, indicating no Fe toxicity per se.

Supplemental dietary Fe reduces the potential of gossypol poisoning of swine fed diets containing high levels of cottonseed meal (Smith and Clawson 1965) and overcomes Fe deficiency in pigs fed a high level of I (Newton and Clawson 1974).

Iron and Disease Resistance

Iron is required for bacterial growth, and unless Fe is bound by carriers such as transferrin, susceptibility to infection is increased. Klasing et al. (1980) and Knight et al. (1983) concluded that parenteral administration of Fe in amounts exceeding the minimum amount required to prevent anemia should be avoided to minimize Fe that is not tightly bound to transferrin. Severity of diarrhea and mortality rate of *Escherichia coli*-challenged baby pigs was increased when 200 mg of Fe was administered orally but not when the same amount of Fe was administered intramuscularly as Fe-dextran (Kadis et al. 1984). Iron given parenterally as Fe-dextran is quickly taken up by the reticuloendothelial system (Ku et al. 1983), and there is minimal loss of parenteral Fe into the alimentary tract (Ku et al. 1981). Transferrin is not saturated following parenteral Fe administration (Ku et al. 1983) or during Fe mobilization from the liver (Furugouri 1974). Anemic pigs are more susceptible to the lethal action of bacterial endotoxins (Osborne and Davis 1968) or transmissible gastroenteritis virus (Parsons et al. 1977) than their littermates that received Fe supplementation. There appears to be little likelihood of enhancing infection when parenteral Fe administration to prevent baby pig anemia is limited to 200 mg of Fe.

COPPER

Copper has been recognized as an essential element in the diet of swine for over 50 years (Elvehjem and Hart 1932) and as a growth promoter at high levels in the diet of growing pigs for over 30 years (Barber et al. 1955a).

Copper Functions

Many of the essential functions of Cu in metabolism have been elucidated, including the following:

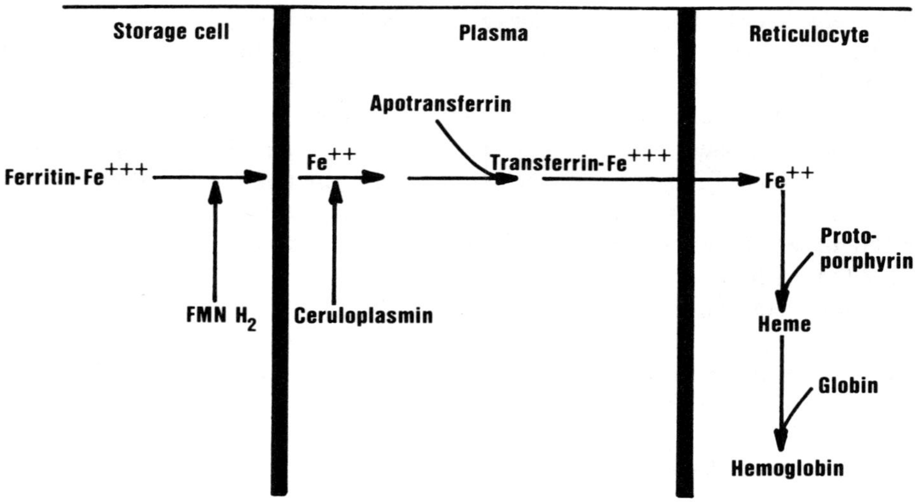

FIGURE 15.1 *Steps in the release of iron from liver storage cells to transferrin in the plasma and then to reticulocytes for hemoglobin synthesis.*

1. ceruloplasmin for ferroxidase activity to release hepatic Fe to transferrin for incorporation into hemoglobin in erythropoiesis (Figure 15.1),
2. lysyl oxidase activity for synthesis of desmosine and isodesmosine for proper collagen and elastin cross-linking,
3. cytochrome oxidase for myelin formation and proper functioning of the central nervous system,
4. tyrosinase for melanin formation and proper pigmentation,
5. superoxide dismutase for conversion of superoxide to peroxide and the proper microbicidal activity of phagocytes, and
6. both cytochrome oxidase and lysyl oxidase for proper cardiovascular functioning (Underwood 1977; Miller et al. 1979).

Copper Deficiency

Copper deficiency in young growing pigs is manifested by microcytic hypochromic anemia, low ceruloplasmin levels, reduced erythrocyte life span, crooked legs with bone disorders, poor appetite, retarded growth, cardiac hypertrophy, aortic rupture, and ataxia (Teague and Carpenter 1951; Carnes et al. 1961; Shields et al. 1982; and reviews of Miller et al. 1979; Whitehair and Miller 1986; ARC 1981). Hill et al. (1983a) were able to readily produce a Cu deficiency in pigs from sows that were fed a high-Zn diet during gestation and lactation.

Copper Requirement

The Cu requirement of swine is influenced by several dietary factors, including levels of Fe, Zn, and S and source of protein (Miller et al. 1979). The Cu requirement of young pigs fed milk or milk protein diets appears to be about 5 ppm (Teague and Carpenter 1951; Lahey et al. 1952; Manners and McCrea 1964; Okonkwo et al. 1979; Hill et al. 1983a) and is reported to be 3 to 6 ppm by the NRC (1988) and 4 ppm by the ARC (1981). Hedges and Kornegay (1973) concluded that 7 ppm of Cu was adequate for normal Fe metabolism in 9-week-old pigs receiving a diet containing 101 ppm of Fe. Feeding 5000 ppm of ZnO to gilts and sows fed corn-soybean meal diets containing 15 ppm of Cu resulted in Cu deficiency including osteochondrosis and very low levels of serum Cu (Hill et al. 1983b).

High Copper Feeding

Copper as a growth stimulant was first reported by Barber et al. (1955a,b,c) and has been reviewed by Braude (1967, 1975), Wallace (1967), Hays and Muir (1979), Omole (1980), and Cromwell et al. (1981). Diets of starting pigs (5 to 20 kg body weight) and growing pigs (20 to 60 kg body weight) supplemented with 250 ppm of Cu from $CuSO_4 \cdot 5H_2O$ consistently resulted in increased growth rate. Supplementing these diets with 500 ppm of S from Na_2S or FeS resulted in growth promotion without excessive build-up of liver Cu concentration (Cromwell et al. 1981). Growth promotion from high Cu feeding of starting and growing pigs is primarily due to the microbicidal effect of Cu in the intestinal tract (Shurson et al. 1986).

Copper Availability

A corn-soybean meal diet without supplemental Cu will meet the nutritional Cu requirement providing that interfering factors, such as a high Zn level, are not included in the diet. Usually, a Cu salt (CuO or $CuSO_4 \cdot 5H_2O$) are incorporated into the trace mineral premix that is supplemented to add about 10 ppm of Cu to the diet. Copper sulfate and CuO have quite high Cu availability (see Chapter 20), while CuS has very low Cu availability to the pig. Copper from $CuSO_4 \cdot 5H_2O$ at 125 to 250 ppm is most effective in growth promotion.

Copper Toxicity

When Cu is supplemented as $CuSO_4 \cdot 5H_2O$ to add 250 ppm of Cu to the diet and is fed throughout the starting, growing, and finishing periods, pigs may develop a Cu toxicity unless 100 ppm of Fe and Zn or 500 ppm of S as Na_2S or FeS is added to the diet. Thus, the margin of safety between the growth promotion level and the toxic level is quite narrow unless the precautions of including additional Zn, Fe, or S are followed. Signs of Cu toxicity are inappetence, generalized jaundice, anemia, and bloody feces. At necropsy there is discoloration of the liver (yellow-orange), internal hemorrhage, ulceration of the esophageal zone of the stomach, and pulmonary edema (Whitehair and Miller 1986).

ZINC

In the first three editions of the National Research Council's *Recommended Nutrient Allowances for Swine* and *Nutrient Requirements of Swine* (NRC 1944, 1950, 1953), it was noted that Zn was believed to be necessary for swine but that data on quantitative dietary requirements were lacking. In the fourth edition (NRC 1959), the work of Tucker and Salmon (1955), Luecke et al. (1956, 1957), Lewis et al. (1956, 1957), and Stevenson and Earle (1956) had been reported, and a dietary Zn requirement of 50 ppm was established with the caution that higher Zn levels may be needed if excess Ca is used in the diet. Zinc is now added to all commercially manufactured and farm-processed feeds for swine receiving grain-plant protein diets in the important commercial swine production areas of the world (Miller and Kornegay 1983).

Zinc Functions

Zinc functions in the body as a component of many enzymes, including dehydrogenases, phosphatases, kinases, ribonucleases, peptidases, and carbonic anhydrase, and as a component of insulin. As such, Zn influences protein, amino acid, nucleic acid, carbohydrate, lipid, and vitamin A metabolism. Zinc plays a role in diverse functions such as taste and smell acuity, immunocompetence, growth, reproduction, lactation, and behavior (see review of Miller et al. 1979).

Zinc Deficiency

Zinc deficiency is manifested by parakeratosis, anorexia, retarded growth, depleted fat depots, serous atrophy of fat, atrophy of thymus, depletion of thymocytes, and keratinization of tongue, esophagus, and cardia of the stomach (see review of Miller et al. 1979).

Nutritionally, parakeratosis is unique to Zn deficiency and even in moderately severe cases of parakeratosis, lesions disappear in 10 to 14 days following Zn supplementation. Parakeratosis is primarily a disease of the epidermal layer of the skin. Early clinical signs are small circumscribed erythematous areas and papules in the skin of the ventral abdominal wall and medial surface of thighs, followed by a circumscribed elevated area 3 to 5 mm in diameter, which is soon overlain with scales and keratinous crusts. The lesion fails to extend much beyond its original locus in some pigs, but in most cases it spreads until it affects a large area of the body (Whitehair and Miller 1986).

The histopathologic changes in parakeratosis are confined to the skin and are subacute to chronic noninflammatory (Kernkamp and Ferrin 1953). A characteristic feature is the presence in the outer layer of the epithelium of many nuclei and collections of keratohyalin granules. Another important alteration is an increase in the number and length of the rete pegs that dip down into the derma portion of the skin.

In Zn deficiency there is atrophy of the thymus of young pigs with a reduced percentage of lymphocytes in the differential leukocyte counts and an elevated percentage of band neutrophils (Miller et al. 1968). The thymus is important in immunological competence (via the T cell) and Zn is essential for proper T cell helper function (Luecke et al. 1978).

Recently, Kalinowski and Chavez (1984) observed a greatly lengthened parturition time for Zn-deficient sows ($\bar{x} = 4.54$ hours) as compared with control sows ($\bar{x} = 2.08$ hours). This effect of Zn deficiency had been observed by Bunce et al. (1985) in pregnant rats, in which they also found diminished gap junction formation in uterine tissue. Bunce et al. proposed that this prevented the timely establishment of estrogen dominance and impaired the transition steps necessary for the onset and efficient completion of labor.

Zinc Requirement

Zinc requirement of swine is influenced by factors that influence Zn absorption, including dietary calcium (Ca), Cu, Co, and cadmium (Cd) levels, phytic acid, level and type of protein, and level of histidine. Intestinal infections, such as with transmissible gastroenteritis virus, greatly reduce Zn absorption (Whitenack et al. 1978). The requirement of growing pigs fed corn-soybean meal diets ranges from 50 to 100 ppm (NRC 1988). The Zn requirement is much lower on casein-glucose diets (Smith et al. 1962; Shanklin et al. 1968). The Zn requirement is higher for developing boars and gilts than for barrows (Liptrap et al. 1970).

Zinc Availability

It has already been noted that a high level of Ca in a corn-soybean meal diet results in poor Zn absorption. This is due to the phytic acid from the corn and soybean meal forming a Ca-Zn-phytate complex in the digestive tract. This complex is insoluble and greatly reduces Zn availability. Zinc salts vary in the availability of their Zn when included in the diet. The Zn in $ZnSO_4 \cdot H_2O$, $ZnCO_3$, $ZnCl_2$, and Zn metal dust is highly available. Zinc is less available from ZnO and is poorly available from ZnS. Zinc from grains and plant proteins has low availability, while Zn is quite available from some of the animal protein sources. Zinc in milk is highly available due to the properties of the Zn-binding ligand found in milk (Lonnerdal et al. 1980).

Zinc Toxicity

Zinc toxicity in growing pigs is manifested by growth depression, arthritis, hemorrhage in axillary spaces, gastritis, and death (Brink et al. 1959). These pigs were fed a corn-soybean meal diet supplemented with 2000 to 4000 ppm of Zn from $ZnCO_3$. These levels of Zn from ZnO in the diet were not toxic to growing pigs (Hsu et al. 1975; Cox and Hale 1962; Hill et al. 1983b). Pigs fed a diet containing 1000 ppm of Zn as Zn lactate became lame and unthrifty within 2 months (Grimmett et al. 1937), while pigs fed a diet containing 1000 ppm of Zn from $ZnSO_4 \cdot H_2O$ showed no signs of Zn toxicity during a 7-month experimental period (Kulwich et al. 1953). Sows fed 5000 ppm of Zn from ZnO for two parities became lame and weaned lightweight pigs, indicating reduced milk production (Hill et al. 1983b).

MANGANESE

Manganese has long been recognized as an activator of metabolic enzymes that requires a nonspecific divalent cation. These nonspecific Mn^{+2}-activated enzymes include hydrolases, kinases, decarboxylases, and transferases. There are certain enzymes, such as succinic dehydrogenase, which are Fe-containing enzymes but which require Mn specifically for activation. Other enzymes, such as pyruvate carboxylase, require both Mn^{+2} and Mg^{+2}. Arginase activity depends heavily on Mn^{+2}.

Manganese Functions

The principal function of Mn is in connective tissue synthesis. Manganese does not play a role in the calcification process of bone formation, but it does play a role in the synthesis of the organic matrix. Specifically, Mn is essential for mucopolysaccharide synthesis, particularly that of chondroitin sulfate (Leach and Muenster 1962). There is a requirement for Mn^{+2} by glycosyl transferase enzymes in this synthesis (Leach 1971). In view of the importance of the chondroitin sulfate-protein complex in the maintenance of the rigidity of connective tissue, the skeletal deformities that occur with Mn deficiency seem logical.

Manganese Deficiency

Manganese deficiency results in skeletal and postural defects in many species. In Mn-deficient pigs, the skeletal abnormalities are characterized by lameness and enlarged hock joints with crooked and shortened legs (Underwood 1981). In addition, Plumlee et al. (1956) observed reduced skeletal growth and an accompanying skeletal or muscular weakness, increased fatness, irregular estrual cycles of gilts, and resorption of fetuses or birth of small, weak pigs that could neither stand nor walk properly (neonatal ataxia).

Manganese Requirement

The dietary requirement of Mn for growth is quite low, probably no more than 4 ppm (Johnson 1943, 1944; Grummer et al. 1950; Plumlee et al. 1956; Liebholz et al. 1962; Kayongo-Male et al. 1975; Svajgr et al. 1969; NRC 1988). The requirement for good reproductive performance of gilts and sows is higher, probably about 10 ppm (ARC 1981; NRC 1988; Grummer et al. 1950; Plumlee et al. 1956; Johnson 1943).

Manganese Availability

In chickens, high dietary levels of Ca and P reduce the availability of Mn (Caskey and Norris 1939). Manganese and Fe compete for the same intestinal absorption site (Matrone et al. 1959). The availability of Mn from natural feed sources is quite low (Underwood 1981). The relative biological values of Mn salts with $MnSO_4 \cdot H_2O$ at 100 as a standard are 100 for $MnCl_2$, 66 for MnO, 40 for $MnCO_3$, and <30 for MnO_2 (see Chapter 20).

Manganese Toxicity

Grummer et al. (1950) noted decreased food intake and growth, and limb stiffness of pigs fed 500 ppm Mn from $MnSO_4$. Liebholz et al. (1962) noted depressed growth rate of Mn at 2000 to 4000 ppm in the diet of growing pigs. Below these levels the pig is able to maintain Mn tissue levels by low absorption efficiency (2%) and by excretion in bile and by the pancreas.

IODINE

Early studies by Kalkus (1920) in Washington, Welch (1928) in Montana, Hart and Steenbock (1918) in Wisconsin, and later by Andrews et al. (1948) and Slatter (1955) in Indiana demonstrated that the Great Lakes region, the Northwestern United States, and British Columbia are areas of hypothyroidism in swine due to low-I feedstuffs produced on I-deficient soil.

Iodine Functions

The only known role of I is in the synthesis of the thyroid hormones thyroxine (T_4) and triiodothyronine (T_3). These thyroid hormones are under the control of the thyroid stimulating hormone (TSH) of the pituitary, which in turn is released under the action of the thyrotropin releasing factor (TRF) of the hypothalamus. Adequate circulating levels of T_4 and T_3 inhibit release of both TRF and TSH (Underwood 1977). The thyroid hormones function in regulating metabolic rate and, indirectly, cell differentiation and growth, particularly in early life. Thus, there is a vital role of I in reproduction.

Iodine Deficiency

Production of hairless pigs with thickened skin and subcutaneous edema by sows on goitrous feeds is characteristic of I deficiency (Kalkus 1920; Welch 1928; Hart and Steenbock 1918). Myxedema is usually present and makes the pigs at birth appear larger than normal. Most pigs are born alive but die within a few hours. An enlarged thyroid (goiter) is not evident externally. However, on necropsy the gland is enlarged and hemorrhagic. The only observed sign in a borderline I deficiency is weakness in a few pigs or possibly the entire litter. Litters from sows in the same environment and given the same feed vary considerably.

Andrews et al. (1948) found a high incidence of hyperplasia of the follicular epithelium of the thyroid of baby pigs from unsupplemented sows. Protein-bound I levels in plasma of I-deficient pigs was reduced (Sihombing et al. 1974). A number of studies have been conducted to produce a hypothyroid condition by feeding goitrogens. Beeson et al. (1947) fed thiouracil, Braude and Cotchin (1949) fed thiourea and methylthiouracil, Sihombing et al. (1974) fed 1-methyl-2-mercaptoimidazole, and Cromwell et al. (1975) fed potassium thiocyanate. In hypothyroidism, pigs appeared stunted, leg bones were shorter than normal, there was labored breathing, and pigs were lethargic and reluctant to move.

Iodine Availability

Iodine is quite available from NaI or KI. However, I in these salts may be lost by volatilization. Calcium iodate and potassium iodate ($Ca(IO_3)_2 \cdot H_2O$ and KIO_3) are more stable forms in trace mineral premixes or complete feeds. Pentacalcium orthoperiodate ($Ca_5(IO_6)_2$) is also a stable form. Availability of I is good from each of these I compounds. Iodine requirement may be increased by other dietary minerals, including excessive levels of arsenic, fluoride, cobalt, calcium, and sodium chloride (Underwood 1981).

Iodine Toxicity

Frape et al. (1958) reported that 4 ppm of I as KI in the diet of young pigs depressed performance. However, Newton and Clawson (1974) found no depression of performance of growing pigs receiving up to 400 ppm of I as calcium iodate in their diet. At levels of 800 or 1600 ppm of dietary I, they found depressed growth rate, feed intake, hemoglobin level, and liver Fe concentration. Pig performance and hemoglobin level were improved by increasing dietary Fe. Increased serum I levels and increased thyroid weight were observed as I was increased. Arrington et al. (1965) fed sows up to 2500 ppm of dietary I as NaI or KI during the final 30 days of pregnancy without influence on litter size, weight, survival, or growth during lactation. Hart and Steenbock (1918) did not observe adverse effects from feeding 50 mg I daily during pregnancy and 83 mg daily during lactation as 2% iodized calcium carbonate.

INTERACTIONS OF IRON, COPPER, AND ZINC

The study of Tucker and Salmon (1955) not only demonstrated that parakeratosis was due to Zn deficiency, it also demonstrated that high dietary Ca level was involved in this nutritional disease. Luecke et al. (1956) and others demonstrated that increasing dietary Zn overcame the antagonism of elevated dietary Ca. O'Dell et al. (1964) demonstrated that elevated dietary Ca in the presence of phytate in the diet formed an insoluble Ca-Zn-phytate complex, lowering Zn availability. Hoefer et al. (1960) and Wallace et al. (1960) observed that high dietary levels of Cu (125 or 250 ppm) reduced the incidence and severity of parakeratosis of pigs fed low-Zn diets. Later, this was observed by Ritchie et al. (1963) and DeGoey et al. (1971). On the other hand, Smith et al. (1962), Hoekstra (1964), and Miller et al. (1968) found no protection from Zn deficiency when 125 ppm of Cu was added to an isolated soy protein-glucose diet, and O'Hara et al. (1960) and Suttle and Mills (1966b) found that adding 250 ppm of Cu to low-Zn diets increased the incidence and severity of the skin lesions of Zn deficiency.

Wallace et al. (1960), O'Hara et al. (1960), Ritchie et al. (1963), Suttle and Mills (1966b), and Hanrahan and O'Grady (1968) observed Cu toxicosis with diets supplemented with 250 ppm of Cu. Ritchie et al. (1963), Suttle and Mills (1966a,b), Hanrahan and O'Grady (1968), and DeGoey et al. (1971) prevented Cu toxicosis by including 100 to 150 ppm of Zn or similar levels of Zn and Fe to growing pigs' diets containing 250 ppm or more of Cu. Suttle and Mills (1966b) concluded that occasional occurrences of toxicity in pigs fed 250 ppm of Cu as a growth stimulant are probably due to its use in diets low in Zn and Fe and high in Ca. The studies of Bremner (1976) and Bremner and Young (1976) led to the conclusion that Cu and Zn occur in liver in the form of mixed (Cu and Zn) thioneins and that Zn may be essential for stabilization of the metal-binding protein in this fraction of liver Cu.

On a corn-fish meal-dried skim milk diet, Gipp et al. (1967) doubled liver Cu storage by feeding 150 ppm of Cu, which was unaffected by 20 ppm of molybdenum (Mo), 1000 ppm of sulfate, or 63 ppm of Zn. There was no evidence of a Cu-Mo-sulfate interrelationship or a Cu-Zn interaction. Kline et al. (1972) added 250 or 500 ppm of Cu to a corn-soybean meal diet fed to growing-finishing pigs. Growth rate was stimulated by the 250-ppm addition, but both growth rate and hemoglobin level were reduced when 500 ppm of Cu was added. High levels of liver Cu were found in pigs fed the diet supplemented with 500 ppm of Cu that was not diminished by additional levels of Zn or Fe. This is in agreement with the results of Kulwich et al. (1953), Cox and Hale (1962), and Gipp et al. (1967).

The diverse results obtained in different studies of the Cu-Zn interaction present an interesting dilemma that begs an explanation. On the one hand, Allen et al. (1958), Barber et al. (1960), Ritchie et al. (1963), Hanrahan and O'Grady (1968), and DeGoey et al. (1971) obtained a significant reduction in swine liver Cu levels with supplementary Zn. On the other hand, Kulwich et al. (1953), Cox and Hale (1962), Gipp et al. (1967), and Kline et al. (1972) did not find reduced liver Cu levels in pigs when they added Zn to the basal diet. The explanation would appear to be that in situations where supplemental Zn produced a definite reduction in liver Cu level, the basal diet was deficient or borderline in meeting the dietary Zn requirement. Under such conditions, it appears that added Zn may decrease Cu absorption, increase Cu excretion, or partially replace Cu in liver metallothionein storage.

Both high levels of Cu (Bunch et al. 1963; Suttle and Mills 1966b; Gipp et al. 1973a,b; Hedges and Kornegay 1973; Hanrahan and O'Grady 1968) and high levels of Zn (Cox and Hale 1962; Hedges and Kornegay 1973) in the diet reduced liver Fe. High dietary levels of Cu tend to depress hemoglobin level (Bunch et al. 1961, 1963; Wallace et al. 1960; Ritchie et al. 1963; Kline et al. 1972; Miller et al. 1969a; DeGoey et al. 1971; Gipp et al. 1973a,b; Hedges and Kornegay 1973) without significantly affecting serum Zn levels, but they tend to increase liver Zn levels (DeGoey et al. 1971; Gipp et al. 1973a,b).

Kulwich et al. (1953) found that adding 1000 ppm of Mo to pig diets significantly increased liver Cu accumulation, and dietary Zn did not appear to be involved in Cu-Mo imbalance. Hays and Kline (1969) and Kline et al. (1971) observed that 200 ppm of Mo and 10,000 ppm of sulfate were not effective in reducing the liver uptake of Cu in growing pigs. Thus, the Cu-Mo-sulfate interrelationships that are important to the ruminant (Matrone 1970) are not of great consequence in the diet of the pig. The addition of 500 ppm of sulfur (S) as ferrous sulfide to diets containing 250 ppm of Cu reduced liver Cu stores from 278 to 21 ppm, a level approaching that of the pigs on the control diet (Ribeiro de Lima et al. 1981). Cromwell et al. (1978) and Kline et al. (1973) showed similar effectiveness of 450 ppm of sodium sulfate in high-Cu diets in reducing Cu stores in the liver.

The fact that Cu deficiency produces anemia in pigs (Hill et al. 1983a) provides evidence for an interaction between Cu and Fe. In pigs suffering from Cu-deficiency anemia, there was low serum Fe, decreased Fe uptake for hemoglobin synthesis, and low liver Fe (Gubler et al. 1952). Furthermore, the erythrocyte life span was 20% that of controls (Jensen et al. 1956; Bush et al. 1956). The principal form of Cu in plasma is that of ceruloplasmin, a metalloprotein containing eight atoms of Cu per molecule. Ceruloplasmin has ferroxidase activity, which plays a vital role in the movement of Fe out of the storage form (ferritin) to the transport form (transferrin) and in the incorporation into hemoglobin of developing erythrocytes, as shown in Figure 15.1.

In Hill's studies (1983b) of 5000 ppm of Zn from Zn oxide in the gestation and lactation diet of gilts and sows, low tissue and plasma Cu levels were noted in offspring. Normally, the fetal pig stores a reserve of Cu in the liver, which after birth leaves the liver and enters the circulation, raising serum levels from a low value at birth to a sixfold increase within 2 weeks of birth (Ullrey et al. 1967). With the high level of Zn in the dam's diet there was very little storage of Cu by the fetus, and plasma Cu levels at birth and during the nursing period remained low (Hill 1983c). This Zn-induced Cu deficiency in the baby pig was used in studying the Cu requirement of the baby pig (Hill et al. 1983a). Since one of the subclinical signs of Cu deficiency is anemia due to poor utilization of Fe for erythropoiesis, a true Zn-Cu-Fe interaction was demonstrated. Doubtless, there are many other interrelationships of these elements.

These interactions of Fe, Cu, and Zn are indicative of the multitude of interrelationships among the trace elements and between individual essential elements and other nutrients and nonnutrient components of the diet. These interactions also point to the dynamic state of the animal body and the dynamic role that seemingly insignificant traces of inorganic elements play in the well-being and productivity of the pig.

REFERENCES

Allen, M.M., et al. 1958. *Proc. Nutr. Soc.* 17:12.
Ammerman, C.B., et al. 1974. *J. Anim. Sci.* 38:52.
Anderson, T.A., et al. 1974. *J. Nutr.* 104:619.
Andrews, F.N., et al. 1948. *J. Anim. Sci.* 7:298.
Arpi, T., and G. Tollerz. 1965. *Acta. Vet. Scand.* 6:360.
Arrington, L.R., et al. 1965. *J. Nutr.* 87:394.
Barber, R.S., et al. 1955a. *Chem. Ind.* 21:601.
Barber, R.S., et al. 1955b. *Chem. Ind.* 21:1954.
Barber, R.S., et al. 1955c. *Br. J. Nutr.* 9:378.
Barber, R.S., et al. 1955d. *Vet. Rec.* 67:348.
Barber, R.S., et al. 1960. *Br. J. Nutr.* 14:499.
Beeson, W.M., et al. 1947. *J. Anim. Sci.* 6:482.
Behrens, H. 1958. *J. Am. Vet. Med. Assoc.* 132:169.
Blandford, T.B., and G.A. Lodge. 1966. *Vet. Rec.* 78:117.
Brady, P.S., et al. 1978. *J. Anim. Sci.* 47:1135.
Brag, S. 1958. *Proceedings of the 8th Nordic Veterinary Congress.* p. 98. Stockholm: State Veterinary Medicine Institute.
Braude, R. 1967. *World Rev. Anim. Prod.* 3:69.
Braude, R. 1975. *Proceedings of Copper in Farming Symposium.* London: Copper Development Association.
Braude, R., and E. Cotchin. 1949. *Br. J. Nutr.* 3:171.
Bremner, I. 1976. *Br. J. Nutr.* 35:245.
Bremner, I., and B.W. Young. 1976. *Biochem. J.* 155:361.
Brink, M.F., et al. 1959. *J. Anim. Sci.* 18:836.
Brownlie, W.M. 1955. *Vet. Rec.* 67:350.
Bunce, G.E., et al. 1985. TEMA 5 Proceedings. p. 201. London: CAB.
Bunch, R.J., et al. 1961. *J. Anim. Sci.* 20:723.
Bunch, R.J., et al. 1963. *J. Anim. Sci.* 22:56.
Bush, J.A., et al. 1956. *J. Exp. Med.* 103:701.
Campbell, E.A. 1961. *Aust. Vet. J.* 78:83.
Carnes, W.H., et al. 1961. *Fed. Proc.* 20:118.
Caskey, D.C., and L.C. Norris. 1939. *Proc. Soc. Exp. Biol. Med.* 40:590.
Cox, D.H., and O.M. Hale. 1962. *J. Nutr.* 77:225.
Cromwell, G.L., et al. 1975. *J. Anim. Sci.* 41:813.
Cromwell, G.L., et al. 1978. *J. Anim. Sci.* 46:692.

Cromwell, G.L., et al. 1981. *Feedstuffs*. Nov. 2, p. 30.
Cunha, T.J. 1977. *Swine Feeding and Nutrition*. New York: Academic Press.
DeGoey, L.W., et al. 1971. *J. Anim. Sci.* 33:52.
Ducsay, C.A., et al. 1982. *Biol. Reprod.* 26:729.
Ducsay, C.A., et al. 1984. *J. Anim. Sci.* 59:1303.
Elvehjem, C.A., and E.B. Hart. 1932. *J. Biol. Chem.* 95:363.
Frape, D.L., et al. 1958. *J. Anim. Sci.* 17:1225.
Furugouri, K. 1972. *J. Anim. Sci.* 34:573.
Furugouri, K. 1974. *Jpn. J. Vet. Sci.* 36:255.
Furugouri, K. 1981. *Pig News Inform.* 2:279.
Gipp, W.F., et al. 1967. *J. Anim. Sci.* 26:727.
Gipp, W.F., et al. 1973a. *J. Anim. Sci.* 36:91.
Gipp, W.F., et al. 1973b. *J. Nutr.* 103:713.
Grimmett, R.E.R., et al. 1937. *N. Z. J. Agric.* 54:216.
Grummer, R.H., 1950. *J. Anim. Sci.* 9:170.
Gubler, C.J., et al. 1952. *J. Hematol.* 7:1075.
Hanrahan, T.J., and J.F. O'Grady. 1968. *Anim. Prod.* 10:423.
Harmon, B.G., et al. 1967. *J. Anim. Sci.* 26:1051.
Hart, E.E., and H. Steenbock. 1918. *Wisconsin Agricultural Experiment Station Bulletin 279.* Madison: University of Wisconsin.
Hays, V.W., and R.D. Kline. 1969. *Feedstuffs* 41:18.
Hays, V.W., and W.M. Muir. 1979. *Can. J. Anim. Sci.* 59:447.
Hedges, J.D., and E.T. Kornegay. 1973. *J. Anim. Sci.* 37:1147.
Hill, G.M., et al. 1983a. *J. Nutr.* 113:867.
Hill, G.M., et al. 1983b. *J. Anim. Sci.* 57:114.
Hill, G.M., et al. 1983c. *J. Anim. Sci.* 57:130.
Hoefer, J.A., et al. 1960. *J. Anim. Sci.* 19:249.
Hoekstra, W.G., et al. 1964. *Fed. Proc.* 23:1068.
Hsu, F.S., et al. 1975. *J. Nutr.* 105:112.
Jensen, W.N., et al. 1956. *J. Exp. Med.* 103:415.
Johnson, S.R. 1943. *J. Anim. Sci.* 2:14.
Johnson, S.R. 1944. *J. Anim. Sci.* 3:136.
Kadis, S., et al. 1984. *Am. J. Vet. Res.* 45:255.
Kalinowski, J., and E.R. Chavez. 1984. *Can. J. Anim. Sci.* 64:749.
Kalkus, J.W. 1920. *Washington Agricultural Experiment Station Bulletin 156.* Pullman: Washington State University.
Kayongo-Male, H., et al. 1975. *East Afr. Agric. Forest. J.* 41:157.
Kernkamp, H.C.H., and E.F. Ferrin. 1953. *J. Am. Vet. Med. Assoc.* 123:217.
Klasing, K.C., et al. 1980. *J. Nutr.* 110:1914.
Kline, R.D., et al. 1971. *J. Anim. Sci.* 33:771.
Kline, R.D., et al. 1972. *J. Anim. Sci.* 34:393.
Kline, R.D., et al. 1973. *J. Anim. Sci.* 37:936.
Knight, C.D., et al. 1983. *J. Anim. Sci.* 57:387.
Kornegay, E.T. 1972. *J. Anim. Sci.* 34:569.
Ku, P.K., et al. 1981. *Michigan Agricultural Experiment Station Research Report 487.* p. 90. East Lansing: Michigan State University.
Ku, P.K., et al. 1983. *J. Anim. Sci.* 57:638.
Kulwich, R., et al. 1953. *Proc. Soc. Exp. Biol. Med.* 84:487.
Lahey, M.E., et al. 1952. *J. Hematol.* 7:1053.
Lannek, N., et al. 1962. *Nature* 195:1006.
Leach, R.M., Jr. 1971. *Fed. Proc.* 30:991.
Leach, R.M., Jr., and A.M. Muenster. 1962. *J. Nutr.* 78:51.
Lewis, P.K., et al. 1956. *J. Anim. Sci.* 15:741.
Lewis, P.K., et al. 1957. *J. Anim. Sci.* 16:578.

Leibholz, J.M., et al. 1962. *J. Anim. Sci.* 21:772.
Liptrap, D.O., et al. 1970. *J. Anim. Sci.* 30:736.
Lonnerdal, B., et al. 1980. *J. Nutr.* 110:2414.
Luecke, R.W., et al. 1956. *J. Anim. Sci.* 15:347.
Luecke, R.W., et al. 1957. *J. Anim. Sci.* 16:3.
Luecke, R.W., et al. 1978. *J. Nutr.* 108:881.
Manners, M.J., and M.R. McCrae. 1963. *Br. J. Nutr.* 17:495.
Matrone, G.E., et al. 1959. *J. Nutr.* 67:309.
Matrone, G.E., et al. 1960. *J. Nutr.* 72:459.
Matrone, G.E. 1970. *TEMA 1 Proceedings.* p. 354. London: E.S. Livingstone.
McDonald, F.F., et al. 1955. *Br. Vet. J.* 111:403.
McGowan, J.P., and A. Crichton. 1923. *Biochem. J.* 17:204.
Miller, E.R. 1978. *Feedstuffs* 50:20.
Miller, E.R. 1981. *Anim. Nutr. Health* 36:14.
Miller, E.R. 1985. *J. Anim. Sci.* 60:1500.
Miller, E.R., and E.T. Kornegay. 1983. *J. Anim. Sci.* 57:315.
Miller, E.R., et al. 1961. *J. Anim. Sci.* 20:890.
Miller, E.R., et al. 1968. *J. Nutr.* 95:278.
Miller, E.R., et al. 1969a. *J. Anim. Sci.* 29:140.
Miller, E.R., et al. 1969b. *Michigan Agricultural Experiment Station Research Report 99.* p. 38. East Lansing: Michigan State University.
Miller, E.R., et al. 1979. *Copper and Zinc in Animal Nutrition.* Des Moines, IA: NFIA.
Miller, E.R., et al. 1981. *J. Anim. Sci.* 52:783.
Miller, E.R., et al. 1982. *J. Anim. Sci.* 54:106.
Newton, G.L., and A.J. Clawson. 1974. *J. Anim. Sci.* 39:879.
Nilsson, P.O. 1960. *Nord. Vet. Med.* 12:113.
NRC. 1944. *Recommended Nutrient Allowances for Swine.* Washington, DC: National Research Council.
NRC. 1950. *Recommended Nutrient Allowances for Swine.* Washington, DC: National Research Council.
NRC. 1953. *Nutrient Requirements of Swine.* Washington, DC: National Research Council.
NRC. 1959. *Nutrient Requirements of Swine.* Washington, DC: National Research Council.
NRC. 1979. *Nutrient Requirements of Swine.* 8th ed. Washington, DC: National Research Council.
NRC. 1980. *Mineral Tolerances of Domestic Animals.* Washington, DC: National Research Council.
NRC. 1988. *Nutrient Requirements of Swine.* 9th ed. Washington, DC: National Research Council.
O'Dell, B.L., et al. 1964. *Poult. Sci.* 43:415.
O'Donovan, P.B., et al. 1963. *J. Anim. Sci.* 22:1075.
O'Hara, P.J., et al. 1960. *Aust. Vet. J.* 36:225.
Okonkwo, A.C., et al. 1979. *J. Nutr.* 109:939.
Oksannen, H.E. 1967. In: *Selenium in Biomedicine.* Westport, CT: AVI Publishing Co.
Omole, T.A. 1980. *Livestock Prod. Sci.* 7:253.
Osborne, J.C., and J.W. Davis. 1968. *J. Am. Vet. Med. Assoc.* 152:630.
Parsons, M.P., et al. 1977. *Michigan Agricultural Experiment Station Research Report 343.* p. 10. East Lansing: Michigan State University.
Parsons, M.P., et al. 1979a. *Michigan Agricultural Experiment Station Research Report 386.* p. 14. East Lansing: Michigan State University.
Parsons, M.P., et al. 1979b. *Michigan Agricultural Experiment Station Research Report 386.* p. 104. East Lansing: Michigan State University.
Patterson, D.S.P., et al. 1967. *Biochem. J.* 104:2.
Patterson, D.S.P., et al. 1969. *Zentralbl. Veterinarmed.* 16:199.
Patterson, D.S.P., et al. 1971. *Zentralbl. Veterinarmed.* 18:453.

Pickett, R.A., et al. 1960. *J. Anim. Sci.* 19:1284.
Plumlee, M.P., et al. 1956. *J. Anim. Sci.* 15:352.
Pollman, D.S., et al. 1983. *J. Anim. Sci.* 56:640.
Pond, W.G., et al. 1961. *J. Anim. Sci.* 20:747.
Ramirez, C.G., et al. 1963. *J. Anim. Sci.* 22:1068.
Ritchie, H.D., et al. 1963. *J. Nutr.* 79:117.
Shanklin, S.H., et al. 1968. *J. Nutr.* 96:101.
Shields, G.C., et al. 1962. *Am. J. Pathol.* 41:603.
Shurson, G.C., et al. *J. Anim. Sci.* 63(Suppl. 1):266.
Sihombing, D.T.H., et al. 1974. *J. Anim. Sci.* 39:1106.
Slatter, E.R. 1955. *J. Am. Vet. Med. Assoc.* 127:149.
Smith, F.H., and A.J. Clawson. 1965. *J. Nutr.* 87:317.
Smith, W.H., et al. 1962. *J. Anim. Sci.* 21:399.
Stevenson, J.W., and I.P. Earle. 1956. *J. Anim. Sci.* 15:1036.
Suttle, N.F., and C.F. Mills. 1966a. *Br. J. Nutr.* 20:135.
Suttle, N.F., and C.F. Mills. 1966b. *Br. J. Nutr.* 20:149.
Svajar, A.J., et al. 1969. *J. Anim. Sci.* 29:439.
Teague, H.S., and L.E. Carpenter. 1951. *J. Nutr.* 43:309.
Thoren-Tholling, K. 1975. *Acta. Vet. Scand. Suppl.* 54:1.
Towlerton, R.G. 1968. *Vet. Rec.* 82:497.
Tucker, H.F., and W.D. Salmon. 1955. *Proc. Soc. Exp. Biol. Med.* 88:613.
Ullrey, D.E., et al. 1960. *J. Nutr.* 70:187.
Ullrey, D.E., et al. 1961. *J. Anim. Sci.* 20:954.
Ullrey, D.E., et al. 1967. *J. Anim. Sci.* 26:1024.
Ullrey, D.E., et al. 1973. *Michigan Agricultural Experiment Station Research Report 232*. p. 34. East Lansing: Michigan State University.
Underwood, E.J. 1977. *Trace Elements in Human and Animal Nutrition*. 4th ed. New York: Academic Press.
Underwood, E.J. 1981. *The Mineral Nutrition of Livestock*. 2d ed. New York: Academic Press.
Venn, J.A.J., et al. 1947. *J. Comp. Pathol. Ther.* 57:314.
Wallace, H.D., et al. 1960. *J. Anim. Sci.* 19:1153.
Wallace, H.D. 1967. New York: International Copper Research Association, Inc.
Weiser, S., and A. Zaitchek. 1932. *Bied. Zentralbl. Tiernahrung* 4:476.
Welch, H. 1928. *Montana Agricultural Experiment Station Bulletin 214*. Bozeman: Montana State University.
Whitehair, C.K., and E.R. Miller, 1986. In: *Diseases of Swine*. 6th ed. p. 746. Ames, IA: Iowa State University Press.
Whitenack, D.L., et al. 1978. *Am. J. Vet. Res.* 1447.

Chapter 16

Fiber Utilization by Swine

C.C. Calvert

Research on the effects of fiber in swine diets, since the report of Scheunert (1906) that pigs could digest cellulose, has established how well pigs can perform on diets high in fiber, the limitations of feeding various fiber sources, the interactions of fiber with other nutrients, and to a very limited extent, how performance might be improved by including a fiber source in swine diets. This literature has been reviewed extensively by Trautmann and Asher (1941), Forbes and Hamilton (1952), Cranwell (1968), and Rerat (1978). Recently, Varel (1987) published a comprehensive review on fiber-degrading microorganisms in the gut of the pig that covers fiber utilization.

This chapter is not a comprehensive review of the literature on fiber utilization by swine, but it provides references allowing entry into the literature for anyone interested in a more thorough review of this subject. More specifically, this chapter discusses factors dealing with the definition of fiber, its chemical and physical properties, and the various methods currently being used for its analysis. The effects of fiber on pig and sow performance, the amounts of total fiber and fiber components utilized by swine, their effects on nutrient utilization and rate of digesta passage also are reviewed.

DEFINITION OF FIBER

Fiber, as defined by Trowell (1972), may be characterized as those components in plant cell walls that are resistant to all digestive enzymes secreted by any animal. This definition is acceptable to most animal nutritionists, but it should be recognized that there are concerns that this definition is restrictive, since materials not in plant cell walls are also resistant to digestive enzymes. Cummings (1981) has proposed a somewhat less restrictive definition of fiber, which states that fiber includes all nonstarch polysaccharides plus lignin. Asp and Johansson (1984) have been more definitive and have identified those components that might be included in a definition of fiber. By their reasoning, cellulose, hemicellulose, pectins, gums, mucilages, and lignins would be classified as fiber. Cutins and waxes, indigestible proteins and lipids, insoluble starches, inorganic elements, silicates, trace amines or polyamines, lignans, and phenolic monomers would not be considered as fiber components.

Van Soest's procedure (Goering and Van Soest 1970) adds neutral detergent fiber (NDF) and acid detergent fiber (ADF) to the list of components included as fiber. These are two additional fiber fractions derived during the determination of cellulose, hemicellulose, and lignin. Figure 16.1 presents a schematic outline of the Van Soest method for fiber analysis and how NDF and ADF values fit into the scheme of fiber analysis and its definition.

There will continue to be some controversy regarding the definition of fiber, but for purposes of this discussion on fiber in swine nutrition, the sum of the following components will be considered as defining dietary fiber: NDF or ADF, cellulose, hemicellulose, and lignin.

CHEMICAL AND PHYSICAL PROPERTIES OF FIBER

This is no simple chemical description of fiber, since it consists of a variety of chemical constituents that vary widely depending on the origin of the fiber source. No attempt

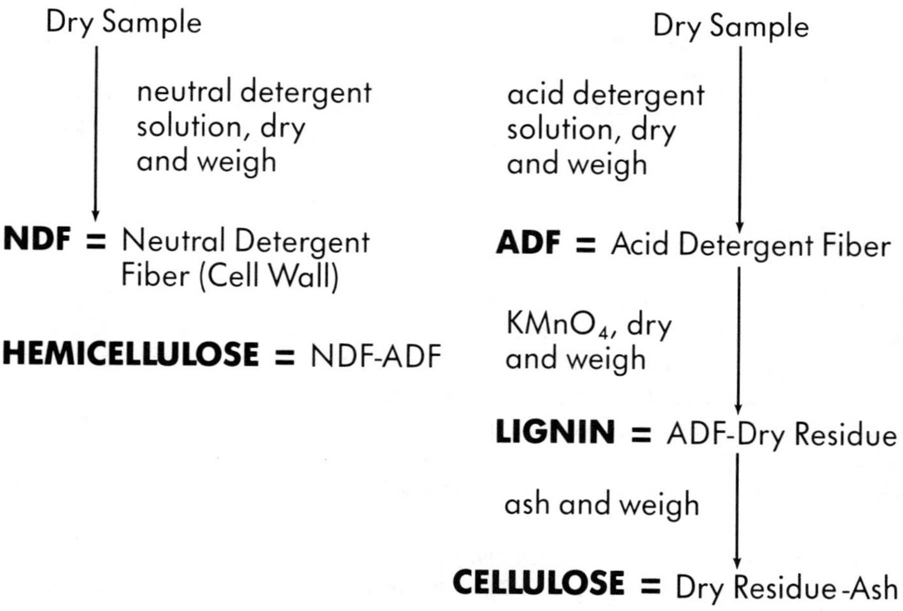

FIGURE 16.1 *Procedures for fiber analysis.*

is made in this chapter to discuss all the chemical constituents, but some of the general categorizations suggested by scientists active in the field of fiber chemistry are briefly considered.

According to Eastwood and Kay (1979) and Selvendran (1983), fiber constituents may be grouped into four major chemical categories: celluloses, hemicelluloses, pectins, and lignins. These four groups include most of the fiber components of major concern to animal scientists. Because of effects on animal health and performance, Jung and Fahey (1983) and Horwitz and Walker (1984) suggest that phenolic monomers and lignans should be added to the four categories.

Southgate (1978) has also suggested a chemical categorization that divides fiber constituents into two major groupings: (1) structural, including noncellulosic polysaccharides, cellulose, and lignins, and (2) nonstructural, including pectins, gums, algal polysaccharides, and modified celluloses. Southgate has included some xylans, mannans, and galactans, classified as noncellulosic polysaccharides, some sulfonated galactans from algal polysaccharides, and some cross-linked ethers and esters as modified celluloses. It does appear that the two categorizations are similar and that the differences between the two are more a matter of degree than of substance.

Physically, fiber varies according to the botanical origin of the plant or forage being used as a fiber source in the animal diet. Additionally, the stage of plant maturity, physical treatment of forage plants (i.e., drying, grinding, or pelleting), chemical treatment, including ensiling or addition of acid, bases, or organic chemicals, all contribute to the physical form of the fiber source and possibly the fiber components as well. The treatment of the fiber and fiber source is of considerable importance in the utilization of fibrous feeds for both ruminant and nonruminant livestock. Much of the evidence for the effects of physical form of fiber comes from work conducted with ruminants, and in some instances the effects would be similar for nonruminants. For example, Nuzback et al. (1984) demonstrated that the utilization of dry matter (DM), digestible energy (DE), cellulose, NDF, and ADF was greater in sows fed alfalfa meal with a particle size of 6.25 mm when compared with sows fed 12.5-mm meal. In general, a similar effect occurs in ruminants except that particles may become so small as to pass out of the rumen before they can be digested by rumen bacteria. Smaller particle size also improved utilization of fiber and fiber components in growing pigs fed oats (Crampton and Bell 1946), barley (Lawrence 1970), and sorghum (Owsley et al. 1981). Nuzback et al. (1984) also reported that cellulose digestibility in sows was improved by pelleting diets containing alfalfa meal, but that other fiber component digestibility was unaffected.

There is considerable practical evidence that ensiled plant materials, especially corn and alfalfa, may be fed and successfully utilized by gestating, but not lactating, sows. For more detail Cunha (1977) and Emsminger and Olentine (1980) should be consulted. The other physical changes produced by chemical treatment or grinding and chopping have not been specifically studied with swine, but the evidence that these factors may affect utilization of fibrous feeds has been well documented in ruminants. Barring evidence to the contrary, there is no reason not to believe that they may influence fiber digestion as well as other nutrient utilization in swine.

METHODS FOR ANALYSIS OF FIBER AND FIBER COMPONENTS

Currently there are three general methods used for determining the fiber and fiber component composition of food and feedstuffs: (1) the Weende, or so-called "crude fiber" method, (2) the detergent method, and (3) the enzyme-insoluble procedures. These analytical procedures are particularly important because each one defines a different end-product, making the comparison of experiments using different analytical procedures very difficult. For example, it would be difficult to compare a study in which the crude fiber method was used to define fiber with one in which a variety of fiber components were determined by detergent analytical procedures. There are no common ingredients defined by the two different procedures. For more detail on methodology than can be provided here, the reviews of Southgate (1969, 1978), Monte and Vaughan (1982), Asp and Johansson (1984), and Moore (1986) should be consulted.

The mainstay of fiber analysis has been the "crude fiber" method. This method involves digestion of a fiber-containing sample with acid followed sequentially with alkali. This treatment results in the isolation of an acid- and base-insulated residue composed almost exclusively of cellulose and lignin. This procedure is still used by some feed manufacturers and researchers who are dealing with samples or feedstuffs that contain relatively small quantities of soluble fiber components. With such samples, this method is quite useful as long as its limitations are recognized and taken into account.

In 1970, research on a method designed to extract fiber components in neutral or acid-detergent solutions by Van Soest and associates culminated in the publication of a report (Goering and Van Soest 1970) detailing the procedures of this new method of defining dietary fiber in feeds and food. The principal components determined by this method, as outlined in Figure 16.1, are widely used in estimating dietary fiber in both human and animal food and feed. The NDF residue, in many instances, is very similar to the crude fiber value in feedstuffs that contain low levels of soluble fiber components. The difference between NDF and ADF is used as an estimate of hemicellulose, and the ADF fraction after treatment with acid or permanganate is used to estimate cellulose and lignin. A criticism of this procedure is that it underestimates total fiber since pectins and other components are soluble in NDF and are not recoverable for an accurate determination. Another problem, residual starch encountered in high-grain diets, has been resolved by amylase digestion during the NDF extraction (Robertson and Van Soest 1977).

Hellendorn et al. (1975) described one of two enzyme methods for fiber analysis. This procedure involves sample digestion with pepsin-pancreatin and the separation of the insoluble residue remaining after digestion. A modification of this method was proposed by Furda (1981) in which ethanol was used to precipitate soluble polysaccharides. Total dietary fiber in this instance is enzyme-insoluble fiber plus fiber precipitated by ethanol. Prosky et al. (1985) have conducted two collaborative studies using a combination of enzymatic and gravimetric procedures, as described above, which has been adopted as an official first action by the Association of Official Analytical Chemists (AOAC). These methods result in some protein contamination, but Prosky et al. (1985)

utilize protease to alleviate some of this difficulty. These enzymatic methods estimate *total* fiber and do not give any estimation of amounts of any of the various components in fiber sources.

As is evident from the preceding discussion, the fiber source and target animal will dictate the analytical procedure used to formulate diets for humans or livestock or evaluate how well a particular animal species utilizes total fiber or specific fiber components. There is no "best" method of fiber analysis, there are just those methods that "best" fit a given set of circumstances in the conduct of a particular experiment or the preparation of food or feed for use in human or livestock diets.

UTILIZATION OF FIBER AND FIBER COMPONENTS

Fiber utilization in growing swine is dependent on level of fiber fed, source of fiber, stage of forage maturity, levels of other nutrients in the diet, and plane of nutrition (Forbes and Hamilton 1952; Teague and Hanson 1954; Keys et al. 1970; Farrell 1973; Keys and DeBarthe 1974a,b; Kass et al. 1980b). Most, if not all, fiber digestion occurs in the cecum and large intestine of swine and is a microbial fermentation process. Volatile fatty acids from fiber fermentation serve as an energy source for pigs and provide from 5% to 28% of the energy requirements of the growing pig (Friend et al. 1963; Farrell and Johnson 1972; Imoto and Namioka 1978a,b; Kass et al. 1980a).

For purposes of the following discussion, "utilization" will be defined as the conversion of fiber by growing pigs and gestating and lactating sows into

1. growth, as expressed by increases in body weight in pigs;
2. weight gain in pregnant sows;
3. body weight changes in lactating sows;
4. reproductive performance as measured by number of pigs farrowed, newborn mortality, birth weight, and number and weight of pigs weaned.

Growing Pigs

As stated by Kass et al. (1980a), the general view regarding growing pigs is that fiber, in excess of 7% to 10% of the diet, has an inhibitory effect on growth. This has been amply demonstrated by a number of researchers, including Whatley et al. (1951), Axelsson and Ericksson (1953), Coey and Robinson (1954), Crampton et al. (1954), Teague and Hanson (1954), Bohman et al. (1955), Merkel et al. (1958), Jensen et al. (1959), Hochstetler et al. (1959), and Pond et al. (1962). The extent of the growth-depressing effect may vary according to the fiber source. According to Hochstetler et al. (1959), dietary wheat bran and alfalfa inhibited growth in pigs but oats did not. Crampton et al. (1954) reported that wheat bran at 25% of the diet did not affect growth rate but a mixture of 12.5% each of alfalfa or oats or wheat bran did decrease weight gain.

Energy dilution is one ready explanation of the effect of fiber on pig growth. Jensen et al. (1959) confirmed that dietary corn oil reversed the effect of feeding oat hulls, and when DE intakes were held constant, corn cobs, wheat bran, alfalfa, cellulose, or oat hulls did not decrease weight gain in pigs (Troelson and Bell 1962). Similarly, Baird et al. (1970) demonstrated that if metabolizable energy (ME) intakes did not decrease, rice mill feed, wheat bran, or cottonseed hulls did not reduce rate of gain in pigs. Other research that demonstrates the effect of energy dilution by fiber and the inability of the growing pig to consume enough of high-fiber diets to overcome the effect of energy dilution has been reported by Kornegay (1978 and 1981) with soybean hulls, Powley et al. (1981) with incremental amounts of alfalfa meal, Drewry (1981) with wheat bran, oats, and alfalfa, and Moser et al. (1982a) with solka floc.

Other reasons for decreasing growth rates in pigs fed high-fiber diets include fiber-mineral interactions, decreased nitrogen and energy utilization, and increased ingesta rate of passage. These factors have effects other than that of decreasing growth rate in pigs and for that reason will be considered later in this chapter.

Sows

Experiments with fiber diets in sow nutrition have dealt primarily with the effect of a variety of fiber sources on reproductive performance traits. These reports indicate few adverse effects of fiber on sow performance parameters including pigs farrowed, birth weight, mortality, and farrowing weight (Cunha et al. 1944; Teague 1955; Seerley and Wahlstrom 1965; Danielson and Noonan 1975; Pollmann et al. 1979, 1981; Kornegay 1981).

In experiments on digestibility of fiber components and other nutrients in sows fed high-fiber diets, Pollman et al. (1979) reported that as fiber content of sow diets increased, fiber, energy, and nitrogen digestibilities decreased. Kornegay (1981) found, however, that when feeding soybean hulls to sows, digestion coefficients for DM, energy, and crude protein increased with increasing levels of fiber, but NDF, ADF, cellulose, and lignin coefficients declined. Nuzback et al. (1984) reported that smaller particle size increased fiber utilization but pelleting had no effect over that of the smaller particle size. Calvert et al. (1985) confirmed the observations of Pollman et al. (1979) and Nuzback et al. (1984) with respect to fiber component digestibility, but also observed that DM, fiber component, energy, and protein digestibility decreased markedly during the last 3 weeks of gestation. Table 16.1 illustrates these effects. These observations have been confirmed by Bray et al. (1987) in sows fed diets containing 50% soybean hulls. This work also showed that DE content of soybean hulls was lower in sows near the end of gestation (100 days). Danielson and Noonan (1975), Pollman et al. (1979), and Calvert et al. (1985) reported that sow weight gain during gestation was reduced in sows fed higher levels of fiber from alfalfa. Reproductive performance as measured by numbers of live pigs farrowed and birth weight was unaffected. Danielson and Noonan (1975) and Calvert et al. (1985) fed sows 95% alfalfa diets during gestation and observed no effects on reproductive performance. In fact, Danielson's experiments extended over three parities with no adverse effects, but he

Table 16.1 Effect of Level of Dietary Alfalfa and Stage of Gestation on Digestibility of Dry Matter, Ash, Fiber Components, Energy, and Protein in Sows

		Diet			
Item (%)	*Days Gestation*	*5% Alfalfa*	*50% Alfalfa*	*95% Alfalfa*	*SE*[c]
Dry matter[a,b]	60	90.4	73.1	59.9	
	100	88.1	67.8	44.7	2.0
Ash[b]	60	52.4	54.2	53.3	
	100	43.6	48.2	39.9	3.0
Neutral detergent fiber[a,b]	60	65.9	44.8	44.0	
	100	60.5	33.9	21.2	3.8
Acid detergent fiber[a,b]	60	59.5	37.3	40.9	
	100	57.0	27.5	18.8	4.2
Hemicellulose[a,b]	60	70.5	57.8	52.6	
	100	63.0	45.0	27.8	3.4
Cellulose[a,b]	60	66.5	44.5	46.4	
	100	63.4	36.0	27.1	3.9
Digestible energy[a,b]	60	92.1	74.7	61.1	
	100	89.8	68.3	44.4	2.0
Digestible protein[a,b]	60	90.8	72.0	63.3	
	100	87.4	65.9	51.6	1.9

[a] Significant diet effect ($P < .05$).
[b] Significant day of gestation effect ($P < .05$).
[c] Pooled SE.
(Adapted, by permission, from Calvert et al. 1985 and Calvert and Steele 1985.)

did not feed alfalfa during the 42-day lactations. Calvert's study showed that when high levels of fiber (95% alfalfa meal) were fed during lactation, weaning weight of sows and pigs was markedly reduced.

In summary, pig growth is reduced or unaffected by fiber additions to the diet. Inclusion of no more than 5% of most common fiber sources would probably have little or no effect on growing pig performance. Both level of fiber and source are factors in determining the ultimate effect on growing pig performance. The evidence suggests that level of fiber has a greater effect on pig growth than does source when common sources such as alfalfa, soybean hulls, oats, and wheat bran are considered. In sows, tolerance of fiber levels from a number of sources is much greater. In some instances, sows have been maintained, without adverse effect on reproductive performance, on all-forage diets even though there were reductions in digestibiity of fiber, energy, and protein. Swine producers are more concerned with decreasing weight gain in sows, and overall performance of sows may be improved by the inclusion of moderate levels of dietary fiber. High-quality silages and forages like alfalfa, soybean hulls, and grass hays may be important ingredients in diets of gestating sows in many parts of the United States, but it is unlikely that dietary fiber will play any positive role during lactation. Dilution of energy intake during lactation has too much of a negative impact during this stage of the reproductive cycle to allow any more than a very low level of fiber in the diet of the lactating sow.

FIBER AND MINERAL UTILIZATION

Because high-fiber diets do not support maximum productivity in growing pigs, there has been relatively little research effort on the influence of fiber on mineral and trace metal utilization in this nonruminant species. In general, as reported by Partridge (1978a,b), Moser et al. (1982a,b), Ravindran et al. (1984), Newton et al. (1983), Dintzis and Watson (1985), and Lindemann et al. (1986), the effects that have been observed are quite varied and present a somewhat confused picture. To avoid a rather lengthy discussion of the various observations, it may be said that dietary mineral level, dietary fiber levels, fiber source, fiber processing, and mineral source probably contribute to the observed effect of fiber on dietary mineral utilization. Whether the effects of fiber on mineral utilization can account for part of the reduced performance in growing pigs has not been determined.

Mature swine, unlike the growing pig, can utilize high levels of fiber. The gestating sow can be fed as much as 95% alfalfa without affecting reproductive performance, but mineral balance and retention have not been extensively investigated. Holtzgraefe et al. (1985) reported that calcium, phosphorus, magnesium, sodium, and potassium metabolism in gestating sows, as measured by percent retention at 40 and 80 days of gestation, were not affected when sows were fed alfalfa-orchardgrass hay diets containing 37% to 40% NDF. There was a significant day of gestation effect on sodium retention in that sodium retention increased at 80 days of gestation. As shown by Calvert and Steele (1985) in Table 16.2, there was a decrease ($P < .05$) in calcium, phosphorus, and copper balance from 60 to 100 days gestation but there was no overall effect on mineral balance as level of dietary fiber increased. Since there were no

Table 16.2 Effect of Level of Dietary Alfalfa and Stage of Gestation on Calcium, Phosphorus, and Copper Balance in Sows

		Diet		
Item	*Days Gestation*	*5% Alfalfa*	*50% Alfalfa*	*95% Alfalfa*
Calcium balance (g/d)[a]	60	5.0	3.8	6.8
	100	1.8	3.4	0.9
Phosphorus balance (g/d)[b]	60	3.2	3.8	4.6
	100	1.0	3.8	0.5
Copper balance (mg/d)[b]	60	8.3	7.3	7.3
	100	3.9	0.5	−3.4

[a]Diet difference ($P < .05$).
[b]Day of gestation difference ($P < .05$).
(Reprinted, by permission, from Calvert and Steele 1985.)

adverse effects of diet on reproductive performance, it would appear that the observed effects on mineral utilization were of little consequence in this study.

Fiber content of the diet has variable effects on any number of minerals or trace metals in the diets of growing pigs or gestating sows. The mechanisms responsible for the effects of fiber on mineral utilization may result from mechanical or physical movement of minerals or mineral sources more rapidly through the digestive system, or physical or chemical absorption or adsorption of minerals on fiber components. Conventional thinking would suggest that the effect would be a decrease in mineral utilization as a result of quick transit of nutrients through the digestive system. It is also possible that some adhering minerals could be retained longer with a delayed release after bacterial or chemical degradation, resulting in an increase in mineral balance and retention. If there is any trend, the results in the literature would suggest that higher levels of dietary fiber have a negative effect on mineral balance, but the variables listed above must be considered before any definitive conclusions can be drawn.

FIBER AND RATE OF DIGESTA PASSAGE

As a general rule, in nonruminant animals, the inclusion of fiber in the diet increases the rate of food passage through the digestive system. Eastwood and Kay (1979) suggest that increasing feed passage most likely accounts for the decrease in feed utilization observed in monogastric animals fed high-fiber diets. Source and level of fiber must also be considered when the effects of fiber on rate of passage are being evaluated (Stanogias and Pearce 1985). Soybean hulls and wheat bran did not affect rate of passage when fed at levels from 7% to 15%, but feed transit time increased when pigs were fed these fiber sources at dietary levels of 22% to 30%. With less degradable fibrous materials such as ground corn cobs and alfalfa stems, digesta passage increased as a level of intake increased. As different sources of fiber, easily degraded versus less easily degraded, pass through the digestive tract, there may be differential retention accounting for differences in rates of passage. Coarse fiber particles (Ehle et al. 1982) may be retained in the cecum longer than more finely ground particles of the same fiber source. Conflicting results were reported by Farrell and Johnson (1972) and DeBarthe and Kane (1980) in studies that suggested that finely ground cellulose (wood pulp) was retained in the cecum or large intestine and reduced digesta passage time. Moore (1986) points out that either meal feeding or restricted feeding techniques may affect fiber utilization and feed passage. It is very possible that rate of passage and utilization of fibrous material is different in pigs fed the same feedstuff ad libitum or as a once-a-day meal. This specific experiment has not been conducted, but these factors must be taken into account when comparing the effects of fiber sources in different experiments. This would also be true when comparing effects of fiber on feed passage between sows (meal-fed) and growing pigs (ad libitum-fed).

Other references that discuss rate of passage in pigs and other nonruminants that were not referred to above are as follows: Castle and Castle (1956, 1957); Seerely et al. (1962); Kass et al. (1980a); Fioramonti and Bueno (1980); Low et al. (1985); Alimon and Farrell (1980); Darcy et al. (1980); Fleming and Lee (1983); Bell (1960); and Lindemann et al. (1986).

The general effect of high levels of fiber in the diet of growing pigs and sows is to increase the rate at which feed passes through the digestive tract. A number of qualifications to that general statement have been discussed, and these must be considered when evaluating the potential effects of various fiber constituents and fiber sources. A thorough review of the suggested references is recommended for anyone seriously interested in the effects of fiber on rate of digesta passage.

SUMMARY

There is an incentive to include fibrous feed ingredients in both growing pig and gestating sow diets. The incentives to use fiber include the value of certain fiber sources or fiber components as energy sources after fermentation in the cecum and large intestine, the use of nondegradable fiber as a dilutent in gestating sow diets, the use of certain fibrous feeds such as alfalfa meal as a protein source, and the opportunity for a feed manufacturer or swine producer to use a variety of alternate feed resources to reduce feed costs. There are also some disincentives for the use of fiber in feeds that often preclude their use in diets during certain phases of swine production. There is no question that as levels of fiber increase in the diets of growing pigs the utilization of a variety of nutrients decreases, resulting in either a reduction in overall performance of the pig or a compensation mechanism in which the animal consumes more feed in order to maintain performance. Since feed and energy intake are crucial during lactation, dilution of feed with fiber sources is not advisable because baby pig performance and sow weight gain are adversely affected. Mineral balance may also be affected in growing pigs and sows, but whether this adversely affects performance is not absolutely clear. In almost all instances, adverse effects on performance occur when fiber is fed at levels above 7% to 10% of the diet, but it is unlikely that adverse effects will occur when any fiber source is fed at levels below 5% of the diet. When fiber sources are used in moderation, the positive incentives outweigh the negative aspects observed with the use of higher levels of fibrous feedstuffs.

REFERENCES

Alimon, A.R., and D.J. Farrell. 1980. *Aust. J. Agric. Res.* 31:615.
Asp, N.G., and C.G. Johansson. 1984. *Nutr. Abst. Rev.* 54A:736.
Axlesson, J., and S. Ericksson. 1953. *J. Anim. Sci.* 12:881.
Baird, D.M., H.C. McCampbell, and J.R. Allison. 1970. *J. Anim. Sci.* 31:518.
Bell, J.M. 1960. *Can. J. Anim. Sci.* 40:71.
Bohman, V.R., J.E. Hunter, and J.A. McCormick. 1955. *J. Anim. Sci.* 14:499.
Bray, R.E., J.V. DeBarthe, and C.C. Calvert. 1987. *J. Anim. Sci.* 65(Suppl. 1):310.
Calvert, C.C., and N.C. Steele. 1985. *J. Anim. Sci.* 61(Suppl. 1):305.
Calvert, C.C., N.C. Steele, and R.W. Rosebrough. 1985. *J. Anim. Sci.* 61:595.
Castle, E.J., and M.E. Castle. 1956. *J. Agric. Sci. (Camb.)* 47:196.
Castle, E.J., and M.E. Castle. 1957. *J. Agric. Sci. (Camb.)* 49:106.
Coey W.E., and K.L. Robinson. 1954. *J. Agric. Sci. (Camb.)* 45:41.
Crampton, E.W., and J.M. Bell. 1946. *J. Anim. Sci.* 5:200.

Crampton, E.W., G.C. Ashton, and L.E. Lloyd. 1954. *J. Anim. Sci.* 13:327.
Cranwell, P.D. 1968. *Nutr. Abstr. Rev.* 38:721.
Cummings, J. 1981. *Br. Med. Bull.* 37:65.
Cunha, T.J. 1977. *Swine Feeding and Nutrition.* New York: Academic Press.
Cunha, T.J., et al. 1944. *J. Anim. Sci.* 3:415.
Danielson, D.M., and J.J. Noonan. 1975. *J. Anim. Sci.* 41:94.
Darcy, B., J.P. Laplace, and P.A. Villiers. 1980. *Ann. Zootechnie.* 29:147.
DeBarthe, J.V., and J.D.H. Kane, III. 1980. *Proceedings of Maryland Nutrition Conference.* p. 31. College Park: University of Maryland.
Dintzis, F.R., and P.R. Watson. 1984. *J. Agric. Food Chem.* 32:1331.
Drewry, K.J. 1981. *J. Anim. Sci.* 52:197.
Eastwood, M.A., and R.M. Kay. 1979. *Am. J. Clin. Nutr.* 32:364.
Ehle, F.R., et al. 1982. *J. Anim. Sci.* 55:1071.
Ensminger, M.E., and C.G. Olentine. 1980. *Feeds and Nutrition—Complete.* Clovis, CA: Ensminger Publishing Co.
Farrell, D.J. 1973. *Anim. Prod.* 16:43.
Farrell, D.J., and K.A. Johnson. 1972. *Anim. Prod.* 14:209.
Fioramonti, J., and L. Bueno. 1980. *Br. J. Nutr.* 43:155.
Fleming, S.E., and B. Lee. 1983. *J. Nutr.* 113:592.
Forbes, R.M., and T.S. Hamilton. 1952. *J. Anim. Sci.* 11:480.
Friend, D.W., H.M. Cunningham, and J.W.G. Nicholson. 1963. *Can. J. Anim. Sci.* 43:156.
Furda, I. 1981. In: *The Analysis of Dietary Fiber in Food.* James, W.P.T., and O. Theander (Eds.). pp. 163–172. New York: Marcel Dekker.
Goering, H.K., and P.J. Van Soest. 1970. *Agric. Handbook No. 379.* Washington, DC: ARS, United States Department of Agriculture.
Hellendoorn, E.W., M.G. Noordhoff, and J. Slagman. 1975. *J. Sci. Food Agric.* 26:1461.
Hochstetler, L.N., et al. 1959. *J. Anim. Sci.* 18:1397.
Holzgraefe, D.P., et al. 1985. *J. Anim. Sci.* 60:1247.
Horwitz, C., and A.R.P. Walker. 1984. *Nutr. Cancer* 6:73.
Imoto, S., and S. Namioka. 1978a. *J. Anim. Sci.* 47:467.
Imoto, S., and S. Namioka. 1978b. *J. Anim. Sci.* 47:479.
Jensen, A.H., D.E. Becker, and S.W. Terrill. 1959. *J. Anim. Sci.* 18:1356.
Jung, H.G., and G.C. Fahey, Jr. 1983. *J. Anim. Sci.* 57:206.
Kass, M.L., P.J. Van Soest, and W.G. Pond. 1980a. *J. Anim. Sci.* 50:192.
Kass, M.L., et al. 1980b. *J. Anim. Sci.* 50:175.
Keys, J.E., Jr., and J.V. DeBarthe. 1974a. *J. Anim. Sci.* 39:53.
Keys, J.E., Jr., and J.V. DeBarthe. 1974b. *J. Anim. Sci.* 39:57.
Keys, J.E., Jr., P.J. Van Soest, and E.P. Young. 1970. *J. Anim. Sci.* 31:1172.
Kornegay, E.T. 1978. *J. Anim. Sci.* 47:1272.
Kornegay, E.T. 1981. *J. Anim. Sci.* 53:138.
Lawrence, T.L.J. 1970. *Anim. Prod.* 12:139.
Lindemann, M.D., E.T. Kornegay, and R.J. Moore. 1986. *J. Anim. Sci.* 62:412.
Low, A.G., R.L. Pittman, and R.J. Elliott. 1985. *Br. J. Nutr.* 54:437.
Merkel, R.A., et al. 1958. *J. Anim. Sci.* 17:3.
Monte, W.C., and L.A. Vaughan. 1982. *J. Appl. Nutr.* 34:46.
Moore, J.M. 1986. "The Effect of High-Fiber Diets on Nutrient Utilization and Intestinal Morphology of Growing Pigs." Ph.D. diss., Virginia Polytechnic Institute and State University, Blacksburg.
Moser, R.L., et al. 1982a. *J. Anim. Sci.* 54:800.
Moser, R.L., et al. 1982b. *J. Anim. Sci.* 54:1181.
Newton, G.L., O.M. Hale, and C.O. Plank. 1983. *Can J. Anim. Sci.* 63:399.
Nuzback, L.J., D.S. Pollmann, and K.C. Behnke. 1984. *J. Anim. Sci.* 58:378.
Owsley, W.F., D.A. Knabe, and T.D. Tanksley, Jr. 1981. *J. Anim. Sci.* 52:557.
Partridge, I.G. 1978a. *Br. J. Nutr.* 39:527.

Patridge, I.G. 1978b. *Br. J. Nutr.* 39:539.
Pollmann, D.S., D.M. Danielson, and E.R. Peo, Jr. 1979. *J. Anim. Sci.* 48:1385.
Pollmann, D.S., et al. 1981. *J. Anim. Sci.* 51:295.
Pond, W.G., R.S. Lowrey, and J.H. Maner. 1962. *J. Anim. Sci.* 21:692.
Powley, J.S., et al. 1981. *J. Anim. Sci.* 53:308.
Prosky, L., et al. 1985. *J. Assoc. Off. Anal. Chem.* 68:677.
Ravindran, V., E.T. Kornegay, and K.E. Webb, Jr. 1984. *J. Anim. Sci.* 59:400.
Rerat, A. 1978. *J. Anim. Sci.* 46:1808.
Robertson, J.B., and P.J. Van Soest. 1977. *J. Anim. Sci.* 44(Suppl. 1):254.
Scheunert, A. 1906. Hoppe Seylers Ztschr. 48:9. Cited by P.D. Cranwell. 1968. *Nutr. Abstr. Rev.* 38:721.
Seerley, R.W., and R.C. Wahlstrom. 1965. *J. Anim. Sci.* 24:448.
Seerley, R.W., E.R. Miller, and J.A. Hoefer. 1962. *J. Anim. Sci.* 21:834.
Selvendran, R.R. 1983. In: *Dietary Fibre.* Birch, G.G., and K.J. Parker (Eds.). pp. 95–148. London: Applied Science Publishers.
Southgate, D.A.T. 1969. *J. Sci. Food Agric.* 20:331.
Southgate, D.A.T. 1978. *J. Plant Foods* 3:9.
Stanogias, G., and G.R. Pearce. 1985. *Br. J. Nutr.* 53:513.
Teague, H.S. 1955. *J. Anim. Sci.* 14:621.
Teague, H.S., and L.E. Hanson. 1954. *J. Anim. Sci.* 13:206.
Trautman, A., and T. Asher. 1941. Tierernahrung. 13:545. Cited by P.D. Cranwell. 1968. *Nutr. Abst. Rev.* 38:721.
Troelsen, J.E., and J.M. Bell. 1962. *Can. J. Anim. Sci.* 42:63.
Trowell, H. 1972. *Am. J. Clin. Nutr.* 25:926.
Varel, V.H. 1987. *J. Anim. Sci.* 65:488.
Whatley, J.A., et al. 1951. *J. Anim. Sci.* 10:1031 (Abstr.)

Chapter 17

Antimicrobial Agents

G.L. Cromwell

Antimicrobial agents are compounds that, at low concentrations, suppress or inhibit the growth of microorganisms. This class of compounds includes the antibiotics (naturally occurring substances produced by yeasts, molds, and other mircoorganisms) and the chemotherapeutics (substances that are chemically synthesized). In addition, the mineral element copper has antibacterial properties when present in high concentrations.

Antimicrobial agents have been used widely as feed additives for swine since the early 1950s. They are used at low (subtherapeutic) levels in feed for growth promotion, improvement of feed utilization, reduction of mortality, and improvement of reproductive efficiency. Approximately 88% of the total use of antibiotics is for subtherapeutic usage (IOM 1988). Antibacterial agents also are used at moderate-to-high (prophylaxis) levels for the prevention of disease in exposed animals and at high (therapeutic) levels for the treatment of certain swine diseases.

The discovery of the growth-stimulating effects associated with the feeding of antibiotics was made in the late 1940s as a result of research involving vitamin B_{12}. Stokstad et al. (1949) fed the fermentation products of the microorganism *Streptomyces aureofaciens* to chicks to assay the amount of vitamin B_{12} and found that the growth rate of the chicks was more than could be accounted for on the basis of the vitamin content. Similar growth responses from fermentation media were subsequently demonstrated in studies with pigs (Cunha et al. 1949, 1950; Jukes et al. 1950; Lepley et al. 1950; Luecke et al. 1950). Stokstad and Jukes identified the agent in the original fermentation media as the antibiotic chlortetracycline.

Soon after the benefits of antibiotics were discovered, swine producers readily accepted them as an integral part of their feeding programs. By 1963, approximately 1 million kg of antibiotics were being used annually in animal feeds (Figure 17.1). In 1988, approximately 13 million kg of antibiotics and chemotherapeutics were produced and 4.65 million kg were sold in the United States, and about one half of these amounts were for feed additive use (U.S. International Trade Commission 1989).

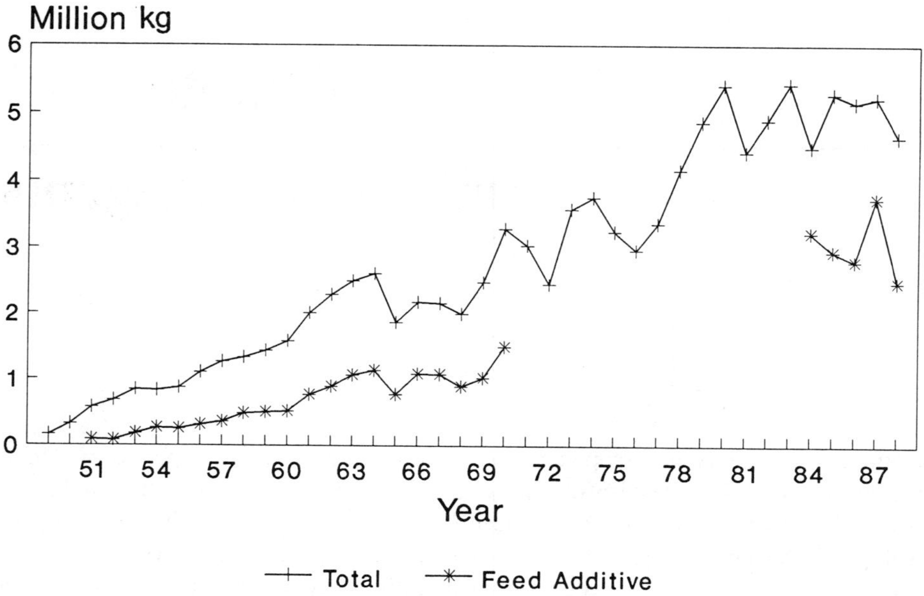

FIGURE 17.1 *Sales of antibiotics for medicinal and nonmedicinal (feed additive) usage in the United States from 1949 to 1988. (Data from United States Tarriff Commission Reports, 1950–1957; United States International Trade Commission Reports, 1958–1989).*

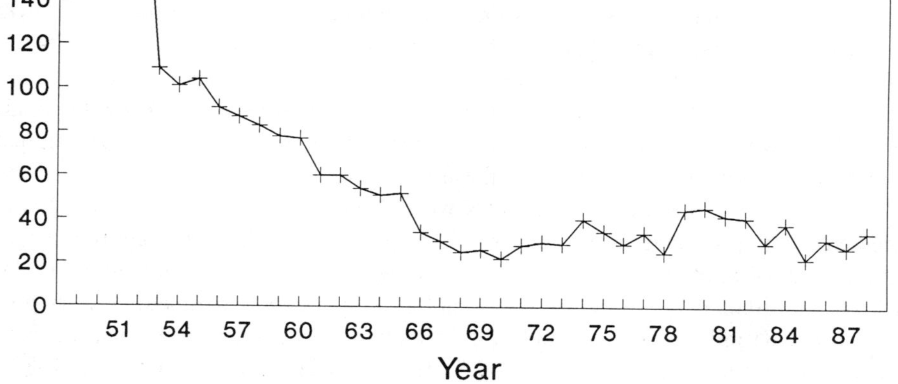

FIGURE 17.2 *Average price of antibiotics for nonmedicinal (feed additive) usage from 1951 to 1988. (Data from United States Tarriff Commission Reports, 1950–1957; United States International Trade Commission Reports, 1958–1989).*

Approximately 85% to 95% of all pig starter feeds, 75% to 80% of all grower feeds, 55% to 60% of finisher feeds, and 20% to 30% of sow feeds contain antimicrobial agents.

In the early years following the discovery of antibiotics, the average cost of feed-grade antibiotics was $200 to $220 per kg (Figure 17.2). By the mid 1960s, the average cost of antibiotics decreased to one tenth of the initial cost, and their cost has remained between $20 and $40 per kg during the 1970s and 1980s.

Currently, 21 antimicrobial agents (13 antibiotics, 8 chemotherapeutics) are cleared by the Food and Drug Administration (FDA) for use in swine feeds, and these are listed in Table 17.1 (Feed Additive Compendium 1990). Certain of these antimicrobial agents are cleared for combination usage (e.g., chlortetracycline-sulfamethazine-penicillin, neomycin-oxytetracycline), while others cannot be used in combination with other drugs. Several other antibiotics (avilamycin, efrotomycin, salinomycin, nosiheptide, and thiopeptin) appear to have potential as growth promoters (Cromwell 1987), but as yet these have not been approved by the FDA for use in swine feeds.

The antimicrobials that are effective in improving performance in pigs have one thing in common: their ability to suppress or inhibit the growth of certain microorganisms. The chemical composition and bacterial spectrum of the antimicrobials vary widely. Some are readily absorbed (e.g., tetracyclines, sulfonamides), while others are largely nonabsorbed (e.g., bacitracin, bambermycins). Some are excreted more rapidly than others (e.g., sulfathiazole versus sulfamethazine). While chemical composition, bacterial spectrum, and absorption-excretion patterns influence the bactericidal and bacteriostatic properties and effectiveness against specific systemic pathogens, these characteristics are less readily associated with the ability of a given antimicrobial agent to stimulate growth.

Table 17.1 Antimicrobial Agents Approved for Swine

Antibiotics	*Chemotherapeutics*
Apramycin	Arsanilic acid
Bacitracin zinc	Carbadox
Bacitracin methylene disalicylate	Furazolidone
Bambermycins	Nitrofurazone
Chlortetracycline	Roxarsone
Lincomycin	Sodium arsanilate
Neomycin	Sulfamethazine
Oxytetracycline	Sulfathiazole
Penicillin	
Streptomycin	
Tiamulin	
Tylosin	
Virginiamycin	

(Adapted, by permission, from Feed Additive Compendium 1990.)

ANTIMICROBIALS AS GROWTH PROMOTERS

The efficacy of antibiotics in improving the rate and efficiency of growth in pigs is well documented in numerous research studies (Hays 1977; CAST 1981; Zimmerman 1986; Cromwell and Dawson 1990). Table 17.2 summarizes data from 1194 experiments conducted in the United States from 1950 to 1985. In studies involving young pigs from 7 to 25 kg, antibiotics improved growth rate by an average of 16.4% and reduced the amount of feed required per unit of gain by 6.9%. In studies with slightly heavier pigs (from 17 to 49 kg), antibiotics improved growth rate by 10.6% and feed efficiency by 4.5%. Over the entire growing-finishing period (from 24 to 89 kg), growth rate was improved by 4.2% and feed efficiency by 2.2% when antibiotics were fed.

Even though some antibiotics have now been used for nearly four decades, they still are as effective as they were in the early years following their discovery. A comparison of data from the first 28 years of antibiotic usage (1950 to 1977) and for the subsequent 8 years (1978 to 1985) indicates that the overall effectiveness of antibiotics has not diminished (Table 17.3).

The benefits from antibiotics, such as those listed in Tables 17.2 and 17.3, are derived mostly from controlled experiments conducted at universities and other research stations. Antibiotics are likely even more beneficial when used at the farm level. The data listed in Table 17.4 indicate that responses to antibiotics under farm conditions may be twice as great as those occurring in a research station environment, where the facilities are generally cleaner, the disease load is less, and the environment is less stressful.

Since most of the data in Tables 17.2 and 17.3 are based primarily on experiment station studies, the relative benefits from subtherapeutic usage of antibiotics are probably underestimated. In actuality, antibiotics may improve growth rate at the farm level by as much as 25% to 30% and feed efficiency by 12% to 15% in weanling pigs. In growing-finishing pigs, improvements in rate and efficiency of gain may be improved by as much as 8% to 10% and by 4% to 5%, respectively, when antibiotics are included in the feed.

In addition to growth enhancement, the use of antibiotics in swine feeds has been found to reduce mortality and morbidity, particularly in young pigs. A summary of 67 field trials conducted over a 22-year period indicates that antibiotics reduced mortality by one half (4.3% to 2.0%) in young pigs (Table 17.5). The reduction in mortality was even greater under high-disease conditions and environmental stress (15.6% versus 3.1%; Table 17.5).

Although not generally classified as an antimicrobial, the mineral element copper has antibacterial properties when present at high concentrations. The initial reports on improved pig performance resulting from high dietary copper were by Evvard et al. (1928) at Iowa State University and Braude (1945) in England. Table 17.6 illustrates that the responses in growth rate and efficiency of feed utilization to high dietary copper (250 ppm) are similar in magnitude to those resulting from antibiotic feeding. Also, the responses to copper and antibiotics appear to be additive in the young pig (Table 17.7).

Table 17.2 Efficacy of Antibiotics as Growth Promoters for Pigs

Stage	*Control*	*Antibiotic*	*Improvement (%)*
Starter phase (7–25 kg)			
Daily gain (kg)	0.39	0.45	16.4
Feed/gain	2.28	2.13	6.9
Growing phase (17–49 kg)			
Daily gain (kg)	0.59	0.66	10.6
Feed/gain	2.91	2.78	4.5
Growing-finishing phase (24–89 kg)			
Daily gain (kg)	0.69	0.72	4.2
Feed/gain	3.30	3.23	2.2

(Data from 453, 298, and 443 experiments, involving 13,632, 5783, and 13,140 pigs for the three phases, respectively. Adapted, by permission, from Hays 1977 and Zimmerman 1986.)

Table 17.3 Efficacy of Antibiotics from 1950 to 1977 and from 1978 to 1985

	1950–1977[a]	*1978–1985*[b]
Stage	*Improvement from Antibiotics (%)*	
Starter phase		
Daily gain	16.1	15.0
Feed/gain	6.9	6.5
Growing-finishing phase		
Daily gain	4.0	3.6
Feed/gain	2.1	2.4

[a] Data from 378 and 279 experiments, involving 10,023 and 5666 pigs for the two phases, respectively; Hays 1977.

[b] Data from 75 and 164 experiments, involving 3609 and 7474 pigs for the two phases, respectively; Zimmerman 1986.

Table 17.4 Efficacy of Antibiotics in Research Station (University) Tests Versus Farm Tests

		Improvement from Antibiotics (%)	
Location	*No. of Trials*	*Daily Gain*	*Feed/Gain*
Summary 1[a]			
Research station tests	128	16.9	7.0
Farm tests	32	28.4	14.5
Summary 2[b]			
Research station tests	9	13.2	4.7
Farm tests	67	25.5	10.0

[a] Data on 12,000 pigs from 7 to 26 kg. Chlortetracycline-sulfamethazine-penicillin, tylosin-sulfamethazine, tetracycline, and carbadox; Hays 1977.

[b] Data on 3321 pigs from 8 to 20 kg. Chlortetracycline-sulfamethazine-penicillin, NCR-89 1984; H.M. Maddock, unpublished data, 1985.

Table 17.5 Effects of Antibiotics[a] on Performance and Mortality of Young Pigs in Commercial Field Tests

	Control	*Antibiotics*	*Improvement (%)*
Summary 1[b]			
Daily gain (kg)	0.31	0.40	26
Feed/gain	2.48	2.23	10
Mortality (%)	4.3	2.0	
Summary 2[c]			
Daily gain (kg)	0.30	0.38	26
Feed/gain	3.07	2.50	19
Mortality	15.6	3.1	

[a] Chlortetracycline-sulfamethazine-penicillin or tylosin-sulfamethazine.

[b] Sixty-seven field trials from 1960 to 1982, 1597 pigs.

[c] Five field trials under high disease level, 638 pigs, 8–31 kg.

(Data from H.M. Maddox [unpublished] 1985.)

Table 17.6 Effects of Copper Sulfate on Performance of Weanling and Growing-Finishing Pigs

	Added Copper (ppm)[a]		
Stage	*0*	*250*	*Improvement (%)*
Starting period (7–14 kg)[b]			
Daily gain (kg)	0.23	0.28	24.0
Feed/gain	2.04	1.86	9.7
Growing period (18–56 kg)[c]			
Daily gain (kg)	0.67	0.71	6.9
Feed/gain	2.80	2.70	3.6
Growing-finishing period (18–93 kg)[c]			
Daily gain (kg)	0.71	0.74	3.1
Feed/gain	3.18	3.10	2.5

[a] The 250 ppm level is in addition to the copper (6–12 ppm) in the trace mineral mix. Copper added as $CuSO_4 \cdot 5H_2O$.

[b] Summary of twelve, 28-day experiments with 462 pigs weaned at 28 days of age; forty-four replicates of four to eight pigs per treatment conducted at the University of Kentucky from 1978 to 1983.

[c] Summary of eighteen experiments; eighty-four replicates of four pigs per treatment conducted at the University of Kentucky from 1970 to 1980.

Responses to copper are influenced by feeding level of the mineral and by its chemical form. In weanling pigs, 250 ppm copper seems to be the most efficacious level; 100 to 125 ppm copper results in about 75% to 80% of the maximum response (Cromwell et al. 1989). The sulfate, carbonate, and chloride salts are efficacious forms of copper (Wallace 1967), but the oxide and sulfide salts are not (Cromwell 1983; Cromwell et al. 1989). High levels of copper (500 ppm) should be avoided because of the chances of copper toxicity in pigs, resulting from the marked accumulation of copper in the liver (Cromwell 1983).

Table 17.7 Effects of Single and Combined Additions of Antibiotics and Copper Sulfate on Performance of Weanling Pigs[a]

	Antibiotics			
	−	+	−	+
	Copper (250 ppm)			
	−	−	+	+
Daily gain (kg)	0.259	0.300	0.309	0.340
Daily feed (kg)	0.540	0.581	0.590	0.631
Feed/gain	2.10	1.95	1.91	1.84

[a]Summary of fourteen experiments involving 1700 pigs (7 to 18 kg) conducted at six stations.

(Data from Beames and Lloyd 1965; Mahan 1980; Stahly et al. 1980; Edmonds et al. 1985; Hagen et al. 1987; Burnell et al. 1988.)

ANTIMICROBIALS AND REPRODUCTIVE EFFICIENCY

Antibiotics are not as commonly used in diets for breeding animals as for growing pigs; however, they are quite effective when fed during certain critical stages of the reproductive cycle, such as at the time of breeding. A summary of nine studies involving 1931 sows shows that the feeding of a high level (0.5 to 1 g/sow daily) of an absorbable antibiotic at the time of breeding improves conception rate by about 7% and improves litter size by nearly one half pig at the subsequent farrowing (Table 17.8).

Table 17.8 Effects of Antimicrobial Agents in the Feed at Breeding on Reproductive Performance of Sows[a]

Researcher	Agent	No. of Sows	Farrowing Rate (%)[b] −[c]	Farrowing Rate (%)[b] +[c]	Live Pigs Born/Litter −[c]	Live Pigs Born/Litter +[c]
Dean and Tribble, 1962	OTC, CTC	59	—	—	7.1	9.7
Mayrose et al., 1964	Ty	192	93.8	91.7	11.0	11.3
Messersmith et al., 1966	CTC	377	68.5	82.9	9.8	10.0
Ruiz et al., 1968	ASP	96	87.5	95.8	9.0	10.3
Myers and Speer, 1973	CTC	249	66.9	75.4	9.9	10.3
Soma and Speer, 1975	CTC	239	70.8	72.3	10.2	10.5
Hays et al., 1978	ASP	182	60.9	70.0	9.8	10.0
Johnson et al., 1985	CTC	112	77.0	96.0	10.7	11.0
Maxwell et al., 1987	CTC	425	84.0	85.0	10.2	10.7
Total and average (weighted)		1931	75.4	82.1	10.0	10.4

Abbreviations: OTC, oxytetracycline; CTC, chlortetracycline, Ty, tylosin; ASP, combination of chlortetracycline, sulfamethazine, and penicillin.

[a]In most instances, antimicrobial agent fed at 0.5 to 1.0 g/day for 1 week before and 2 to 3 weeks after breeding.

[b]100 × (No. of sows that farrowed/no. of sows exposed to boar).

[c]Without (−) or with (+) antimicrobial agents in the feed at breeding.

Table 17.9 Effects of Antimicrobial Agents in the Prefarrowing and Lactation Diet on Reproductive Performance of Sows[a]

Researcher	*Agent*	*No. of Sows*	*Live Pigs Born/ Litter*		*No. of Pigs Weaned/ Litter*[c]		*Survival to Weaning (%)*[c]		*Weaning Weight (kg)*[c]	
			−[b]	+[b]	−[b]	+[b]	−[b]	+[b]	−[b]	+[b]
Sewell and Carmon, 1958	CTC	136	8.0	8.6	5.8	7.0	72.1	80.8	4.80	4.90
Wallace and Combs, 1962	Ty	88	10.1	10.4	8.8	9.0	87.1	86.7	3.41	3.53
Jordan and Waitt, 1963	Ty	291	—	—	—	—	93.6	98.0	5.03	4.92
Wallace and Combs, 1964	OTC,CTC	143	11.2	11.8	9.8	10.3	87.8	87.5	3.26	3.34
Mayrose et al., 1964	Ty	178	11.0	11.3	8.1	8.8	73.1	77.3	3.99	3.99
Wallace et al., 1966	Cu	50	12.0	12.1	10.0	10.3	83.7	85.4	3.28	3.39
Combs and Wallace, 1969	Bac	91	9.4	9.8	7.8	8.4	83.0	85.7	3.63	3.47
Wallace et al., 1974	ASP	149	10.6	11.0	9.3	9.4	88.0	85.3	3.80	3.75
Lillie and Frobish, 1978	Cu	32	8.6	8.5	6.7	7.0	78.4	82.2	4.61	4.94
Johnson et al., 1985	CTC, ASP	97	9.8	9.8	8.5	8.8	86.7	89.2	5.13	5.48
Maxwell et al., 1987	CTC	850	10.5	10.7	8.1	8.3	85.5	87.0	5.28	5.36
Total or average (weighted)		2105	10.3	10.6	8.2	8.6	84.9	87.1	4.65	4.70

Abbreviations: CTC, chlortetracycline; Ty, tylosin; OTC, oxytetracycline; Cu, copper sulfate; Bac, bacitracin zinc; ASP, combination of chlortetracycline, sulfamethazine, and penicillin.

[a] In most instances an antimicrobial agent was added at a high dietary level (110 to 275 mg/kg) from 3 to 7 days before farrowing and during a 14- to 21-day lactation period.

[b] Without (−) or with (+) antimicrobial agents in the prefarrowing and lactation diet.

[c] Weaning age was 21 days in the Sewell and Carmon (1958), Jordan and Waitt (1963), Lillie and Frobish (1978), and Johnson et al. (1985) studies and 14 days in all others.

Table 17.10 Effects of Long-Term Antibiotic Withdrawal in a Swine Herd on Reproductive Performance[a]

Item	*Antibiotics (1963–1972)*	*No Antibiotics (1972–1985)*
No. of litters	398	688
Conception rate (%)	91.4	82.6
No. of pigs born/litter	10.8	10.2
Live pigs born/litter	9.8	9.3
Avg. birth weight (kg)	1.29	1.38
No. of pigs weaned (21 d)	8.8	7.5
Avg. weaning weight (kg)	5.67	5.37
Survival of live born (%)	89.7	80.9
Incidence of MMA (%)	<10	66[b]

Abbreviation: MMA: mastitis, metritis, agalactia.

[a]Closed, specific-pathogen-free herd at the University of Kentucky. Antibiotics were used in breeding, lactation, starter, grower, and finisher diets from 1963 to 1972. Antibiotics were not used in the feed or for treatment purposes from 1972 to 1985.

[b]For the period 1972 to 1975 only.

Antibiotics also have been shown in some experiments to be beneficial at farrowing and during early lactation. In some instances, high levels of antibiotics in the sow feed have reduced the incidence of agalactia and uterine infections that occasionally occurs shortly after farrowing (Langlois et al. 1978a). The data in Table 17.9, based on eleven studies and 2105 litters, indicate a slight improvement in survival and weight gains of nursing pigs when antibiotics are included in the prefarrowing and lactation diet.

Long-term withdrawal of antibiotics from a swine herd has been shown to be associated with a reduction in reproductive performance (Table 17.10).

MODE OF ACTION OF ANTIMICROBIAL AGENTS

The mechanisms by which antibiotics and other antimicrobial agents stimulate growth in animals are not well understood. The proposed modes of action generally are grouped into three categories: (1) a metabolic effect, (2) a nutritional effect, and (3) a disease control effect (Hays 1978).

Metabolic Effect

This mode of action implies that antibiotics may have a direct influence on certain metabolic processes in the animal. Braude and Johnson (1953) demonstrated that chlortetracycline affected water and nitrogen excretion in pigs. Brody et al. (1954) reported that fatty acid oxidation in liver mitochondria was inhibited by tetracyclines. Weinberg

(1957) likewise showed, in bacteria, that phosphorylation and oxidation reactions requiring magnesium ions were inhibited by tetracyclines. Hash et al. (1964) demonstrated that protein synthesis was affected by tetracyclines. Similarly, results of studies by Moser et al. (1980) indicate that carbadox increases protein synthesis in pig muscle cells.

Although numerous studies have shown that antibiotics may have metabolic effects, the tissue levels of antibiotics that result from feeding subtherapeutic levels of antibiotics to pigs probably are not high enough to account for the growth-enhancing effects that occur when antibiotics are fed. Furthermore, a metabolic effect certainly does not explain the action of those antibiotics that are not absorbed from the gut.

Nutritional Effect

This proposed mechanism has a considerable amount of support. Certain microbes that inhabit the intestinal tract synthesize vitamins and amino acids that are essential to animals, while other microbes compete with the host animal for vitamins, amino acids, and other essential nutrients. Shifts in bacterial populations that are associated with the feeding of antibiotics could account for a greater availability of nutrients for the host animal.

Moore et al. (1946) found that streptomycin stimulated the growth of yeasts, and Anderson et al. (1952) found that penicillin increased the numbers of certain intestinal coliforms. Such organisms synthesize nutrients that are essential for the animal. If a diet is nutritionally inadequate in certain vitamins, the deficiency could be partially corrected by microbial synthesis.

A depression in growth of certain organisms that could be considered as competitors with the host animal for nutrients has been shown when antibiotics are fed. In early studies, tetracycline was found to inhibit the growth of lactobacilli, microorganisms that require amino acids in about the same proportions as does the pig (March and Biely 1952; Kellogg et al. 1964). Studies have shown that levels and sources of protein that support maximum growth in pigs are near optimum for the multiplication of lactobacilli in the tract. A reduction in the numbers of these competing microorganisms could be beneficial when diets that are marginally deficient in amino acids or vitamins are fed to pigs.

Studies by Henderickx et al. (1981) have shown that the feeding of virginiamycin results in a shift in the bacterial populations of the intestinal tract, which, in turn, leads to (1) a reduction in ammonia and amine production and (2) a reduction in volatile fatty acid (VFA) and lactic acid production. Hedde (1981) also reported a reduction in lactate and VFA production in the small intestine when this antibiotic was fed to pigs. Since these metabolites represent potential losses of protein and energy, the results of these studies suggest that virginiamycin spares both energy and amino acids for the host animal. Results of studies by Yen et al. (1976) and Moser et al. (1980) also indicate improved utilization of dietary protein when carbadox was fed to pigs.

Another significant change that occurs when antibiotics are fed to animals is a reduction in the thickness of the intestinal wall and an overall decrease in the total gut mass (Braude et al. 1955; Taylor and Harrington 1955; Yen et al. 1985). Increased gut wall thickness is thought to be caused by the inhabitant bacteria, which either damage intestinal tissue or produce toxins that, in turn damage the tissues. Greater ammonia production occurs in the gut when antibiotic-free diets are fed, and the ammonia (an irritant) also may contribute to the increased gut wall thickness and overall mass (Visek 1978).

A thinner gut wall could result in greater nutrient absorption, as suggested in studies by Catron et al. (1953) and Henderickx et al. (1981). Additionally, the gut has a high metabolic rate and has been suggested to contribute significantly to total body heat production (Webster 1981; Koong et al. 1982). The reduced mass of the gut in animals fed antibiotics could mean a greater diversion of energy and other nutrients away from heat production and toward body growth.

If one accepts the concept that certain antibiotics spare energy and protein, it would seem that the dietary requirement for amino acids might be less in pigs fed antibiotics. Early studies by Catron et al. (1952) with chlortetracycline and more recently by Yen et al. (1979) and Moser et al. (1980) with carbadox provide evidence that the pig's dietary protein requirement may be reduced when antibiotics are fed.

Disease Control Effect

This mode of action is probably the most widely accepted theory on how antibiotics function to improve growth in animals. Pigs and other animals are continually exposed to an unfriendly environment of microorganisms that cause varying degrees of nonspecific, subclinical disease. This, in turn, reduces the animal's overall performance. The feeding of antibiotics suppresses the hostile microorganisms and allows the host animal to perform more closely to its maximum genetic potential.

There are several pieces of evidence to support this mechanism of action. The response to antibiotics is greater in young animals than in older animals, as illustrated in Table 17.2. Young pigs are more susceptible to disease organisms, in that their immunological protection is quite low. The immunoglobulins acquired from the sow's colostrum reach minimal levels in the pig's serum by the time they reach 3 to 5 weeks of age (Miller et al. 1961). This corresponds approximately to the same time as weaning, which adds further stress to the pigs. Pigs' ability to synthesize antibodies is poor, so immune protection remains low until 6 to 8 weeks of age. As pigs become older, they develop higher levels of blood immunoglobulins (Miller et al. 1961), which better equip them to cope with the unfriendly organisms in their environment.

Additional evidence to support the disease control mode of action is that the degree of response is strongly influenced by cleanliness of the environment and the disease load of the animals involved. As previously discussed, and as illustrated in Tables 17.4 and 17.5, responses to antibiotics generally are minimal when tested in a clean and less stressful environment. Table 17.11 shows that antibiotics were more effective in a "dirty" nursery building than in a "clean" one (Hays and Speer 1960). Table 17.12 summarizes experiments in which antibiotics were tested with slow-growing and fast-growing pigs (Braude et al. 1953). Improvements were considerably greater when

Table 17.11 Effects of Cleanliness of Environment on Responses of Young Pigs to Antibiotics[a]

Item	*Control*	*Antibiotics*[b]	*Improvement (%)*
Gain (kg)			
Clean building	8.1	10.4	28
Dirty building	4.8	7.5	55
Feed/gain			
Clean building	1.90	1.74	8
Dirty building	2.89	2.05	29

[a] Data on 615 pigs initially averaging 5.7 kg; 4- to 5-week trials; from Hays and Speer 1960.
[b] Spiramycin, chlortetracycline, or oxytetracyline.

Table 17.12 Effects of Overall Thriftiness in Pigs on Response to Antibiotics

	Daily Gain (kg)		
No. of Trials	*Control*	*Antibiotics*	*Improvement (%)*
4 slowest growers	0.09	0.25	161
12	0.18	0.34	85
16	0.27	0.45	65
12	0.36	0.50	38
16	0.45	0.57	26
32	0.55	0.63	15
48	0.64	0.71	12
22 fastest growers	0.73	0.79	9

(Adapted, by permission, from Braude et al. 1953.)

antibiotics were fed to slow-growing pigs. Again, the greater response to antibiotics in the poor environment and/or in unthrifty pigs is attributed to the fact that antibiotics suppress the bacteria that are responsible for reduced animal performance because of subclinical disease.

PROPER USAGE—RESIDUE AVOIDANCE

Antibacterial drugs should be used only in approved combinations and at approved levels, as outlined in the Feed Additive Compendium (1990). Certain drugs require withdrawal from the feed for a prescribed period prior to slaughter so that residues do not occur in edible tissue. Those requiring withdrawal include apramycin, the arsenicals (arsanilic acid, sodium arsanilate, roxarsone), carbadox, lincomycin, neomycin, the nitrofurans (furazolidone, nitrofurazone), and the sulfonamides (sulfamethazine, sulfathiazole). Proper use levels and withdrawal times are imperative for the production of residue-free pork.

The most common residue found in pork in recent years has been sulfamethazine. The sulfa residue problem stems from the fact that only trace amounts of sulfamethazine

(2 ppm) in the feed will cause a high incidence of residues in liver tissue (Cromwell et al. 1981). Using improper mixing procedures or failure to prevent contamination of "clean" feed with sulfa-containing feed can result in finishing feed having sufficient levels of sulfa to cause a violative residue (0.1 ppm) in liver or muscle tissue. The sulfonamides have electrostatic properties, and they tend to accumulate in feed dust, which can contaminate other batches of feed. The granulated forms of sulfamethazine are less apt to contribute to cross contamination than powdered sulfamethazine (Cromwell et al. 1982).

SAFETY OF ANTIBIOTICS

Not long after the antibiotics were discovered and accepted into feeding programs for livestock and poultry, questions were raised relative to their safety. The greatest concern today is whether the widespread usage of antibiotics in animal feeds contributes to a reservoir of drug-resistant enteric bacteria that are capable of transferring their resistance to pathogenic bacteria (such as the salmonella), thereby causing a potential public health hazard (Smith 1962; Falkow 1975; Linton 1977). The greatest concern is in regard to penicillin and the tetracyclines, since they also are used in human medicine.

Although transfer of R plasmids occurs rapidly in vitro, the extent to which it occurs in the animal, and between animal bacteria and human bacteria, is not well documented. Animal bacteria do not colonize very effectively in humans unless extremely large doses are consumed; and even then, they are transient (Smith 1969).

Steps were taken in the early 1970s in Great Britain to restrict the use of certain drugs (those used in human medicine and those capable of cross-resisting with drugs used in human medicine) to a prescription basis (Swann 1969). A similar plan was proposed by the FDA in the mid-1970s (Kennedy 1977) but was never implemented. Shortly after a report by Holmberg et al. (1984), which attempted to link several cases of salmonellosis in humans with the consumption of beef from cattle that had been exposed to antibiotics, a petition was filed by the National Resources Defense Council to declare an immediate ban on penicillin and tetracyclines, claiming that they constitute an imminent hazard to public health. After extensive hearings, however, it was concluded that a ban was not justified, and the peitition was denied.

In 1987, the FDA asked the Institute of Medicine to conduct an independent review of the human health consequences and to make a quantitative risk assessment associated with the use of penicillin and the tetracyclines at subtherapeutic levels in animal feeds. The committee was unable to find a substantive body of direct evidence that established the existence of a definite health hazard in humans that could be associated with the use of subtherapeutic concentrations of penicillin and the tetracyclines in animal feeds (IOM 1988).

Whether restricting or even banning the use of certain antibiotics would have a significant influence on the pool of drug-resistant microorganisms is questionable. Action taken by the British government to limit the use of certain drugs to a prescription basis has not reduced the overall usage of tetracyclines, nor has it influenced

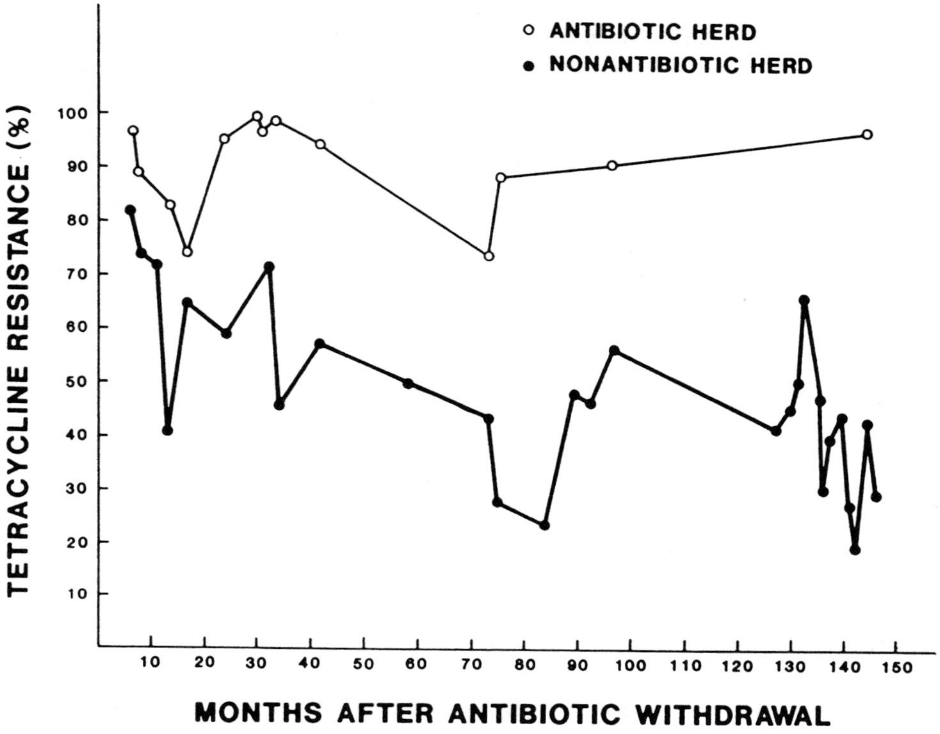

FIGURE 17.3 *Tetracycline resistance of fecal coliforms isolated from pigs in a herd not exposed to antibiotics since 1972 (nonantibiotic herd) and in a herd fed chlortetracycline continuously since 1972 (antibiotic herd). (Reprinted, by permission, from Langlois et al. 1986.)*

the resistance patterns in enteric bacteria of pigs in Britain (Smith 1975, 1977; Braude 1978).

The studies by Langlois et al. (1978a,b; 1986) lend further evidence that even a complete ban on subtherapeutic use of all antibiotics would have only minor influences on antimicrobial resistance levels and patterns. Figure 17.3 illustrates that a rather large percentage of enteric microbes in pigs are resistant to tetracycline, even after 13 years of no antibacterial exposure in a closed swine herd. Multiple resistance also was relatively high in pigs having no exposure to antibacterials for 13 years (Figure 17.4; Table 17.13). Factors such as animal age, type of housing, and transportation stress were found by these researchers to have as much impact on shedding of resistant organisms as the presence of antibiotics in the feed (Table 17.14).

The question of whether antimicrobial resistance constitutes a significant threat to human health will continue to be debated in the scientific community as well as in the political arena. While the incidence of antimicrobial resistance in the human population is quite high, there is no evidence that the levels or patterns have changed over the past

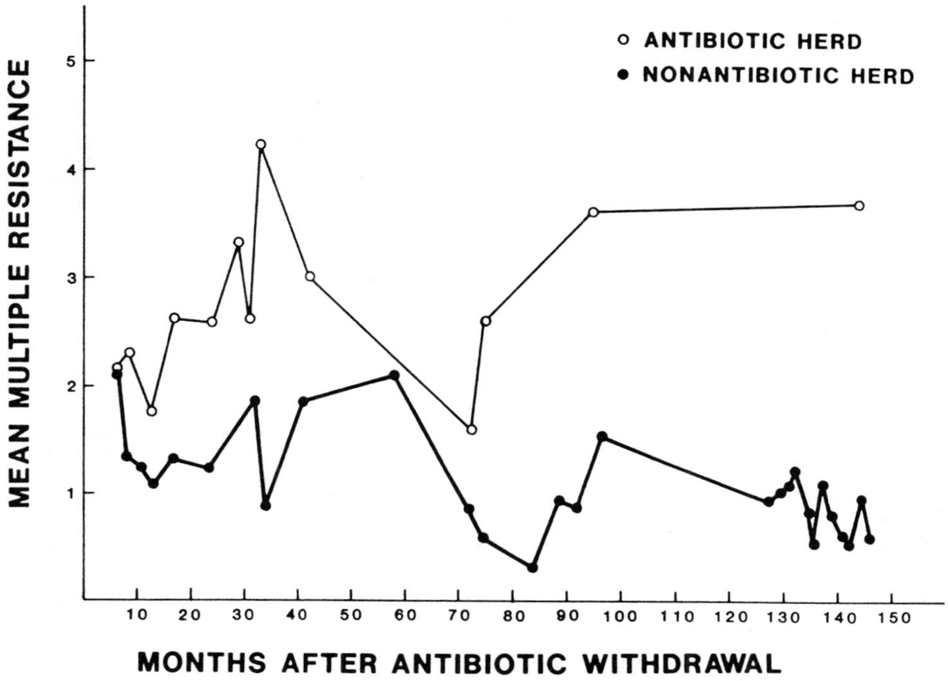

FIGURE 17.4 *Mean multiple resistance to ten antimicrobial agents of fecal coliforms isolated from pigs in a herd not exposed to antibiotics since 1972 (nonantibiotic herd) and in a herd fed chlortetracycline continuously since 1972 (antibiotic herd). (Reprinted, by permission, from Langlois et al. 1986.)*

Table 17.13 Resistance of Fecal Coliform Isolates from Herds Having No Exposure or Continuous Exposure to Antibiotics for Thirteen Years

	Antibiotic Exposure	
	Continuous[a]	*None*
No. of isolates	1761	4886
% Isolates resistant to the following:		
Ampicillin	25	7
Kanamycin	39	<1
Neomycin	30	<1
Streptomycin	62	20
Sulfisoxazole	32	23
Tetracycline	92	46
Avg. no. of agents to which coliforms were resistant	2.87	1.00

[a] Less than 3% of the isolates from the pigs having antibiotic exposure were resistant to cephalothin, chloramphenicol, gentamicin, and nalidixic acid.

(Data from Langlois et al. 1986.)

Table 17.14 Effects of Age, Housing System, and Moving Stress on Tetracycline Resistance of Fecal Coliforms from Pigs Not Exposed to Antibiotics for Thirteen Years

Item	*No. of Isolates*	*Coliforms Resistant to Tetracycline (% of Total)*	*Multiple Resistance*[a]
Age of pig (mo)			
<2	1069	70	1.52
2–6	1110	64	1.38
7–11	719	24	0.50
12–23	1648	33	0.69
>24	340	29	0.61
Housing			
Farrowing house	464	50	1.11
Feeding floor	1326	69	1.47
Pasture	2421	29	0.62
Moving stress			
Unmoved	4886	46	1.00
After moving 300 km	696	82	2.21

[a] Average number of antimicrobials (of 10 tested) to which fecal coliforms were resistant.
(Reprinted, by permission, from Langlois et al. 1986.)

10 to 15 years (Lorian 1986). Antibiotics have been fed for nearly 40 years to literally billions of animals, yet there is no convincing evidence that there are any unfavorable health effects in humans that can be directly linked to the feeding of subtherapeutic levels of antibiotics to animals.

ECONOMIC BENEFITS OF ANTIBIOTICS

The economic returns to the swine producer using antibiotics in the feeding program are influenced by a number of factors, including the degree of response to the particular antibiotic (i.e., improvement in rate and efficiency of growth, improvement in reproductive performance, reduction in mortality and morbidity, the cost of the antibiotic, the cost of feed and other production variables, and the market price of hogs). Based on average figures, the total benefit from antimicrobial usage was calculated by Zimmerman (1986) to be $2.64 per marketed pig.

The ultimate beneficiary from increased production efficiency is, of course, the consumer. In 1981 it was estimated that the use of antimicrobial agents in animal production resulted in a $3.5 billion annual savings in meat costs to the consumer in the United States (CAST 1981). Likely, this savings is even greater today.

REFERENCES

Anderson, G.W., J.D. Cunningham, and S.J. Slinger. 1952. *J. Nutr.* 47:175.
Beames, R.M., and L.E. Lloyd. 1965. *J. Anim. Sci.* 24:1020.

Braude, R. 1945. *J. Agric. Sci.* 35:163.
Braude, R. 1978. *J. Anim. Sci.* 46:1425.
Braude, R., and B.C. Johnson. 1953. *J. Nutr.* 49:505.
Braude, R., H.D. Wallace, and T.J. Cunha. 1953. *Antibiot. Chemother.* 3:271.
Braude, R., et al. 1955. *Br. J. Nutr.* 9:363.
Brody, T.M., M.R. Hurwitz, and J.A. Bain. 1954. *Antibiot. Chemother.* 4:864.
Burnell, T.W., G.L. Cromwell, and T.S. Stahly. 1988. *J. Anim. Sci.* 66:1100.
CAST. 1981. "Antibiotics in animal feeds." In: *Report No. 88.* Ames, IA: Council for Agricultural Science and Technology.
Catron, D.V., et al. 1952. *J. Anim. Sci.* 11:221.
Catron, D.V., et al. 1953. *Antibiot. Chemother.* 3:571.
Combs, G.E., and H.D. Wallace. 1969. *Florida Animal Science Mimeograph Series No. 69–11.* Gainesville: University of Florida.
Cromwell, G.L. 1983. *Proceedings of the NFIA Mineral Nutrition Institute.* Des Moines, IA: National Feed Ingredient Association.
Cromwell, G.L. 1987. *Proceedings of the Georgia Nutrition Conference.* pp. 146–149. Athens: University of Georgia.
Cromwell, G.L., and K.A. Dawson. *Antibiotic Growth Promotants. Emerging Agricultural Technology: Issues for the 1990's.* Office of Technology Assessment, U.S. Congress, Washington, D.C. (in press).
Cromwell, G.L., R.I. Hutagalung, and T.S. Stahly. 1982. *J. Anim. Sci.* 55(Suppl. 1):267.
Cromwell, G.L., T.S. Stahly, and H.J. Monegue. 1989. *J. Anim. Sci.* 67:2996.
Cromwell, G.L., et al. 1981. *J. Anim. Sci.* 53(Suppl. 1):95.
Cunha, T.J., et al. 1949. *Arch. Biochem.* 23:324.
Cunha, T.J., et al. 1950. *J. Anim. Sci.* 9:653.
Dean, B.T., and L.F. Tribble. 1962. *J. Anim. Sci.* 21:207.
Edmonds, J.S., O.A. Izquierdo, and D.H. Baker. 1985. *J. Anim. Sci.* 60:462.
Evvard, J.M., V.E. Nelson, and W.E. Sewell. 1928. *Proc. Iowa Acad. Sci.* 35:211.
Falkow, S. 1975. *Infectious Multiple Drug Resistance.* London: Pion Ltd.
Feed Additive Compendium. 1990. Minneapolis, MN: Miller Publishing Co.
Hagen, C.D., et al. 1987. *Nutr. Rep. Int.* 35:1083.
Hash, J.H., M. Wishnick, and P.A. Miller. 1964. *J. Biol. Chem.* 239:2070.
Hays, V.W. 1977. *Effectiveness of Feed Additive Usage of Antibacterial Agents in Swine and Poultry Production.* Washington, DC: Office of Technology Assessment, U.S. Congress. (Edited version: Hays, V.W. 1981. *The Hays Report.* Long Beach, CA: Rachelle Laboratories, Inc.)
Hays, V.W. 1978. "The role of antibiotics in efficient livestock production." In: *Nutrition and Drug Interrelations.* New York: Academic Press.
Hays, V.W., and V.C. Speer. 1960. *J. Anim. Sci.* 19:938.
Hays, V.W., et al. 1978. *J. Anim. Sci.* 46:884.
Hedde, R.D. 1981. *Proceedings of the Growth Promotion Mode-of-Action Symposium.* pp. 10–20. Philadelphia: SmithKline Corp.
Henderickx, H.K., et al. 1981. *Proceedings of the Growth Promotion Mode-of-Action Symposium.* pp. 3–9. Philadelphia: SmithKline Corp.
Holmberg, M.D., et al. 1984. *N. Engl. J. Med.* 311:617.
IOM. 1988. *Human Health Risks with the Subtherapeutic Use of Penicillin or Tetracyclin in Animal Feed.* Institute of Medicine, National Academy of Sciences. Washington, DC: National Academy Press.
Johnson, D.D., et al. 1985. *J. Anim. Sci.* 61(Suppl. 1):437.
Jordan, C.E., and W.P. Waitt. 1963. *J. Anim. Sci.* 22:838.
Jukes, T.H., et al. 1950. *Arch. Biochem.* 26:324.
Kellogg, R.F., et al. 1964. *J. Anim. Sci.* 23:1089.
Kennedy, D.F. 1977. *HEW News,* April 15. Rockville, MD: U.S. Department of Health, Education and Welfare.

Koong, L.J., et al. 1982. *J. Nutr.* 112:1638.
Langlois, B.E., G.L. Cromwell, and V.W. Hays. 1978a. *J. Anim. Sci.* 46:1369.
Langlois, B.E., G.L. Cromwell, and V.W. Hays. 1978b. *J. Anim. Sci.* 46:1383.
Langlois, B.E., et al. 1986. *J. Anim. Sci.* 62(Suppl. 3):18.
Lepley, K.C., D.V. Catron, and C.C. Culbertson. 1950. *J. Anim. Sci.* 9:608.
Luecke, R.W., W.N. McMillan, and F. Thorp, Jr. 1950. *Arch. Biochem.* 26:326.
Lillie, R.J., and L.T. Frobish. 1978. *J. Anim. Sci.* 46:678.
Linton, A.H. 1977. In: *Antibiotics and Antibiosis in Agriculture.* Woodbine, M. (Ed.). pp. 315–343. Woburn, MA: Butterworths.
Lorian, V. 1986. *J. Anim. Sci.* 62(Suppl. 3):49.
Mahan, D.C. 1980. *Ohio Swine Research and Industry Report No. 80-2.* p. 1. Columbus: Ohio State University.
March, B., and J. Biely. 1952. *Poult. Sci.* 31:177.
Maxwell, C.V., et al. 1987. *J. Anim. Sci.* 65(Suppl. 1):312.
Mayrose, V.B., et al. 1964. *J. Anim. Sci.* 23:737.
Messersmith, R.E., et al. 1966. *J. Anim. Sci.* 25:752.
Miller, E.R., et al. 1961. *J. Anim. Sci.* 20:31.
Moore, P.R., et al. 1946. *J. Biol. Chem.* 165:437.
Moser, B.D., E.R. Peo, Jr., and A.J. Lewis. 1980. *Nutr. Rep. Int.* 22:949.
Myers, D.J., and V.C. Speer. 1973. *J. Anim. Sci.* 36:1125.
NCR-89 Committee on Confinement Management of Swine. 1984. *J. Anim. Sci.* 58:801.
Ruiz, M.E., et al. 1968. *J. Anim. Sci.* 27:1602.
Sewell, R.F., and J.L. Carmon. 1958. *J. Anim. Sci.* 17:752.
Smith, H.W. 1962. *Proceedings of the University of Nottingham Ninth Easter School in Agricultural Science.* p. 374. London: Butterworths.
Smith, H.W. 1969. *Lancet* 1:1174.
Smith, H.W. 1975. *Nature* 258:628.
Smith, H.W. 1977. In: *Antibiotics and Antibiosis in Agriculture.* Woodbine, M. (Ed.). pp. 344–357. Woburn, MA: Butterworths.
Soma, J.A., and V.C. Speer. 1975. *J. Anim. Sci.* 41:100.
Stahly, T.S., G.L. Cromwell, and H.J. Monegue. 1980. *J. Anim. Sci.* 51:1347.
Stokstad, E.L.R., et al. 1949. *J. Biol. Chem.* 180:647.
Swann, M.M. 1969. *Report of the Joint Committee on the Use of Antibiotics in Animal Husbandry and Veterinary Medicine.* London: Her Majesty's Stationery Office.
Taylor, J.H., and G. Harrington. 1955. *Nature* 175:643.
U.S. International Trade Commission. 1989. *USITC Publication No. 2219,* Washington, DC.
Visek, W.J. 1978. *J. Anim. Sci.* 46:1447.
Wallace, H.D. 1967. *High Level Copper in Swine Feeding.* New York: International Copper Research Association, Inc.
Wallace, H.D., and G.E. Combs. 1962. *Florida Animal Science Mimeograph Series. No. 63-3.* Gainesville: University of Florida.
Wallace, H.D., and G.E. Combs. 1964. *Florida Animal Science Mimeograph Serise. No. 64–14.* Gainesville: University of Florida.
Wallace, H.D., R.H. Hauser, and G.E. Combs. 1966. *Florida Animal Science Mimeograph Series No. 66-12.* Gainesville: University of Florida.
Wallace, H.D., D.D. Thieu, and G.E. Combs. 1974. *Florida Animal Science Mimeograph Series No. 74-6.* Gainesville: University of Florida.
Webster, A.J.F. 1981. *Proc. Nutr. Soc.* 40:121.
Weinberg, E.D. 1957. *Bacteriol. Rev.* 21:46.
Yen, J.T., T.L. Veum, and R. Lauxen. 1979. *J. Anim. Sci.* 49(Suppl. 1):257.
Yen, J.T., et al. 1976. *J. Anim. Sci.* 42:375.
Yen, J.T., et al. 1985. *J. Nutr.* 115:970.
Zimmerman, D.R. 1986. *J. Anim. Sci.* 62(Suppl. 3):6.

Chapter 18

Water: The Forgotten Nutrient

A.J. Thulin and M. C. Brumm

IMPORTANCE OF WATER

Water is one of the most important nutrients required by swine to meet their metabolic needs. It is an integral part of the structure of the soft tissues of the body in that the cell contents (cytoplasm) are lyophilic gels. Thus, they readily take up and release water as a part of metabolism. Water accounts for about 53% of a 90-kg pig (whole body weight less gastrointestinal tract contents) and as much as 82% of the empty body weight of the newborn pig (Shields et al. 1983). Water plays a classical role in the reactions of energy-yielding nutrients in the body. Most digestive changes in dietary carbohydrates, fats, and proteins entail the addition of water to the substrate. For example, practically all enzyme-catalyzed reactions in the body involve (1) addition or subtraction of water, (2) addition of oxygen or removal of hydrogen, (3) addition or removal of phosphoric acid, or (4) splitting or formation of a carbon-carbon linkage.

Water has several unique properties that are very important to swine production. The specific heat of water is considerably higher than that of any other liquid. This makes water indispensable for dispersing the heat produced by some of the chemical reactions in metabolism. Because of this, water is important in the adjustment of body temperature to environmental temperatures as water gives up its latent heat during evaporation by panting (respiration) or sweating (perspiration). About 580 calories of heat are released when 1 g of water changes from liquid to vapor.

Water is also important for the movement of nutrients to the cells of body tissues and for the removal of metabolic end products from the cells. It is important for lubrication of joints, for providing protective cushioning for the nerve system, for the production of milk, and for growth and reproduction.

WATER TURNOVER

Pigs meet their needs for water primarily by three sources: (1) drinking water; (2) moisture received from the content of feed (about 10% to 12% of air dry feed); and

(3) metabolic water formed during metabolism. The oxidation of 1 kg of fat, carbohydrate, or protein produces 1190, 560, or 450 kg of water, respectively (NRC 1981). Total water turnover in the body may be quite large. Although a portion of the water that is secreted from various tissues may be reabsorbed at other points, there is considerable loss that must be replaced by ingested fluid or metabolic water from the diet. Water losses are principally through the urine, feces, and evaporation from the respiratory tract and the body surface.

The amount of water excreted in the urine is highly variable. The kidneys regulate the volume and composition of body fluids by excreting more or less water, depending on intake and outgo through other mechanisms and the amounts of catabolic products such as waste salts and urea, for which water serves as a solvent. Water intake can therefore be increased when diets containing greater amounts of minerals and protein are fed. The larger the amount of protein in the diet, the greater the water loss, and thus the greater the water requirement, accordingly. In addition, when a high-protein diet is fed, there is less metabolic water formed in protein catabolism than is the case for carbohydrate or fats. This also enhances the need for increased water consumption. Schmidt-Nielsen (1964) has reported that in dry climates, carbohydrates supply more net metabolic water then either proteins or fats. Similarly, increased intake of salt results in increased water intake and concomitant increase in urine output. Research has shown that water:feed ratio of 2:1 was increased linearly by dietary salt content to 3.5:1 when diets containing from 0.1% to 3.0% NaCl were fed to growing-finishing pigs (Sinclair 1939).

In certain pathological conditions, excess water is retained in the tissues and body cavities, causing edema. In addition, conditions such as diarrhea from enteritis can result in large losses of water, and serious dehydration can result if these conditions persist. However, fecal water excretion is little affected by variations in intake of drinking water (Agricultural Research Council 1981). The losses through the gut vary with the nature of the diet. They increase with the level of fiber intake and with the intakes of other feeds that have laxative qualities. In general, the greater the proportion of undigested material, the greater the water loss (Maynard and Loosli 1969).

Although perspiration water loss is a major means of dissipation of heat in the regulation of body temperature in some species, swine depend more on the respiratory than the cutaneous route for heat dissipation (NRC 1981). Expired air is saturated by water and, even for an animal at rest in a cool environment, represents a substantial loss. This loss is greatly increased with the effective surface area of the body, by physical activity and by temperature and environmental conditions that increase pulmonary exchange. Losses of water vapor from the lungs and skin for 1-, 45-, and 90-kg pigs were reported to be 86 g, 1.3 kg, and 2.1 kg/day, respectively (Mitchell and Kelly 1938).

WATER REQUIREMENT

While the metabolic water requirements of swine are well defined, the practical estimates of daily water intakes are less clearly understood. In addition to metabolic needs, pigs of all sizes consume water to meet a variety of needs, including physical and social. Factors such as body size, feed intake, lactation, ambient temperature, type and amount of feed ingredients and chemical substances (including medications and flavors) ingested, general state of health, stress, and individual animal differences influence the pig's absolute requirement for water (CAST 1982).

For planning purposes, estimates of water needs for various weight groupings of pigs are listed in Table 18.1 for pigs fed a dry diet with ad libitum access to a water device (Gadd 1988; Weckowicz et al. 1978). A review of estimates of water needs for the various classes of swine indicates that much variation exists in current estimates. These estimates do not, however, indicate the type of watering device and its possible role in water intake.

Brooks et al. (1984), in a study using 3- to 7-week-old weaning pigs, concluded that daily feed intake was the best single predictor of ad libitum water intake for ad libitum-fed pigs. The relationship was described by the equation:

$$\text{Water intake (L/day)} = 0.149 + (3.053 \times \text{kg daily dry feed intake})$$

A combination of feed intake and metabolic body weight was given as the best overall predictor equation:

$$\text{Water intake (L/day)} = 0.788 + (2.23 \times \text{kg daily dry feed intake}) + (0.367 \times \text{kg body weight}^{.6})$$

At environmental temperatures around 25 °C, Yang et al. (1981) concluded that growing pigs have a daily water turnover of 120 to 130 ml/kg live weight or about 250 ml/kg$^{.82}$ when fed dry pellets at the rate of 4% to 5% of body weight daily. This turnover rate is higher than that of the donkey, sheep, goat, and camel and lower than that of cattle (Macfarlane 1976).

Mount et al (1971) discussed the impact of temperature on water consumption in a general way. Ingram and Stephens (1979) demonstrated that at an ambient temperature of 21 °C to 24 °C, warming the hypothalamus of 15- to 35-kg pigs for 10 minutes increased water intake approximately 40%, while cooling for a similar period reduced intake by 70%. Neither scrotal heating nor spinal cord heating or cooling had

Table 18.1 Daily Ad Libitum Drinking Water Estimates

Pig Age (d) or Class	*Approximate Body Weight (kg)*	*L/d*
Piglets to 55	5–30	2.8
55–95	30–50	8
96–156	50–85	12
157–230	85–110	20
Gilts	150	16
Pregnant sows	180	22
Suckling sows	180	27
Boars	180	20

(Adapted, by permission, from Weckowicz et al. 1978.)

as much effect as hypothalamus temperature modification. Osmotic stimuli through infusion of various NaCl solutions was similarly effective in modifying water intake. The NRC (1988) included an extensive literature review on factors influencing water intake.

Olsson and Andersson (1985), using nose-operated drinker devices, concluded that water consumption at feeding for growing-finishing pigs has a distinct periodicity with a peak at the beginning and at the end of the feeding period. Water consumption between feeding periods peaked 2 hours after the morning feeding and 1 hour after the afternoon feeding. These results support the conclusions of Yang et al. (1981, 1984) that growing pigs have a tendency, when feed intake is restricted, to increase the total amount of water ingested, possibly due to a desire for abdominal fill. In general, their results suggested that water for abdominal fill was taken during the afternoon when food was restricted. Brooks et al. (1984) reported a diurnal pattern to water intake for weaned pigs housed under conditions of constant light, with increased consumption recorded from 0830 to 1700 as compared with the 1700 to 0830 time period.

Consideration of water availability must also include those factors that influence the rate of water availability from noncup-type devices. Water flow rates vary considerably due to design, manufacturing, and installation differences. Partial plugging due to mineral deposits or feed particle deposits affect the ultimate delivery rate.

Nienaber and Hahn (1984), in a 4-week trial, concluded that nipple water flow rates between 100 and 1100 ml/minute had no measurable effect on body weight gain, feed intake, or feed conversion for pigs weaned at 4.5 weeks of age. However, as flow rate increased, water use (disappearance) increased. At a flow rate of 100 ml/minute, the time spent drinking was nearly fourfold higher than the average time spent at the higher flow rates.

In more recent work, Thulin et al. (1990) demonstrated no differences in 4-week growth performance for weaned pigs given access to nipple waterers set to deliver water at 70 or 700 ml/minute and penned 6 or 12 pigs per pen. However, when flow rate was reduced from 700 ml/minute to 70 ml/minute, nipple-waterer contact was increased nearly threefold for 6 pigs and over twofold for 12 pigs per pen stocking density.

Similarly, Barber et al. (1988) reported no difference in gain, feed intake, or conversion for growing-finishing pigs given access to Arato-80 drinkers set to deliver 300 or 900 ml/minute. However, water use at 900 ml/minute was 105% greater than that at 300 ml/minute. They also noted that apparent drinking time at the lower delivery rate was significantly greater than at the higher rate.

Carlson and Peo (1980), while not directly reporting flow or delivery rates, reported no differences in gain for weaned pigs (four pigs per pen) given access to nipple drinkers with 1- versus 3-mm orifices. However, feed conversion was 6% better for pigs given access to the 3-mm orifice drinker. In a subsequent trial in the same facility (Carlson and Peo 1982), no differences in performance was reported for weaned pigs given access to nipple drinkers with 2- or 2.5-mm orifices. However, water use (disappearance) was greater in pens with nipples pointing upward at a 45° angle than in pens with nipples pointing down at a 45° angle.

For both growing-finishing swine and weaned pigs, Carlson and Peo (1979) reported that water use increased from cup versus nipple drinkers. These investigators concluded that water waste due to play activity was a major factor in the apparent difference in use.

Recommendations on water delivery rates and stocking densities must take into account diet ingredients and feeding regimens. While English et al. (1988) suggest a water:feed ratio of 2.5 L of water for each kilogram of meal for wet feeding systems, Brooks et al. (1986) demonstrated improved performance at ratios up to 3.5:1. They suggest that the physiological and ethological needs of the pigs can only be satisfied by the provision of an unrestricted supply of water at all times.

Because of the costs associated with water delivery and subsequent waste disposal, Europeans have been very interested in water delivery devices in recent years. Olsson and Andersson (1985) concluded that for growing-finishing pigs the water system capacity should reach 0.25 L/minute/pig. Water delivery capacity in an individual nose-operated drinking delivery valve should be at least 1.0 to 1.5 L/minute when water is available on an intermittent time basis.

This delivery rate compares with suggested rates for nipple drinkers in the United States of 0.25 L/minute for 5- to 15-kg pigs, 0.5 L/minute for 15- to 35-kg pigs, and 0.6 L/minute for finishing pigs. For lactating sows with unlimited water access, the delivery rate minimum was suggested as 1.0 L/minute.

While general recommendations are available for density of pigs at drinker spaces (MWPS 1982), research data are limited. Brumm and Shelton (1986), using 3- to 4-week-old weaned pigs, reported a slight reduction in average daily gain (0.19 versus 0.32 kg) and an increase in weight variation within pens of 16 pigs given access to one versus two nipple drinkers for 5 weeks postweaning. They concluded that when drinker space (access) is limited, average performance suffers only slightly. However, weight variation within a pen of pigs increases.

Generally, for groups larger than ten pigs in a nursery and fifteen to twenty pigs in a growing-finishing facility, a minimum of two water delivery devices per group is recommended (MWPS 1982; Brumm and Reese 1986), although Olsson (1983) recommends one bite valve per five finishing pigs.

WATER QUALITY

A common belief is that water is reasonably safe for livestock if it looks clean and is readily consumed. However, water quality surveys show that even if water looks clean, it may contain substances that may have detrimental effects on livestock. The question is, at what levels do these substrates become unsafe for livestock? There is no simple answer, since quality standards are difficult to define due to the many factors that affect the response of a group of animals to a specific water source. Factors that can influence water quality are pH, salinity (salt content of water), nitrates and nitrites, toxic inorganic chemicals, organic toxins, and microbial contamination.

The pH is a measure of acidity or alkalinity of the water. While a low pH (e.g., 2) would represent extremely high acidity, a high pH (e.g., 12) would indicate high alkalinity. The pH of water consumed by pigs normally ranges from 6 to 8. Alkalinity is sometimes confused with salinity as it is a part of salinity. It represents the buffering capacity of the minerals in saline water. Alkaline water contains primarily sodium and potassium carbonate.

Water hardness is caused by mineral salts of calcium and magnesium and is reported in equivalent amounts of calcium carbonate ($CaCO_3$) in grains per gallon (gpg) or milligrams per liter (mg/L), which is the same as parts per million. Low levels of strontium, iron, aluminum, zinc, and magnesium salts are not detrimental to pig health, since hogs can tolerate and utilize these minerals. Concentrations of these salts are seldom too high to be tolerated (NAS 1980). However, very high levels of calcium in the water may require that higher levels of phosphorus be fed to avoid a dietary calcium-phosphorus imbalance. The hardness of domestic water, according to Durfor and Becker (1964), is classified in Table 18.2.

Concentrations of all constituents dissolved in water is referred to as ''total dissolved solids'' (TDS). The term *salinity* is synonymous with TDS as an indication of the total ionic concentration in fresh water. Salinity (salt content of water) commonly involves calcium, magnesium, and sodium in the bicarbonate, chloride, or sulfate form. Water containing <5000 ppm sulfate and 6000 ppm TDS may cause temporary diarrhea and increased daily water intake, although health and performance are not greatly affected. Patterson et al. (1979) offered water containing 3320 ppm sulfate and 5060 ppm TDS to gilts and sows and reported no significant effect on reproduction. The addition of up to 4400 ppm sulfate and 6000 ppm TDS to water offered to weaned pigs has resulted in no effect on growth performance or feed efficiency. However, there was reported increased water intake, temporary mild diarrhea, and less firm feces with pigs offered the higher sulfate and TDS levels in their water (Embry et al. 1959; Anderson and Stothers 1978; Patterson et al. 1978). Water containing over 7000 ppm TDS should not be offered for swine consumption. Water with TDS greater than this may present a health risk for pregnant or lactating sows or stressed pigs (NAS 1974). Much of the research to date conducted to evaluate the effects of sulfate and nitrates on pig performance has involved the use of tap water (for human consumption) with added salts. This may not necessarily emulate the water conditions on a farm, since water may contain any number of substances, such as toxic inorganic chemicals, organic toxins, and microbial contamination, which may have a detrimental effect on pig consumption and performance. Table 18.3 describes the acceptable TDS levels for swine.

Table 18.2 Water Hardness

Hardness Range ($CaCO_3$, *ppm)*	*Description*
0–60	Soft
61–120	Moderately hard
121–180	Hard
>180	Very hard

(Adapted, by permission, from Durfor and Becker 1964.)

Table 18.3 A Guide for Use of Saline Waters for Swine

TDS (ppm)	*Use Recommendations*
<3000	These waters should be satisfactory for swine. May cause temporary, mild diarrhea in pigs not accustomed to them.
3000–5000	Generally satisfactory. Temporary diarrhea and water refusal initially when pigs not accustomed to them. May cause increased water consumption.
5000–7000	May be used with reasonable safety for growing-finishing pigs. Should avoid the use of these approaching the higher levels for pregnant or lactating sows.
>7000	Considerable risk may exist with pregnant or lactating sows, or with pigs subjected to heat stress, water loss, or disease conditions.

Abbreviation: TDS, total dissolved solids.
(Adapted, by permission, from National Academy of Sciences 1974.)

Nitrates are widely dispersed in our environment and can cause health hazards when significant amounts enter drinking water. While the concentration of the nitrate ion (NO_3) commonly found in drinking water is well tolerated by swine, nitrite (NO_2, the reduced form of nitrate) is readily absorbed and can be toxic. At toxic levels, nitrite oxidizes the iron in hemoglobin to form methemoglobin, thus reducing the oxygen-carrying capacity of the blood. Frequently, nitrates found in the water supply indicate a bacterial contamination. Bacterial reduction of nitrate to nitrite is promoted as pH level increases in the intestines. Bacteria in water sources contaminated with feed and bedding can convert nitrate to nitrite. Seerley et al. (1965) reported that levels of nitrate providing up to 300 ppm NO_3-N in the drinking water had no adverse effect on weight gain or reproductive performance in swine. In addition, adding 100 ppm NO_2-N to drinking water provided to swine gave measurable but small increases in methemoglobin without obvious detrimental effect on performance or liver vitamin A as determined after 105 days on treatment. Recommended limits of concentration for potentially toxic substances in water are shown in Table 18.4.

The general sanitary quality of a water sample may be determined by bacterial examination. While the term *coliforms* is used to indicate the presence of organisms, it does not tell anything about pathogens. Fecal streptococci or fecal coliforms may be of more significance to livestock. The U.S. Environmental Protection Agency (1973) proposed that acceptable limitations for water to be used directly by livestock should not exceed 5000 coliforms/100 ml. However, if pigs are allowed to drink surface waters, the proposed limits would be unenforceable and of doubtful value. Coliforms and other bacteria in water may offer a significant source of infection to pigs. In addition, there are many diseases affecting swine that are transmitted via water. A veterinarian should be contacted for an evaluation should bacteria be found in the water supply.

Pesticides may enter ground water from many sources such as industrial spills, faulty disposal, surface runoff, and rainfall. Unfortunately, because of the great num-

Table 18.4 Recommended Limits for Concentration of Potentially Toxic Substances in Drinking Water for Livestock

	Safe Upper Limit of Concentration (mg/L)	
Substance	*NAS*[a]	*CAST*[b]
Arsenic	0.2	0.5
Boron	NE	10.0
Cadmium	0.05	0.5
Chromium	1.0	5.0
Cobalt	1.0	1.0
Copper	0.5	0.5
Fluoride	2.0	3.0
Iron	NE	NE
Lead	0.1	0.1
Mercury	0.01	0.01
Nickel	1.0	NE
Nitrate	440.0	1320.0
Nitrite	33.0	33.0
Selenium	NE	0.1
Vanadium	0.1	1.0
Zinc	25.0	25.0

Abbreviation: NE, not established.

[a]Recommended by National Academy of Sciences 1974.

[b]Recommended by the Council of Agricultural Science and Technology (CAST). *Report No. 26. Quality of Water for Livestock.* 1974.

ber of toxic compounds and the limited information available on experimentally determined toxicity levels, good judgment is necessary when applying information reported in the literature to practical production situations. Usually, many conditions are involved in the decision of whether or not certain levels of toxicants will cause harm. Table 18.5 provides the U.S. Environmental Protection Agency's recommended guidelines for human drinking water, which may provide some insight into toxic levels of various pesticides.

In summary, ample quantity and quality of water is necessary for optimum swine production. The producer is typically very interested in the performance of his hogs, the control of disease within the herd, and the acceptability of his product to the consumer. Water quality can greatly influence these factors and, consequently, the viability of the swine enterprise. Because of this, routine water analyses should be conducted at least once per year.

Water may become suspect in chronic poor performance that is unresponsive to changes in management, nutrition, environment, and health programs. Analyses of water quality should be conducted in this case. Where treatment of water is needed, it is important to have a good water analysis before purchasing equipment. Tests related to common problems such as hardness and nitrate content can be performed by the health department or the equipment supplier. Potentially toxic substances analysis can also be made by many laboratories. Commercial equipment is available to solve water

Table 18.5 Maximum Concentrations of Pesticides for Human Drinking Water

Pesticide	*Maximum Concentration (mg/L)*
Aldrin	0.001
Chlordane	0.003
DDT	0.05
Dieldrin	0.001
Endrin	0.0002
Heptachlor/heptachlor epoxide	0.0001
Lindane	0.004
Methoxychlor	0.1
Toxaphene	0.005
2,4-D	0.1
2,4,5-T	0.1

Reprinted, by permission, from U.S. Environmental Protection Agency. *Drinking Water Standards.* 1975.

quality problems. However, the cost may be prohibitive in the cases of highly mineralized well water. An alternative source of water may be justified in this case.

REFERENCES

Agricultural Research Council. 1981. *The Nutrient Requirements of Pigs.* Slough, England: Commonwealth Agricultural Bureaux.

Anderson, D.M., and S.C. Stothers. 1978. *J. Anim. Sci.* 47:900.

Barber, J., et al. 1988. *Proceedings of the British Society of Animal Producers, Winter Meeting, No. 127.*

Brooks, P.H., S.J. Russell, and J.L. Carpenter. 1984. *Vet. Rec.* 115:513.

Brooks, P.H., et al. 1986. *Diss and Caythrope Pig Conference.* London: Meat and Livestock Commission.

Brumm, M.C., and D.E. Reese. 1986. *University of Nebraska Neb Guide G86–821.* Lincoln: University of Nebraska.

Brumm, M.C., and D.P. Shelton. 1986. *Nebraska Swine Report. University of Nebraska Publication No. EC86–219.* Lincoln: University of Nebraska.

Carlson, R., and E.R. Peo, Jr. 1979. *Nebraska Swine Report. University of Nebraska Publication No. EC79–219.* Lincoln: University of Nebraska.

Carlson, R., and E.R. Peo, Jr. 1980. *Nebraska Swine Report. University of Nebraska Publication No. EC80–219.* Lincoln: University of Nebraska.

Carlson, R.L., and E.R. Peo, Jr. 1982. *Nebraska Swine Report. University of Nebraska Publication No. EC82–219.* Lincoln: University of Nebraska.

CAST. 1974. *Report No. 26. Quality of Water for Livestock.*

Durfor, C.M., and E. Becker. 1964. *USGS Water-Supply Paper 1812.* Washington, DC: U.S. Government Printing Office.

Embry, L.B., et al. 1959. *South Dakota Agricultural Experiment Station Bulletin 481.*

English, P.R., et al. 1988. In: *The Growing and Finishing Pig: Improving Efficiency.* Ipswich, U.K: Farming Press.

Gadd, J. 1988. *Pig Farming.* May, 1988. Ipswich, U.K.: Farming Press.

Ingram, D.L., and D.B. Stephens. 1979. *J. Physiol.* 293:501.

Lloyd, L.E., et al. 1978. *Fundamentals of Nutrition.* 2nd Ed. San Francisco: Freeman and Co.

Macfarlane, W.V. 1976. ''Adaptation to climate zones and the ecophysiology of ruminants.'' In: *Progress in Biometerology.* Division B, Vol. 1, Part 1. Johnson, J.E. (Ed.). Amsterdam: Swetz and Zeitlinger.

Maynard, L.A., and J.K. Loosli. 1969. *Anim. Nutr.* 6th ed. New York: McGraw-Hill.

Meyer, V.M., et al. 1988. Building Materials and Equipment for Swine Facilities. *Pork Industry Handbook 32.* West Lafayette, IN: Purdue University.

Midwest Plan Service. 1982. *Swine Housing and Equipment Handbook. Publication No. MWPS-8.* Ames, IA: Iowa State University.

Ministry of Agriculture, Fisheries and Food. 1985. *Codes of Recommendations for the Welfare of Livestock: Pigs. Leaflet 702.*

Mitchell, H.H., and M.A.R. Kelly. 1938. *J. Agric. Res.* 56:811.

Mount, L.E., et al. 1971. *Anim. Prod.* 13:561.

National Academy of Sciences. 1974. *Nutrients and Toxic Substances in Water for Livestock and Poultry.* Washington, DC: National Academy Press.

National Academy of Sciences. 1980. *Mineral Tolerance of Domestic Animals.* Washington, DC: National Academy Press.

National Research Council. 1981. *Effect of Environment on Nutrient Requirements of Domestic Animals.* Washington, DC: National Academy Press.

National Research Council. 1988. *Nutrient Requirements of Swine.* 9th ed. Washington, DC: National Academy Press.

Nienaber, J.A., and G.L. Hahn. 1984. *J. Anim. Sci.* 59:1423.

Olsson, O. 1983. *Trans. ASAE* 26:1495.

Olsson, O., and T. Andersson. 1985. *Acta Agric. Scand.* 35:55.

Patterson, D.W., et al. 1979. *J. Anim. Sci.* 49:664.

Schmidt-Nielsen, K. 1964. *Desert Animals, Physiology Problems of Heat and Water.* Oxford, England: Oxford University Press.

Seerley, R.W., et al. 1965. *J. Anim. Sci.* 24:1014.

Shields, R.G., Jr., et al. 1983. *J. Anim. Sci.* 57:43.

Sinclair, R.D. 1939. *Sci. Agric.* 20:109.

Thulin, A.J., et al. 1990. *J. Anim. Sci.* 68(Suppl 1):483.

U.S. Environmental Protection Agency. *Environmental Reporter* 4(16):663. August 17, 1973.

Wechowicz, E., et al. 1978. Biuletyn Informacyjny, Instytut Zootechniki, Zaklad Informacji, Zootechnicznej, Warsaw, Poland. 16:3.

Yang, T.S., B. Howard, and W.V. Macfarlane. 1981. *Appl. Anim. Ethol.* 7:259.

Yang, T.S., et al. 1984. *Appl. Anim. Behavior Sci.* 12:103.

PART IV

Factors Influencing Swine Nutrition

Chapter 19

Bioavailability of Amino Acids in Feedstuffs for Swine

D.A. Knabe

A major goal of the swine nutritionist is to formulate diets from a variety of feedstuffs to provide, at minimum cost, the correct amounts and balance of the essential amino acids needed to support a specified level or type of performance. To do this effectively, the nutritionist must know the amounts of amino acids in feedstuffs that are biologically available to the pig. The primary factors affecting bioavailability are the efficiencies of protein digestion and amino acid absorption and the efficiency of using amino acids at the tissue level after absorption. Common causes of reduced digestion of protein in feedstuffs are excessive heat treatment during processing, indigestible cell walls, which prevent the proteases from entering the cell, and the presence of antinutritional factors in feedstuffs (such as trypsin inhibitors, tannins, and gossypol). Possible causes of lowered utilization of amino acids after digestion are differences in rates of amino acid absorption among feedstuffs (e.g., crystalline amino acids versus native protein) and amino acid antagonisms. Because utilization of amino acids in feedstuffs varies, formulation of diets on a bioavailable amino acid basis should be more accurate than formulation on a total amino acid basis. Correct formulation of diets is important for efficient swine production; incorrect formulations result in lowered performance or unnecessarily expensive diets.

This chapter reviews the in vivo methods used to estimate bioavailability of amino acids, presents a summary of amino acid bioavailabilities, and discusses how amino acid bioavailabilities may be used in applied diet formulation. Other reviews in these areas are those of Zebrowska (1978), Low (1982), Sauer and Ozimek (1986), and Sibbald (1987). For information on the in vitro methods of estimating bioavailability and indirect in vivo methods, such as plasma amino acid levels and a mobile nylon bag technique, the reader is referred to the review of Sibbald (1987).

Two terms need to be defined before proceeding. The terms *digestibility* and *availability* have often been used interchangeably to describe the portion of an amino acid in a feedstuff that is utilized by the pig. In a strict sense, these terms have different meanings, and their definitions are related to the experimental procedures used. Digestibility measures the portion of an amino acid in a feedstuff that disappears from the digestive tract, the common assumption being that disappearance is synonymous with absorption. Availability, on the other hand, has been defined as the portion of an amino acid in a feedstuff that can be utilized by the pig for growth, development, and maintenance, and as such, measures the net result of digestion, absorption, and metabolism. Availabilities are usually determined from growth assays using the slope-ratio method.

DIGESTIBILITY OF AMINO ACIDS

Digestibilities are determined from digestion trials in which a diet is fed and the corresponding excreta (feces or ileal digesta) are collected. Samples of the diet and excreta are analyzed for amino acid content. When total collection of excreta is possible, apparent digestibility is calculated as follows:

$$((\text{amount of amino acid consumed} - \text{amount of amino acid excreted})/\text{amount of amino acid consumed}) \times 100$$

Apparent digestibility is a measure of total amino acid absorption and does not take into account the amino acids in feces or ileal digesta of endogenous origin. Endogenous amino acids are derived from proteins secreted into the digestive tract; examples are digestive enzymes and proteins in sloughed intestinal cells. True digestibility is similar to apparent digestibility, except that amino acids of endogenous origin are estimated and included in the calculation:

$$((\text{amount of amino acid consumed} - (\text{amount of amino acid excreted} - \text{amount of endogenous amino acid}))/\text{amount of amino acid consumed}) \times 100$$

True digestibilities are always higher than apparent digestibilities.

Endogenous amino acid excretion is estimated either by feeding a protein-free diet and measuring the amino acids in feces or ileal digesta or by feeding graded levels of protein from the test feedstuff and calculating fecal or ileal amino acid content at zero protein intake (Carlson and Bayley 1970). Unfortunately, the measures of endogenous amino acid excretion may not reflect the actual endogenous excretion of pigs fed diets containing a variety of feedstuffs. For example, when protein-free diets are fed, the type and level of dietary fiber affects the type and amount of endogenous secretions (Taverner et al. 1981a; Green et al. 1987). Because of the difficulties in determining endogenous amino acid excretion, apparent digestibility, although imperfect, appears to be more useful in applied swine nutrition. Also, apparent digestibility may be more meaningful because it represents the net amounts of amino acids, irrespective of origin, that are absorbed from the digestive tract.

Amino acid digestibilities were first determined over the total digestive tract (fecal digestibilities), and digestibilities in a wide range of feedstuffs have been determined using this method (Dammers 1964; Eggum 1973). Fecal amino acid digestibilities have been used, particularly in the Scandinavian countries, in formulating diets.

Fecal amino acid digestibilities are affected by degradation and synthesis of amino acids by microorganisms in the large intestine. The microflora of the large intestine can ferment most amino acids to ammonia and amines (Michel 1966). Early studies (Zebrowska 1973) showed that protein infused into the terminal ileum of pigs fed a protein-free diet was almost completely digested and absorbed from the large intestine, but nitrogen retention was not increased, the absorbed nitrogen being excreted in the urine. These studies, plus those of others (Hodgdon et al. 1977; Gargallo and Zimmerman 1981; Just et al. 1981), have led to the conclusion that the large intestine, for all practical purposes, is not a site of amino acid absorption.

The extent of fermentation in the large intestine is also not constant for all feedstuffs nor for all amino acids within a feedstuff. For example, coarsely ground wheat was more completely degraded in the large intestine than finely ground wheat (Sauer et al. 1977a), and underheated soyflakes were more completely degraded than properly heated soyflakes (Vandergrift et al. 1983). In general, feeds with lower digestibility at the end of the small intestine undergo greater fermentation in the large intestine than feeds with high digestibility at the end of the small intestine. Thus, fermentation in the large intestine tends to equalize digestibilities across feedstuffs. The action of microflora on individual amino acids within the same feed is also not constant. Of the essential amino acids, threonine and tryptophan are generally degraded to a greater extent than the other amino acids, and often there is net synthesis of methionine (Tanksley and Knabe 1984).

Because amino acids that enter the large intestine are not used by the pig for protein synthesis, and because microbial action in the large intestine differs among feedstuffs, digestibilities determined near the end of the small intestine (ileal digestibilities) are a better measure of amino acid absorption by the pig.

To collect digesta routinely from the small intestine, surgically modified pigs are needed. Four different types of surgical modification have been used. In the first method, pigs are fitted with a re-entrant cannula in the terminal ileum. Digesta passing the proximal cannula is collected and sampled, and the remaining digesta is returned through the distal cannula. The distal cannula may be placed either in the terminal ileum or in the cecum. This method allows total collection of digesta, but blockage of flow through the cannula is a practical problem, particularly when fibrous feeds are fed. This method of cannulation also requires transection of the small intestine, and some researchers feel that this alters normal gut motility and function. In the second method, a simple, open T-cannula is installed in the terminal ileum. Total collection is not possible and digestibilities must be calculated from the changes in concentration of an indigestible marker (usually chromic oxide). The surgery needed for T-cannulas is simpler than for re-entrant cannulas, and problems of blockage of the cannula are minimal unless extremely fibrous feeds are fed. The third method, developed by French workers (Darcy et al. 1980), is called the ileocolic postvalvar method. In this method, a cannula is installed past the ileocecal valve, and all digesta flows out of the cannula. The digesta is then returned via another cannula in the large intestine. The surgical procedure is difficult, but the method preserves the function of the ileocecal valve and allows evaluation of fibrous diets. The most recent method of collecting ileal digesta is to establish an ileorectal anastomosis, which allows the collection of ileal digesta from the anus. The terminal ileum is transected, and the anterior end is attached to the distal colon. This procedure has been modified by completely isolating the large intestine and installing a drainage cannula from the large intestine (Green et al. 1987).

Because four different methods have been used to determine ileal amino acid digestibilities, it is important to know whether the method affects the results obtained. In general, comparisons of re-entrant and T-cannulas indicate that digestibilities are similar for both methods (Zebrowska et al. 1978; Taverner et al. 1983). Picard et al. (1984) have indicated that ileorectal anastomosis and ileocecal re-entrant cannulas yield similar digestibilities.

Other factors that can affect digestibilities include fineness of grinding of feedstuffs, time and duration of ileal digesta collection in relation to feeding intervals, and frequency and amount of feed per day. A common practice is that of limit-feeding pigs during digestion trials, and the question arises whether values obtained under limit-feeding protocols are applicable to pigs fed ad libitum. Results of trials in which feed intake varied from approximately 1.4% of body weight per day to ad libitum intake (5.4% of body weight per day) indicate that level of feed intake has little or no effect on apparent ileal digestibilities (Jorgensen et al. 1981; Haydon et al. 1984).

Summaries of apparent ileal digestibilities of protein and selected essential amino acids in cereal grains, grain by-products, and high-protein feeds are given in Tables 19.1 and 19.2. In addition to the means, the standard deviation is reported when more than two samples have been evaluated. A comprehensive summary of ileal amino acid digestibilities has been published by Heartland Lysine, Inc., Chicago.

Several wheat and barley samples have been evaluated, but the number of samples for corn, sorghum, and oats is small. Comparisons among these latter grains should thus be made with caution. Wheat consistently has higher digestibilities than does barley. Corn and sorghum appear to have essentially the same lysine digestibility, but sorghum has higher threonine and tryptophan digestibility. The values for sorghum are for low-tannin sorghums; high-tannin sorghum would be expected to have lower digestibilities (Cousins et al. 1981). Oats has the lowest amino acid digestibility, possibly due to its higher fiber content. Excluding oats (64%), absolute differences in average lysine digestibility among the grains are small (72% to 75%).

There are substantial differences among samples of the same grain, as indicated by the large standard deviations. For example, in five samples of corn, the digestibility of lysine ranged from 57% to 82% and had a standard deviation of 9. Undoubtedly, some of this variation is due to differences in experimental procedures among the trials. Because these are apparent digestibilities and because the grains are low in these amino acids, small changes in endogenous secretions can have a large impact on apparent digestibilities. This is particularly true for threonine because of the high concentration of this amino acid in endogenous secretions (Low 1979). Other factors that may affect digestibilities are the variety of the grain and agronomic practices that influence the structure and nutrient content of the grain. Also, fineness of grinding has been shown to affect apparent digestibilities (Sauer et al. 1977a; Owsley et al. 1981).

Table 19.1 Apparent Ileal Digestibility of Protein and Selected Amino Acids in Cereal Grains and Grain By-Products

Feedstuff	*Reference*[a]	*No of Samples*[b]	*Protein*	*Lys*	*Thr*	*Trp*	*Ile*
Barley	3,4,5,8,9,12,14	10(1)	75±3[c]	73±4	69±5	73	78±3
Corn	3,5,7,12,14	5(2)	78±4	72±9	71±5	72	83±5
Oats	6,8	2(1)	62	64	54	59	73
Sorghum	5,14	2(1)	81	75	78	80	88
Wheat	1,2,3,4,5,8,12,14	16(1)	82±5	75±6	73±7	81	85±4
Brewers' dried grain	10,13	3	70±3	68±4	67±4	71±3	79±2
Corn gluten feed	11,13	3	52±6	41±11	47±5	33±6	59±7
Oat groats	14	1	84	82	78	81	86
Wheat bran	8	1	62	74	55		
Wheat middlings	10,13,14	6	67±3	72±3	60±3	72±5	70±5

Abbreviations: Lys, lysine; Thr, threonine; Trp, tryptophan; Ile, isoleucine.

[a]References are as follows: 1, Ivan and Farrell 1976; 2, Sauer et al. 1977a; 3, Sauer et al. 1977b; 4, Sauer et al. 1981; 5, Taverner et al. 1981b; 6, Zebrowska et al. 1981; 7, Adeola et al. 1985; 8, Just et al. 1985; 9, Moughan and Smith 1985; 10, Knabe et al. 1986a; 11, Knabe et al. 1986b; 12, Green et al. 1987; 13, La Rue et al. 1987; 14, Lin et al. 1987.

[b]Number of observations for tryptophan digestibility in parentheses when the number differs from the total number of observations.

[c]Standard deviation.

Table 19.2 Apparent Ileal Digestibility of Protein and Selected Amino Acids in Protein Feedstuffs

Feedstuff	*Reference*[a]	*No. of Samples*[b]	*Protein*	*Lys*	*Thr*	*Trp*	*Ile*
Blood meal, ring-dried	20	3	87±2[c]	93±2	87±2	89±4	70±10
Canola meal	9,20	3(1)	70±1	74±1	67±2	71	76±1
Casein	2,4,16	3(1)	89±4	95±2	86±3	91	90±3
Corn gluten meal	20	1	88	80	86	72	92
Cottonseed meal, glanded	4,5,6,18,20	6(4)	75±5	56±11	59±7	72±5	65±7
Cottonseed meal, glandless	6,15	2	83	82	78	81	85
Feather meal, hydrolyzed	20	1	63	40	66	60	75
Fish meal	8,10,12,13,20	7(5)	78±6	84±6	79±5	74±3	83±6
Meat and bone meal	3,5,13,14,20	13(11)	66±6	68±8	61±8	54±10	69±8
Peanut meal	19,20	4(3)	76±7	70±9	65±11	71±5	78±7
Poultry by-product meal	20	4	76±2	86±2	75±3	79±3	80±2
Rapeseed meal	9,14	2	70	75	67		78
Skim milk, dried	14	1	86	94	84		
Soybeans, extruded	11,20	2	74	80	69	70	74
Soybean meal, hulled	2,5,6,11,15,20	7	79±4	85±3	75±3	80±4	82±2
Soybean meal, dehulled	1,3,9,11,13,14,17,18,19	12(6)	80±2	86±3	76±3	78±1	84±3
Sunflower meal	7,13,14,19,20	6(2)	74±1	73±3	70±3	76	78±2

Abbreviations: Lys, lysine; Thr, threnonine; Trp, tryptophan; Ile, isoleucine.

[a]References are as follows: 1, Holmes et al. 1974; 2, Zebrowska et al. 1977; 3, Zebrowska and Tanskley 1979; 4, Haydon et al. 1981; 5, Tanksley et al. 1981a; 6, Tanksley et al. 1981b; 7, Atwal and Stothers 1982; 8, Darcy et al. 1982; 9, Sauer et al. 1982; 10, Poppe et al. 1983; 11, Rudolph et al. 1983; 12, Darcy-Vrillon and LaPlace 1984; 13, Jorgensen et al. 1984; 14, Just et al. 1985; 15, LaRue et al. 1985; 16, Kies et al. 1986; 17, Chang et al. 1987; 18, Garren et al. 1987; 19, Green et al. 1988; 20, Knabe et al. 1989.

[b]Number of observations for tryptophan digestibility in parentheses when the number differs from the total number of samples.

[c]Standard deviation.

Among the grain by-products, digestibilities are highest for oat groats, lowest for corn gluten feed, and intermediate for brewers' dried grains and wheat middlings. As noted for the grains, there is a large amount of variation among samples of the same feedstuff. The low digestibility of corn gluten feed may reflect its higher fiber content and the heat applied during drying. Wheat middlings, a common feedstuff used in commercial diets, has lysine and tryptophan digestibilities similar to corn.

In general, the apparent digestibilities of amino acids in high-protein feeds are highest for ring-dried blood meal, casein, corn gluten meal, dried skim milk, fish meal, poultry by-product meal, soybean meals, and extruded soybeans. Values are intermediate for canola meal, meat and bone meal, peanut meal, rapeseed meal, and sunflower meal. Glanded cottonseed meal and feather meal have the lowest digestibilities.

Between hulled and dehulled soybean meal, very small differences are found in amino acid digestibility, although most values are 1 to 2 percentage units higher for dehulled meal. The amount of heat treatment is the major factor known to affect amino acid digestibilities of soybean products. Underheating does not adequately inactivate trypsin inhibitors, resulting in lowered digestibility (Vandergrift et al. 1983), and overheating damages the protein and lowers digestibility (Garren 1987). With commercially processed soybean meals, the degree of heat treatment appears to be relatively consistent and of little practical concern (Chang et al. 1987). This may be the reason that variation in apparent digestibilities of the soybean meals is small, even when measured across a number of trials using different methodologies.

Differences in the raw material and the severity of heat treatment are probably responsible for some of the variation in digestibilities found among samples of meat and bone meal. In a recent study, Knabe et al. (1989) evaluated ten meat and bone meals processed with different types of commercial equipment. They found that meat and bone meals processed with modern equipment, which apply less heat, had higher digestibilities than meals processed by traditional methods, which apply more heat. Amino acid digestibilities of two of the meals were essentially equal to those of soybean meal and supported greater pig performance than meals with lower digestibility (Knabe et al. 1987). Differences in heat treatment during processing may also be responsible for some of the variation found in fish meals.

Poultry by-product meal has been evaluated at one research station only, so the results may not be representative of all meals. However, in contrast to the meat and bone meals, poultry by-product meal appears to have uniformly high digestibility. It should be noted that the blood meals evaluated were ring-dried, a process that uses minimal heat. Vat-dried blood meal would be expected to have much lower digestibilities (Waibel et al. 1977).

The low digestibilities for glanded cottonseed meal are probably caused by the formation of indigestible gossypol-amino acid complexes during processing. Chlorogenic acid is a constituent of sunflower seed and has been shown to bind with proteins and amino acids during processing. Whether these compounds lower digestibility is uncertain. The causes of the relatively lower digestibilities of canola, rapeseed, and peanut meal are not evident.

AVAILABILITY OF AMINO ACIDS

Amino acid availabilities are determined from growth assays. Some type of slope-ratio method is the most common procedure (Batterham et al. 1979; Baker 1978). A basal diet is formulated to be adequate in all nutrients except the amino acid under investigation. Two series of diets are used. In one series, the crystalline amino acid is added in incremental amounts to the basal diet, and in the other series, the test feedstuff is added in incremental amounts to provide the same amounts of the test amino acid as in the first series. These substitutions are usually made at the expense of starch. The diets are fed and pig performance (e.g., weight gain, feed efficiency, or carcass gain) for each series of diets is regressed on intake of the test amino acid, thus creating two regression lines. The regression line from the first series of diets describes the response in performance due to the addition of the crystalline amino acid. The other regression line describes the response due to the addition of the amino acid from the test feedstuff. The ratio of the two slopes (test feedstuff:crystalline amino acid) represents the availability value. For the slope-ratio method to be valid, the levels of amino acid fed must result in a linear response in performance, and the two regression lines must have a common intercept.

Some basic assumptions of the slope-ratio assay are that the crystalline amino acid is 100% available, and that the response in performance from adding the test feedstuff is due only to its content of the test amino acid. The second assumption has received the most criticism. The inclusion of the test feedstuff alters the dietary concentrations of many nutrients, and the response in performance may be due to nutrient interactions or some other nonnutritive factor in the feedstuff. Baker (1978) and Sato et al. (1987) have proposed that the best estimates of availability are obtained when the diets used to establish the standard curve contain additional crystalline amino acids to obtain the same amino acid excesses found from the additions of the test feedstuff.

Amino acid availabilities are superior to amino acid digestibilities in that they measure, indirectly, both amino acid digestibility and utilization after absorption from the digestive tract. They are also appealing because the response that is measured is a trait of economic importance in swine production. However, the labor and costs of conducting these assays limit their usefulness for surveying differences in amino acid availability across a large number of feedstuffs. A summary of amino acid availabilities measured in swine is presented in Table 19.3.

USE OF BIOAVAILABLE AMINO ACIDS IN DIET FORMULATION

Each of the three methods of estimating amino acid bioavailability has advantages and limitations for diet formulation. Fecal digestibilities are the simplest to determine, and some researchers (Just 1980; Lennis 1983) contend that the effects of fermentation in the large intestine are not large enough to invalidate this method. Ileal digestibilities measure amino acid absorption more accurately than fecal digestibilities, but they are more difficult to determine. A complete data base of ileal-digestible amino acid con-

Table 19.3 Availabilities of Lysine and Tryptophan in Feedstuffs Determined Using the Slope-Ratio Method with Pigs[a]

	Lysine[b]			*Tryptophan*[c]		
Feedstuffs	*No. of Samples*	*Mean*	*Reference*[d]	*No. of Samples*	*Mean*	*Reference*[d]
Blood meal, ring-dried	2	108	4			
Corn				1	94	5
Cottonseed meal, glanded	2	41	1,2	1	81	5
Dried skim milk	1	85	1			
Meat or meat and bone meal	7	67±17	1,4	1	82	5
Peanut meal	1	57	3			
Rapeseed meal	2	87	2			
Sorghum				1	86	5
Soybean meal	3	90±7	1,3	1	95	5
Sunflower meal	3	60±6	2			

[a] Values are means ± standard deviation.

[b] Availability is based on feed:carcass gain.

[c] Availability is based on weight gain.

[d] References are as follows: 1, Batterham et al. 1979; 2, Batterham et al. 1981; 3, Batterham et al. 1984; 4, Batterham et al. 1986; 5, Sato et al. 1987.

tents for feeds is not currently available, but research continues to develop such a data base. Just et al. (1985) reported that ileal-digestible protein and amino acids had slightly higher correlations to deposited protein than fecal-digestible protein and amino acids. Examination of the lysine availabilities in Table 19.3 and lysine digestibilities in Table 19.2 shows, in general, that both methods rank the feedstuffs in the same order. Because of the increased precision of ileal digestibilities over fecal digestibilities and because of the greater ease of determining ileal amino acid digestibilities than availabilities, it appears that ileal digestibilities are, for the present, the most useful means of estimating amino acid bioavailabilities for use in diet formulation.

Formulation of diets on an ileal-digestible amino acid basis should be more accurate than formulation on a total amino acid basis when the following conditions are found:

1. Ileal digestibilities of amino acids in the feedstuffs are reasonably well known and vary among feedstuffs.
2. Associative effects are minimal.
3. Differences in ileal digestible amino acid content of diets result in comparable differences in pig performance.

From the preceding section it is evident that large differences in ileal amino acid digestibility exist among some feedstuffs, but other differences are relatively small. The differences among the cereal grains are not large, with the exception of oats, and these differences alone will have minimal impact on diet formulation due to the low content of the limiting amino acids in grains. Use of grain by-products, on the other hand, will have a greater impact due to the larger differences in amino acid digestibility and their higher amino acid content. The greatest variation exists among the high-protein feeds, and formulation on a digestible amino acid basis will have its greatest impact when feeds such as meat and bone meal, peanut meal, sunflower meal, and glanded cottonseed meal are used to replace soybean meal in diets. Another important use of bioavialability data is when crystalline amino acids, which are essentially 100% digestible (Huisman et al. 1986; Leibholz 1986; Shipley et al. 1987), are added to replace a portion of the protein feeds in pig diets. The digestible amino acid requirements of swine have not been determined, and this limits the routine use of formulation on a digestible amino acid basis. It is possible, however, to survey the existing literature on amino acid requirements and calculate the digestible amino acid requirements using the average digestibility values of the dietary ingredients. Until more research is reported, these estimates will have to suffice.

In the majority of trials determining ileal digestibilities, the test feedstuff is fed as the only source of dietary protein. Use of these values in diet formulation is not valid if feeding a mixture of feeds alters the digestibility of amino acids in the individual ingredients. This possibility has not been investigated thoroughly, but the limited data (Garren 1987; Imbeah et al. 1988) suggest that associative effects are minimal.

It is difficult to verify that differences in dietary ileal-digestible amino acid contents result in corresponding differences in pig performance. Tanksley and Knabe (1984) and Knabe et al. (1985, 1987) have reported the results of growth trials comparing diets with the same total lysine or tryptophan contents but with different digestible lysine or tryptophan contents. They also evaluated the effects of equalizing digestible lysine or tryptophan content of the diets through the addition of crystalline lysine or tryptophan. A consistent finding in all trials was that performance was poorer on diets having a lower digestible lysine or tryptophan content. The addition of crystalline lysine or tryptophan to the diets with lower digestible contents improved performance in most instances. Although this type of data indicates that differences in digestible amino acid content caused differences in performance, it is not possible to determine if the effect was specifically caused by the differences in content of digestible lysine or tryptophan. This is because the diets that differed in digestible amino acid content were composed of different feedstuffs and the addition of crystalline amino acids increased both digestible and total content. Leibholz (1985) suggested that differences in ileal-digested lysine can be used as an indicator of lysine utilization by the pig. Utilization in that study was based on retention of ileal-digestible lysine in the carcass.

SUMMARY

Knowledge of the proportion of the essential amino acids in feedstuffs that are bioavailable to the pig is essential to accurate diet formulation. This proportion has been estimated through digestion trials, which estimate amino acid absorption, and by the slope-ratio method, which combines the effects of digestion, absorption, and metabolism. Digestibilities are reported as either apparent or true, the latter correcting for endogenous amino acid output. Because of the difficulties of accurately measuring endogenous amino acid output, apparent digestibilities are more useful in practical swine feeding. Digestibilities determined near the end of the small intestine (ileal digestibilities) are superior to digestibilities determined over the total tract (fecal digestibilities) because they are determined prior to the microbial action in the large intestine. Availabilities determined from valid slope-ratio assays probably measure differences among feedstuffs in their ability to supply amino acids used for protein synthesis more accurately than do digestibilities. The labor and cost involved in availability assays limits the usefulness as part of a diet formulation system.

The apparent ileal digestibilities of a number of feedstuffs have been reported. Cereal grains do not differ greatly in digestibility of lysine, the most limiting amino acid in most swine diets. Grain by-products and high-protein feeds have a wider range in digestibility. Formulation of diets on a digestible amino acid basis should be more accurate than formulation on a total amino acid basis when feedstuffs that differ greatly in amino acid digestibility are used or when crystalline amino acids are added to lower the content of protein feeds in the diet and simultaneously reduce the cost of production.

REFERENCES

Adeola, O., et al. 1985. *Ontario Swine Res. Rev.* p. 2.

Atwal, A.S., and S.C. Stothers. 1982. *Proceedings of the Nutrition Conference Feed Manufacturers.* pp. 59–65. University of Guelph.

Baker, D.H. 1978. *Proceedings of the Georgia Nutrition Conference.* pp. 1–12. Atlanta. Athens: University of Georgia.

Batterham, E.S., R.D. Murison, and L.M. Andersen. 1984. *Br. J. Nutr.* 51:85.

Batterham, E.S., R.D. Murison, and C.E. Lewis. 1979. *Br. J. Nutr.* 41:383.

Batterham, E.S., R.D. Murison, and R.F. Lowe. 1981. *Br. J. Nutr.* 45:401.

Batterham, E.S., et al. 1986. *Br. J. Nutr.* 55:427.

Carlson, K., and H.S. Bayley. 1970. *J. Nutr.* 100:1353.

Chang, C.J., et al. 1987. *J. Anim. Sci.* 65:1273.

Cousins, B.W., et al. 1981. *J. Anim. Sci.* 53:1524.

Dammers, J. 1964. "Verteringgsstudies bij het varken. Faktoren van invloed op de vertering der veevoeder-componenten en de verteerbaarheid der aminozuren." Ph.D. thesis, Institut Veevoedingsonderzoek, Leuven, Belgium.

Darcy, B., J.P. LaPlace, and P.H. Duee. 1982. *Ann. Zootech. (Paris)* 31:279.

Darcy, B., J.P. LaPlace, and P.A. Villiers. 1980. *Ann. Zootech. (Paris)* 29:147.

Darcy-Vrillon, B., and J.P. LaPlace. 1984. *Ann. Zootech. (Paris)* 33:467.

Eggum, B.O. 1973. "A study of certain factors influencing protein digestibility in rats and pigs." Ph.D. thesis, National Institute of Animal Science, Copenhagen, Denmark.

Gargallo, J., and D. Zimmermann. 1981. *J. Nutr.* 111:1390.

Garren, J.B. 1987. "Formulation of swine diets based on apparent digestible amino acid values determined at the end of the small intestine in pigs." M.S. thesis, Texas A&M University, College Station.

Green, S., et al. 1987. *J. Sci. Food Agric.* 41:29.

Green, S., et al. 1988. *J. Sci. Food Agric.* 42:119.

Haydon, K.D., D.A. Knabe, and T.D. Tanksley, Jr. 1981. *Proceedings of Swine Short Course, Texas Animal Agriculture Conference.* pp. 82–89. College Station: Texas A&M University.

Haydon, K.D., D.A. Knabe, and T.D. Tanksley, Jr. 1984. *J. Anim. Sci.* 59:717.

Hodgdon, E.S., F.D. Horney, and H.S. Bayley. 1977. *Can. J. Anim. Sci.* 57:832 (Abstr.).

Holmes, J.H.G., H.S. Bayley, and P.A. Leadbeater. 1974. *Br. J. Nutr.* 32:479.

Huisman, J., et al. 1986. *J. Anim. Physiol. Anim. Nutr.* 55:267.

Imbeah, M., W.C. Sauer, and R. Mosenthin. 1988. *J. Anim. Sci.* 66:1409.

Ivan, M., and D.J. Farrell. 1976. *Anim. Prod.* 23:111.

Jorgensen, H., W.C. Sauer, and A. Just. 1981. *J. Anim. Sci.* 53(Suppl. 1):249 (Abstr.).

Jorgensen, H., W.C. Sauer, and P.A. Thacker. 1984. *J. Anim. Sci.* 58:926.

Just, A. 1980. In: *Current Concepts of Digestion and Absorption in Pigs.* Low, A.G., and I.G. Partridge (Eds.). pp. 66–77. Reading, U.K.: National Institute for Research in Dairying.

Just, A., H. Jorgensen, and J.A. Fernandez. 1981. *Br. J. Nutr.* 46:209.

Just, A., H. Jorgensen, and J.A. Fernandez. 1985. *Livest. Prod. Sci.* 12:145.

Kies, A.K., P.J. Moughan, and W.C. Smith. 1986. *Anim. Feed Sci. Technol.* 16:169.

Knabe, D.A., and T.D. Tanksley, Jr. 1985. *J. Anim. Sci.* 61(Suppl. 1):323 (Abstr.).

Knabe, D.A., D.C. LaRue, and G. Martinez. 1987. *J. Anim. Sci.* 65(Suppl. 1):299 (Abstr.).

Knabe, D.A., et al. 1986a. *J. Anim. Sci.* 63(Suppl. 1):279 (Abstr.).

Knabe, D.A., et al. 1986b. *J. Anim. Sci.* 63(Suppl. 1):278 (Abstr.).

Knabe, D.A., et al. 1989. *J. Anim. Sci.* 67:441.

LaRue, D.C., D.A. Knabe, and T.D. Tanksley, Jr. 1985. *J. Anim. Sci.* 64:95.

LaRue, D.C., D.A. Knabe, and T.D. Tanksley, Jr. 1987. *J. Anim. Sci.* 65(Suppl. 1):126 (Abstr.).

Leibholz, J. 1985. *Br. J. Nutr.* 53:615.

Leibholz, J., et al. 1986. *Anim. Feed Sci. Tech.* 15:141.
Lennis, N.P. 1983. *Fourth International Symposium of Protein Metabolism and Nutrition.* pp. 385–389. Cleremont-Ferrand, France. Paris: Institut National de la Recherche Agronomique.
Lin, F.D., D.A. Knabe, and T.D. Tanksley, Jr. 1987. *J. Anim. Sci.* 64:1655.
Low, A.G. 1979. *Br. J. Nutr.* 41:147.
Low, A.G. 1982. *Livest. Prod. Sci.* 9:511.
Michel, M.C. 1966. *Ann. Biol. Anim. Biochem. Biophys.* 6:33.
Moughan, P.J., and W.C. Smith. 1985. *N.Z. J. Agric. Res.* 28:365.
NRC. 1988. *Nutrient Requirements of Swine.* 9th ed. Washington, DC: National Academy Press.
Owsley, W.F., D.A. Knabe, and T.D. Tanksley, Jr. 1981. *J. Anim. Sci.* 52:557.
Picard, M., et al. 1984. *J. Rech. Porcine Fr.* 16:355.
Poppe, S., et al. 1983. *Arch. Tiernahrung* 33:155.
Rudolph, B.C., et al. 1983. *J. Anim. Sci.* 57:373.
Sato, H., et al. 1987. *J. Anim. Sci.* 64:191.
Sauer, W.C., R. Cichon, and R. Misir. 1982. *J. Anim. Sci.* 54:292.
Sauer, W.C., and L. Ozimek. 1986. *Livest. Prod. Sci.* 15:367.
Sauer, W.C., S.C. Stothers, and R.J. Parker. 1977a. *Can. J. Anim. Sci.* 57:775.
Sauer, W.C., S.C. Stothers, and G.D. Phillips. 1977b. *Can. J. Anim. Sci.* 57:585.
Sauer, W.C., et al. 1981. *Can. J. Anim. Sci.* 61:793.
Shipley, T.M., D.A. Knabe, and G. Martinez. 1987. *J. Anim. Sci.* 65(Suppl. 1):297 (Abstr.).
Sibbald, I.R. 1987. *Can. J. Anim. Sci.* 67:221.
Tanksley, T.D., Jr., and D.A. Knabe. 1984. In: *Recent Advances in Animal Nutrition-1984.* Haresign, W., and D.J.A. Cole (Eds.). pp. 75–95. London: Butterworths.
Tanksley, T.D., Jr., et al. 1981a. *Proceedings of Swine Short Course, Texas Animal Agriculture Conference.* pp. 71–81. College Station: Texas A&M University.
Tanksley, T.D., Jr., et al. 1981b. *J. Anim. Sci.* 52:769.
Taverner, M.R., D.M. Curic, and C.J. Rayner. 1983. *J. Sci. Food Agric.* 34:122.
Taverner, M.R., I.D. Hume, and D.J. Farrell. 1981a. *Br. J. Nutr.* 46:149.
Taverner, M.R., I.D. Hume, and D.J. Farrell. 1981b. *Br. J. Nutr.* 46:159.
Vandergrift, W.L., D.A. Knabe, T.D. Tanksley, Jr. 1983. *J. Anim. Sci.* 57:1215.
Waibel, P.E., et al. 1977. *J. Agric. Food Chem.* 25:171.
Zebrowska, T. 1973. *Rocz. Nauk. Rolnic.* 95B:85.
Zebrowska, T. 1978. *Feedstuffs* 50:15, 43.
Zebrowska, T., and T.D. Tanksley, Jr. 1979. *Proceedings of Swine Short Course, Texas Animal Agriculture Conference,* pp. 67–75. College Station: Texas A&M University.
Zebrowska, T., L. Buraczewska, and S. Buraczewski. 1977. *Fifth International Symposium on Amino Acids.* pp. 1–3. Budpest, Hungary.
Zebrowska, T., L. Buraczewska, and H. Zebrowska. 1981. *Sixth International Symposium on Amino Acids.* Seroc, Poland.
Zebrowska, T., et al. 1978. *Rocz. Nauk Rolnic.* 99B:75.

Chapter 20

Bioavailability of Minerals and Vitamins

D.H. Baker

Minerals and vitamins present in feed ingredients, and even from crystalline sources, are generally not fully available when compared with a common and generally well-utilized source of the mineral or vitamin in question. Mineral elements may be bound in phytate complexes or attached to fiber, and vitamins often exist as either precursor compounds or as coenzymes that may also be bound or complexed in some manner. Hence, gut processes are required to release or convert both minerals and vitamins to absorbable chemical entities.

The literature on mineral and vitamin bioavailability is much more extensive for chicks and rats than for swine. Indeed, in several instances no data whatsoever exist for bioavailability estimates made using swine. This review will cover pertinent aspects of mineral and vitamin bioavailability, with an emphasis on swine. Laboratory animal data will nonetheless be used in those cases where limited pig data are available.

MINERAL BIOAVAILABILITY

Several excellent reviews are available that deal with comparative mineral bioavailability (Nelson 1964; Ammerman and Miller 1972; Peeler 1972; Cantor et al. 1975a, 1975b; Hays 1976; Harms et al. 1976; Peo 1976; Miller 1978; O'Dell et al. 1979; Harmon 1979; Cromwell 1979; Miller 1980). Most of these have dealt with relative bioavailability of inorganic rather than organic (i.e., feed) sources of mineral elements.

Calcium

Other than the recent data from Cromwell's laboratory (Cromwell et al. 1983; Ross et al. 1984; Cromwell et al. 1985), no definitive information is available on calcium

(Ca) bioavailability for swine. The Kentucky work showed that limestone, oyster shell, gypsum, marble dust, and aragonite were essentially 100% available as sources of Ca, relative to a $CaCO_3$ precipitate used as a standard. Calcium bioavailability in dolomitic limestone, however, was lower, ranging from 51% to 78%. Ross et al. (1984) also established that particle size of the Ca sources evaluated had no effect on the bioavailability of Ca. Only one feed ingredient, alfalfa meal, was evaluated by Cromwell et al. (1983). Using slope-ratio analyses (bone breaking strength regressed on Ca intake), Ca in dehydrated alfalfa meal was only 21% available relative to Ca in the $CaCO_3$ precipitate standard.

Based on poultry data reviewed by Harms et al. (1976) and Peeler (1972), it can be generalized that 100% bioavailability of Ca exists in dicalcium phosphate, tricalcium phosphate, defluorinated rock phosphate, Ca gluconate, Ca citrate, Ca lactate, Ca sulfate, and bone meal. Little work has been done on Ca bioavailability in protein- and energy-furnishing feed ingredients in any species. It is nonetheless generally assumed that Ca availability in meat and fish meals is equivalent to that in feed-grade limestone. Plant-source Ca is probably not fully available, although except for University of Kentucky work on alfalfa meal, quantitative estimates are not available.

Phosphorus

A summary of phosphorus (P) bioavailability estimates in various inorganic and organic feed ingredients for swine and poultry is contained in the review article by Miller (1980). Current thinking regarding turkey nutrition is that relative to commercial mono-dicalcium phosphate (i.e., $Ca(H_2PO_4)_2$ set at 100%), P availability in commercial dicalcium phosphate is about 90%, and that in defluorinated rock phosphate is about 80% (Waibel et al. 1984). Those familiar with the commercial feed-grade phosphate industry generally assume that all feed-grade dicalcium phosphates are actually mixtures of $Ca(H_2PO_4)_2$ and $CaHPO_4$, and both compounds are variable in water of hydration, e.g., $CaHPO_4{\cdot}H_2O$ or $CaHPO_4{\cdot}2H_2O$ (T.S. Nelson, personal communication). Thus, Ca or P analysis is perhaps the only accurate means of establishing the ratio of $CaHPO_4$ (23% Ca, 18.5% P) to $Ca(H_2PO_4)_2$ (16% Ca and 21% P). A rule of thumb for swine formulation would consist of setting the P availability in the purchased feed-grade phosphate source at 100% (regardless of whether labeled dicalcium or mono-dicalcium phosphate) and then assuming that P bioavailability in commercial defluorinated phosphate is 90%.

Plant-source P is relatively unavailable (Nelson 1967), although some feed ingredients (e.g., wheat and barley) contain phytase, which may improve P availability somewhat. Most swine nutritionists consider the P contained in corn-soybean meal combinations used in commercial diets to be 30% bioavailable, primarily because 60% to 70% of the P in corn-soybean combinations is present as phytate-P (Erdman 1979; Cromwell 1985). Cromwell (1985) estimated the bioavailability of P in corn to be only 12% and that in soybean meal 25% to 39%, relative to $CaHPO_4$. He further estimated that the P in wheat and wheat by-products was 35% to 50% available, that in rice bran, 25%, cottonseed meal, 0%, and peanut meal, 12%. He considered the P contributed by fish meal and alfalfa meal to be 100% bioavailable. It should be noted that high-moisture corn contains up to four times the bioavailable P content of dry number-2 yellow corn (Cromwell 1985).

Fermentation-derived P is highly available because much of the P in yeast, distillers' solubles, etc., is in the form of nucleic acid-P, most of which is RNA. Research using chicks has established that the P in RNA is close to 100% bioavailable relative to KH_2PO_4 used as a standard (Burns and Baker 1976). Meat- and fish-source P is likewise generally considered 100% bioavailable as compared with commercial dicalcium phosphate.

Phytate

There is much confusion regarding effects of phytates on not only P bioavailability but on the trace mineral status of animals. Phytates added to various research diets are generally provided as phytic acid or as the sodium (Na) or Ca salt of phytic acid. These compounds are not the same as the mixed calcium-magnesium-potassium (Ca-Mg-K) salt of phytic acid generally found in plant-source feed ingredients (Nelson 1967; Erdman 1979). Moreover, the negative effects of added phytates on trace mineral utilization are affected significantly by dietary Ca level (O'Dell et al. 1964; Hendricks et al. 1969; Bafundo et al. 1984a). Research in our laboratory using chicks, for example, has shown that the zinc (Zn) antagonizing effect of 1.2% supplemental Na phytate when added to a typical corn-soybean meal broiler diet is evident only when Ca is provided in the diet in a quantity at least twice the National Research Council (NRC) recommended level (NRC 1984; Bafundo et al. 1984a).

Knowledge of where phytate occurs in plant-source feedstuffs is important to proper interpretation of effects of such ingredients on mineral bioavailability (Erdman 1979). Corn is unique among the cereal grains because 90% of the phytate present is located in the germ portion of the kernel. Wheat and rice germ also contain considerable phytate, but the hull portion is also rich. Thus, wheat and rice bran are extremely rich in phytate (Halpin and Baker 1987). Soybeans, too, are different from most other oilseeds in that phytic acid is contained in protein bodies distributed throughout the seed. Hence, protein isolates have been found to be richer in phytate than is soybean meal (Erdman 1979). Phytic acid in peanuts, cottonseed, and sunflower seeds is concentrated only in crystaloid and globoid substructures. Diekert et al. (1962) isolated two protein-rich fractions from peanuts and found one to contain 0.5% phytic acid and the other, 5.7%.

Potassium

Definitive information on K bioavailability from various K sources is lacking. Corn-soybean meal diets for swine are rich in K, making K bioavailability a subject of primarily academic interest. Peeler (1972) predicted that K_2CO_3, $KHCO_3$, K_2HPO_4, K acetate, and K citrate would be 100% available, relative to the K in KCl.

E.R. Miller and co-workers recently addressed the subject of K bioavailability in various K sources for young pigs (Combs et al. 1985; Combs and Miller 1985). Among response criteria examined, that is, blood K, urinary K, and K retention, only K retention (balance trials) responded linearly to K intake for all K sources examined. Based on slope-ratio methodology and within the realm of experimental error, K from K_2CO_3, $KHCO_3$, corn, and soybean meal was judged essentially 100% bioavailable relative to K acetate, which was used as the standard.

Magnesium

Judging from Peeler's review (1972) and from field observation of Mg deficiency, Mg bioavailability is probably more of a problem in ruminant nutrition than in nonruminant nutrition. Miller (1980) estimated that the Mg supplied by feed-grade sources of MgO, $MgSO_4$, and $MgCO_3$ was 100% bioavailable for swine relative to the Mg in reagent-grade MgO. He also estimated that grains and concentrates would have Mg bioavailabilities of 50% to 60% as compared with MgO. Cook's (1973) research using rats appears to be the only nonruminant study in which bioavailability of Mg was determined directly, rather than estimated. He found oxide, chloride, carbonate, phosphate, sulfate, and silicate salts of Mg to be equally bioavailable.

Sodium and Chloride

There appears to be no good evidence on the relative utilization of Na and chlorine (Cl) from various sources. Using information from requirement studies, one can generalize that NaCl, Na_2SO_4, $NaHCO_3$, Na acetate, and Na citrate are equal in bioavailable Na activity and that NaCl, KCl, NH_4Cl, and $CaCl_2 \cdot 2H_2O$ are equivalent in bioavailable Cl activity. Because Na and Cl (also K) are so intimately involved in acid-base balance and in urinary excretion of cations and anions, suitable bioassays of availability are difficult to develop. Defluorinated phosphates are generally rich in Na, and this ingredient is not uncommon in swine diets. Miller (1980) estimated that Na in this product is 83% available relative to the Na in NaCl.

Iron

Baby pigs are uniquely susceptible to iron (Fe) deficiency anemia due to their rapid growth rate, confinement rearing (little access to soil), and lack of placental or mammary iron transfer from dam to offspring. Thus, it has become standard practice to give newborn piglets Fe injections during the first few days of life. Braude et al. (1962) and Miller et al. (1973) demonstrated that over 90% of the Fe from Fe-dextran (100- or 200-mg injections) is incorporated into hemoglobin over the ensuing 4 weeks. Later, Harmon (1974), Cornelius and Harmon (1976), Thoren-Tolling (1975), and Schmitz and Miller (1973) observed that similar Fe-dextran doses administered orally during the first 12 hours after birth (prior to gut closure) likewise promote efficient Fe incorporation into hemoglobin.

There is no effective means of increasing placental or mammary transfer of Fe from the sow to her offspring. Work at Cornell University showed conclusively that whether Fe sources are administered to dams orally or via injection, neither piglet Fe stores at birth nor Fe concentration in milk is increased sufficiently to prevent anemia in the offspring (Pond et al. 1961). Iron sources fed to lactating sows at high levels do elicit hemoglobin responses in the nursing piglets, but this has been shown to be more due to Fe consumption from the Fe in the dam's feces than to an increased concentration of Fe in the dam's milk.

Pig studies on Fe bioavailability have revealed essentially 100% availability of Fe in $FeSO_4 \cdot 2H_2O$, $FeSO_4 \cdot 7H_2O$, Fe citrate, and Fe choline citrate (relative to Fe in $FeSO_4 \cdot H_2O$), and the chick and rat data of Fritz et al. (1970) have largely confirmed these findings (Miller et al. 1977; Miller 1978; Harmon et al. 1967; Ullrey et al. 1973; Furugouri and Kawabata 1975). Chick and rat data indicate that Fe ammonium citrate, $FeCl_2$, Fe fumarate, and Fe gluconate are also 100% bioavailable, while $FeCl_3$, $Fe_2(SO_4)_3$, and Fe carbonate are less available. Oxides of Fe are almost totally unavailable, while carbonates are variable in availability, depending on from where they were mined (Harmon et al. 1969; Ammerman et al. 1974).

Commercial dicalcium and defluorinated phosphates are rich in Fe, which constitutes from 1.0% to 1.5% of these ingredients. Bioavailability of Fe in these products generally ranges from 35% to 85% (Ammerman and Miller 1972; Kornegay 1972; Miller 1978; Czarnecki-Maulden 1990).

It is conventional in human nutrition circles to categorize Fe sources as heme or nonheme in nature. However, this categorization often leads to misinterpretation, since many nutritionists unwittingly conclude that all animal sources of Fe are heme Fe, when in fact they are generally a mixture of heme (highly available), ferritin (less available), and hemosiderin (poorly available) cf. Layrisse et al. (1975) and Bogunjoko et al. (1983). To illustrate the confusion, liver (fresh or dried) is rich in Fe but the Fe present therein is about 10% heme Fe and 90% nonheme Fe. Thus, liver Fe may be lower in availability than the Fe in poultry by-product meal or meat meal (Chausow 1987). While Fe in commercial blood meal would be expected to be highly available, values ranging from 40% to 50% (relative to $FeSO_4 \cdot 7H_2O$) were listed by Miller (1980) for flash-dried blood meal and only 22% was reported by Chausow and Czarnecki-Maulden (1988a). It is probable, therefore, that the drying process influences the bioavailability of Fe in dried blood meals.

The Fe in grains and oilseed meals may be largely bound to or complexed with phytate, fiber, or protein. As such, its bioavailability would be expected to be lower than that of $FeSO_4 \cdot H_2O$. Data on availability of Fe in these sources are limited. Without definitive data, one should probably assume that cereal grain and oilseed Fe sources are no more than 50% available relative to $FeSO_4 \cdot H_2O$.

Chausow (1987) and Chausow and Czarnecki-Maulden (1988a,b) have recently evaluated the utilization of several Fe sources (relative to $FeSO_4 \cdot 7H_2O$) in chicks, cats, and dogs. Based on their chick bioavailability results where hemoglobin of Fe-depleted chicks was regressed on Fe intake, dried blood meal was assigned an Fe bioavailability value of 22%, while meat and bone meal, poultry by-product meal, feather meal, and fish meal were assigned values of 48%, 68%, 39%, and 32%, respectively. Among plant-source feed ingredients evaluated, Fe bioavailabilities of 96%, 77%, 65%, 45%, and 20%, respectively, were found for sesame meal, rice bran, alfalfa meal, dehulled soybean meal, and yellow corn (Czarnecki-Maulden 1990).

Zinc

Little swine data exist on Zn bioavailability, although Miller et al. (1981) have reported a high bioavailability in Zn dust as compared with ZnO for young pigs. Work in our laboratory has revealed that plasma Zn, plasma alkaline phosphatase, and soft tissue stores of Zn are often misleading criteria of bioavailable Zn concentration. Thus, these criteria do not respond linearly to incremental intakes of Zn in chicks (Halpin 1986). Weight gain and bone Zn accumulation are probably the best criteria of Zn bioavailability (Fordyce et al. 1987; Wedekind and Baker 1990).

Zinc, like many other trace elements, is poorly utilized by nonruminant animals fed conventional corn-soybean meal diets. Indeed, the dietary requirement for Zn is often threefold or fourfold higher in animals fed these diets than in those fed casein-dextrose diets. Also, in the presence of phytate and fiber, excess Ca decreases Zn utilization. Work in our laboratory has established that while excess Zn can exacerbate copper (Cu) and Fe deficiency states, excesses of either Cu or Fe have minimal effects on Zn utilization (Bafundo et al. 1984b; Southern and Baker 1983a).

Based on estimates made by Edwards (1959) and Sullivan (1961), and the reviews of Ammerman and Miller (1972) and O'Dell et al. (1979), the Zn present in ZnO, $ZnSO_4 \cdot H_2O$, $ZnSO_4 \cdot 7H_2O$, $ZnCO_3$, $ZnCl_2$, and Zn metal (dust) is highly available relative to technical-grade ZnO. However, a recent chick study that compared feed-grade ZnO (Waelz process) and Zn-methionine (Zn-Met) to feed-grade $ZnSO_4 \cdot H_2O$ (the standard) yielded bioavailability values of 61% for ZnO and 124% for Zn-Met based on weight gain, but 44% for ZnO and 176% for Zn-Met based on tibia Zn accumulation (Wedekind and Baker 1990). It is probably gratuitous to even attempt quantification of Zn bioavailability in protein- and energy-furnishing feed ingredients, except to generalize that utilization is low in plant-source ingredients and probably higher in animal-source ingredients. The observation of Baker and Halpin (1988) that addition of 10% fish meal to a casein-dextrose diet containing either 68 or 318 mg Zn/kg diet would materially depress Zn levels in bone, liver, and pancreas of chicks provides evidence that even some animal-source products may contain factors that can antagonize Zn utilization. Whether this would have occurred had fish meal been added to a corn-soybean meal diet is problematic.

Copper

Copper bioavailability, like that of Zn, is difficult to quantify accurately. Hence, Cu accumulation in tissues (primarily liver) increases only slightly (and curvilinearly) between deficient levels and a dietary level of about 250 mg Cu/kg diet. Beyond this level, Cu accumulates rapidly, and generally in a linear fashion. Relative to $CuSO_4 \cdot 5H_2O$, Miller (1980) suggests good utilization of the Cu in CuO, $CuCl_2$, and $CuCO_3$, and poor utilization in CuS. More recent pig work by Cromwell et al. (1989), confirmed in our laboratory with chicks, has shown that the Cu in CuO is almost totally unavailable for absorption from the gut. The Cu in grains and concentrates would be expected to be utilized poorly. Copper ingested from fecal material or manure is utilized no better than 30% relative to that provided as $CuSO_4 \cdot 5H_2O$ (Izquierdo and Baker 1986). Cu absorption from the gut is reduced substantially if either Na_2S (Barber et al. 1961; Cromwell et al. 1978) or roxarsone (i.e., 3-nitro) is co-administered (Czarnecki and Baker 1985; Edmonds and Baker 1986).

Manganese

Manganese (Mn) is a species mineral problem (i.e., poultry) and is therefore of only minor interest to swine nutritionists. The recent studies from Ammerman's laboratory (Black et al. 1984, 1985; Henry et al. 1986) and from our own laboratory (Southern and Baker 1983b, 1983c; Halpin and Baker 1986a, 1986b; Halpin et al. 1986c; Halpin and Baker 1987; Baker et al. 1986) have provided considerable information on Mn bioavailability. Tissues (primarily bone) accumulate Mn in a linear fashion, and this fact can be used as a basis for assessing Mn bioavailability. Relative to $MnSO_4 \cdot H_2O$, Mn availability is approximately 100% in $MnCl_2$, 66% in MnO, 40% in $MnCO_3$, and <30% in MnO_2. Availability of Mn in a protein-Mn or a methionine-Mn chelate has been observed in our laboratory to be at least as high as that in $MnSO_4 \cdot H_2O$ (Baker and Halpin 1988; Fly et al. 1989). The Mn in corn, soybean meal, wheat bran, and fish meal should probably be considered totally unavailable for poultry and swine (Baker et al. 1986), while the (considerable) Mn present in rice bran should be considered only minimally bioavailable. In practice, excesses of either Fe or cobalt in corn-soybean meal diets have minimal effects on Mn utilization, although considerable excesses of Mn do reduce Fe absorption from the gut. Excess dietary P (inorganic or phytate) reduces Mn utilization substantially (Baker and Wedekind 1988).

Even with a highly available source of Mn such as $MnSO_4 \cdot H_2O$, gut absorption of Mn by chicks is only about 1.6% of the ingested dose. Elimination of all fiber and phytate from the diet increases the absorption efficiency to 2.4% (Halpin et al. 1986).

Selenium

Based on studies by Mathias (1967), Miller et al. (1972), Cantor (1975a, 1975b), Hitchcock (1975), Mahan and Moxon (1978), and Gabrielson and Opstvedt (1980), as reviewed by Miller (1980), selenium (Se) in Na_2SeO_3 and Na_2SeO_4 is well utilized, while that existing as selenomethionine is probably utilized somewhat less efficiently (except that based on Se accumulation in tissues, selenomethionine would be judged over 100% available relative to Na_2SeO_3). Selenium seems to be well utilized from cereal grains (60% to 80%) and extremely well utilized from alfalfa meal (>100%), but utilization is poor from fish and poultry by-product meals (10% to 40%). Poultry data have provided Se bioavailability estimates in soybean meal of only 18% for restoration of glutathione peroxidase activity (Gabrielson and Opstvedt 1980) but 60% for prevention of exudative diathesis (Cantor et al. 1975b).

Selenium absorption from the gut is relatively efficient, that is, 63% of an administered dose was found to be absorbed by pigs (Wright and Bell 1966). A variety of arsenic compounds as well as cysteine, methionine, Cu, tungsten, mercury, cadmium, and silver have been reported to decrease the efficiency of inorganic Se absorption from the gut (Baker and Czarnecki-Maulden 1987; Lowry and Baker 1989a).

Iodine

Little definitive work on I availability has been carried out in any species. What does exist is primarily rat research in which bioavailability assessment was not the primary objective. Nonetheless, Miller (1980) estimated that (relative to NaI), the I in KI, $Ca(IO_3)_2 \cdot 2H_2O$, KIO_3, and CuI was 100% bioavailable. It seems reasonable to assume, also, that the I present in iodized salt is 100% available relative to NaI.

VITAMIN BIOAVAILABILITY

There are really two primary concerns regarding vitamin bioavailability in modern swine diets and premixes: (1) stability in vitamin and vitamin-mineral premixes as well as in diets and supplements, and (2) utilization efficiency from plant- and animal-source feed ingredients. Readers are referred to the reviews of Schneider (1986), McGinnis (1986), and Wornick (1968), as well the recent research of Zhuge and Klopfenstein (1986) for details of factors affecting the stability of crystalline vitamins in diets and premixes. Regarding vitamin bioavailability in feed ingredients, a paucity of pig research data exists, and even considering chick and rat data, few feed ingredients have been evaluated.

There are many pitfalls in vitamin (and mineral) bioavailability assessment. Body stores often preclude developing a distinct deficiency during the course of a conventional growth trial. Even if a frank deficiency can be produced within the framework of available funding, one must deal with the vexing question of whether the responding parameter (usually weight gain) increased because of the vitamin being supplied or perhaps because of increased diet intake that results from adding the unknown ingredient to an often less than voraciously palatable purified diet.

Our chick work in the area of vitamin bioavailability has caused us to come to certain conclusions concerning the proper bioassay methodology for maximum efficacy and extrapolative value of results:

1. Pretest periods to obtain desired deficiency states are generally necessary.
2. Activity of a key enzyme of which the vitamin is a component or cofactor is generally a less desirable dependent variable than is weight gain.

3. Precursor materials (e.g., methionine for choline; tryptophan for niacin) must be carefully considered.
4. Use of specific vitamin inhibitors may assist in establishing veracity of assessed bioavailability values.

Because water-soluble B vitamins respond better insofar as growth is concerned, they are, in many respects, easier to evaluate than are fat-soluble vitamins. Certainly, one of the more difficult, water-soluble vitamins to study is biotin.

Biotin

Commercial D-biotin has no specific unit of activity. Thus, 1 g of D-biotin equals 1 g of activity. Pelleting or heat have little effect on biotin activity in feeds, but oxidative rancidity severely reduces biotin bioavailability. Avidin, a glycoprotein found in egg albumen, binds biotin and makes it totally unavailable. Proper heat treatment of egg white will denature avidin and prevent it from binding biotin. Based on bioassay results using biotin-depleted chicks, it is apparent that among the cereal grains, bioavailability of biotin in corn is high (≥ 100%) while that in wheat, barley, and sorghum is lower (about 50%) cf. Anderson and Warnick (1970), Frigg (1976), and Anderson et al. (1978). Bioavailable biotin concentrations of 0.11 mg/kg (corn), 0.08 mg/kg (barley), 0.09 mg/kg (sorghum), and 0.04 mg/kg (wheat) were estimated by Anderson et al. (1978). Feedstuff ingredient tables generally list the biotin concentration in soybean meal as 0.30 mg/kg. Buenrostro and Kratzer reported that biotin is 100% available in soybean meal and 86% available in meat and bone meal for laying hens. Hence, with considerable bioavailable biotin present in corn-soybean meal diets, growing-finishing pigs fed such diets have generally not been found to respond to supplemental biotin. With sows, Bryant et al. (1985a, 1985b) have provided evidence that under some conditions supplemental biotin may improve conception rate, decrease the weaning to estrus interval, and improve both foot health and hair coat, particularly in advanced parities.

Biotin may be the only vitamin where a good test exists to assess the veracity of the bioavailability assay. Thus, growth responses to ingredients added to a biotin-free purified diet can be measured in the presence and absence of crystalline avidin. When we did this, growth rate of biotin-depleted chicks was doubled by supplementation with 20% corn, but it was not significantly increased when the same quantity of corn was fed in the presence of 3.81 mg avidin/kg diet. Similar results occurred when barley was evaluated (Anderson et al. 1978). These results, therefore, provide rather convincing evidence that the growth responses observed from feed grain supplementation of the biotin-free purified diet resulted from the available biotin per se furnished by the grains.

Niacin

The term *niacin* is the generic descriptive term for pyridine 3-carboxylic acid and derivatives delivering nicotinamide activity. Thus, pyridine 3-carboxylic acid per se is properly referred to as nicotinic acid (Anonymous 1979). Niacin is a very stable vitamin when added to feed or premixes, being little affected by heat, oxygen, moisture, or light. In plant-source feed ingredients, much of the niacin activity, mostly nicotinamide nucleotides, is bound and therefore unavailable (Yen et al. 1977). Ghosh et al. (1963) estimated that 85% to 90% of the niacin activity in cereal grains and 40% in oilseeds is in a bound unavailable form. Alkaline hydrolysis is the only means by which niacin can be efficiently released from its bound state in these ingredients. Meat and milk products, on the other hand, contain no bound niacin, but instead contain free nicotinic acid and nicotinamide.

Because excess tryptophan is converted to nicotinic acid and because all common feed ingredients contain tryptophan as well as nicotinic acid, there is no good way to assess the bioavailability of niacin per se. Thus, 50 mg of tryptophan yields 1 mg of nicotinic acid (Baker et al. 1973; NRC 1979; Czarnecki et al. 1983). Does excess leucine in corn-soybean meal swine diets antagonize tryptophan or nicotinic acid or does it impair the metabolic conversion of tryptophan to nicotinic acid? This subject is controversial (Anonymous 1986) and data exist to support both points of view. Our recent chick studies suggest that excess leucine has no effect on either tryptophan conversion to niacin or niacin bioavailability (Lowry and Baker 1989b).

Niacin activity can be purchased as either free nicotinic acid or free nicotinamide. Relative to nicotinic acid, nicotinamide has been observed to be roughly 120% bioavailable in delivering niacin bioactivity (Baker et al. 1976). Other work, however, has suggested niacin and nicotinamide to be equal in biopotency for chicks (Bao-Ji and Combs 1986; Ruiz and Harms 1988).

Riboflavin

This vitamin is relatively labile, being reduced in bioactivity by light, alkali, and oxygen. In feedstuffs, it exists primarily as nucleotide coenzymes, in which form the bioavailability is probably less than 100%. Chung and Baker (1990) estimated that riboflavin bioavailability in a corn-soybean meal diet is 60% for chicks relative to crystalline riboflavin. Klopenstein and Zhuge (1986) reported that crystalline riboflavin loses activity in vitamin-mineral premixes over time and that high-temperature storage enhances the loss. Gadient (1986), however, suggested that riboflavin activity in feeds is little affected by heat and oxygen and only slightly affected by moisture and light. He observed 95% to 100% retention of riboflavin bioactivity in pelleted feeds stored for 3 months at room temperature.

Pantothenic Acid

This B vitamin is generally sold as either D- or DL-Ca pantothenate, and only the D-isomer has bioactivity (Staten et al. 1980). Thus, 1 g of D-Ca pantothenate equals 0.92 g pantothenic acid (PA) activity and 1 g DL-Ca pantothenate equals 0.46 g of PA activity. Crystalline PA is relatively stable to heat, oxygen, and light, but it can lose activity rapidly when exposed to moisture. Gadient (1986) concluded that PA should retain at least 80% of its activity after 3 months when present in pelleted feed or vitamin-mineral premixes.

Feed ingredients contain PA in the form of coenzyme A, and in this form it may not be fully available for gut absorption. Our chick bioassay work suggested that the PA in corn and soybean meal is 100% bioavailable, while that in barley, wheat, and sorghum is about 60% available (Southern and Baker 1981). "Processed" feed ingredients may exhibit losses in PA bioavailability, although definitive animal data are lacking on this subject. Sauberlich (1985) estimated that PA in the typical adult American diet was only 50% bioavailable. He further suggested that processing (freezing, canning, refining, etc.) may decrease bioavailability further.

Vitamin B_{12}

Cyanocobalamin, or B_{12}, is available in crystalline form, where 1 United States Pharmacopeia (USP) unit is considered equivalent to 1 μg of the vitamin. Vitamin B_{12} is essentially devoid in plant-source feed ingredients, existing instead in animal-source proteins and fermentation products, where it is considered (but not proved) to be 100% available. As in humans, but unlike in sheep and in horses, an "intrinsic" factor is required for gut absorption of B_{12} in swine. Gadient (1986) considers vitamin B_{12} to be quite stable in feeds and premixes.

Choline

In mammalian but not avian species, the dietary need for choline can be replaced by excess methionine. In crystalline form, choline chloride (87% choline) is hygroscopic, and therefore it is considered a stress agent to other vitamins in a vitamin-mineral premix. Crude plant oils (e.g., corn and soybean oil) contain choline as phospholipid-bound phosphatidyl choline. The bioavailability of choline in this form is not known. Refined plant oils generally have been subjected to alkaline treatment and "bleaching," and these processes almost totally remove the phospholipid-bound choline (Reiners and Gooding 1975). Crystalline choline is considered quite stable in animal feeds and premixes.

The choline present in soybean meal ranges from 60% to 75% in bioavailability for chicks (Molitoris and Baker 1976a). Also in chicks, excess dietary protein has been observed to materially increase the dietary requirement for choline (Molitoris and Baker 1976b). Minimizing liver lipid content may require a higher level of dietary choline than that required to maximize rate and efficiency of weight gain (Anderson et al. 1979). Betaine can probably spare some of the choline need, although recent chick work in our laboratory with purified diets has shown that the majority of the choline requirement is for choline per se, rather than for its metabolic oxidation product, betaine (Lowry and Baker 1987).

As with nicain, for which tryptophan serves as a precursor, choline bioavailability assessment would be difficult, if not impossible, in pigs, because all common feed ingredients would supply both choline and methionine. Therefore, it would be difficult to separate responses from one or the other, although use of the transmethylation inhibitor, ethionine, or the inhibitor of methionine methylation of aminoethanol in choline biosynthesis, that is, 2-amino-2-methyl-1-propanol, might prove useful in this endeavor (Molitoris and Baker 1976a; Anderson et al. 1979; Lowry and Baker 1987).

Corn-soybean meal swine grower diets often do not respond to choline supplementation, probably because soybean meal is so rich in choline content (NCR-42 1980).* Swine pregnancy has been shown to benefit from choline addition to corn-soybean meal diets (Stockland and Blaylock 1974; NCR-42 1976).

Vitamin B_6

This vitamin is not generally added in supplemental crystalline form to practical-type diets for swine because both corn and soybean meal are plentiful in this B vitamin. Our work suggests that vitamin B_6 is about 40% bioavailable in corn and about 60% bioavailable in soybean meal (Yen et al. 1976). Moderate heat treatment (80 °C to 120 °C) of corn seems to enhance B_6 bioavailability, while greater heat treatment (160 °C) decreases availability. Most of the vitamin B_6 activity in corn exists as pyridoxal and pyridoxamine, forms that are more heat-labile than is pyridoxine (Schroeder 1971). Even with the reduced bioavailability of vitamin B_6 in corn and soybean meal relative to crystalline pyridoxine·HCl, a surfeit of available B_6 would still be present in practical-type diets for swine, thus precluding a response to supplemental vitamin B_6 if added to these diets.

In premixes, vitamin B_6 can lose bioactivity, particularly when minerals in the form of carbonates or oxides are present (Verbeeck 1975). High temperatures enhance loss of activity. Adams (1982) found 76% retention of B_6 activity after 3 months of storage at room temperature, but only 45% retention after 3 months of storage at 37 °C. Loss of B_6 activity in stored pelleted complete feeds averages about 20% during 3 months of storage at room temperature (Gadient 1986).

Thiamin

Thiamin is available to the food and feed industries as thiamin·HCl (89% thiamin) or thiamin·NO_3 (92% thiamin). One international unit of thiamin activity is equivalent to 3 μg of crystalline thiamin·HCl. Because it contains a free amino group, heat processing can rapidly destroy thiamin bioactivity via the Maillard reaction. Likewise, any processing procedure that involves alkaline treatment leads to loss of thiamin activity.

---

*Failure of corn-soybean meal swine and poultry diets to respond to vitamin supplementation is not unique to choline (among those generally supplemented). Unpublished work in our laboratory has shown that these diets also fail to respond consistently to either nicotinic acid or PA. Choline, nicotinic acid, and PA should nonetheless be included in swine vitamin mixtures to provide a margin of safety against environmental and stress conditions that might manifest in a swine production operation.

Some raw ingredients (e.g., fish) contain thiaminase, which can destroy thiamin in diets to which it may be added. While thiaminase is of particular concern in the nutrition of cats and fur-bearing animals, it is of little consequence in modern swine feeding. Thiamin in fish meal is lost to the fish solubles fraction when fish meal is made. Thus, fish meal has essentially no bioavailable thiamin. Likewise, due to the high-temperature processing, meat meals contain very little bioavailable thiamin activity.

Pelleting results in some loss of thiamin activity, as does premix storage in the presence of minerals (Gadient 1986). Adams (1982) found 48% and 95% retention of thiamin activity when stored in the form of the HCl and NO_3, respectively, in a premix for 21 days at 40 °C and 85% relative humidity. In a complete feed stored under similar conditions, thiamin·HCl retained only 21% of its activity, while thiamin·NO_3 retained 97% of its activity. Thus, the mononitrate form of thiamin would seem to be the more stable form when storage in hot environments is anticipated.

Grains and soybean meal are sufficiently rich in thiamin that even with considerable losses of bioactivity due to heat or lengthy storage, seldom would there be a case where practical-type diets for swine would respond to supplementation with this vitamin.

Folacin

The term *folacin* is the officially accepted generic term for folic acid and related compounds exhibiting "folacin activity." Over 150 forms of folacin have been found to exist in foods (McGinnis 1986). Like thiamin, folic acid has a free amino group, and thus it is very sensitive to losses in activity due to heat treatment. It is also light-labile. Adams (1982) reported only 38% retention of activity in a mineral-free premix stored for 3 weeks at 45 °C. At room temperature, 57% of original activity was present after 3 months. Verbeeck (1975) observed that losses are even greater when minerals are present in the premix.

Most of the folacin present in feed ingredients is bound as polyglutamate conjugates, which require intestinal action by conjugases to be made available for absorption. Bioavailability estimates of bound folacin in foods and feeds are not available, but it is generally assumed that bound forms of folacin are lower in bioavailability than are free folic acid forms.

Vitamin C

There is little concern about the bioavailability of vitamin C (ascorbic acid) because swine are capable of synthesizing this vitamin. Nonetheless, vitamin C is often included in vitamin premixes for use in purified swine diets because of its antioxidant and putative antistress properties. Adams (1982) observed considerable losses of vitamin C activity in stored layer rations. Coating ascorbate with ethylcellulose minimized the loss of potency. Gadient (1986) noted that both pelleting and extruding can markedly reduce the bioactivity of supplemental ascorbate added to feeds or premixes. Losses due to oxidation are well known, as ascorbic acid (reduced form) can be reversibly oxidized to dehydroascorbic acid, which in turn can be further irreversibly oxidized to diketogulonic acid. While both reduced and oxidized forms of ascorbate retain scurvy-preventing ascorbate activity, diketogulonic acid has no activity.

Vitamin A

Vitamin nomenclature policy dictates that the term *vitamin A* be used for all B-ionone derivatives, other than provitamin A carotenoids, exhibiting the biological activity of all-*trans* retinol (i.e., vitamin A alcohol or vitamin A_1). Esters of all-*trans* retinol should be referred to as retinyl esters.

Vitamin A is present in animal tissues, while most plant materials contain only provitamin A carotenoids, which must be split in the intestinal tract to form vitamin A. In blood, vitamin A is transported as retinol, but it is stored, primarily in the liver, as retinyl palmitate. Absorption efficiency of vitamin A is relatively constant over a wide range of doses (Olson 1984), but higher doses of carotenoids are absorbed much less efficiently than are lower doses (Erdman et al. 1988).

Vitamin A esters are more stable in feeds and premixes than is retinol. The hydroxyl group as well as the four double bonds on the retinol side chain are subject to oxidative losses. Thus, esterification of vitamin A alcohol does not totally protect this vitamin from oxidative losses. Current commercial sources of vitamin A are generally "coated" esters (e.g., acetate or palmitate) that contain an added antioxidant such as ethoxyquin or butylated hydroxytoluene (BHT).

The water content of premixes and feedstuffs has a negative effect on vitamin A stability. Moisture causes vitamin A beadlets to soften and become more permeable to oxygen (Schneider 1986). Thus, both high humidity and presence of free choline chloride (hygroscopic) enhance vitamin A destruction. Trace minerals also exacerbate vitamin A losses in premixes exposed to moisture. For maximum retention of vitamin A activity, premixes should be as moisture-free as possible and should be made to have a pH above 5. Low pH causes isomerization of all-*trans* vitamin A to less potent *cis* forms and also results in de-esterification of vitamin A esters to retinol (De Ritter 1976). Likewise, heat processing, especially extrusion, can reduce vitamin A bioavailability (Harper 1988). Crystalline beta-carotene is absorbed from the gut more efficiently than beta-carotene existing in foods and feeds (Rao and Rao 1970). Some of the beta-carotene in foods is complexed with protein. Fiber components of feeds, especially pectins, have been shown to reduce beta-carotene absorption from the gut in chicks (Erdman et al. 1986).

Ullrey (1972) reviewed the bioavailability aspects of vitamin A precursor materials for swine and reported that pigs were far less efficient than rats in converting carotenoid precursors to active vitamin A. Thus, bioefficacies (weight/weight) ranging from 7% to 14% were observed for corn carotenes in pigs relative to all-*trans* retinyl palmitate. Thus, at best, carotenoid precursors in corn (also corn gluten meal) have no more than 261 IU/mg vitamin A activity when consumed by swine. This is decidedly less than the theoretical potency of 1667 IU/mg (assuming all the carotenoids are all-

trans-beta carotene), which is assumed for the rat. Corn carotenoids that have provitamin A activity consist of about 50% cryptoxanthin, 25% beta-zeacarotene, and 25% beta-carotene (Ullrey 1972).

Vitamin D

The term *vitamin D* is appropriate for all steroids having cholecalciferol biological activity. Cholecalciferol, itself, is synonymous with vitamin D_3, as distinguished from ergocalciferol, which is also called vitamin D_2. Commercially, vitamin D_3 is available as a spray-dried product or (frequently in combination with vitamin A) as gelatin-coated beadlets; one international unit is equal to 0.025 μg of cholecalciferol. These products are quite stable if stored as the vitamin itself at room temperature. In complete feeds and mineral-vitamin premixes, Schneider (1986) has observed activity losses up to 10% and 30%, respectively, after either 4 or 6 months of storage at 22 °C.

Vitamin D precursors are present in plant (ergosterol) and animal (7-dehydrocholesterol) feedstuffs, but they require ultraviolet irradiation for conversion into active D_2 and D_3, respectively. Although D_2 and D_3 have long been considered equal in biological activity for pigs, the recent findings of Horst et al. (1982) suggest that D_3 may be more bioactive than D_2.

Vitamin E

Vitamin E is the generic term for all tocol and tocotrienol derivatives having alpha-tocopherol biological activity. There are eight naturally occurring forms of vitamin E: alpha-, beta-, gamma-, and delta-tocopherols and alpha-, beta-, gamma-, and delta-tocotrienols. Among these, D-alpha-tocopherol possesses the greatest biological activity (Bieri and McKenna 1981). One international unit of vitamin E is the activity of 1 mg of DL-alpha-tocopheryl acetate. All racemic or DL-alpha-tocopherol has about 70% of the activity of pure D-alpha-tocopherol. Bieri and McKenna (1981) consider beta-tocopherol and gamma-tocopherol to have only 40% and 10% of the activity, respectively, of alpha-tocopherol (set at 100%). The only other natural form to possess activity is alpha-tocotrienol, which on the rating scale used above was listed by Bieri and McKenna (1981) as containing a biopotency of 25%.

Plant-source ingredients are richer in vitamin E bioactivity than are animal-source feed ingredients. Plant oils are particularly rich in bioactive vitamin E, although corn and corn oil contain about six times more gamma-tocol than alpha-tocol (Ullrey 1981). Fat-extracted soybean meal has very little vitamin E activity.

Vitamin E is subject to destruction by oxidation, and this process is accelerated by heat, moisture, unsaturated fat, and trace minerals. Losses of 50% to 70% have been observed to occur in alfalfa hay stored at 32 °C for 12 weeks; losses up to 30% have been known to occur during dehydration of alfalfa (Livingston et al. 1968). Treatment of high-moisture grains with organic acids also greatly enhances vitamin E destruction (Young et al. 1975, 1977, 1978). However, even mildly alkaline conditions of vitamin E storage are also very detrimental to vitamin E stability (Schneider 1986). Thus, finely ground limestone or MgO coming in direct contact with vitamin E can markedly reduce its bioavailability.

Vitamin K

This fat-soluble vitamin exists in three series: phylloquinones (K_1) in plants, menaquinones (K_2) formed by microbial fermentation, and menadiones (K_3), which are synthetic. All three forms of vitamin K are biologically active. Only water-soluble forms of menadione are used to supplement swine diets. The commercially available forms of K_3 supplements are menadione sodium bisulfite (MSB), menadione sodium bisulfate complex (MSBC), and menadione dimethyl pyrimidinol bisulfite (MPB). Stability of these K_3 supplements in premixes and diets is impaired by moisture, choline chloride, trace elements, and alkaline conditions. Coated K_3 supplements are generally more stable than are uncoated supplements. MPB has been found to be more bioactive than either MSB or MSBC for chicks (Griminger 1965; Charles and Huston 1972). Seerley et al. (1976) also found MPB to be effective for swine. Although certain feed ingredients are known to be rich in vitamin K activity for swine, for example, alfalfa meal (Fritschen 1971), little quantitative information exists on the bioavailability of vitamin K in swine feedstuffs.

REFERENCES

Adams, C.R. 1982. *Proceedings of the NFIA Nutrition Institute.*
Ammerman, C.B., and S.M. Miller. 1972. *J. Anim. Sci.* 35:681.
Ammerman, C.B., et al. 1974. *J. Anim. Sci.* 38:52.
Anderson, J.O., and R.E. Warnick. 1970. *Poult. Sci.* 49:569.
Anderson, P.A., D.H. Baker, and S.P. Mistry. 1978. *J. Anim. Sci.* 47:654.
Anderson, P.A., et al. 1979. *J. Anim. Sci.* 49:522.
Anonymous. 1979. *J. Nutr.* 109:8.
Anonymous. 1986. *Nutr. Rev.* 44:26.
Bafundo, K.W., D.H. Baker, and P.R. Fitzgerald. 1984a. *Poult. Sci.* 63:2430.
Bafundo, K.W., D.H. Baker, and P.R. Fitzgerald. 1984b. *J. Nutr.* 114:1306.
Baker, D.H. 1986. *Proceedings of the BASF Technical Symposium.* p. 13.
Baker, D.H., and G.L. Czarnecki-Maulden. 1987. *J. Nutr.* 117:1003.
Baker, D.H., and K.M. Halpin. 1988. *Nutr. Res.* 8:213.
Baker, D.H., and K.J. Wedekind. 1988. *Proceedings Maryland Nutritional Conference.* p. 29.
Baker, D.H., N.K. Allen, and A.J. Kleiss. 1973. *J. Anim. Sci.* 36:299.
Baker, D.H., et al. 1976. *Nutr. Rep. Int.* 14:115.
Baker, D.H., et al. 1983. *Poult. Sci.* 62:133.
Baker, D.H., et al. 1986. *Proceedings of the Arkansas Nutrition Conference.* p.1.
Bao-Ji, C., and G.F. Combs. 1986. *Poult. Sci.* 65(Suppl. 1):24 (Abstr.)
Barber, R.S., et al. 1961. *Br. J. Nutr.* 15:189.
Bieri, J.G., and M.C. McKenna. 1981. *Am. J. Clin. Nutr.* 34:289.
Black, J.R., et al. 1984. *Poult. Sci.* 63:1999.
Black, J.R., et al. 1985. *Poult. Sci.* 64:688.
Bogunjoko, F.E., R.J. Neale, and D.A. Ledward. 1983. *Br. J. Nutr.* 50:511.
Braude, R., et al. 1962. *Br. J. Nutr.* 16:427.

Buenrostro, J.L., and F.H. Kratzer. 1980. *Poult. Sci.* 63:1563.

Burns, J.M., and D.H. Baker. 1976. *Poult. Sci.* 55:2447.

Cantor, A.H., M.L. Scott, and T. Noguchi. 1975b. *J. Nutr.* 105:96.

Cantor, A.H., et al. 1975a. *J. Nutr.* 105:106.

Charles, O.W., and T.M. Huston. 1972. *Poult. Sci.* 51:1421.

Chausow, D.G. 1987. "Selected Aspects of Mineral Nutrition of the Cat and Dog with Special Emphasis on Magnesium and Iron." Ph.D. thesis, University of Illinois, Urbana.

Chausow, D.G., and G.L. Czarnecki-Maulden. 1988a. *Nutr. Res.* 8:175.

Chausow, D.G., and G.L. Czarnecki-Maulden. 1988b. *Nutr. Res.* 8:1041.

Chung, T.K., and D.H. Baker. 1990. *Poult. Sci.* 69:1357.

Combs, N.R., and E.R. Miller. 1985. *J. Anim. Sci.* 60:715.

Combs, N.R., E.R. Miller, and P.K. Ku. 1985. *J. Anim. Sci.* 60:709.

Cook, D.A. 1973. *J. Nutr.* 103:1365.

Cornelius, S.G., and B.G. Harmon. 1976. *J. Anim. Sci.* 42:1351.

Cromwell, G.L. 1979. *Proceedings of the Distillers Feed Research Council.* p. 40.

Cromwell, G.L. 1985. *Proceedings of Alltech 1st Annual Symposium.* Lexington, KY.

Cromwell, G.L., V.W. Hays, and T.L. Clark. 1978. *J. Anim. Sci.* 46:692.

Cromwell, G.L., R.D. Ross, and T.S. Stahly. 1985. *Proceedings of the Guelph Nutrition Conference.* p. 88. Guelph, Ontario, Canada.

Cromwell, G.L., T.S. Stahly, and H.J. Monegue. 1983. *J. Anim. Sci.* 57(Suppl. 1):242.

Cromwell, G.L., T.S. Stahly, and H.J. Monegue. 1989. *J. Anim. Sci.* 67:2996.

Czarnecki-Maulden, G.L. 1990. *Proceedings of the Guelph Nutrition Conference.* p. 73. Guelph, Ontario, Canada.

Czarnecki, G.L., and D.H. Baker. 1985. *J. Anim. Sci.* 60:440.

Czarnecki, G.L., K.M. Halpin, and D.H. Baker. 1983. *Poult. Sci.* 62:371.

DeRitter, E. 1976. *Food Technol.* 30:48.

Diekert, J.W., et al. 1962. *J. Food Sci.* 27:321.

Edmonds, M.S., and D.H. Baker. 1986. *J. Anim. Sci.* 63:533.

Edwards, H.M. 1959. *J. Nutr.* 69:306.

Erdman, J.W. 1979. *J. Am. Oil Chem. Soc.* 56:736.

Erdman, J.W., G.C. Fahey, and C.B. White. 1986. *J. Nutr.* 116:2415.

Fly, A.D., et al. 1989. *Nutr. Res.* 9:901.

Fordyce, E.J., et al. 1987. *J. Food. Sci.* 52(Suppl. 2):440.

Fritschen, R.D., O.D. Grace, and E.R. Peo. 1971. *Nebraska Swine Report E.C. 71-219.* p. 22.

Fritz, J.C., et al. 1970. *Agric. Food Chem.* 18:647.

Furugouri, K., and A. Kawabata. 1975. *J. Anim. Sci.* 41:1348.

Gadient, M. 1986. *Proceedings of the Maryland Nutrition Conference.* p. 73.

Ghosh, H.P., P.K. Sarkar, and B.C. Guha. 1963. *J. Nutr.* 79:451.

Griminger, P. 1965. *Poult. Sci.* 44:210.

Halpin, K.M. 1986. "Factors Affecting Manganese Homeostasis in the Chick." Ph.D. thesis. University of Illinois, Urbana.

Halpin, K.M., and D.H. Baker. 1986a. *Poult. Sci.* 65:995.

Halpin, K.M., and D.H. Baker. 1986b. *Poult. Sci.* 65:1371.

Halpin, K.M., and D.H. Baker. 1987. *Poult. Sci.* 66:332.

Halpin, K.M., D.G. Chausow, and D.H. Baker. 1986. *J. Nutr.* 116:1747.

Harmon, B.G. 1979. *Proceedings of the Georgia Nutrition Conference.* p. 98. Athens: University of Georgia.

Harmon, B.G., D.E. Becker, and A.H. Jensen. 1967. *J. Anim. Sci.* 26:1051.

Harmon, B.G., et al. 1974. *J. Anim. Sci.* 39:699.

Harmon, B.G., et al. 1969. *J. Anim. Sci.* 29:706.

Harms, R.H., et al. 1976. *Calcium in Broiler, Layer and Turkey Nutrition.* West Des Moines, IA: NFIA.

Harper, J.M. 1988. In: *Nutritional Evaluation of Food Processing.* 3rd ed. Karmas, E., and R.S. Harris (Eds.). New York: Van Nostrand Reinhold Co.

Hays, V.W. 1976. *Phosphorus in Swine Nutrition.* West Des Moines, IA: NFIA.
Hendricks, D.G., et al. 1969. *J. Anim. Sci.* 28:342.
Hitchcock, J.P. 1975. Ph.D. thesis. East Lansing: Michigan State University.
Horst, R.L., J.L. Napoli, and E.T. Littledike. 1982. *Biochem. J.* 204:185.
Izquierdo, O.A., and D.H. Baker. 1986. *Can. J. Anim. Sci.* 66:1145.
Kornegay, E.T. 1972. *J. Anim. Sci.* 34:569.
Layrisse, M., et al. 1975. *Blood* 45:689.
Livingston, A.L., J.W. Nelson, and G.O. Kohler. 1968. *J. Agric. Food Chem.* 16:492.
Lowry, K.R., and D.H. Baker. 1987. *Poult. Sci.* 66(Suppl. 1):135 (Abstr.).
Lowry, K.R., and D.H. Baker. 1989a. *J. Anim. Sci.* 67:959.
Lowry, K.R., and D.H. Baker. 1989b. *FASEB J.* 3:A666 (Abstr.).
Mahan, D.C., and A.L. Moxon. 1978. *J. Anim. Sci.* 47:456.
Mathias, M.M., D.E. Hogue, and J.K. Loosli. 1967. *J. Nutr.* 93:14.
McGinnis, C.H. 1986. *Proceedings of the NFIA Nutrition Institute.*
Miller, E.R. 1978. *Feedstuffs* 50:20.
Miller, E.R. 1980. *Proceedings of the Minnesota Nutrition Conference.* p. 144.
Miller, E.R., J.P. Hitchcock, and D.E. Ullrey. 1973. *Michigan Agricultural Experiment Station Report 232.* p. 39. East Lansing: Michigan State University.
Miller, E.R., P.K. Ku, and D.E. Ullrey. 1977. *Michigan Agricultural Experiment Station Report 343.* East Lansing: Michigan State University.
Miller, E.R., et al. 1981. *J. Anim. Sci.* 52:312.
Molitoris, B.A., and D.H. Baker. 1976a. *J. Anim. Sci.* 42:481.
Molitoris, B.A., and D.H. Baker. 1976b. *J. Nutr.* 106:412.
NCR-42 Committee on Swine Nutrition. 1976. *J. Anim. Sci.* 42:1211.
NCR-42 Committee on Swine Nutrition. 1980. *J. Anim. Sci.* 55:403.
Nelson, T.S. 1967. *Poult. Sci.* 46:862.
Nelson, T.S., and A.C. Walker. 1964. *Poult. Sci.* 43:94.
NRC. 1979. *Nutrient Requirements of Swine.* Washington, DC: National Academy of Sciences.
NRC. 1984. *Nutrient Requirements of Poultry.* Washington, DC: National Academy of Sciences.
O'Dell, B.L., E.R. Miller, and W.J. Miller. 1979. *Copper and Zinc in Poultry, Swine and Ruminant Nutrition.* West Des Moines, IA: NFIA.
O'Dell, B.L., J.M. Yoke, and J.E. Savage. 1964. *Poult. Sci.* 43:415.
Olson, J.A. 1984. "Vitamin A." In: *Handbook of Vitamins.* Machlin, L.J. (Ed.). p. 1. New York: Marcel Dekker, Inc.
Peeler, H.T. 1972. *J. Anim. Sci.* 35:695.
Peo, E.R. 1976. *Calcium in Swine Nutrition.* West Des Moines, IA: NFIA.
Pond, W.G., et al. 1961. *J. Anim. Sci.* 20:747.
Rao, N., and B.S.N. Rao. 1970. *Am. J. Clin. Nutr.* 23:105.
Reiners, R.A., and C.M. Gooding. 1975. In: *Corn, Culture, Processing, Products.* Inglett, G.E. (Ed.). p. 241. Westport, CT: AVI Publishing Co.
Ross, R.D., G.L. Cromwell, and T.S. Stahly. 1984. *J. Anim. Sci.* 59:125.
Ruiz, N., and R.H. Harms. 1988. *Br. Poult. Sci.* 29:491.
Sauberlich, H. 1985. *Prog. Food Nutr. Sci.* 9:1.
Schmitz, H., and A. Muller. 1973. *Schweiz Arch Tierheilkd* 115:391.
Schneider, J. 1986. *Proceedings of the NFIA Nutrition Institute.*
Schroeder, H.A. 1971. *Am. J. Clin. Nutr.* 24:562.
Seerley, R.W., et al. 1976. *J. Anim. Sci.* 42:599.
Southern, L.L., and D.H. Baker. 1981. *J. Anim. Sci.* 53:403.
Southern, L.L., and D.H. Baker. 1983a. *J. Nutr.* 113:688.
Southern, L.L., and D.H. Baker. 1983b. *J. Nutr.* 113:172.
Southern, L.L., and D.H. Baker. 1983c. *Poult. Sci.* 62:642.
Staten, F.E., et al. 1980. *Poult. Sci.* 59:1673.
Stockland, W.L., and L.G. Blaylock. 1974. *J. Anim. Sci.* 39:1113.
Sullivan, T.W. 1961. *Poult. Sci.* 40:340.

Thoren-Tolling, K. 1975. *Acta Vet. Scand.* Suppl. 54.
Ullrey, D.E. 1972. *J. Anim. Sci.* 35:648.
Ullrey, D.E. 1981. *J. Anim. Sci.* 53:1039.
Ullrey, D.E., et al. 1973. *Michigan Agricultural Experiment Station Report 232.* p. 34. East Lansing: Michigan State University.
Verbeeck, J. 1975. *Feedstuffs* 9:8, p. 45.
Waibel, P.E., et al. 1984. *Poult. Sci.* 63:730.
Warnick, R.C. 1968. *Feedstuffs* 40:25.
Wedekind, K.J., and D.H. Baker. 1990. *J. Anim. Sci.* 68:684.
Wright, P.L., and M.C. Bell. 1966. *Am. J. Physiol.* 211:6.
Yen, J.T., A.H. Jensen, and D.H. Baker. 1976. *J. Anim. Sci.* 42:866.
Yen, J.T., A.H. Jensen, and D.H. Baker. 1977. *J. Anim. Sci.* 46:269.
Young, L.G., et al. 1975. *J. Anim. Sci.* 40:495.
Young, L.G., et al. 1977. *J. Anim. Sci.* 45:1051.
Young, L.G., et al. 1978. *J. Anim. Sci.* 47:639.
Zhuge, Q., and C.F. Klopfenstein. 1986. *Poult. Sci.* 65:987.

Chapter 21

Appetite and Feeding Behavior

K.A. Houpt and T.R. Houpt

There are a variety of factors that influence feeding in pigs, some short-term, others long-term; still others are operational only in emergency situations. Taste can either stimulate or inhibit intake. Taste factors have been used to increase intake of newly weaned pigs. Gastric factors, particularly gastric fill, can suppress feeding. Changes within the intestinal tract such as an increase in osmotic pressure and release of the hormone cholecystokinin can bring a meal to an end, thus inhibiting intake. These are all short-term factors. The long-term controls of feeding in which intake is controlled as part of the regulation of body weight or body fat are obviously operational in pigs, because they respond appropriately to manipulation of the caloric density of their diet. However, the mechanisms underlying long-term control remain unknown. Eating in response to lack of metabolizable glucose is an emergency mechanism that is probably not involved in meal-to-meal initiation of eating. Increasing blood levels of glucose does not suppress feeding. When food is freely available, pigs eat many meals a day, the number decreasing with the size of the pig. Water drinking is associated with eating. Under these circumstances, initiation of a meal is probably a response to waning of the satiety signals. These signals are integrated in the brain, where a variety of neurotransmitters and anatomical sites are involved in feeding. The finding that depressants introduced into the brain stimulate feeding reinforces the concept that hunger occurs when satiety signals weaken.

APPETITE

Hunger is aroused by a physiological need. Appetite is aroused by a different type of motivation: a desire, rather than a drive, to repeat a pleasurable experience. Hunger can be satisfied by calories; appetite is satisfied by palatability. Animals will defend a lean body mass no matter how unpalatable the diet, but a different and higher body weight will be defended and a greater amount of food eaten when a palatable diet is offered. Palatability is mostly a function of the taste and texture of food, for removing the sense of smell does not reduce food intake in pigs (Baldwin and Cooper 1979). The importance of increasing appetite is confirmed by Pekas' (1983, 1985) finding that pigs gain more weight when overfed intragastrically than when eating ad libitum. That means that neither gastrointestinal fill nor rate of passage limit intake; the pig's appetite does.

FOOD PREFERENCES

The taste responses of pigs, like those of other animals, can be divided into preferences, aversions, and tastes that are not differentiated from water. Taste preferences have been investigated more fully than aversions, usually with the goal of increasing intake of newly weaned pigs.

Sweetness

When preferences for pure chemicals were tested, the strongest preference was for sucrose (Kare et al. 1965). Kennedy and Baldwin (1972) found that pigs would consume up to 17 L of sucrose solution in 12 hours. Care must be taken in assuming that what tastes sweet to humans also tastes sweet to pigs. Most humans, for example, report that both the artifical sweeteners saccharin and cyclamate taste sweet. However, pigs show a preference for saccharin, but they are indifferent to cyclamate (Kennedy and Baldwin 1972). All of the studies mentioned so far involved preferences for solutions. The pigs demonstrated preference either by consuming more of the solution than of water or by pushing a panel to obtain a reward of sweetened fluid. Pigs also show a preference for sucrose in solid food. When presented a cafeteria of various concentrations of sucrose, they preferred the feed with the highest concentration (20%). Baby pigs gain more weight and are more efficient on sucrose-supplemented starter diets (Lewis et al. 1955) than on nonsupplemented ones.

Stimulating Intake in the Weanling Pig

Preference for sweet taste is apparently innate, for newborn piglets that have not yet suckled show preferences for saccharin solutions (Foster 1968). Bottle-raised piglets showed preference (over water) for sucrose, lactose, and fructose, in that order (Houpt and Houpt 1976). Despite strong sweet preferences, inclusion of sugar, an expensive feedstuff, in starter rations does not appear to increase total intake when young pigs (<1 month old) are stressed by the weaning process (Diaz et al. 1956).

Social facilitation can increase intake in adult pigs (see Hunger: Environmental Factors), that is, pigs will eat more when housed in groups than when housed singly. A similar phenomenon appears to be operating in suckling pigs; playing a recording of piglet nursing calls can also be used to stimulate intake in early weaned pigs (Csermely and Wood-Gush 1981).

Just as an aversion can be learned (see Learned Food Aversions: Laboratory Learning), satiety can be learned. A flavor can be introduced into the sow's diet that will flavor the milk, and the piglets should learn that the flavor is paired with well-being. Later they should eat more of a similarly flavored feed; however, use of this technique has had inconsistent effects on feed intake of newly weaned pigs (Ogunbameru et al. 1979; Campbell 1976).

INNATE FOOD AVERSIONS

Sodium Chloride

Many species, particularly herbivores that consume a sodium-deficient diet, show a preference for salt solutions, but pigs do not (Kare et al. 1965) unless they have been adrenalectomized (Lustgarden et al. 1973). The aversion to concentrated NaCl solutions is not very strong and can be overcome by thirst; therefore, salt poisoning can occur in pigs whose only source of fluid is contaminated with salt (Smith 1975).

Bitter

Pigs show an aversion to quinine, the chemical typically used as a bitter tastant (Kare et al. 1965; Yang et al. 1981; Leamaster and Cheeke 1979), but pigs do not show an aversion to bitrex, a compound that tastes extremely bitter to humans (Blair and Fitz-Simons 1970). There are feedstuffs that are nutritionally adequate, but that pigs reject because of their taste. For example, rapeseed meal contains glucosinolate, which pigs apparently find unpalatable (Lee et al. 1984). The saponins in alfalfa also suppress intake (Leamaster and Cheeke 1979).

LEARNED FOOD AVERSION

Laboratory Learning

Reactions to sweet and bitter are innate, but some taste preferences and, in particular, aversions can be learned. Pigs can learn to avoid a taste of a food that they normally prefer if the taste of that food is followed by illness. This phenomenon, taste aversion learning, is similar to other kinds of learning in that a conditioned stimulus is paired with an unconditioned stimulus, but it differs in three ways. First, the unconditioned stimulus must be illness, not pain; nausea is the best stimulus. Second, the salient feature of the conditioned stimulus is the taste or odor of food, not the location where the illness occurred. Third, the illness does not have to be closely paired in time with the ingestion of the food. Pigs are able to form taste aversions to such normally preferred tastes as maple syrup and honey if the taste is paired with nausea produced either by systematically administered apomorphine or intestinally administered lithium chloride (Anika et al. 1981). Suckling pigs can learn to form an aversion to teats flavored with maple syrup if suckling from the flavored teat was paired with illness (Houpt et al. 1979).

Amino Acid Imbalance or Protein Deficiency

The depression of food intake in pigs fed an imbalanced diet, particularly one imbalanced with respect to amino acids, or a protein-free diet, is probably also a form of taste aversion learning (Devilat et al. 1970; Robinson 1974, 1975; Robinson et al. 1974). The pig learns that it feels ill while eating the poor diet and decreases its intake, but because it has no other choice of diet, it eats enough to maintain itself.

MEAL PATTERNS

Normal Feeding and Drinking Patterns

A number of investigators have studied meal patterns in pigs. Most studies have been of young, 2 to 4-month-old pigs. These pigs eat approximately 12 meals per day (Friend 1973; Montgomery et al. 1978; Baldwin and Cooper 1979; Auffray and Marcilloux 1980). Auffray and Marcilloux (1983) found that mature pigs (250 kg) ate only two to five meals per day. Most meals were eaten during the day, indicating that, at least under conditions of domestication, the pig is a diurnal animal. Wangsness et al. (1980) found that obese Ossabaw Island pigs ate a greater number of smaller meals than did lean Yorkshire pigs of the same age. The Ossabaw pigs also ate more slowly.

Thirst and its stimuli have been studied in pigs. Pigs will drink in response to water deprivation, to an increase in osmolality of their blood, and to an increase in environmental temperature (Ingram and Stephens 1979; Anderson and Houpt 1990), but most drinking in pigs is associated with feeding rather than with changes in plasma osmolality or volume (Houpt and Anderson 1990). Twenty-five percent of water intake occurs before meals, 30% during meals, and 20% after meals. Only 25% of water drinking occurs more than 10 minutes before or after feeding (Bigelow and Houpt 1988). The same physiological mechanisms that stimulate gastric secretion (histamine, gastrin, and cholinergic agents) stimulate water drinking (Houpt et al. 1986), suggesting that gastric secretion just before and perhaps during and after a meal acts as a stimulus of such drinking. Just as most food intake appears to occur without a major change in body energy balance, most drinking occurs without a change in body fluid balance. The osmotic and volume depletion stimuli to drinking appear to be emergency mechanisms to restore body water under life-threatening conditions.

Changes of Feeding and Drinking Schedules with Age

Young pigs (10 to 15 kg) eat twelve meals per day. As they mature, meal size increases and the number of meals decreases, leveling off to seven meals per day as the pigs reach 60 kg. As the pigs grow, more food is eaten per day in a smaller number of larger meals. Increase in meal size is achieved primarily by increasing the rate of eating, apparently because larger pigs have larger mouths. There is no consistent increase in the length or duration of meals (Bigelow and Houpt 1988). The mechanics of chewing also change as the pig matures (Herring 1977). The ratio of water:food and the pattern of water intake does not change during development in pigs over 10 kg.

One of the major problems with early-weaned pigs may be drinking. Brooks et al. (1984) found that piglets weaned at 21 days drank virtually nothing until 2 days after weaning. They then drank a great deal before leveling off. The piglets drank more during the day than at night even when their cages were lighted for the entire 24 hours.

HUNGER

Normal Hunger: The Absence of Satiety

When food is freely available, pigs eat a large number of meals, as discussed previously. There does not appear to be a hunger signal that precedes the onset of feeding. This and the evidence that most of the experimental depressants of feeding act through or in conjunction with sympathetic arousal has led to the hypothesis that hunger is not the active process, satiety is. Animals eat when the satiety signals wane rather than ceasing to eat when the hunger signals wane. Exceptions to this are thermostatic eating, in which eating is in response to the cold, and glucostatic eating, in which the response is to a lack of metabolizable glucose.

Hypoglycemia and Glucoprivation

A decrease in the amount of utilizable brain glucose will stimulate feeding in pigs. This stimulation can be produced either by hypoglycemia as the result of insulin injection (Houpt and Houpt 1977) or by injection of the glucose analogue 2-deoxy-D-glucose, which enters the cell and is phosphorylated, but which cannot be metabolized beyond the glucose-6-phosphate step (Stephens 1980a). Depriving the brain of glucose locally by intraventricular administration of deoxyglucose also stimulates feeding (Parrott and Baldwin 1978).

Glucostatic feeding does not appear to be present in suckling pigs; although piglets eat in response to deprivation of sow's milk, they do not increase their intake in response to insulin (Houpt, Houpt, and Pond 1977). Pekas et al. (1959), using piglets weaned at 2 weeks, also found that neither tolbutamide nor insulin stimulated intake or weight gain.

Environmental Factors

Social Facilitation

It has long been known that pigs will eat more when housed in groups than when housed separately (Cole 1967). Hsia and Wood-Gush (1982) have demonstrated this more directly. This effect—the act of eating by one animal stimulating another to eat—is called social facilitation of feeding.

Central Nervous System Depressants as Stimulants of Appetite

The pig is not well-suited to intracranial manipulation because of the rapid growth and individual variation of cranial structures. However, a reliable means of stimulating the central nervous system has been intracerebral ventricular injection. Barbiturates, calcium, magnesium, and deoxyglucose injected into the lateral ventricle stimulate intake (Baldwin et al. 1975; Parrott and Baldwin 1978). Similarly, direct application of pentobarbital to the ventromedial hypothalamus stimulates intake (Khalaf and Robinson 1972b). The common feature of these diverse substances is that they inhibit cerebral function either directly by anesthesia (barbiturate and magnesium) or glucoprivation (deoxyglucose) or by altering the electrolyte concentration (calcium). The mechanism of action of neuropeptide Y in stimulating intake in pigs is not clear (Parrott et al. 1986), but the peptide is widely distributed in the central nervous system.

SATIETY

Satiety is more than an absence of hunger. First, it is anticipatory in that eating during a meal ceases before body energy stores can be repleted by digestion and absorption of the ingested food. Satiety may be signaled by humoral or neural means, or, most likely, by both. Second, satiety is not necessarily a pleasant sensation; there may be an aversive component to satiety that prevents overeating, even in the presence of abundant, palatable feed.

Humoral Correlates of Satiety

Feeding changes the plasma concentrations of a variety of metabolites and hormones. Changes in one or more of these factors may provide the cue that food is being ingested and cause reduction of hunger before all the ingested calories have been absorbed. Corticosteroids decrease with feeding, indicating that fasting is a stress (Houpt, K.A., et al. 1983a). Further, corticotropin releasing factor administered centrally can depress intake, presumably because of a rise of cortisol (Parrott 1990). Free fatty acid concentrations also fall with feeding as metabolism shifts from lipolyis and transport of fatty acids to liver for oxidation during the fast to fat synthesis after feeding. Glucose levels rise as it is absorbed. Plasma glucose and intestinal glucose stimulate insulin release so that hormone also rises in the plasma (Houpt, K.A. et al. 1983a). Triiodothyronine, the metabolically most active thyroid hormone, also increases with feeding (Dauncey et al. 1983). Increasing a thermogenic hormone may be a way of dissipating excess energy in the form of heat. Of all the changes that accompany feeding, few are seen following spontaneous meals in free-feeding pigs (Houpt, K.A. et al. 1983b). The exception is the response of free fatty acids. Free fatty acid concentrations fall significantly following consumption even of a spontaneous meal (Houpt, Reimers, and Boyd 1986).

Pigs eat less when they are in estrus and at the same time expend more time walking (Friend 1973; Altmann 1941). These responses can be used to detect estrus in the absence of a boar. They presumably are due to the well-known changes in concentrations of the sexual hormones.

Gastrointestinal Factors in Satiety

If the size of a meal is to be matched with nutrient needs, rapid initiation of satiety signals to the CNS could be used while the meal is in progress to inhibit feeding after an appropriate amount of feed has been ingested (Figure 21.1). Obvious effects of food injected within the tract that might initiate such satiety signals are distention, hyper-

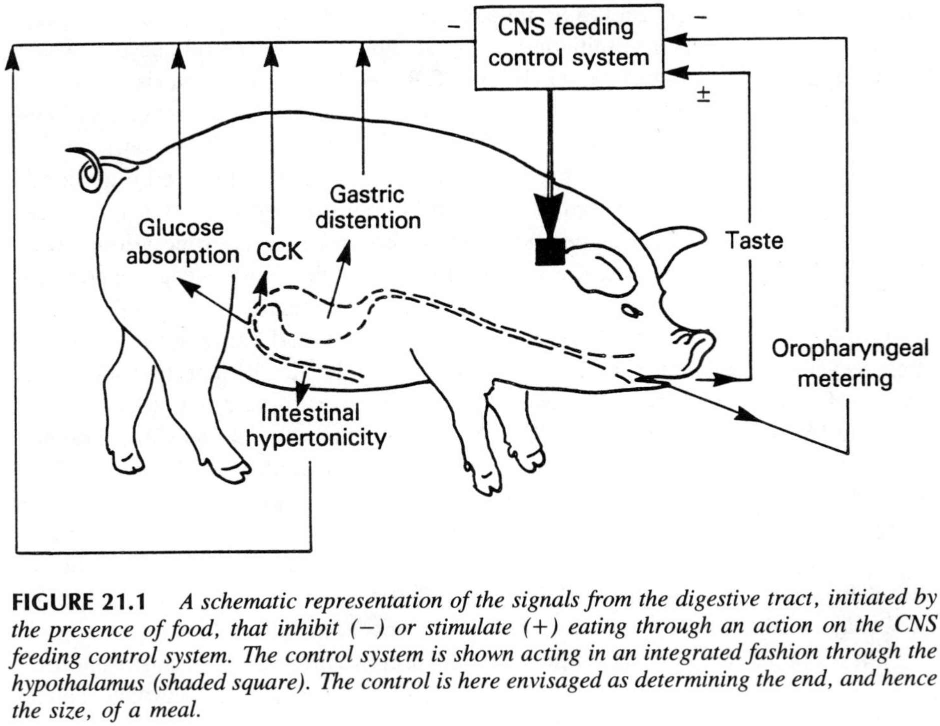

FIGURE 21.1 *A schematic representation of the signals from the digestive tract, initiated by the presence of food, that inhibit (−) or stimulate (+) eating through an action on the CNS feeding control system. The control system is shown acting in an integrated fashion through the hypothalamus (shaded square). The control is here envisaged as determining the end, and hence the size, of a meal.*

tonicity, and the presence of specific nutrients such as glucose, amino acids, and fatty acids. To some degree, the role of each of these stimuli in control of eating during a meal has been investigated in young weaned pigs.

Distention is the most nonspecific result of food ingestion. The likelihood that gastric and intestinal stretch inhibit eating seems high, but it has not been investigated thoroughly in the pig. We have found that intragastric pressure rises slightly immediately upon initiation of a meal from a fasted pressure of about 5 cm H_2O to 8 to 10 cm H_2O, then gradually rises during the meal to a pressure of 18 to 22 cm H_2O when eating stops. Typically, an immediate slight fall of pressure occurs, followed by a gradual fall as digestion proceeds (Houpt 1985). The correlation between a mean pressure of approximately 20 cm H_2O and cessation of eating suggests a causal relationship. Pressure changes presumably reflect distention, but the reflex receptive relaxation of the stomach confuses this pressure-distention relationship. There is also evidence that distention of the small intestine by only a few centimeters H_2O will effectively inhibit eating (Houpt 1982).

A rise in osmolality of gastrointestinal content is also a relatively nonspecific result of food ingestion. Presumably, the hypertonicity reflects the solubility of the food and its digestibility, and a rough correlation between hyperosmolality and nutrient value of the food would be expected. Sensory receptor systems seem most sensitive in the duodenum, as compared with the stomach and lower intestine, and it is here that the osmotic satiety control has been studied. Infusion of a hypertonic solution of an absorbable compound into the duodenum causes immediate inhibition of eating, and the strength of the inhibition varies with the degree of hypertonicity of the infused solution. The inhibitory control appears to be initiated primarily by hypertonic solutions penetrating the intestinal mucosa, initiating neuronal signals to the central nervous system (Houpt et al. 1979; Stephens 1980b; Houpt, T.R., et al. 1983a). Such rises do occur after ingestion of nutrient meals with an appropriate time course of osmotic rise in the duodenum to serve as an intrameal satiety stimulus (Houpt, T.R., et al., 1983b). Finally, certain of the specific nutrients resulting from the ingestion and digestion of food of high quality have been implicated in satiety controls. However, thus far glucose has not been shown to have a specific satiety effect from the intestine (Houpt et al. 1979; Stephens 1985); in fact, the satiety effects to both intraduodenal glucose and NaCl solutions of equiosmotic strength appear to be identical (Houpt et al. 1979).

One of the most striking effects of certain amino acids and fatty acids is the release of cholecystokinin (CCK) from the duodenal mucosa. Besides its digestive role, CCK has been found in other species to have a satiety effect, and there is similar evidence in the pig (Anika et al. 1981). The CCK appears to act not directly on the central nervous system, but rather at a site in the distal stomach or duodenum (Houpt 1983). It should be noted, however, that CCK can have a general sedative-type action. For example, when CCK is administered as a bolus injection rather than as a continuous infusion, operant responses for food, water, and heat are reduced, indicating a nonspecific depression (Baldwin et al. 1982). Nevertheless, the evidence that endogenous CCK plays a role in satiety continues to mount (Ebenezer et al. 1990).

These are the satiety signals initiated by the presence of food in the gastrointestinal tract that have been investigated in the pig. Many other hormonal and neuronal changes associated with the presence of food in the tract have been suggested as possible satiety signals for determination of meal size, but there have been few or no studies of these in pigs.

Suckling piglets also respond to gastrointestinal factors. All the experiments have involved administration of loads by gavage, that is, through an orally inserted catheter that is passed into the stomach. Isotonic glucose and lactose solutions were more effective in suppressing subsequent intake than milk, cream, or a protein hydrolysate (Houpt et al. 1977; Stephens 1975; Houpt et al. 1983b).

Blood-Borne Satiety Factors

Some of the metabolites that are obvious candidates for a humoral satiety factor, for example, glucose, seem not to have any effect on feeding in pigs (Stephens and Baldwin 1974; Houpt et al. 1979). Although high, unphysiological levels of insulin stimulate feeding by depressing blood glucose concentration, there is also some evidence that low levels of insulin may inhibit intake (Anika et al. 1980). The possible role of glucose availability and of insulin in the immediate control of eating is unclear.

Environmental Factors

Heat

Pigs eat less in the heat, just as they eat more in the cold (Ingram and Legge 1974). When faced with a high environmental temperature, the pig apparently attempts to avoid hyperthermia, which would occur when triiodothyronine stimulates heat production after feeding.

Social

Pigs can suffer undernourishment despite the fact that a well-balanced diet is available in adequate amounts if other pigs keep them from the food. This is most apt to occur when limited amounts are fed and/or too little trough space is available (Baldwin and Meese 1979; Hansen et al. 1982; Hsia and Wood-Gush 1982). This is the converse of social faciliation, and it is due to the dominance of some members of the group over others. Social facilitation can be used to encourage feeding without sparking competition by providing individual feeding stalls that allow only one pig to enter, but that allow visual and auditory contact with other pigs.

Central Neural Involvement in Satiety

Anatomical Site

Classically, lesions of the ventromedial hypothalamus cause an increase in food intake and body weight, whereas lesions of the lateral hypothalamus cause anorexia and a loss in body weight in a variety of animals. The ventromedial hypothalamus, therefore, would be involved in bringing meals to an end, thereby limiting weight gain. This appears to be true of pigs as well (Auffray 1969; Khalaf 1969; Khalaf and Robinson 1972a).

Neurotransmitters and Modulators

The number of neurotransmitters and neuromodulators now identified has greatly increased our estimation of the complexity of the brain. This has made any search for a particular chemical or combination of chemicals that will cause satiety or feeding or any other behavior more difficult, but a few attempts have been made in pigs. The hormone CCK, which suppresses intake when administered peripherally, is also present in the brain of pigs (Muller et al. 1977). When exogenous CCK is injected into the cerebral ventricles, food intake is suppressed (Baldwin et al. 1982). A related hormone, bombesin, had the same effect in pigs, but the effect in this case appeared to be nonspecific because water intake was also suppressed and the majority of the pigs vomited (Parrott and Baldwin 1982).

Another category of brain peptides that appears to be involved in ingestive behavior is that of the opiates. The opiate antagonist naloxone does not, however, affect feeding in pigs; rather, it suppresses water intake (Baldwin and Parrot 1985).

REFERENCES

Altmann, M. 1941. *J. Comp. Psychol.* 31:481–498.
Anderson, C.R., and T.R. Houpt. 1990. *Am. J. Physiol.* 258:R149–R154.
Anika, S.M., T.R. Houpt, and K.A. Houpt. 1980. *Physiol. Behav.* 25:21–23.
Anika, S.M., T.R. Houpt, and K.A. Houpt. 1981. *Am. J. Physiol.* 240:R310–R318.
Auffray, P. 1969. *Ann. Biol. Anim. Biochim. Biophys.* 9:513–526.
Auffray, P., and J.C. Marcilloux. 1980. *Reprod. Nutr. Develop.* 20:1625–1632.
Auffray, P., and J.C. Marcilloux. 1983. *Reprod. Nutr. Develop.* 23:517–524.
Baldwin, B.A., and T.R. Cooper. 1979. *Appl. Anim. Ethol.* 5:153–159.
Baldwin, B.A., and G.B. Meese. 1979. *Anim. Behav.* 27:947–957.
Baldwin, B.A., and R.F. Parrott. 1985. *Pharm. Biochem. Behav.* 22:37–40.
Baldwin, B.A., T.R. Cooper, and R.F. Parrott. 1982. *Proc. Nutr. Soc.* 41:119–121.
Baldwin, B.A., et al. 1975. *Pharm. Biochem. Behav.* 3:915–918.
Bigelow, J.A., and T.R. Houpt. 1988. *Physiol. Behav.* 43:99–109.
Blair, R., and J. FitzSimons. 1970. *Anim. Prod.* 12:529–530.
Brooks, P.H., S.J. Russell, and J.L. Carpenter. 1984. *Vet. Rec.* 115:513–515.
Campbell, R.G. 1976. *Anim. Prod.* 23:417–419.
Cole, D.J.A., J.E. Duckworth, and W. Holmes. 1967. *Anim. Prod.* 9:141–148.
Csermely, D., and D.G.M. Wood-Gush. 1981. *Biol. Behav.* 6:159–165.
Dauncey, M.J., et al. 1983. *Horm. Metab. Res.* 15:499–502.
Devilat, J., W.G. Pond, and P.D. Miller. 1970. *J. Anim. Sci.* 30:536–543.
Diaz, F., et al. 1956. *Anim. Sci.* 15:315–319.
Ebenezer, I.S., C. DeLaRiva, and B.A. Baldwin. 1990. *Physiol. Behav.* 47:145–148.
Foster, R. 1968. *Psychonom. Sci.* 10:83–84.
Friend, D.W. 1973. *J. Anim. Sci.* 37:1137–1141.
Hansen, L.L., A.M. Hagelso, and A.M. Madsen. 1982. *Appl. Anim. Ethol.* 8:307–333.
Herring, S.W. 1977. *J. Dental Res.* 56:1377–1382.
Houpt, K.A. 1982. *Neurosci. Biobehav. Rev.* 6:145–164.

Houpt, K.A., and T.R. Houpt. 1976. *Chem. Senses Flavour* 2:219–228.
Houpt, K.A., and T.R. Houpt. 1977. "The neonatal pig: A biological model for the development of taste preferences and controls of ingestive behavior." In: *Taste and Development: The Genesis of Sweet Preference*. Weiffenbach, J.M. (Ed.). pp. 86–98. Bethesda, MD: U.S. Department of Health, Education, and Welfare.
Houpt, K.A., et al. 1983a. *Am. J. Physiol.* 244:R279–R284.
Houpt, K.A., T.R. Houpt, and W.G. Pond. 1983b. *J. Anim. Sci.* 57:413–417.
Houpt, K.A., T.R. Houpt, and W.G. Pond. 1977. *Am. J. Physiol.* 232:E510–E514.
Houpt, K.A., T.J. Reimers, and R.D. Boyd. 1986. *Physiol. Behav.* 37:573–576.
Houpt, K.A., et al. 1979. *Vet. Sci. Commun.* 3:165–169.
Houpt, T.R. 1983. *Physiol. Behav.* 31:693–698.
Houpt, T.R. 1985. *Proc. Nutr. Soc.* 44:323–330.
Houpt, T.R., and C.R. Anderson. 1990. *Am. J. Physiol.* 258:R143–R148.
Houpt, T.R., S.M. Anika, and K.A. Houpt. 1979. *Am. J. Physiol.* 236:R328–R337.
Houpt, T.R., B.A. Baldwin, and K.A. Houpt. 1983a. *Physiol. Behav.* 30:787–795.
Houpt, T.R., K.A. Houpt, and A.A. Swan. 1983b. *Am. J. Physiol.* 245:R181–R189.
Houpt, T.R., L.C. Weixler, and D.W. Troy. 1986. *Am. J. Physiol.* 251:R157–R164.
Hsia, L.C., and D.G.M. Wood-Gush. 1982. *Appl. Anim. Ethol.* 8:410.
Ingram, D.L., and K.F. Legge. 1974. *Comp. Biochem. Physiol.* 8:573–581.
Ingram, D.L., and D.B. Stephens. 1979. *J. Physiol.* 293:501–512.
Kare, M.R., W.C. Pond, and J. Campbell. 1965. *Anim. Behav.* 13:265–269.
Kennedy, J.M., and B.A. Baldwin. 1972. *Anim. Behav.* 20:706–718.
Khalaf, F. 1969. *Res. Vet. Sci.* 10:514–517.
Khalaf, F., and D.W. Robinson. 1972a. *Res. Vet. Sci.* 13:1–4.
Khalaf, F., and D.W. Robinson. 1972b. *Res. Vet. Sci.* 13:5–7.
Leamaster, B.R., and P. Cheeke. 1979. *Can. J. Anim. Sci.* 59:467–469.
Lee, P.A., S. Pittam, and R. Hill. 1984. *Br. J. Nutr.* 52:159–164.
Lewis, C.J., et al. 1955. *J. Anim. Sci.* 14:1103–1115.
Lustgarten, C., G.D. Bottoms, and J.R. Shaskas. 1973. *Am. J. Vet. Res.* 34:279–282.
Montgomery, G.W., D.S. Flux, and J.R. Carr. 1978. *Physiol. Behav.* 20:693–698.
Muller, J.E., E. Straus, and R.S. Yalow. 1977. *Proc. Natl. Acad. Sci. USA* 74:3035–3037.
Ogunbameru, B.O., et al. 1979. *Nutr. Rep. Int.* 20:455–460.
Parrott, R.F. 1990. *Physiol Behav.* 47:519–524.
Parrott, R.F., and B.A. Baldwin. 1978. *Physiol. Behav.* 21:329–331.
Parrott, R.F., and B.A. Baldwin. 1982. *Physiol. Behav.* 28:521–524.
Parrott, R.F., R.P. Heavens, and B.A. Baldwin. 1986. *Physiol. Behav.* 36:523–525.
Parrott, R.F., et al. 1988. *Am. J. Physiol.* 255:R248–R251.
Pekas, J.C. 1983. *Appetite* 4:23–30.
Pekas, J.C. 1985. *Growth* 49:19.27.
Pekas, J.C., et al. 1959. *J. Anim. Sci.* 18:1282–1291.
Robinson, D.W. 1974. *Br. Vet. J.* 130:522–527.
Robinson, D.W. 1975. *Br. Vet. J.* 131:595–600.
Robinson, D.W., J.H.G. Holmes, and H.S. Bayley. 1974. *Br. Vet. J.* 130:361–365.
Smith, D.L.T. 1975. "Sodium salt poisoning." In: *Diseases of Swine. 4th ed.* Dunne, H.W., and A.D. Leman (Eds). pp. 854–860. Ames, IA: Iowa State University Press.
Stephens, D.B. 1975. *J. Comp. Physiol. Psychol.* 88:796–805.
Stephens, D.B. 1985. *Q. J. Exp. Physiol.* 70:129–135.
Stephens, D.B. 1980a. *Physiol. Behav.* 25:691–699.
Stephens, D.B. 1980a. *J. Physiol.* 299:453–463.
Stephens, D.B., and B.A. Baldwin. 1974. *Physiol. Behav.* 12:923–929.
Wangsness, P.J., J.L. Gobble, and G.W. Sherritt. 1980. *Physiol. Behav.* 24:407–410.
Yang, T.S., B. Howard, and W.V. Macfarlane. 1981. *Appl. Anim. Ethol.* 7:259–270.

Chapter 22

Physical Forms of Feed: Feed Processing and Feeder Design and Operation

D.O. Liptrap and M.G. Hogberg

Approximately 55% to 65% of the total cost of producing a market hog can be attributed to feed. Consequently, it is important to evaluate methods of improving nutrient utilization of feedstuffs by various processing methods. Through proper processing, some feedstuffs that seemingly have little value can be converted to useful sources of energy and essential nutrients for pigs. Thus, the real purpose of feed processing is to alter a feedstuff to improve its usefulness in supplying available nutrients to the pig.

Feed processing can alter the physical or chemical properties of a feedstuff through mechanical, chemical, thermal, or bacterial treatments. These processes can improve (1) the digestibility of the nutrients that provide energy, (2) the bioavailability of amino acids, vitamins, or essential elements, (3) diet palatability, and (4) destruction of toxins. Although a laboratory conducted nutrient analysis of a feedstuff may not be changed by a processing method, the digestibility or bioavailability of nutrients may be enhanced or hindered. Thus, nutrient analysis, coupled with an understanding of the effects of feed processing, is important in obtaining optimum productive performance.

Feed processing methods that have been used in preparation of swine diets include grinding, pelleting, liquid feeding, paste feeding, roasting, steam flaking, micronizing, and extruding. Most feeds are processed in some form before distribution and consumption (Table 22.1)

FEED PROCESSING METHODS

Grinding

Swine are quite capable of chewing corn and other grains in which most kernels are partially broken down into smaller particles. Small, hard kernels are more difficult to break into smaller particles during mastication, allowing some kernels to pass through

Table 22.1 Effects of Processing Feedstuffs or Complete Diets on Pig Performance

Processing Method	Type of Grain, Other Feedstuff, or Complete Diet	Change in			Comments
		Growth Rate	*Feed Intake*	*Feed Conversion*	
Grinding	Corn	Improved 3–5%	No effect	Improved 3–5%	Medium screen (1/4–3/8 in); generally most acceptable.
	Grain sorghum	Improved	No effect	Improved	Grinding too fine may reduce palatability.
Pelleting	Corn Grain sorghum Barley Oats	Improved 3–6%	Reduced 1–3%	Improved 5–8%	
	Alfalfa Wheat	Improved 3–6%	Reduced 1–3%	Improved 7–10%	Greater improvement with higher fibrous materials.
Paste	Corn	Improved 10–15%	Increased 10–15%	No change	Feed:water ratio of 1.2–5:1; advantage with G-F pigs but not weanlings.
Liquid	Corn	Improved	Increased	Improved	Water:feed ratio 2:1; advantages with limit-fed systems; full-fed levels fail to improve performance.

Roasting	Corn	No change	No change	Slightly improved	Processing cost greater than improvement return.
	Soybeans	No change	Decreased 4–6%	Improved	Necessary for adequate performance: Comparisons made with SBM.
Steam flaking	Corn	No change	No change	No change	
	Grain sorghum	No change	No change	No change	
Micronizing	Corn	No change	No change	No change	Availability of amino acids may be reduced.
	Grain sorghum	No change	No change	No change	
Extruding	Wheat	No change	No change	No change	
	Grain sorghum	No change	No change	No change	
	Soybeans	No change	Decreased	Improved 4–6%	Comparison made with SBM necessary for adequate performance.

Abbreviation:: SBM, soybean meal.

Source: Hogberg et al. 1980. National Pork Industry Handbook, no. 71.

the alimentary tract underutilized. Grinding reduces particle size and increases the surface area, exposing a larger area to the digestive enzymes in the alimentary tract. Wu and Allee (1984) reported surface area to decrease linearly as particle size increased. Normally, finely ground feeds pass through the digestive tract slightly faster than do more coarsely ground feeds (Hogberg et al. 1980).

When feeding a total mixed ration, it is important to grind ingredients to a uniform particle size to prevent sorting by the pig. Normally, the grinding of feedstuffs is classified as fine, medium, or coarse. Generally, when feedstuff particles pass through a 1/8- to 3/16-inch hammer mill screen, the feed is classified as finely ground. Feed that passes through a 1/4- to 3/8-inch hammer mill screen is classified as medium ground. Coarsely ground feed is that which passes through a 1/2-inch or larger screen. Using only screen size to classify the fineness of grind can be somewhat misleading. Other factors that determine fineness of grind include hammer mill speed and area of the screen through which the feed passes.

Young pigs appear to perform better on finely ground feed. Wu and Allee (1984) found that feed intake decreased and feed efficiency improved as particle size decreased. Similar results have been reported for growing-finishing swine. Holden (1981) summarized data in which little effect on growth rate was noted when the particle size of the diet varied from coarse to fine grind.

Feed efficiency is generally improved as feeds are ground more finely. Pig performance on grains such as wheat and sorghum generally is enhanced by feeding ground as compared with feeding the whole grain. However, Luce et al. (1970) and Ohh et al. (1983) showed that reducing particle size of sorghum did not improve pig performance. Conversely, Owsley et al. (1981) showed that digestibilities of dry matter, starch, gross energy, and nitrogen were improved by feeding finely ground sorghum as compared with a medium or coursely ground sorghum. They concluded that increasing the fineness of grind improves digestibility of nutrients in sorghum by growing-finishing pigs. Grinding wheat too finely can reduce palatability, thus reducing feed intake (Hogberg et al. 1980).

Increasing the fineness of grind can result in several other production problems. Bridging in self-feeders increases dramatically with finely ground diets (Jensen 1978). An increase in incidence of gastric ulcers is also noted as feeds become more finely ground (Newer et al. 1965; Mahan et al. 1966). Excessively dusty conditions in confinement facilities can be attributed largely to finely ground feed. Using a medium grind is generally recommended to take advantage of improvement in feed efficiency while minimizing potential gastric ulcer problems in the pigs.

Feedstuffs with increased fiber content may also benefit from grinding. Nuzback et al. (1982) showed that decreasing particle size of sun-cured alfalfa increased the utilization of dry matter and digestable energy (DE) by gestating sows. This would indicate that alfalfa can be better utilized by gestating sows if particle size is reduced.

Pelleting

Pelleting is used extensively in commercially prepared diets, since a more uniform product can be delivered to the producer. Pelleting greatly reduces the "settling out" of fine particles during transportation. To begin the pelleting process, feed is ground to a fine or medium texture then steamed and formed into a pellet by extrusion through a die. The use of steam in the process increases the pellet durability and produces less starch damage in the grain. Pellets can be made in varying lengths, diameters, and degrees of hardness. When given a preference, nursing and newly weaned pigs prefer a pelleted diet over a meal diet (Jensen 1966). Crumbled feeds are preferred over pellets (Vanschoubroek et al. 1971). Additionally, this same age pig decreased feed intake by 6% to 9% and improved feed utilization by 5.9% to 7.4% with no effect on growth rate when fed a pelleted diet rather than a meal diet. Size of pellet can play a major role in feed acceptability, especially with small pigs. Aumaitre and Salmon-Legagneur (1961) found that smaller pigs prefer a small pellet (2.5 mm in diameter) over a larger pellet (5 to 7 mm in diameter).

Hardness of pellet can also affect intake. Jensen (1966) reported that hardness of pellet affects acceptance by the young pig. Pellets made from wheat-based diets usually result in a hard pellet. Grinding sorghum can cause a powdery texture that reduces acceptability by the pig. Pelleting the ground sorghum-based diet results in gains and efficiency of gains similar to those achieved using pelleted corn-based diets (Jensen 1966).

Jensen (1966) summarized thirty trials concerning pelleting of diets for growing-finishing swine. Although variable results were noted, average growth rate, feed intake, and gain per feed were improved by 6.2%, 1.2%, and 4.9%, respectively, when diets were pelleted.

More recently, the NCR-42 Committee (1969) reported no effect on growth rate and a significant improvement in efficiency of gain by pelleting the diets of growing-finishing swine. Vanschoubroek et al. (1971) reported a 2.1% decrease in feed intake and concomitant improvement in weight gain and efficiency of gain in swine. This coincides with data from North Carolina State University, where Clawson and Otto (1965) reported a 1.1% decrease in feed intake associated with feeding a pelleted diet. Hoefer et al. (1958) and Vanschoubroek (1971) reported that pelleting high-fiber feeds results in greater pig performance. This is especially true for diets containing high levels of alfalfa. Pelleting meal diets containing 0%, 20%, and 40% oats increased daily gain by 10%, 12%, and 28%, respectively (Hoefer et al. 1958). Daily gain was the same for all pelleted diets, while the gains decreased as the oat level increased in the meal rations.

Pelleting of feed increases the passage rate through the digestive tract. Seerley et al. (1962b) found average retention time of pelleted diets to be 29.3 hours as compared with 35.8 hours for the same diet fed in meal form. Troelsen and Bell (1962) noted a marked increase in DE intake due to higher digestibility of the energy fraction following the pelleting of a diet. This is assumed to be due to an increase in the soluble starch, which allows starch to be more readily attacked by amylase (Vanschoubroek et al. 1971). Reground pellets improve efficiency over the same diet in an unpelleted form (Holden 1981), suggesting that the moist heat and/or pressure produced in the pelleting process may increase the digestibility of the starch fraction of the diet. Pelleting high-fiber diets increases DE by 10% to 15%. No improvement in protein digestibility in pelleted diets has been observed (Seerley et al. 1962a).

Hogberg et al. (1980) mention other advantages and disadvantages in feeding a pelleted diet. Advantages include reduced dustiness, reduced storage space, less feed wastage, less wind loss, and reduced sorting of the diet by the pig. Crane et al. (1972) reported a marked decrease in the incidence of salmonella when pigs were fed pelleted feed. Disadvantages of pelleting swine diets include increased cost, reduced acceptance of hard pellets by young swine, and difficulty in pelleting diets containing fat levels of ≥6%.

Liquid Feeding

Various commercial feeding systems are available to provide liquid-feed mixtures for all phases of swine production. Each system operates differently, but the principle of providing feed is similar. The feed and water are combined either prior to or at the time of delivery to the trough. Systems can be operated either on a limit-fed or full-fed basis. Pond and Maner (1984) suggest that a 2:1 water to feed ratio will provide the best results.

Although water is provided in the mixture at the trough, it is essential for pigs to have continual access to additional water. Pigs adapt readily to liquid feeding systems with few problems (Hogberg et al. 1980). To get pigs to eat during the initial phase of liquid feeding, it may be advantageous to restrict water intake. Feed wastage is minimized when equipment is properly adjusted. The use of feed-water mixtures can reduce feed dust accumulation in a building.

Much of the research on feeding a liquid diet to growing-finishing pigs was summarized by Speer (1969). When swine are limit-fed, growth rate and feed conversion are improved when they are fed a liquid diet as compared with a dry diet. A summary of industry and university trials shows growth rate to increase by 0.8% and gain per unit of feed to increase by 5.9% when ad libitum liquid diets are compared with dry diets. Liquid feeding was shown to have no effect on farm-to-market shrink, cooler shrink, meat quality, or carcass measurements (Speer 1969).

Paste Feeding

Paste feeding is similar to liquid feeding, but water and feed are mixed at a ratio of 1.1 to 1.5:1.0, forming a paste material. This material is delivered on demand through a self-feeder. Performance is generally improved in growing-finishing pigs fed a paste diet as compared with a dry diet. No benefits have been observed for feeding a paste diet to weanling pigs (Hogberg et al. 1980). Average daily gain and feed intake are substantially increased (10% to 15%) with little improvement noted in feed conversion when feeding a paste diet to growing pigs (Teague et al. 1970).

Heating Feed Ingredients

Cereal grains and many feed by-products are not normally heat processed before mixing into swine diets, except to prepare them for safe, long-term storage. Grains, such as corn, are often dried with heated air to reduce moisture content to a level that will allow the grain to be stored without spoilage. Normal drying temperatures will not have a negative effect on feed value or pig performance. In a study reported by Jensen et al. (1960), corn dried at 140 °F, 180 °F, and 220 °F did not affect average daily gain or feed conversion when fed to weanling pigs and growing-finishing pigs. Drying grains at temperatures greater than 300 °F, however, reduces the acceptability of the corn when fed to finishing pigs. Drying temperature does not affect the content of carotene (vitamin A precursor), riboflavin, or niacin, but pantothenic acid and thiamin may be decreased. If, during the harvesting and/or handling process, the grain kernel is cracked and then dried, nutrient destruction is increased. This destruction is particularly true for carotene and vitamin E (Hogberg et al. 1980).

Heating some feedstuffs has been shown to improve pig performance by eliminating certain toxins, destroying enzyme inhibitors, or making certain nutrients more available to the pig. Most processing methods include either heat; heat and moisture; or heat, moisture, and pressure. Excessive heat can cause reducing carbohydrates such as glucose to react with free amino groups to form a bond (Maillard reaction) that is not hydrolyzed by digestive enzymes (Pond and Maner 1984). Since the digestive enzymes cannot release the bonded amino acids, such as lysine, they become unavailable to the pig. Consequently, the time and temperature of the heating process may affect the digestibility and availability of the amino acids.

Roasting

Roasting corn can influence palatability and efficiency of feed conversion. Jensen (1978) reported a study where weanling pigs were given their choice of corn passed through a roaster (passage time, 30 to 75 seconds) at temperatures of 175 °F, 212 °F, 250 °F, 280 °F, and 320 °F. Pigs showed a preference for corn roasted at 212 °F. There was a tendency for increased weight gain per unit of roasted feed consumed with no effect on average daily gain. Jensen (1978) also reported that efficiency of ration utilization was decreased when corn at 14% moisture was roasted at 300 °F. Similar effects were noted when 23%-moisture corn was roasted at 250 °F. Considering the cost of roasting corn and its small effect on pig performance, there has been little interest in this processing method. Veum et al. (1972) reported that pigs fed roasted milo had improved average daily gain and gain per unit of feed. This improvement in feed conversion was thought to be due partially to the reduction in water content of the roasted milo.

Some feedstuffs must be heat-treated to be effectively used by swine. Soybeans are a good example. The major objectives in the processing of soybeans for use by swine are (1) to destroy the trypsin inhibitor, (2) to destroy the urease enzyme, (3) to inactivate the toxic hemaggluten, and (4) to increase the nutrient availability. Achieving these objectives requires a wide range of processing conditions. The primary factors involved are cooking temperature and time, moisture content of the seeds, particle size, and equipment used to process the beans. For further information on the processing and use of whole soybeans in swine nutrition see Chapter 35.

Steam Flaking and Micronizing

Steam flaking is a process by which grain is heated to approximately 200 °F in a steam chamber for 20 minutes and then flattened through rollers. Micronizing consists of dry heating grain to 300 °F for 20 seconds before rolling and converting it into flakes. The dry heat is supplied by infrared radiation. The micronizing process ruptures the cell wall and causes partial gelatinization of the starch, which increases its availability.

Tanksley and Osbourn (1972) reported that pigs fed steam-flaked sorghum displayed improved feed efficiency with no effect on average daily gain. Energy and protein digestibility of sorghum were significantly improved with steam flaking.

Steam flaking has generally not improved pig performance. Ly et al. (1966) reported no improvement in performance of pigs fed steam-flaked milo. Consequently, this method has had little use in the industry. However, micronizing certain hard-shelled grains, such as milo, may improve pigs' growth rate and feed efficiency. Early trials by Yang et al. (1975) indicated that micronizing sorghum increased growth rate from 6% to 18% and improved feed efficiency. In other studies reported by Sasse et al. (1975), growth rate was reduced with no effect on feed efficiency when micronized sorghum was fed. Luce et al. (1974) reported that growing-finishing pigs fed reground micronized milo had improved feed conversion with no effect on daily gain. Ewan (1979) was unable to see any added effect on pig performance from feeding micronized corn to weanling pigs.

Extrusion

Extrusion is the process of forcing feedstuffs through a restricting die under pressure that generates heat from friction. Little research has been conducted to compare the nutritional value of extruded corn with that of ground corn. Allee (1976) reported that extruding milo did not improve growth rate or feed efficiency in weanling pigs.

FEEDING METHODS

The most common method of feeding swine in the United States is ad libitum with the use of a self feeder. Early self feeders were constructed by the farmer and used primarily to feed protein supplements and grains in separate compartments (Ashbrook and Gonger 1917; Carmichael 1918). Modern self feeders are available from many different companies in many styles and materials. Stainless steel, fiberglass, and plastic are preferred materials for feeders in confinement swine houses because of their durability and ease of sanitation.

Free-Choice Versus Complete Feeds

In free-choice feeding, different components of the diet, such as grain and protein supplement fortified with minerals and vitamins, are offered in separate compartments of a self feeder. The pig is allowed to eat as much of each component as it desires, thereby balancing its dietary nutrient needs. This method of feeding was popular for many years and was supported by research. Data comparing free-choice with complete mixed rations for pigs fed on concrete (nine trials) and pasture (ten trials) showed a 3% advantage in feed conversion for free-choice feeding. Pigs fed a complete mixed diet grew 4% faster on concrete and 8% faster on pasture than did pigs fed free-choice (Conrad 1958).

Earlier work at the University of Illinois comparing complete feeds with free-choice feeding reported 6.4% and 27.6% increases in daily gain in pigs fed complete diets on concrete and pasture (Hutchinson et al. 1956). They did not find any difference in feed conversion between complete and free-choice feeding methods. The reduction in gain with free-choice feeding can be eliminated by feeding a complete diet until pigs reach 60 kg, followed by feeding free-choice (Overfield et al. 1968).

More recent research on free-choice feeding of supplement and high-moisture or dry corn found no difference in growth rate, feed conversion, or carcass traits between pigs fed a complete mixed diet or free-choice (Engelke et al. 1984). However, these researchers concluded that pigs fed free-choice did not consistently regulate their protein intake well.

While free-choice feeding offers greater simplicity to swine producers, more supervision is usually required to ensure adequate intake of all nutrients and optimum performance. Differences in palatibility of dietary components can cause pigs to overeat or undereat these components, thus affecting the level and cost of performance. Since protein supplement is expensive and protein intake is critical to pig performance, producers should monitor supplement intake on a weekly, if not daily, basis to optimize performance with free-choice feeding. Free-choice feeding may be an option for smaller producers. However, most larger producers will choose complete mixed rations to reduce labor and management associated with monitoring supplement intake.

Restricted Feeding

Restricting energy intake, especially in finishing swine, has long been practiced in Europe and Canada to reduce carcass backfat. Price discounts are severe for pigs with excessive backfat in many countries; therefore, producers limit daily feed intake during the finishing phase to improve carcass grade. Table 22.2 provides a summary of the effects on performance of restricted feeding (Braude 1972). Feed restriction reduces growth rate and increases carcass backfat. The effect of feed restriction on feed conversion is less clear, especially in the United States.

Several American researchers reported no difference in feed conversion ratio

Table 22.2 Comparison of Pig Performance on Ad Libitum and Restricted Feeding

Effect of Ad Libitum Feeding[a]	*Growth Rate*	*Feed/Gain Ratio*	*Carcass Quality*
Improvement	88	13	1
Deterioration	—	60	72
None	1	12	10
No information available	—	4	6

[a]Number of experiments reporting the indicated change. (Data from Braude 1972.)

when comparing ad libitum-fed pigs with those restricted to 75% to 80% of ad libitum intake (Klay et al. 1964; Just 1973; Stahly and Wahlstrom 1973; Vandergrift et al. 1985). Another researcher reported decreased feed conversion ratio in pigs restricted to 85% of ad libitum during the late finishing stage as compared with ad libitum-fed pigs (Haydon 1985). Still other American researchers have reported an improvement in gain:feed ratios with feed allowances of 60% to 90% of ad libitum intake (Becker et al. 1964; Meade et al. 1964; Cleveland et al. 1983).

More detailed analysis of American and European data indicates that the relationship between feed and gain:feed ratio is curvilinear. As daily feed intake is reduced, gain:feed ratio improves slightly and then deteriorates. Gain:feed ratio is maximized at intakes of 75% to 90% of ad libitum intake (Vanschoubroek et al. 1967; Davies and Lucas 1972; Kanis 1988). Figure 22.1 illustrates the impact of feed intake on feed conversion ratio and daily live weight gain.

Restricting daily feed intake during the finishing period is a management tool that can be used to improve the lean:fat ratio in pig carcasses. Producers can reduce backfat on market pigs by 2.5 mm by restricting feed intake 10% to 15% during the finishing period. This restriction will result in a 7- to 10-day longer feeding period with no detrimental effect on gain:feed ratio.

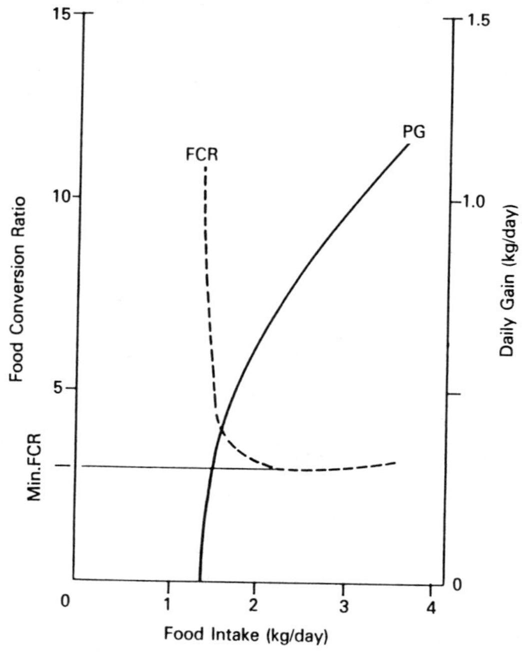

(Adapted, by permission, from Kanis 1988.)

FIGURE 22.1 *Schematic representation of the relationship of feed intake on daily gain (PG) and feed conversion ratio (FCR).*

Meal Feeding Versus Nibbling

Many researchers consider this topic controversial. Research with rats has shown an improvement in feed conversion and reduced body fat with increased frequency of feeding (Cohn and Joseph 1959). A large study conducted at seventeen research stations with 209 pigs per treatment found no difference in daily gain, gain:feed ratio, or carcass traits in pigs fed to scale once or twice daily (Braude et al. 1963). Similar results were reported with pigs fed one or five times daily (Friend and Cunningham 1964) and with pigs fed two, six, or eight times per day (Walker 1970). Feeding frequency of two or five times per day had no effect on DE, metabolizable energy (ME), and net energy for maintenance (NE_m) value of the diet or the efficiency of ME for maintenance (Sharma et al. 1973). They further reported that frequent feeding (five times per day) increased fasting heat production, ME for maintenance, net efficiency of utilization of ME for production, and net energy for growth (NE_g) value of the diet. Frequency of feeding over a long period of time has little influence on performance and carcass parameters in pigs. Romeos et al. (1977) fed pigs one versus four meals every 48 hours for 5.5 months. Meal frequency did not influence body weight gain, body composition, glucose tolerance or plasma glucose, cholesterol, or triglyceride levels. Pigs fed less frequently had elevated malic enzyme activity in adipose tissue, indicating greater lipogenic capacity. These studies indicate that when pigs consume the same quantity of feed daily, the frequency of feeding does not affect pig performance or carcass traits.

FEEDER DESIGN AND MANAGEMENT

Types of Feeders

Growing and finishing pigs consume nearly 75% of the total feed used by the swine herd in a farrow-to-finish operation. Therefore, the type and design of feeders used in the growing-finishing phase of swine production is very important in dispensing feed for optimum pig performance without waste and with ease of adjustment. Dry feeders fall into three types: round, used to feed one pen; rectangular, commonly placed in the pen partition to feed two pens; and time clock design, used to restrict pigs' access to feed and water to three to four meals per day. Very little comparative research has been conducted on these feeders. However, one study has been reported that found no difference in daily gain or gain:feed ratio in pigs fed with a round, rectangular, or time clock-controlled feeder (Hines and Vargas 1985). Another study did report a 4.2% improvement in gain:feed ratio in pigs fed meals with the time clock-controlled feeder (Jones 1988). This study also reported that water usage was 4.2 L/pig/day with meal feeding as compared with 12.4 L/pig/day with ad libitum access to feed and water. This difference in water consumption is important when making recommendations on manure storage and disposal.

Another type of feeder available to swine producers is called a wet feeder. Most commonly, feed is dropped into a pool of water and the pigs mix the feed and water together. Various methods are used to control the water:feed ratio. Studies with early wet feeder designs reported little difference in performance as compared with dry feeders (Teague 1969). Weanling pigs (5 to 20 kg) fed with the same type of feeder as reported by Teague (1969) grew 17% faster with a slight reduction in gain:feed ratio as compared with littermates on dry feeders (Stitzlein et al. 1984). Studies with more recent designs of wet feeders have shown a 4% to 6% improvement in daily growth rate and 0% to 5% improvement in gain:feed ratio with wet feeders as compared with dry feeders (Hines and Vargas 1984, 1985; Patterson 1987). These results are consistent with European reports (Braude 1972) that record improvements in gain and feed conversion ratios with wet feeding. Another design of wet feeder controlled by a computer that limits daily feed allowances to predetermined growth and intake curves was studied by Hirschinger (1986). He found that daily gain was reduced by 5% while gain:feed ratio was improved by 16.9% in pigs fed with the wet feeder compared with pigs fed with a dry feeder. He theorized that the reduction in gain was due to the small restriction in daily feed intake on the wet feeder as compared with ad libitum-fed pigs on a dry feeder.

Feeder Management

Producers have been admonished for years to prevent feed wastage by keeping their feeders properly adjusted. A large study comparing nineteen different feeders in seven trials reported wastage of 1% to 6% for eighteen feeders, and 20% for one feeder, which wasted feed due to faulty design of the agitator mechanism (Horvath and Elliott 1964). Another study reported a linear increase in daily gain due to widening the agitator plate setting from 1.2 to 4.4 cm (Liptrap et al. 1984). Percent of feed wasted increased from 3% to 8.4%; however, the feed conversion ratio did not change. The increase in daily gain of pigs fed with the wider plate settings compensated for the increase in feed waste. These reports indicate that pigs fed a meal ration waste, on the average, 3% to 4% of the feed placed in the self feeder. Variation in eating behavior and the amount of feed wasted between pens of pigs requires the producer to pay attention to individual feeder adjustment to avoid excessive feed wastage. When selecting new feeders, ease of adjustment should be an important consideration.

Feed wastage is also a concern in the gestation and farrowing houses. Individual behavior patterns of sows caused the amount of wasted feed to vary considerably. One study compared several commercially available sow feeders using sows fed 2.3 kg feed per day. The range in feed wasted was 0.1% to 38%, and the investigators concluded that sow feeder design does affect feeding behavior and feed wastage (Taylor and Curtis 1988). They calculated that each 1% in waste from poorly designed sow feeders is equal to 909 kg of feed being wasted per year per 100 sows in the herd.

Feeder space allocation has not been researched extensively. One feeder space per four to five market hogs is the normal recommendation and is considered adequate for ad libitum feeding. No difference in growth rate or feed conversion was observed in nursery-age pigs assigned one feeder cup per one to five pigs (Lindemann et al. 1987). Nursery pigs reportedly need space equivalent to twice the width of the pig's head for each pig attempting to eat at the same time (McGlone et al. 1983). If one assumes that a pig spends 3 hours/day eating and the width of its head is 20 to 25 cm, then 40 to

50 cm of feeder space would feed eight pigs. Because one feeder space is 30 cm, it should be adequate to feed five to six pigs. Therefore, the standard recommendation is adequate with a reasonable margin for error.

REFERENCES

Allee, G.L. 1976. *Kansas State University Report of Progress* 283:24.

Ashbrook, F.G., and R.E. Gonger. 1917. *United States Department of Agriculture Plans, 1-Ag 84F-No. 906.* Washington, DC: United States Department of Agriculture.

Aumaitre, A., and Salmon-Legagneur. 1961. *Ann. Zootech.* 10:197.

Becker, D.E., et al. 1964. *Illinois Swine Grower's Day Report AS-602C.* Urbana: University of Illinois.

Braude, R. 1972. In: *Feeding Methods in Pig Production.* Cole, D.J.A. (Ed.). University Park, PA: The Pennsylvania State University Press.

Braude, R., et al. 1963. *J. Agric. Sci.* 60:389.

Carmichael, W.S. 1918. *University of Illinois Agricultural Experiment Station Bulletin No. 218.* Urbana: University of Illinois.

Clawson, A.J., and C.H. Otto. 1965. *North Carolina Agricultural Experiment Station.* Raleigh: North Carolina State University.

Cleveland, E.R., et al. 1983. *J. Anim. Sci.* 56:570.

Cohn, C., and D. Joseph. 1959. *Am. J. Physiol.* 196:965.

Conrad, J.H. 1958. *Feedstuffs* 30:38.

Crane, F.M., et al. 1972. *Effect of Processing on the Nutritional Value of Feeds.* pp. 72–90. Washington, DC: National Academy of Sciences.

Davies, J.L., and I.A.M. Lucas. 1972. *Anim. Prod.* 15:117.

Engelke, G.L., et al. 1984. *J. Anim. Sci.* 58:1307.

Ewan, R.C. 1979. *Iowa State University 1979 Swine Research Report AS-494J.* Ames, IA: Iowa State University.

Friend, D.W., and H.M. Cunningham. 1964. *J. Nutr.* 83:251.

Haydon, K.D. 1985. *Swine Research Report.* Athens, GA: University of Georgia.

Hines, R.H., and J.V. Vargas. 1984. *Report of Progress 461, Agricultural Experiment Station.* Manhattan, KS: Kansas State University.

Hines, R.H., and J.V. Vargas. 1985. *Report of Progress 486. Agricultural Experiment Station.* Manhattan, KS: Kansas State University.

Hirschinger, C.W. 1986. *Swine Report.* Madison, WI: University of Wisconsin-Madison.

Hoefer, J.A., et al. 1958. *Michigan Swine Research Report A.H. 30.* East Lansing, MI: Michigan State University.

Hogberg, M.G., et al. 1980. "Physical forms of feedprocessing for swine." In: *National Pork Industry Handbook, No. 71.* West Lafayette, IN: Purdue University.

Holden, P. 1981. "Physical forms of feed." *Proceedings of the 1981 Profit Symposium: Essential Elements of Efficiency.* Des Moines, IA: National Pork Producers Council.

Horvath, D.J., and K.C. Elliott. 1964. *West Virginia University Agricultural Experiment Station Bulletin 501T.* Morgantown, WV.

Hutchinson, H.D., et al. 1956. *Illinois Swine Grower's Day Report AS435.* Urbana: University of Illinois.

Jensen, A.H. 1966. *Feedstuff* 38:24.

Jensen, A.H. 1978. *Effects of Certain Processing Methods on Nutritional Value of Feedstuffs for Growing-Finishing Swine.* Mimeo. Urbana: University of Illinois.

Jensen, A.H., et al. 1960. *J. Anim. Sci.* 19:629.

Jones, E.E. 1988. *Animal Science Report No. 243.* Raleigh, NC: North Carolina State University.

Just, A.N. 1973. *J. Anim. Sci.* 36:476.

Kanis, E. 1988. *Anim. Prod.* 46:111.

Klay, R.F., et al. 1964. *J. Anim. Sci.* 23:598.
Lindemann, M.D., et al. 1987. *J. Anim. Sci.* 64:8.
Liptrap, D.O., et al. 1984. *Progress Report No. 284. University of Kentucky Agricultural Experiment Station.* Lexington, KY: University of Kentucky.
Luce, W.G., et al. 1970. *Oklahoma Animal Science Research Report.* p. 60. Stillwater: Oklahoma State University.
Luce, W.G., et al. 1974. *Oklahoma Animal Science Research Report.* p. 179. Stillwater: Oklahoma State University.
Ly, C.-C., et al. 1966. *Bulletin 493. Kansas State University Agricultural Experiment Station.* p. 77. Manhattan, KS: Kansas State University.
Mahan, D.C., et al. 1966. *J. Anim. Sci.* 25:1019.
McGlone, J.J., et al. 1983. *J. Anim. Sci.* 57:140.
Meade, R.J., et al. 1964. *J. Anim. Sci.* 23:1201.
Newer, A.J., et al. 1965. *J. Anim. Sci.* 24:113.
NRC-42 Committee on Swine Nutrition. 1969. *J. Anim. Sci.* 29:927.
Nuzback, L.J., et al. 1982. *Report of Progress 422. Kansas State University Agricultural Experiment Station.* Manhattan, KS: Kansas State University.
Ohh, S.J., et al. 1983. *Report of Progress 442. Kansas State University Agricultural Experiment Station.* Manhattan: Kansas State University.
Overfield, J.R., et al. 1968. *Progress Report No. 176. University of Kentucky Agricultural Experiment Station.* Lexington, KY: University of Kentucky.
Owsley, W.F., et al. 1981. *J. Anim. Sci.* 52:557.
Patterson, D.C. 1987. *Br. Soc. Anim. Prod.* 44:489.
Pond, W.G., and J.A. Maner. 1984. *Swine Production and Nutrition.* Westport, CT: AVI Publishing Co.
Romsos, D.R., et al. 1978. *Proc. Soc. Exp. Biol. Med.* 157:528.
Sasse, C.E., et al. 1975. *Proceedings of the 23rd Annual Swine Shortcourse. Agricultural Science Technology Report No. T-5-111.* Lubbock, TX: Texas Tech University.
Seerley, R.W., et al. 1962a. *J. Anim. Sci.* 21:829.
Seerley, R.W., et al. 1962b. *J. Anim. Sci.* 21:834.
Sharma, V.D., et al. 1973. *Can. J. Anim. Sci.* 53:157.
Speer, V.C. 1969. *Feedstuffs* 41:30.
Stahly, T.S., and R.C. Wahlstrom. 1973. *J. Anim. Sci.* 36:1109.
Stizlein, G.A., et al. 1984. *Ohio Swine Research Report.* p. 46. Columbus, OH: Ohio State University.
Tanksley, T.D., Jr., and L.K. Osbourn. 1972. *Swine Research, 1966-70.* p. 12. College Station, TX: Texas A&M Agricultural Experiment Station.
Taylor, I., and S.E. Curtis. 1988. *Nat. Hog Farmer* 33:24.
Teague, H.S. 1969. *Swine-Agronomy Day Report Mimeo.* South Charleston, OH: Western Branch, Ohio Agricultural Research and Development Center.
Teague, H.S., et al. 1970. *Animal Science Mimeo #201.* Columbus, OH: Ohio Agricultural Experiment Station.
Troelson, J.E., and J.M. Bell. 1962. *Can. J. Anim. Sci.* 42:63.
Vandergrift, W.L., et al. 1985. *J. Anim. Sci.* 61:1454.
Vanschoubroek, F., et al. 1967. *Anim. Prod.* 9:67.
Vanschoubroek, F., et al. 1971. *Nutr. Abs. Rev.* 41:1.
Veum, T.L., et al. 1972. *J. Anim. Sci.* 35:1111 (Abstr.).
Walker, N. 1970. *J. Agric. Sci.* 75:241.
Wu, J.F., and G.L. Allee. 1984. *Report of Progress, Agricultural Experiment Station.* Manhattan, KS: Kansas State University.
Yang, S.P., et al. 1975. *Proc. of the 23rd annual swine shortcourse. Agricultural Science and Technology Report No. T-5-111.* Lubbock, TX: Texas Tech University.

Chapter 23

Environment and Management Factors That Influence Swine Nutrition

A.H. Jensen

Numerous pig production systems are successful. Common to all is the awareness of the environmental influences on pig behavior and performance. The extent to which the environment is regulated has been largely determined by economic factors. Optimal environments are seldom achieved under practical conditions, but the awareness of pigs' responses to environment and the provision of appropriate management and housing should help maximize nutritional efficiency.

Systems of swine production range from shade-only field systems to totally enclosed, environmentally regulated buildings. The change from open field to confinement resulted in increased awareness of, and attention to, environmental and management factors affecting pig behavior, performance level, and feed utilization. Indeed, confinement is a biological environment in great contrast to the historical pig habitat. Increased population density has modified behavioral patterns and has presented new management challenges.

ENVIRONMENT

All external factors affecting the development and productivity of pigs are components of environment. Research of the effects of environment on pig productivity has been extensive, and with development of more precise descriptions and control of environments, some of the environment-nutritional interactions have been evaluated. It was recognized early that the reading on the wall thermometer was not a reliable indicator of the confinement "pig environment." The effective environmental temperature (EET), which takes into account the ambient temperature, air speed at pig level,

Table 23.1 A Suggested Total Environment in Pig Housing

Classification	*Components*	*Method of Regulation*
Climatic	Temperature, humidity, air movement, gases and odors, particles, light, and sound	Building design and function—i.e., ventilation, heating, cooling
Structural	Floors, partitions, equipment	Materials and designs
Social	Space per pig; pigs per group; age, size, weight	Husbandry practices

type of flooring, and insulation values of the walls (Curtis 1981), better describes "where the pig is." When the EET is above (upper critical temperature, UCT) or below (lower critical temperature, LCT) thermoneutrality, pig behavior, and feed utilization can be markedly affected. Within limits, pigs compensate for temperatures above or below thermoneutrality by changing metabolic rate, feed ingestion, and heat dissipation. These can alter energetic efficiency and dictate changes in diet formulation.

Of the many components of the pig house environment (Table 23.1), temperature is most readily identified and usually of most concern to the pig producer. However, many other factors, alone or in concert, can affect pig responses.

Temperature and Feed Intake

Temperatures above the UCT will significantly reduce voluntary feed consumption, with subsequent lower gain and usually decreased feed efficiency. A tropical, as compared with a controlled thermoneutral, environment markedly affected metabolism, resulting in decreased feed intake, gain, and gain per feed by individually fed growing-finishing pigs (Christon 1988). Conversely, cold temperatures stimulate feed intake, but this compensatory consumption may be largely used for energy demands of increased metabolic activity (Mount 1968). In severe cold, the stress may modify behavior such that feed intake is actually reduced, increasing the proportion of dietary energy directed to maintaining body warmth (Jensen et al. 1978b).

Based on a review of energy balance studies, Holmes and Close (1977) suggested that for each 1 °C below the LCT, 20-kg pigs need an additional 13 g of feed and 100-kg pigs need an additional 35 g to compensate for the reduction in gain that would result from energy expenditure due to the cold stress. Verstegen et al. (1982) fed a diet containing 3 Mcal metabolizable energy (ME)/kg and 13.4% crude protein to finishing pigs to gain at similar rates in environments of 2 °C or 6 °C below LCT. For each degree Celsius below LCT, the extra feed needed per day was 25 g for 25- to 60-kg pigs and 39 g for 60- to 100-kg pigs.

Table 23.2 Estimates of Increase in Feed Intake in Grams Per Day as Effective Environmental Temperature Decreases

Pig Weight (kg)	*Lower Critical Temperature (°C)*	*Effective Environmental Temperature* 15 °C	10 °C	5 °C
20	18	39	104	169
100	14	0	144	334

(Data from NRC 1981, p. 101.)

Temperature and Nutrient Utilization

Although it is known that environmental extremes affect animal behavior and voluntary feed intake, information concerning specific nutrient requirements of pigs in these extremes is sparse.

Energy

An excellent summary of extensive studies (NRC 1981) showed that various factors, such as pig weight and EET, affect feed and energy needs (Table 23.2).

The degree of cold stress affects response. Usually a modest cold stress will stimulate sufficient increase in feed intake to maintain body weight gain, but if the stress is severe enough, the extra heat demand may exceed the capacity for compensatory feed intake or modify behavior such that feed intake is depressed. A summary of data indicated that growing-finishing pigs in practical conditions required 30 to 40 g of extra feed per day per degree Celsius below LCT. In heat stress environment, growing-finishing pigs reduced feed intake by 30 g and daily gain by 7 g for each degree Celsius above UCT (NRC 1981).

Both environmental temperature and ME intake affected body heat loss (Close and Stanier 1984). For weaned pigs from 14 to 35 days of age, LCT was calculated to decrease from about 27 °C at maintenance feed intake to about 24 °C at twice maintenance. Jordan et al. (1985) reported a LCT of 28 °C for pigs weaned at 17 or 28 days of age. Verhagen et al. (1987) found that group-fed 10-week-old pigs became acclimatized to 15 °C after six days of exposure, then performed comparably to pigs at 25 °C .

Le Dividich and Noblet (1986) fed diets with 3.6 Mcal and 3.1 Mcal digestible energy (DE) per kg to 22-day-old pigs individually caged in temperature-controlled chambers with either 28 °C, 22 °C, or 16 °C ambient temperature. During the 42-day test period, pigs at 16 °C consumed 8% more feed and required 11% more feed per unit of gain than the pigs housed in 22 °C temperature. At 28 °C, feed intake and growth rate decreased 25% and 28%, respectively, as compared with those in 22 °C temperature. At 16 °C, high- and low-energy diets produced comparable performance, but at 28 °C, feed intake, gain, and gain per feed were depressed by the low-energy diet. Noblet et al. (1985) had previously estimated that energy required for maintenance for 50-kg pigs increased 3.7 kcal ME/kg$^{.75}$ for each Celsius decrease in environmental temperature. Campbell and Taverner (1988) estimated the maintenance energy of pigs from 9 to 20 kg to be 1.09 and 0.52 Mcal DE per day at 14 °C and 32 °C, respectively.

Close et al. (1971) and Close (1971) found that heat production was highest in pigs with highest feed intake, and pigs stressed with high temperature had higher body temperature and used energy for heat dissipation (Close and Mount 1978). When feeding diets of lower heat increment character, Seerley et al. (1978) and Stahly and Cromwell (1979) found that fat addition to diets was advantageous during warm seasons. Coffey et al. (1982) found that lower energy diets did not reduce daily gains during cool seasons, but did in warm seasons. High-energy diets gave greater daily gain during warm but not during cool seasons. Gain per feed values were higher with the high-energy diets in both seasons, and highest during warm seasons. Rouse et al. (1986) noted a trend for fat addition (4% soybean oil) to be of greater benefit in summer than in winter. When lysine:energy ratios were the same in the diets, gain was 6% higher and gain per feed 10% higher during the winter season with the higher-energy diet.

Reports of effect of temperature on digestibilities have varied. Fuller and Boyne (1972) suggested that energy digestibility increased 0.12 percentage unit per degree Celsius increase in environmental temperature. However, Holmes (1973, 1974) reported a decrease in digestibility with increase in temperature but found that ME was not significantly affected. At the high temperatures, heat production and maintenance cost increased with fed, but not with fasted, pigs. Phillips (1980) found a 0.27% increase in energy digestibility per degree, as temperature increased from 6 °C to 20 °C. Le Dividich and Noblet (1986) reported digestibilities of energy and protein by individually caged 22-day-old weaned pigs to be similar at 22 °C and 28 °C, and higher than those in a 16 °C environment.

Individually penned sows had lower energy consumption and nitrogen retention in 30 °C than in 20 °C environment, but energy digestibility was not significantly affected (Schoenherr et al. 1986). After reviewing the literature, Verstegen et al. (1987) concluded that sows weighing 140 to 160 kg at mating had a maintenance requirement of 1.7 to 1.85 kg of feed per day (4.87 to 5.30 Mcal ME). For each degree Celsius below thermoneutrality, an additional 4% intake would be required.

Protein

Sorensen (1961) and Sorensen and Moustgaard (1961) found that nitrogen retention in finishing pigs decreased as temperature decreased from 23 °C to 3 °C. Nitrogen retention was also decreased at high temperatures (Holmes and Grace 1975; Gray and McCracken 1974).

Seymour et al. (1964) noted more efficient gains by growing-finishing pigs at 15 °C than at 4.5 °C, and there was evidence of interaction between dietary protein level and temperature. Data of Wahlstrom et al. (1971) supported this, with interaction between dietary protein level and housing on rate of gain.

The results obtained appear to reflect feed intake, not temperature per se. Thus, dietary nutrient manipulation correlated to feed intake level affected by the environmental temperature could meet the pig's needs. Stahly et al. (1979) suggested that the dietary lysine level for maximum growth rate is lower for pigs in temperatures above or below a thermoneutral environment, and that dietary lysine allowances should be adjusted for seasonal environments (Stahly et al. 1986).

Vitamins

Since feed intake by pigs responds to environments, required dietary levels of vitamins essential to metabolic reactions may also change. Mitchell et al. (1950) reported that the riboflavin requirement of growing pigs varied inversely with environmental temperature. Early evaluation of the dietary thiamin requirement was inconclusive (Heidenreich et al. 1961), while Peng and Heitman (1974) suggested an increase in requirement with increase in environmental temperature.

Kornegay et al. (1986) added vitamins C and E to diets for weaned pigs, 7.5 kg, in environments of 27 °C or 19 °C initial temperature, which was reduced 2 °C per week for the 5- to 6-week periods. Vitamin supplementation increased plasma levels of C and E, but did not affect pig performance. Gains were unaffected, but feed intake was higher and gain per feed lower in the cooler environment.

Minerals

Holmes and Grace (1975) found that pigs in a 33 °C environment had higher excretion levels of calcium and potassium than those at 25 °C.

Under uniformly good management, production system has not been shown to significantly affect dietary mineral requirements for growing-finishing pigs (Cromwell et al. 1972; Parker et al. 1974) or for sows (Kornegay et al. 1973; Kornegay and Meachem 1973).

Water

Studies of the relationship between environmental temperature and voluntary water consumption have been inconclusive (Fuller 1965; Close et al. 1971). Mount et al. (1971) reported that average ratios of water:feed intake were between 2.1 and 2.7 at temperatures between 7 °C and 22 °C, and between 2.8 and 5.0 at 30 °C and 35 °C. The range of average daily water intake was from 92 to 184 ml/kg body weight.

Growing pigs with access to 7 °C water gained an average of 63 g more per day than pigs having only unheated—sometimes frozen—water (Altman et al. 1952). Warming water to 13 °C was of no advantage over the 7 °C water. In contrast, Nienaber and Hahn (1984) reported that for 4.5-week-old weaned pigs in a 5 °C environment, heating the drinking water to 30 °C resulted in increase in gain. Holmes (1971) reported that pigs fed whey of 15 °C temperature gained slower and were less efficient than those fed 40 °C whey. Gain increase was 11% in an environment of 16 °C, and 5% in a 22 °C environment. This suggested that warming the ingested cool whey increased the amount of dietary energy available for tissue synthesis.

Fiber

The fiber in corn bran (Stahly et al. 1983), but not that in wheat bran (Turlington et al. 1983), had a higher feeding value for pigs in a cold environment than for those in a warm environment. Dietary fat (10.6%) increased sow milk energy at both 20 °C and 32 °C environments while dietary wheat bran (48.5%) reduced milk energy in 32 °C but not 20 °C environments (Schoenherr et al. 1987).

Humidity

Relative humidity (RH) per se was thought to have little effect on pig performance (Ingram 1965), except when combinations of high RH and high ambient temperatures occurred (Robinson and Lee 1941; Sorensen and Moustgaard 1961). Weight and other factors are likely involved, since Addis et al. (1967) found no significant effect of 30% to 85% RH in a psychometric chamber with 29 °C on pigs from 65 to 84 kg, whereas Pacheco et al. (1981) reported decreased daily gain and feed efficiency in pigs when RH exceeded 80% in 16 °C to 22 °C environments.

Drafts

Younger, smaller pigs are more susceptible to changes in air movement than are older, heavier pigs. The extent of body heat loss will depend on the pig's weight, ambient temperature, and whether pigs are penned individually or in groups. In an unheated building with a range of temperatures from −3 °C to 19 °C, 5-kg pigs, three per group, protected by a hover, gained 6% faster on 25% less feed than did littermates without the benefit of a hover (Muehling and Jensen 1961). In controlled chamber environments, Mount and Ingram (1965) and Verstegen and van der Hel (1977) demonstrated that increasing air movement was equivalent to reducing environmental temperature. The effects were greater at lower temperatures, with lighter-weight pigs, and with individually fed pigs. An increase of 5.3 cm/second air movement increased LCT by 1 °C (Close et al. 1981).

Air Contaminants

Odor and dust levels in confinement buildings vary widely and reflect ventilation efficiency and management practices. Curtis et al. (1975) tested for ammonia, hydrogen sulfide, and dust levels in several commercial units. Levels commonly found were then used singly or in combination in air-pollutant exposure chambers in which growing pigs were confined. These levels did not significantly affect growing pig performance. In additional trials, however, it was found that ammonia levels above 50 ppm reduced feed intake and growth rate, in agreement with observations of Stombaugh et al. (1969).

Carbon monoxide at 300 ppm, but not at 200 ppm, for a 21-day period reduced rate of gain and feed efficiency of weanling pigs (Morris et al. 1985).

Negative air ionization has been used to precipitate air particulate matter in swine housing. Jensen and Curtis (1976) found it had no effect on growing pigs, whereas Zemke and Mehlhorn (1978) suggested there were beneficial effects on sows and litters.

Sound

Pigs reacted to sudden noise, but were apparently quite tolerant for short periods and became conditioned over long periods to sound intensities up to 120 to 135 decibels (Bond et al. 1963). However, in a commercial unit with a combination of noise levels generated by ventilation fans and sirens, decibels of 120 or above resulted in decreased level of pig performance (Ivos and Krsnik 1979).

Light

Early studies on the effects of artificial light environments were inconclusive. Terrill et al. (1950) and Braude and Mitchell (1958) with growing-finishing pigs and Catron and Facto (1960) with baby pigs found no effect on feed intake and efficiency. Dufour and Bernard (1968) noted a nonsignificant decrease in feed required per unit of gain when light-hours per day were reduced. More recently, Yurkov (1985) reported that growing-finishing pigs with a daily cycle of 18 hours light and 6 hours of dark had better performance than did those in a 12:12 cycle. Also, Mabry et al. (1983) studied the effects of 8- to 16-hour daily photoperiods on sows from day 107 of gestation to 28 days postpartum. Piglets in the 16-hour light nursed more often than those in the 8-hour light, and they were heavier at weaning. Although the sows were equally fed during lactation, milk yield tended to be higher, and total milk solids were significantly higher in sows exposed to the greater photoperiod.

MANAGEMENT AND ENVIRONMENT

Management determines total productive efficiency and includes all those decisions necessary for best possible environmental and operational efficiency—it has to do with all controllable factors. Thus, choice of building materials and design and husbandry practices can significantly affect pig behavior and nutritional efficiency.

Housing

Pigs can adapt to a wide range of environments. In controlled environments, Sorensen (1961) and Sorensen and Moustgaard (1961) found that abrupt changes from 19 °C to 3 °C or from 3 °C to 19 °C markedly affected nitrogen retention of growing pigs for 10 days following the temperature change. As measured by growth rate and feed efficiency, adjustment to abrupt change from 19 °C to 3 °C required about 28 days, whereas from 3 °C to 19 °C less time was required.

It was recognized early that housing environment could affect nutritional efficiency. Relief from heat (Jensen 1964; Bowland 1963) and cold stress (Jensen 1964) resulted in more rapid and efficient gains. In the cold environment, the benefits of enclosed housing over portable field units were not solely due to temperature. For example, pigs in central housing had feed and water available continuously, while those in portable units had to go out into the weather for feed and water, the latter on occasion being frozen.

During winter seasons, pigs in heated, enclosed buildings gained significantly faster and more efficiently than did those in unheated and open-front buildings (Jensen et al. 1969; Wahlstrom and Libal 1980). To the extent that housing modified environmental stress, pig gain and efficiency were usually improved.

In a 3-year study, sows housed in either enclosed or open-front buildings had similar reproductive performance, but during winter seasons sows in the open-front required more feed to maintain desired condition (Jensen et al. 1978a). Others have shown similar effects of cold on gestating sows (Lynch 1978; Baxter and Robertson 1980). McGlone et al. (1988) reported that snout coolers (directing cool air to the head) and drip coolers (scheduled dripping of cool water on shoulder and head) can significantly increase feed intake and efficiency of lactating sows.

Floors

Pigs on totally slotted floors were more susceptible to environmental temperatures outside thermoneutrality than were pigs on solid or partially slotted floors (Jensen 1964). Restricting floor space further stressed pigs in high environmental temperatures, markedly reducing feed intake, rate of gain, and feed efficiency. In general, however, in nonstressful environments, performance of growing-finishing pigs on totally or partially slotted floors has been similar (Jensen 1979).

In controlled environmental chamber environments below thermoneutrality, growing pigs on slats grew appreciably slower and required more feed per gain than did pigs with the benefit of straw (Verstegen et al. 1977). Others have demonstrated that flooring materials in commercial productive units can affect efficiency of pig performance in environments above or below thermoneutrality (Ames and Brink 1974; Wilson et al. 1977).

Le Dividich and Aumaitre (1978) pointed out that various interactions, that is, air temperature and feeding level, air temperature and management system (type of floor; pigs individual or group), affect performance efficiency of young pigs. Weight of pig and the sanitation of its environment also affect efficiency of performance. For pigs weaned at 3 to 4 weeks of age, modified (lowered) nocturnal nursery temperature may stimulate feed intake and gain (Brumm and Shelton 1988). Initial cold stress (McConnell et al. 1987) or continuous heat stress will depress feed intake and gain per feed (McConnell et al. 1987; McGlone et al. 1987).

Management decisions in practical situations can minimize environmental stress. For example, in a concrete floor commercial unit, 27-kg pigs were confined in pens without or with a wooden overlay in the sleeping area. Daily average ambient temperatures during the first 14 days ranged from −9 °C to 18 °C (Jensen et al. 1978b). Pigs on the bare concrete huddled together for warmth to the exclusion of venturing to the self-feeder. This resulted in lower feed intake, lower gain, and markedly lower gain per feed as compared with pigs with wooden overlay in the sleeping area. With subsequent increase in body weight, temperature stress decreased and a compensatory growth rate was observed, but gain per feed was still significantly higher for the pigs with wooden overlay.

In a commercial nursery, gain, feed intake, and gain per feed values of cold-stressed pigs were higher in pens with punched stainless steel floor than with steel slat floor, and in pens with solid partitions instead of wire partitions (Jensen 1979). The cumulative effect of pig movement, floor type, and cold stress increased feed required per unit of gain by 4% (Geers et al. 1987).

Group Size and Pig Space

Number of pigs per pen and floor space per pig also affect performance of growing-finishing pigs (Gehlbach et al. 1966; Jensen and Curtis 1976; NCR-89 Committee 1986). In general, increase in number of pigs per pen did not consistently affect daily feed intake and gain, but feed efficiency was significantly greater in the smaller groups. In environments above UCT, increase in number per group and restriction of space would markedly decrease performance and efficiency whereas at environments below LCT, they could prove beneficial because of behavior modified to reduce body heat loss. Other studies (Lindemann et al. 1987; Meunier-Salaum et al. 1987; Yen and Pond 1987; Edmonds and Armsby 1988) showed that crowding consistently adversely affects feed utilization by pigs.

Based on research under controlled conditions, Holmes and Close (1977) estimated LCT for pigs of different weights and housed singly or in groups, and for thin and fat sows (Table 23.3).

Table 23.3 Estimated Lower Critical Temperatures

	Management	
Pig Weight (kg) or Age	*Single*	*Group*
2	29 °C	24 °C
20	17 °C	15 °C
60	16 °C	13 °C
100	14 °C	12 °C
Sow	14 °C (thin)	12 °C (fat)

(Reprinted, by permission, from Holmes and Close 1977.)

Table 23.4 Recommended Management of and Optimum Temperatures for Maximum Nutritional Efficiency

		Minimum Space Per Animal Unit (m^2)				
Animal Unit	*Weight (kg)*	*Solid Floor*	*Partially Slotted Floor*	*Slotted Floor*	*No. of Animals Per Pen*	*Optimum Temperature (°C)*[a]
Breeding females						
Gilt	114–136	1.3	1.1	1.1	12–15	15
Sow	136–227	1.6	1.3	1.3	10–12	15
Gestating females						
Gilt	114–182	1.5	1.2	1.2	12–15	15[b]
Sow	136–227	1.6	1.3	1.3	12–15	15
Lactating sow	—	3.1	3.1	3.1	—	21(32)[c]
Boars	—	6.3	4.5	4.5	1–3	15
Weaned pig	4–11	0.36	0.25	0.25	10–30	27
Growing pig	11–23	0.54	0.27	0.27	10–30	24
	23–45	0.72	0.36	0.36	10–30	21
Finishing pig	45–68	0.90	0.54	0.54	10–15	18
	68–100	1.08	0.72(0.81)[d]	0.72(0.81)[d]	10–15	15

[a] These values could be reduced by 5 °C when bedding is used.

[b] For gilts in individual stalls or tethered, 17 °C.

[c] In piglet sleeping area.

[d] Suggested during very hot weather.

Recommendations

Based on published information, housing and management recommendations have been made (Table 23.4).

REFERENCES

Addis, P.B., et al. 1967. *J. Anim. Sci.* 26:705.

Altman, L.B., Jr., G.C. Ashton, and D.V. Catron. 1952. *Iowa Farm Sci.* 7:41.

Ames, D., and D. Brink. 1974. *Swine Industry Report.* Manhattan, KS: Kansas Agricultural Experiment Station.

Baxter, S.H., and A.M. Robertson. 1980. *Pig News and Inform.* 1:21.

Bond, J., et al. 1963. *USDA Technical Bulletin 1280.* Washington, DC: United States Department of Agriculture.

Bowland, J.P. 1963. *42nd Annual Feeders Day Report.* Edmonton, Canada: University of Alberta.

Braude, R., and K.G. Mitchell. 1958. *Proc. Nutr. Soc.* 17:38.

Brumm, M.C., and D.P. Shelton. 1980. *J. Anim. Sci.* 66:1067.

Campbell, R.G., and M.R. Taverner. 1988. *Livest. Prod. Sci.* 18:287.

Catron, D.V., and L.A. Facto. 1960. *Proc. Dist. Feed Conf.* 15:60.

Christon, R. 1988. *J. Anim. Sci.* 66:3112.

Close, W.H. 1971. *Anim. Prod.* 13:295.

Close, W.H., and L.E. Mount. 1978. *Br. J. Nutr.* 40:413.

Close, W.H., and M.W. Stancer. 1984. *Anim. Prod.* 38:221.

Close, W.H., R.P. Heavens, and D. Brown. 1981. *Anim. Prod.* 32:75.

Close, W.H., L.E. Mount, and I.B. Start. 1971. *Anim. Prod.* 13:285.

Coffey, M.T., et al. 1982. *J. Anim. Sci.* 54:95.

Cromwell, G.L., V.W. Hayes, and D.D. Kratzer. 1972. *J. Anim. Sci.* 35:215 (Abstr.).

Curtis, S.E. 1981. *Animal Environmental Service.* Mahomet, IL.

Curtis, S.E., et al. 1975. *J. Anim. Sci.* 41:735.

Dufour, J., and C. Bernard. 1968. *Can. J. Anim. Sci.* 48:425.

Edwards, S.A., and A.W. Armsby. 1988. *Anim. Prod.* 46:453.

Fuller, M.F. 1965. *Br. J. Nutr.* 19:531.

Fuller, M.F., and A.W. Boyne. 1972. *Br. J. Nutr.* 25:259.

Geers, R., et al. 1987. *Livest. Prod. Sci.* 16:175.

Gehlbach, G.D., et al. 1966. *J. Anim. Sci.* 25:386.

Gray, R., and K.J. McCracken. 1974. *Sixth Symposium on Energy Metabolism. EAAP Publication No. 14.* Hohenheim: Stuttgart University.

Heidenreich, C.J., J.H. Conrad, and F.N. Andrews. 1961. *Purdue Agricultural Experiment Station Mimeo AS 306.* West Lafayette, IN: Purdue University.

Holmes, C.W. 1971. *Anim. Prod.* 13:1.

Holmes, C.W. 1973. *Anim. Prod.* 16:117.

Holmes, C.W. 1974. *Anim. Prod.* 19:211.

Holmes, C.W., and W.H.Close. 1977. In: *Nutrition and the Climatic Environment.* Haresign, W., H. Swan, and D. Lewis (Eds.). London: Butterworths.

Holmes, C.W., and N.D. Grace. 1975. *Anim. Prod.* 21:341.

Ingram, D.L. 1965. *Res. Vet. Sci.* 6:9.

Ivos, J., and B. Krsnik. 1979. *Veterinaria Yugoslavia.* 28:165.

Jensen, A.H. 1964. *J. Anim. Sci.* 23:1185.

Jensen, A.H. 1978. *Proc. Pig. Vet. Soc.* 5:85.

Jensen, A.H., and S.E. Curtis. 1976. *J. Anim. Sci.* 42:8.

Jensen, A.H., et al. 1978a. *J. Anim. Sci.* 47:347.

Jensen, A.H., D.P. Holzgraefe, and B.A. Fisher. 1978b. *Proceedings of the Pork Industry Conference*. Urbana, IL: Illinois Agricultural Experiment Station.
Jensen, A.H., et al. 1969. *J. Anim. Sci.* 29:451.
Jordan, J.W., A. McAllister, and S.T.C. Weatherup. 1985. *Anim. Prod.* 41:425.
Kornegay, E.T., and T.N. Meachem. 1973. *J. Anim. Sci.* 37:506.
Kornegay, E.T., H.R. Thomas, and T.N. Meachem. 1973. *J. Anim. Sci.* 37:493.
Kornegay, E.T., et al. 1986. *J. Anim. Sci.* 63:484.
Le Dividich, J., and A. Aumaitre. 1978. *Livest. Prod. Sci.* 5:71.
Le Dividich, J., and J. Noblet. 1986. *Livest. Prod. Sci.* 14:255.
Lindemann, M.D., et al. 1987. *J. Anim. Sci.* 64:8.
Lynch, P.B. 1978. *Moorepark Pig Farming Conference*. Dublin, Ireland: An Foras Taluntais, p. 18.
Mabry, J.W., M.T. Coffey, and R.W. Seerley. 1983. *J. Anim. Sci.* 57:292.
McConnell, J.C., J.C. Engle, and R.C. Waldorf. 1987. *J. Anim. Sci.* 65:1201.
McGlone, J.J., W.F. Stansbury, and L.F. Tribble. 1987. *J. Anim. Sci.* 65:456.
McGlone, J.J., W.F. Stansbury, and L.F. Tribble. 1988. *J. Anim. Sci.* 66:885.
Meuneir-Salaum, M.C., et al. 1987. *J. Anim. Sci.* 64:1371.
Mitchell, H.H., et al. 1950. *J. Nutr.* 41:317.
Morris, G.L., S.E. Curtis, and T.M. Widowski. 1985. *J. Anim. Sci.* 61:1080.
Mount, L.E. 1968. *The Climatic Physiology of the Pig*. Baltimore: Williams and Williams Co.
Mount, L.E., and D.L. Ingram. 1965. *Res. Vet. Sci.* 6:84.
Mount, L.E., et al. 1971. *Anim. Prod.* 13:561.
Muehling, A.J., and A.H. Jensen. 1961. *Illinois Agricultural Experiment Station Bulletin 670*. Urbana, IL: University of Illinois.
NRC. 1981. *Effect of Environment On Nutrient Requirements of Domestic Animals*. Washington, DC: National Academy Press.
NRC-89. Committee On Confinement Management of Swine. 1986. *J. Anim. Sci.* 62:871.
Nienaber, J.A., and G.L. Hahn. 1984. *J. Anim. Sci.* 59:1423.
Noblet, J., J. Le Dividich, and T. Bikawa. 1985. *J. Anim. Sci.* 61:452.
Pacheco, C.R.V.M., A.R. De Freitas, and E.T. Fialho. 1981. *Pesquisa Agropecuaria Brasilevia* 16:141.
Parker, G., G.L. Cromwell, and V.W. Hayes. 1974. *J. Anim. Sci.* 39:980 (Abstr.).
Peng, C.L., and H. Heitman. 1974. *Br. J. Nutr.* 32:1.
Phillips, P.A., B.A. Young, and J.B. McQuitty. 1980. *Can J. Anim. Sci.* 60:557.
Robinson, K., and D.H.K. Lee. 1941. *J. R. Soc. (Queensland)* 53:145.
Rouse, P., H.W. Jones, and T.R. Cline. 1986. *Purdue University Swine Day Report*. West Lafayette, IN: Purdue University.
Schoenherr, W.D., T.S. Stahly, and G.L. Cromwell. 1986. *J. Anim. Sci.* 63(Suppl 1):276.
Schoenherr, W.D., T.S. Stahly, and G.L. Cromwell. 1987. *J. Anim. Sci.* 65(Suppl. 1):318.
Seerley, R.W., M.C. McDaniel, and H.C. Campbell. 1978. *J. Anim. Sci.* 47:427.
Seymour, E.W., et al. 1964. *J. Anim. Sci.* 23:275.
Sorensen, P.H. 1961. *Aarsberet*. p. 185. Denmark: Institut Sterilitetsforskning.
Sorensen, P.H., and J. Moustgaard. 1961. *VIII International Animal Husbandry Congress*. p. 127. Hamburg, Germany.
Stahly, T.S., and G.L. Cromwell. 1979. *J. Anim. Sci.* 49:1478.
Stahly, T.S., G.L. Cromwell, and M.P. Aviotti. 1979. *J. Anim. Sci.* 49:1242.
Stahly, T.S., G.L. Cromwell, and J.H. Randolph. 1986. *J. Anim. Sci.* 63(Suppl. 1):271.
Stahly, T.S., et al. 1983. *Kentucky Swine Research Report*. Lexington, KY: University of Kentucky.
Stombaugh, D.P., H.S. Teague, and W.L. Roller. 1969. *J. Anim. Sci.* 28:844.
Terrill, S.W., et al. 1950. *Illinois Agricultural Experiment Station Publication No. AS-152*. Urbana, IL: University of Illinois.
Turlington, W.H., T.S. Stahly, and G.L. Cromwell. 1983. *Kentucky Swine Research Report*. Lexington, KY: University of Kentucky.

Verhagen, J.M.F., et al. 1987. *Anim. Prod.* 44:427.
Verstegen, M.W.A., and W. van der Hel. 1977. *Publ. Eur. Assoc. Anim. Prod.* 19:347.
Verstegen, M.W.A., H.A. Brandsma, and G. Mateman. 1982. *J. Anim. Sci.* 55:88.
Verstegen, M.W.A., W. van der Hel, and G. Williams. 1977. *Anim. Prod.* 24:253.
Verstegen, M.W.A., J.M.F. Verhagen, and L.A. den Hartog. 1987. *Livest. Prod. Sci.* 16: 25–89.
Wahlstrom, R.C., and G.W. Libal. 1980. *J. Anim. Sci.* 50:1045.
Wahlstrom, R.C., J.F. Fredrikson, and G.W. Libal. 1971. *J. Anim. Sci.* 32:1138.
Wilson, R.D., et al. 1977. *Texas Technological University Agriculture Report No. T-5-125.* Lubbock, TX: Texas Technological University.
Yen, J.T., and W.G. Pond. 1987. *J. Anim. Sci.* 64:1672.
Yurkov, V. 1985. *Pig News Inform.* 6:17.
Zemke, P., and G. Mehlhorn. 1978. *Pig News Inform.* 1:397.

Chapter 24

Nutritional and Environmental Influences on Immunocompetence

K.W. Kelley and R.A. Easter

Good health is affected by a large number of genetic and environmental variables. There are genetic associations with a number of diseases, particularly those that are autoimmune in origin, and these diseases are linked to genes within the major histocompatibility complex of humans and animals. The gene products of the major histocompatibility complex are expressed on the surface of cells and are critically important for cell-to-cell interactions within the immune system. Environmental factors also affect lymphoid cells, with nutritional, thermal, gaseous, light, particulate, social, and microbial environments simultaneously impinging on domestic livestock. If these conditions combine to overwhelm the host, infection and disease can result. It is therefore important to understand how environmental conditions, acting singly or in combination with other variables, affect the resistance of animals to infectious and noninfectious diseases.

It seems reasonable to view many disease processes as the outcome of a number of interactions, and this concept is known as the doctrine of multiple causation. If an infectious organism is quite virulent or if the animal is given a large dose of a pathogen, clinical symptoms of disease will follow in the absence of any adversive environmental stimulus. Similarly, if an animal is stressed in the absence of an infectious organism, no disease will appear. However, an interaction occurs when the normally nonsusceptible animal is exposed to an adversive environmental situation and is also presented with an appropriate dose of an infectious organism. While neither agent alone is capable of causing disease, the combination of stress and the infectious organism is sufficient to cause disease. The environment is somehow able to enhance pathogenicity of the organism. This concept is significant in view of the chronic, insidious diseases that reduce growth and well-being of domestic animals. For those diseases, good vaccines are generally not available. Therefore, the general recommendation is to improve the animal's environment.

The purpose of this chapter is to provide a brief summary of how a single environmental factor, nutrition, affects the pig's immune system. Emphasis will also be given to interactions between animal management and the immune system. No attempt will be made to exhaustively cover the literature of nutrition and immune function of species other than pigs, but reviews on this broader topic are available (Stinnett 1983; Chandra 1983, 1988; Sheffy and Williams 1982; Gross and Newberne 1980; Beisel 1982; Scarpelli and Migaki 1986).

INFECTION AND DISEASE

A number of microbial organisms cause infectious diseases, and in humans and laboratory animals, autoimmune diseases are also important. The immune system is generally considered to protect animals against infectious diseases because:

- Animals with a congenital absence of the thymus gland, or those that have had a neonatal thymectomy, readily succumb to most bacterial and viral pathogens.
- Passive transfer of either preformed antibodies (e.g., colostrum) or appropriately sensitized lymphoid cells to naive recipients can protect against infectious disease.
- Successful vaccines that stimulate either antibody or cell-mediated immunity can protect animals against clinical signs of many diseases.
- Animals that are born with defects in lymphoid stem cells or in stem cell differentiation (e.g., severe combined immunodeficiency) and therefore cannot develop certain differentiated lymphoid cells are susceptible to many infections.
- Lymphoid cells or antibodies can cause autoimmune disease by directing their attack against host tissues.
- Immunodeficiency states, artificially induced by chemotherapy, radiation, or viruses, reduce disease resistance.

Despite these general relationships between disease processes and host resistance, it is still not known which immune functions are most important for protecting both humans and animals (Marshall 1986). An immune event that may be protective against one type of infectious disease may be detrimental in another disease process. In domestic livestock, it is also generally unknown how an environmentally or genetically induced change in immune events will specifically affect resistance to infectious diseases. Therefore, a number of potential problems exist when trying to relate specific immunological changes to disease susceptibility. However, even though the exact number of antigen-specific cells or amount of specific antibody that is needed to kill or neutralize a fixed number of bacteria or viral particles in vivo is unknown, it is clear that lymphoid and myeloid cells are important in disease resistance. In pigs, for example, removal of the thymus early in life substantially reduces growth rate, increases susceptibility to cutaneous, respiratory, and enteric diseases, and suppresses a number of immune events (Binns et al. 1972, 1977; Binns 1980). Therefore, even though much is unknown about mechanisms of host resistance to infectious diseases in domestic animals, it is reasonable to hypothesize that genetic and environmental factors affect disease processes by affecting lymphoid and myeloid cells.

ENERGY INTAKE

The role of energy intake on specific immune responses of pigs has not been very well studied. However, an indirect effect of cold and heat exposure on passively acquired colostral immunoglobulins has been reported in neonatal pigs. Normally, cold exposure increases energy intake in pigs and other animals, while heat stress has an opposite effect. This situation does not appear to be true for neonatal piglets.

Newborn piglets are born with very low levels of blood-borne immunoglobulins. After ingesting colostrum, blood levels of IgG rise from < 1 mg/ml blood to approximately 30 mg/ml. If piglets are removed from the dam at birth and exposed to a cold-air temperature, the amount of passively acquired immunoglobulin in their blood is significantly reduced (Blecha and Kelley 1981a). This detrimental effect is not caused by cold exposure reducing the amount of immunoglobulin that is localized, internalized, and transported through intestinal epithelial cells and ultimately into the blood (Kelley et al. 1982). Instead, cold exposure of the newborn pig actually reduces the intake of colostrum (LeDividich and Noblet 1981).

These data have been interpreted to indicate that cold exposure results in behavioral changes in piglets that lead to a reduction in either nursing time or nursing vigor (Kelley 1983). This reduction in colostrum consumption reduces the concentration of colostrum-derived antibodies in the blood of newborn piglets. Similarly, heat exposure of sows a few days before and during parturition leads to a significant reduction in the amount of colostral immunoglobulin in the blood of their piglets (Machado-Neto et al. 1987). This detrimental effect may be caused directly by cortisol inhibiting absorption of immunoglobulins, but it is also possible that piglets from heat-stressed sows consume less colostrum. This effect might be caused by either behavioral abnormalities of the sow or piglets, and these indirect effects might account for the reduced levels of passively derived antibodies in the blood of piglets from heat-stressed sows.

In summary, direct effects of feed intake on specific immune events of pigs are generally unknown. Since deficiencies or imbalances of vitamins, minerals, and amino acids generally suppress food consumption, it is sometimes difficult to interpret data on nutritional events and immunocompetence. However, both heat and cold exposure reduce passively acquired antibody immunity in newborn piglets. It is likely that these effects are indirectly caused by a reduction in colostrum intake.

PROTEIN

Most experiments that have been conducted on protein deficiency and immunocompetence in pigs have concentrated on antibody-mediated immunity rather than cell-mediated immune responses. Many of these experiments are difficult to interpret. The ability to synthesize antibody is generally assessed by measuring either antibody titers to a specific antigen or all antibodies within a given isotype in blood serum. If dietary treatments affect blood volume or turnover rate of immunoglobulins in blood, it would be difficult to interpret these studies. This problem could be circumvented by enumerating specific antibody-forming cells in the spleen, but such an approach would require that the animals be killed. Similarly, the measurement of only antibody titers does not indicate the relative affinity of those antibodies for antigen. Furthermore, many investigators have administered antigen in a potent adjuvant, such as Freund's complete adjuvant. Adjuvants act to increase antigen processing by causing infiltration of inflammatory cells and to continuously release antigen over a long time period. Therefore, if dietary treatments affect antigen clearance or processing, these effects would be masked by use of an adjuvant. These potential problems must be considered when evaluating many of the experiments on nutrition and immunocompetence.

Restriction of dietary protein during gestation adversely affects piglet survival and growth rate, and these effects are probably caused by a reduction in milk production of the dam. However, when sows were fed a 9% crude protein (CP) ration during gestation and an 18% CP ration during lactation, there was no effect on the ability of piglets to synthesize antibody (Haye et al. 1981). Similarly, serum levels of IgG, IgA, and IgM in plasma were not affected by the amount of dietary protein fed to the dam. These data show that a moderate restriction of dietary protein in the sow's diet does not affect serum levels of passively derived immunoglobulin or the ability of piglets to synthesize antibodies. When sows were fed only a corn-based diet during gestation, followed by a 16% CP diet during lactation, there was only a moderate, nonsignificant reduction in the capability of the dams to synthesize antibodies and to transport these immunoglobulins into colostrum (Corley et al. 1983). In these experiments, however, particulate and protein antigens were administered in Freund's adjuvant, which may have masked any differences caused by dietary treatments.

The role of dietary protein in antibody synthesis by young pigs has also been studied. McGillivray (1967) observed a linear increase in antibody titers to heat-killed *Salmonella pullorum* when dietary protein was varied from 0% to 35%. Increasing dietary protein also caused a linear increase in percentage of lymphocytes in blood, with a concomitant reduction in the percentage of neutrophils. These experiments were conducted over a time span of 5 weeks. However, even when all the essential amino acids were deleted from the diet, pigs were able to synthesize significant amounts of antibodies.

When sorghum protein is fed to growing and finishing swine, the first- and second-limiting amino acids are lysine and threonine, respectively. Pregnant swine, however, may have a higher threonine requirement. When a corn-soybean meal diet was fed to pregnant gilts and compared with an isonitrogenous fortified basal diet consisting of sorghum grain, there was about a 25% reduction in plasma concentrations of IgG (Cuaron et al. 1984). However, there were no significant changes in the concentration of IgG in either colostrum or plasma from piglets of dams fed the sorghum diet. The reduction in plasma IgG found in gilts fed the sorghum diet was prevented by supplementation with threonine, but not by lysine. Furthermore, gilts fed the threonine-supplemented diet synthesized more antibodies to a protein antigen (bovine serum albumin) than gilts fed only the basal diet (Cuaron 1983). There were also more antibodies specific for bovine albumin in the colostrum of threonine-supplemented gilts. The beneficial effects of threonine were greatly reduced when a T-independent antigen (dextran) was used.

These results with threonine-supplemented sorghum diets are interesting because they indicate that even when the first-limiting amino acid for nitrogen balance (lysine) is inadequate, threonine can restore the IgG response in plasma and also enhance antibody synthesis to a T-dependent antigen. This finding indicates that threonine is the first-limiting amino acid in sorghum for the maintenance of plasma IgG concentrations in pregnant gilts, even though lysine is the first-limiting amino acid as determined by nitrogen retention. The investigators suggested that the higher requirement for threonine may be related to the elevated amount of threonine in immunoglobulin proteins.

Although threonine is important for immunoglobulin synthesis in gravid swine, lysine is more important for productivity (Cuaron 1984). The positive effect of lysine on piglet performance is most clearly observed in suboptimal, moderately cold environments (17 °C). Lysine supplementation in sorghum-based diets improves gestation weight gain, but it does not affect plasma or colostral concentrations of IgG. Furthermore, when pigs from lysine-supplemented sows are farrowed in a warm environment, neither threonine nor lysine affects plasma IgG concentrations. When piglets are farrowed at colder ambient temperatures, plasma immunoglobulin concentrations in piglets and survival to weaning are reduced. However, lysine supplementation of the sow's diet partially ameliorates the detrimental effects of cold exposure on both concentrations of plasma IgG and piglet survival. These data support the idea that cold exposure reduces consumption of colostrum, which decreases plasma levels of piglet IgG shortly after birth. The beneficial effects of lysine are not observed in warm environments, but are manifested only when piglets are cold stressed. This observation indicates that lysine supplementation of sorghum diets may augment acquisition of colostral IgG and subsequent piglet survival by increasing colostrum consumption.

Another amino acid also appears to be quite important in the inhibition of growth of tumor cells that is caused by activated macrophages (Hibbs et al. 1987). In these experiments, serum-free, totally defined tissue culture medium was used. Addition of only L-arginine was sufficient to induce cytotoxic-activated macrophages to inhibit mitochondrial respiration of tumor cells. This type of in vitro approach is an excellent means for studying the specific effects of nutrients on a variety of functions of myeloid cells.

Several independent experiments have demonstrated that early weaning of pigs reduces their ability to synthesize antibodies (Miller et al. 1962; Blecha and Kelley 1981b; Haye and Kornegay 1979) and suppresses cell-mediated immune events both in vivo and in vitro (Blecha et al. 1983, 1986). The earlier that pigs are weaned, the greater are these suppressive effects. It is not known whether immunosuppression is caused by the change from a liquid, milk-based diet to a solid cereal-based diet that occurs at weaning or by other stressful factors present at this time. Recently, Crenshaw et al. (1986) reported that there was no difference in the ability of either 2- or 3-week-old artificially reared pigs to synthesize antibodies or to mount cell-mediated immune reactions in vivo. Furthermore, neither simple nor complex weaning diets affected these immune responses, even though there were large changes in the ability of these diets to support growth of weaned pigs. However, in this experiment, pigs were not compared with nonweaned, sow-reared controls. All of the earlier experiments that studied age at weaning and immune responses used sow-reared, nonweaned controls. Therefore, while the experiment by Crenshaw et al. (1986) does not permit a true comparison between weaned and nonweaned pigs, the data do indicate that vastly different diets for early-weaned (and probably immunosuppressed) pigs do not affect their ability to synthesize antibodies or mount certain cell-mediated immune responses. However, perhaps the immunosuppression that is caused by early weaning can be partially offset by other means. Hennessy et al. (1987) demonstrated that both levamisole and isoprinosine supplementation can reverse the reduction in cell-mediated immune response that occurs when pigs are weaned shortly after birth.

To summarize, the available data indicate that antibody-mediated immune responses are not substantially affected by moderate protein deficiencies. However, as emphasized by Miller (1985), it is probably more important to study how infectious disease processes affect nutritional status of the host. This idea is consistent with the concept of common physiological loops between the immune system and other physiological systems (Kelley 1988). For example, both sheep red blood cells and *Escherichia coli* induce specific changes in protein turnover in chickens, and this leads to protein accretion in the bursa of fabricius and liver and protein loss in muscle (Klasing and Austic 1984a,b). These effects of inflammatory agents on protein turnover may be mediated by a potent cytokine known as interleukin 1 (Klasing and Austic 1984c) or perhaps another monocyte-derived protein known as tumor necrosis factor-alpha. Interleukin 1 and tumor necrosis factor-alpha have important effects on a variety of tissues (Dinarello 1984; Beutler and Cerami 1988), and they are probably responsible for the fever, reduction in feed intake, and drowsiness that accompany many infections. Both interleukin 1 and tumor necrosis factor-alpha are major metabolic hormones, and they are now recognized to be important molecules in human clinical nutrition (Pomposelli et al. 1988). Empirical observations with other cytokines, such as the interferons and interleukin 2, indicate that they can also induce unpleasant and significant side effects. It will be important to understand the role of these cytokines on the nutritional requirements of both human and domestic animals.

POSTWEANING DIARRHEA AND CREEP FEED

Consumption of small amounts of protein (<600 g) before weaning has been proposed to be associated with postweaning diarrhea in pigs (Miller et al. 1984a,b). When pigs were not weaned and had creep feed available continuously, there was no diarrhea even though weaning per se caused the appearance of hemolytic *E. coli* in the intestinal fluids. However, when pigs were offered creep feed for only 3 days before weaning, all of the pigs shed hemolytic *E. coli* and had clinical signs of diarrhea. Abrupt weaning in the absence of creep feeding resulted in only one third of the pigs displaying diarrhea. Furthermore, the investigators could induce diarrhea in nursing pigs by feeding limited amounts of casein followed by weaning onto a casein diet. The diarrhea could be prevented by feeding a hydrolyzed casein diet.

The investigators interpreted these data to indicate that postweaning diarrhea of the early-weaned pig (≤ 3 weeks) may be caused by a hypersensitivity reaction in the small intestine. According to this theory, pigs initially mount an immunological response to small quantities of foreign proteins introduced via the oral route. After a few days, this immunological response to the foreign protein is reduced, and this phenomenon is called immune tolerance. When creep feed is provided continuously, both initial activation and subsequent suppression of the immune response occurs prior to weaning, and therefore little diarrhea is observed. However, if only small amounts of creep feed are consumed prior to weaning, the immune system of the young pig is primed to mount a hypersensitivity response when reexposed to the antigen at weaning. Consumption of protein results in a transient diarrhea that is extinguished after a few days as immune tolerance is developed. A small percentage of those pigs that are not exposed to creep feed before weaning experience diarrhea as they develop immunological tolerance to dietary proteins after weaning. This hypothesis is supported by the induction of diarrhea in pigs that are primed with casein and subsequently fed casein at weaning. Furthermore, reduction of the antigenic burden by hydrolyzing the casein can prevent clinical signs of diarrhea.

One practical problem with the concept of hypersensitivity-induced diarrhea in early-weaned pigs is that baby pigs often consume their mother's diet, which often contains soybean meal. In the United States, pigs are then weaned onto a diet that also contains soy protein. Depending on the amount of protein that is consumed, this situation could predispose weaning pigs to a nutritional, immunologically mediated diarrhea. In an attempt to circumvent this problem, Giesting et al. (1986) fed sows a corn-corn gluten feed-based diet supplemented with only lysine and tryptophan. Pigs from these sows were compared with pigs that received 60 g of soybean meal before weaning or to pigs that were given ad libitum access to soybean meal as a creep feed. Surprisingly, Giesting et al. (1986) found that pigs from all of the dietary treatments mounted hypersensitivity responses to a soluble extract of soy protein. The response was specific for soy protein because this hypersensitivity reaction was greater than that for pig albumin. Kinetics of the hypersensitivity response indicated that it was similar to immediate rather than delayed hypersensitivity, which suggested that antibodies against soy protein might be involved. Subsequent testing revealed that sows from all diets had high titers of antibodies against soy protein in their colostrum. Although pigs were born devoid of antibodies to soy protein, high titers were detected in their blood within a few hours after ingesting colostrum. These data clearly indicate that sows raised on soybean meal-based diets synthesize and transport antibodies to soy protein from their blood and into colostrum. The possible role of these passively derived antibodies to dietary antigens in the development of postweaning diarrhea in early-weaned pigs is currently unknown, but this phenomenon should be more fully explored.

VITAMIN E AND SELENIUM

A substantial amount of research has been reported on the immunomodulatory role of vitamin E and selenium in swine (Nockels 1983) and in a number of other species. Vitamin E inhibits the formation of lipid peroxides that is catalyzed by free radicals, while selenium is an integral component of glutathione peroxidase. When vitamin E and/or selenium are added to nutritionally adequate diets, there is generally an increase in the ability of pigs to synthesize antibodies (Ellis and Vorhies 1976; Peplowski et al. 1981; Blodgett et al. 1986). Newborn pigs have very low levels of plasma tocopherols and glutathione peroxidase, and concentrations of both of these are substantially increased after consumption of colostrum (Loudenslager et al. 1986). Therefore, colostral-derived vitamin E and/or selenium might be important in normal development of antibody synthesis in young pigs.

Vitamin E and selenium have also been reported to augment T cell proliferation in pigs (Larsen and Tollersrud 1981). Since this experiment was conducted using whole blood cultures from pigs, rather than isolated and washed lymphoid cells, this beneficial effect may have been caused by removal of a suppressive factor in the blood of animals that were deficient in vitamin E and selenium (Lessard et al. 1986; Langweiler et al. 1981). However, neither nutrient affected delayed-type hypersensitivity reactions in vivo (Blodgett et al. 1986). In chickens, an augmentation in immune functions caused by vitamin E and/or selenium may be related to direct effects on size or function of the thymus, spleen, or bursa of fabricius (Marsh et al. 1986).

In poultry and rodents, the augmented immune response caused by supplemental vitamin E is also associated with greater resistance to pathogenic bacteria and viruses, although these studies are somewhat limited. In pigs, initial experiments showed that the combination of vitamin E and selenium increased resistance of pigs that were experimentally inoculated with a crude preparation of *Treponema hyodysenteriae* (Teige et al. 1977). Further studies demonstrated that most of this beneficial effect on the resistance of pigs to swine dysentery could be attributed to supplemental selenium rather than vitamin E (Tiege et al. 1978, 1982), although the combination of nutrients generally produced the most beneficial results.

IRON AND IMMUNOCOMPETENCE

A number of studies in humans and rodents have been conducted to determine the role of iron in host resistance to infectious diseases, probably because iron deficiency is one of the most common nutrient deficiencies in both industrialized and developing countries. Although the results are variable between studies, the general pattern that has emerged indicates that iron imbalances, those levels that are either too high or too low, increase susceptibility to a number of bacterial and parasitic infections (Sherman 1984). When iron-deficient diets are fed to gestating and lactating rats, antibody synthesis in the offspring is suppressed (Kochanowski and Sherman 1985a). This suppression in antibody synthesis, as well as certain other effects in the thymus, spleen, and liver, are not reversed by iron repletion (Kochanowski and Sherman 1985b). Therefore, there may be long-lasting effects of iron deficiency on the immune system.

Few studies have been reported to determine the role of iron on specific immune responses of pigs. These studies would be interesting, because activated mononuclear cells of rodents display a large number of specific transferrin receptors, which indicates an important functional role for iron in lymphoid cells. However, because of the low iron content of milk, several studies have been conducted to determine the optimal amount of iron that should be provided to newborn pigs to prevent anemia and to enhance growth. Although most iron is tightly chelated by iron-binding proteins (e.g., transferrin and lactoferrin), iron supplementation at birth can saturate these proteins. The excess unbound iron is then available to bacteria to support their growth. Inflammatory agents normally reduce plasma iron, and this beneficial effect is probably caused by the secretion of interleukin 1 from macrophages (Southern and Baker 1982; Sherman 1984; Klasing 1984; Bolin 1986). It has recently been shown in rats that iron deficiency also reduces the synthesis of interleukin 1 by peritoneal macrophages (Helyar and Sherman 1987). In pigs, addition of iron to milk enhances proliferation of enterotoxigenic *E. coli* both in vitro and in isolated intestinal segments (Klasing et al. 1980). Heat treatment of milk also enhances bacterial multiplication, probably because it destroys iron-binding proteins. Serum from pigs injected with 100 or 200 mg of iron-dextran at 1 to 3 days of age supports enhanced growth of *E. coli* when compared with control pigs (Knight et al. 1983). Similarly, pigs administered excess iron by the oral route have more diarrhea and a greater incidence of mortality when challenged with an enterotoxigenic strain of *E. coli* (Kadis et al. 1984). These differences are not detected when iron is administered intramuscularly, probably because it is rapidly removed by the reticuloendothelial system, which prevents a significant loss of iron into the gastrointestinal tract. Therefore, although it is clear that iron supplementation is necessary to prevent anemia in baby pigs, excess iron administered orally can increase bacterial proliferation in the alimentary tract during the first few days after injection.

VITAMIN A

Vitamin A is well known to support structural and functional integrity of epithelial tissues. A deficiency of this vitamin may cause a reduction in mucociliary function and mucous secretion in the respiratory tract, therefore leading to enhanced colonization, multiplication, and penetration of bacteria. Vitamin A also affects cells of the immune system. However, many of these studies are difficult to interpret because vitamin A deficiency leads to inanition. Some of the earliest research on the effects of vitamin A on immune function was conducted with pigs at Michigan State University. These experiments showed that vitamin A-deficient pigs synthesize less than one tenth of the amount of antibody produced by control pigs fed vitamin A-fortified diets (Harmon et al. 1963a). Other research conducted with rodents supports the concept that vitamin A is needed for antibody synthesis (Cohen and Cohen 1973; Chandra and Au 1981), T cell proliferation (Chandra and Au 1981; Moriguchi et al. 1985; Butera and Krakowka 1986), and phagocytic activity of polymorphonuclear cells (Ongsakul et al. 1985). The latter effect may be caused by an inability of promyelocytes to differentiate into granulocytes in the absence of sufficient amounts of vitamin A (Breitman et al. 1980). Vitamin A deficiency also leads to impaired secretion of IgA into the bile (Puengtomwatanakul and Sirisinha 1986) and impairs the migration of lymphoblasts into the intestine (McDermott et al. 1982). These combined immunological defects contribute to the increase in susceptibility of vitamin A-deficient animals to a number of infectious agents.

ZINC AND IMMUNITY

Zinc has an established role in maintenance of lymphoid cells (Bach 1981) and resistance to some parasitic infections (Fraker et al. 1982). Coccidial and bacterial infections reduce tissue zinc concentrations (Klasing 1984; Southern and Baker 1983), which again shows that the nutritional status of the host is influenced by environmental pathogens. In several animal species, zinc deficiency causes thymic involution (Beach et al. 1980), and this general principle is also true in pigs (Miller et al. 1968). A diet containing 12 ppm zinc leads to a fivefold reduction in thymic size when compared with pair-fed control pigs that receive 100 ppm zinc. Zinc deficiency also leads to leukocytosis, lymphopenia, and adrenal hypertrophy. Since acutely stressful factors that elevate plasma cortisol are associated with thymic involution (Westly and Kelley 1984), and porcine splenocytes have specific receptors for glucocorticoids (as well as catecholamines; Westly and Kelley 1987), perhaps some of the immunological defects caused by zinc deficiency in pigs are mediated by cortisol. However, this does not appear to be the case in rodents (Depasquale-Jardieu and Fraker 1980).

Although the effects of zinc deficiency on functional immune responses of pigs are unknown, a large amount of data with other species has shown that zinc deficiency reduces proliferative responses to T cell lectins, antibody synthesis to T-dependent antigens, and generation of cytotoxic T cells (Bach 1981). Substantial research on zinc and immune function has been reported from the laboratory of Fraker. She has demonstrated that antibody responses of suckling mice are suppressed when the mother is fed a zinc-deficient diet (Fraker et al. 1984). Supplemental zinc can even augment antibody synthesis in lymphoid cells from old mice (Winchurch et al. 1984), although high doses of zinc clearly can lead to toxicity and suppress certain immune events (Anonymous 1985). It is now known that zinc is essential for the biologic activity of a thymic hormone known as thymulin (Iwata et al. 1979; Dardenne et al. 1982), and this could be an important link between immune dysfunction and zinc deficiencies.

OTHER NUTRIENTS AND THE IMMUNE SYSTEM

A deficiency in the B-complex vitamins, pantothenic acid, pyridoxine, or riboflavin, leads to a dramatic reduction in antibody synthesis to *S. pullorum* in pigs (Harmon et al. 1963b). More importantly, this suppression in antibody synthesis remains in pigs that are pair-fed, which demonstrates that the inanition that accompanies diets deficient in B vitamins is not responsible for this suppressive effect.

It is now clear that lymphoid cells communicate with each other, as well as other physiologic systems, by secreting soluble, hormone-like molecules (Westly et al. 1986; Kelley 1988). Monocytes, as well as activated lymphocytes, have receptors for the active form of vitamin D, 1,25-dihydroxyvitamin D_3, or calcitriol (Provvedini et al. 1983). This hormone activates macrophages (Abe et al. 1984; Cohen et al. 1986), but it inhibits T cell proliferation, interleukin-2 synthesis (Tsoukas et al. 1984; Bhalla et al. 1984), and immunoglobulin synthesis (Iho et al. 1986). Synthesis of calcitriol normally occurs in the liver, but it is now known that calcitriol can also be synthesized by alveolar macrophages from normal humans (Reichel et al. 1987) and from patients with sarcoidosis (Adams et al. 1983). Therefore, vitamin D may be a very important immunoregulatory hormone, but its effect on lymphoid cells of pigs is not yet known.

REFERENCES

Abe, E., et al. 1984. *Proc. Natl. Acad. Sci. USA* 81:7112.
Adams, J.S., et al. 1983. *J. Clin. Invest.* 72:1856.
Anonymous. 1985. *Nutr. Rev.* 43:141.
Bach, J.F. 1981. *Immunol. Today* 2:225.
Beach, R.S., et al. 1980. *J. Nutr.* 110:805.
Beisel, W.R. 1982. *Am. J. Clin. Nutr.* 35:(Suppl. 2):417.
Beutler, B., and A. Cerami. 1988. *Endocr. Rev.* 9:57.
Bhalla, A.K., et al. 1984. *J. Immunol.* 133:1748.
Binns, R.M. 1980. *Monogr. Allergy* 16:19.
Binns, R.M., D.E. McFarlin, and J.R. Sugar. 1972. *Nature New Biol.* 238:181.
Binns, R.M., et al. 1977. *Int. Arch. Allergy Appl. Immunol.* 55:96.
Blecha, F., and K.W. Kelley. 1981a. *J. Anim. Sci.* 52:594.
Blecha, F., and K.W. Kelley. 1981b. *J. Anim. Sci.* 53:439.
Blecha, F., D.S. Pollmann, and E.F. Kluber, III. 1986. *Can. J. Vet. Res.* 50:522.
Blecha, F., D.S. Pollmann, and D.A. Nichols. 1983. *J. Anim. Sci.* 56:396.
Blodgett, D.J., G.G. Schurig, and E.T. Kornegay. 1986. *Am. J. Vet. Res.* 47:1517.
Bolin, C.A. 1986. *Am. J. Vet. Res.* 47:1813.
Breitman, T.R., S.E. Selonick, and S.J. Collins. 1980. *Proc. Natl. Acad. Sci. USA* 77:2936.
Butera, S.T., and S. Krabowka. 1986. *Am. J. Vet. Res.* 47:850.
Chandra, R.K. 1983. *Lancet* 1:688.
Chandra, R.K. 1988. *Contemporary Issues in Clinical Nutrition. Nutrition and Immunology.* Vol. 11. pp. 1–342. New York: Alan R. Liss.
Chandra R.K., and B. Au. 1981. *Nutr. Res.* 1:181.
Cohen, B.E., and I.K. Cohen. 1973. *J. Immunol.* 111:1376.
Cohen, M.S., et al. 1986. *J. Immunol.* 136–1049.
Corley, J.R., et al. 1983. *J. Anim. Sci.* 56:108.
Crenshaw, T.D., et al 1986. *J. Anim. Sci.* 63:1845.
Cuaron, J.A. 1984. " Lysine and threonine supplementation of sorghum diets for swine gestation." Ph. D. dissertation. University of Illinois at Urbana-Champaign.
Cuaron, J.A., R.P. Chapple, and R.A. Easter. 1984. *J. Anim. Sci.* 58:631.
Dardenne, M., et al. 1982. *Proc. Natl. Acad. Sci. USA* 79:5370.
Depasquale-Jardieu, P., and P.J. Fraker. 1980. *J. Immunol.* 124:2650.

Dinarello, C.A. 1984. *Rev. Infect. Dis.* 6:51.
Ellis, R.P., and M.W. Vorhies. 1976. *J. Am. Vet. Med. Assoc.* 168:231.
Fraker, P.J., R. Caruso, and F. Kierszenbaum. 1982. *J. Nutr.* 112:1224.
Fraker, P.J., K. Hildebrandt, and R.W. Luecke. 1984. *J. Nutr.* 114:170.
Giesting, D.W., K.W. Kelley, and R.A. Easter. 1986. *J. Anim. Sci.* 63(Suppl. 1):278.
Gross, R.L., and P.M. Newberne. 1980. *Physiol. Rev.* 60:188.
Harmon, B.G., et al. 1963a. *J. Nutr.* 79:263.
Harmon, B.G., et al. 1963b. *J. Nutr.* 79:269.
Haye, S.N., and E.T. Kornegay. 1979. *J. Anim. Sci.* 48:1116.
Haye, S.N., E.T. Kornegay, and D.C. Mahan. 1981. *J. Anim. Sci.* 53:1262.
Helyar, L., A.R. Sherman. 1987. *Am. J. Clin. Nutr.* 46:346.
Hennessy, K.J., et al. 1987. *Am. J. Vet. Res.* 48:477.
Hibbs, J.B., Jr., Z. Vavrin, and R.R. Taintor. 1987. *J. Immunol.* 138:550.
Iho, S., et al. 1986. *J. Immunol.* 136:4427.
Iwata, T., et al. 1979. *Cell. Immunol.* 47:100.
Kadis, S., et al. 1984. *Am. J. Vet. Res.* 45:255.
Kelley, K.W. 1983. *Transactions ASAE* 26:834.
Kelley, K.W. 1988. *J. Anim. Sci.* 66:2095.
Kelley, K.W., F. Blecha, and J.A. Regnier. 1982. *J. Anim. Sci.* 55:363.
Klasing, K.C. 1984. *Am. J. Physiol.* 247:R901.
Klasing, K.C., and R.E. Austic. 1984a. *Proc. Soc. Exp. Biol. Med.* 176:276.
Klasing, K.C., and R.E. Austic. 1984b. *Proc. Soc. Exp. Biol. Med.* 176:292.
Klasing, K.C., and R.E. Austic. 1984c. *Proc. Soc. Exp. Biol. Med.* 176:285.
Klasing, K.C., C.D. Knight, and D.M. Forsyth. 1980. *J. Nutr.* 110:1914.
Knight, C.D., K.C. Klasing, and D.M. Forsyth. 1983. *J. Anim. Sci.* 57:387.
Kochanowski, B.A., and A.R. Sherman. 1985a. *J. Nutr.* 115:279.
Kochanowski, B.A., and A.R. Sherman. 1985b. *Am. J. Clin. Nutr.* 41:278.
Langweiler, M., R.D. Schultz, and B.E. Sheffy. 1981. *Am. J. Vet. Res.* 42:1681.
Larsen, H.J., and S. Tollersrud. 1981. *Res. Vet. Sci.* 31:301.
Le Dividich, J., and J. Noblet. 1981. *Biol. Neonate* 40:167.
Lessard, M., et al. 1986. *Proceeding of the 1st International Veterinary Immunology Symposium University of Guelph.* p. 74. (Abstr.)
Loudenslager, M.J., et al. 1986. *J. Anim. Sci.* 63:1905.
Machado-Neto, R., C.N. Graves, and S.E. Curtis. 1987. *J. Anim. Sci.* 65:445.
Marsh, J.A., et al. 1986. *Proc. Soc. Exp. Biol. Med.* 182:425.
Marshall, E. 1986. *Science* 234:1490.
McDermott, M.R., et al. 1982. *Immunology* 45:1.
McGillivray, J.J. 1967. "Immunological response of the pig as affected by amino acid nutrition." Ph.D. dissertation, University of Illinois at Urbana-Champaign.
Miller, B.G., et al. 1984a. *Res. Vet. Sci.* 36:187.
Miller, B.G., et al. 1984b. *Am. J. Vet. Res.* 45:1730.
Miller, E.R. 1985. *J. Anim. Sci.* 60:1500.
Miller, E.R., et al. 1962. *J. Anim. Sci.* 21:309.
Miller, E.R., et al. 1968. *J. Nutr.* 95:278.
Moriguchi, S., L. Werner, and R.R. Watson. 1985. *Immunology* 56:169.
Nockels, C.F. 1983. *Pig News Inform.* 4:289.
Ongsakul, M., S. Sirisinha, and A.J. Lamb. 1985. *Proc. Soc. Exp. Biol. Med.* 178:204.
Peplowski, M.A., et al. 1981. *J. Anim. Sci.* 51:344.
Pomposelli, J.J., E.A. Flores, and B.R. Bistrian. 1988. *J. Parenter. Enter. Nutr.* 12:212.
Provvedini, D.M., et al. 1983. *Science* 221:1181.
Puengtomwatanakul, S., and S. Sirisinha. 1986. *Proc. Soc. Exp. Biol. Med.* 182:437.
Reichel, H., et al. 1987. *J. Clin. Endocrinol. Metab.* 64:1.
Scarpelli, D.G., and G. Migaki (Eds.). 1986. *Current Topics in Nutrition and Disease.* Vol. 15. pp. 1–582. New York: Alan R. Liss.

Sheffy, B.E., and A.J. Williams. 1982. *J. Am. Vet. Med. Assoc.* 180:1073.
Sherman, A.R. 1984. "Iron, infection, and immunity." In: *Nutrition, Disease Resistance, and Immune Function.* R.R. Watson (Ed.). pp. 251–266. New York: Marcel Dekker, Inc.
Southern, L.L., and D.H. Baker. 1982. *J. Nutr.* 112:2353.
Southern, L.L., and D.H. Baker. 1983. *Poult. Sci.* 62:401.
Stinnett, J.D. 1983. *Nutrition and the Immune Response.* pp.1–150. Boca Raton, FL: CRC Press, Inc.
Teige, J., Jr., K. Nordstoga, and J. Aursjo. 1977. *Acta. Vet. Scand.* 18:384.
Teige, J., Jr., F. Saxegaard, and A. Froslie. 1978. *Acta. Vet. Scand.* 19:133.
Teige, J., Jr., et al. 1982. *Res. Vet. Sci.* 32:95.
Tsoukas, C., D.M. Provvedini, and S.C. Monalagas. 1984. *Science* 224:1438.
Westly, H.J., et al. 1986. *J. Exp. Med.* 163:1589.
Westly, H.J., and K.W. Kelley. 1984. *Proc. Soc. Exp. Biol. Med.* 177:156.
Westly, H.J., and K.W. Kelley. 1987. *Proc. Soc. Exp. Med.* 185:211.
Winchurch, R.A., et al. 1984. *J. Immunol.* 133:569.

Chapter 25

Genetic and Sex Considerations in Swine Nutrition

K.E. Ekstrom

A review of research devoted to establishing the dietary requirement of the pig for any specific nutrient reveals a great deal of variation in results. There are always many potential sources of the variation. Speculation concerning sources of variation almost always includes genetics. This chapter focuses on experimental evidence defining the potential for performance and body composition differences among sex and genetic groups. Research directed toward assessing the impact of these differences on nutrient requirements is presented.

Grummer (1975) reviewed research addressing the influence of sex differences and genetic variance on the nutritional requirements of the pig. The review cited examples of significant interactions of sex, genetics, and diet. However, several studies that found no evidence for such interactions were also cited. Overall, Grummer concluded that there are genetic lines of swine and sex groups that perform differentially as nutrition is varied. The remainder of this chapter deals primarily with research reported since 1975. Emphasis is placed on research defining the scope of the differences and assessing the nutritional implications.

BOARS, GILTS, BARROWS

Before addressing the evidence for differences in nutrient requirements among sex groups, it would be useful to summarize evidence documenting differences that exist in growth rate and efficiency of feed utilization.

Growth and Feed Utilization

Generally, boars grow more rapidly then do gilts. Siers (1975) evaluated the differences among Yorkshire sex groups. In this study, boars grew about 13% faster than gilts. The advantage in growth rate was in part due to larger daily feed intake, but boars also required 7% less feed per unit of gain. Other studies, including those of Bereskin (1983) and Kennedy (1984), have reported similar relationships. However, depending on the population sampled, other relationships may exist. Bereskin and Steele (1986) found that Duroc gilts grew 3% faster than boars, while Yorkshire boars grew 8% faster than gilts. Hertzer and Miller (1972) reported that boars grew significantly faster than gilts within the Yorkshire breed but not within the Duroc breed. Castell et al. (1985) found that crossbred boars and gilts did not differ in growth rate, but gilts consumed 4.5% more feed to give boars a 5% advantage in gain per feed.

Castell et al. (1985) compared Hampshire × (Landrace × Yorkshire) boars, gilts, and barrows. In this study, barrows grew 12% faster than gilts. The faster growth was associated with a similar (13%) increase in feed intake. Consequently, the efficiency of feed utilization was similar for both sex groups. Watkins et al. (1977) evaluated barrows and gilts from several breeds and crosses and found barrows grew 8% faster than gilts. Siers (1975) reported barrows to have a 10% advantage in gain versus gilts. In general, the preceding research indicates that boars grow about 10% faster than gilts. Barrows tend to grow at a rate more similar to that of boars than that of gilts. Differences in feed intake among the sex groups are smaller and more variable than differences in growth rate. The largest and most significant difference in feed efficiency is the advantage of boars over barrows and gilts. Are the differences discussed previously associated with differential responses of sexes to specific levels of nutrient fortification? Several experiments have attempted to address this question with respect to dietary amino acid and energy levels.

Castell et al. (1985) found no sex by diet interactions when comparing performances of boars, gilts, and barrows fed diets calculated to contain either 0.84% or 0.76% lysine. However, these lysine levels are relatively high, and there also were no signficant main effects of diet. Castell and Strain (1985) compared the effects of two diets varying in nutrient density on the performance of Lacombe and Yorkshire boars, gilts, and barrows (Table 25.1). There were no significant diet-sex interactions within the Yorkshire breed. In the Lacombe line, increasing the calculated metabolizable energy (ME) and lysine levels of the diet by approximately 7% resulted in a 15% decrease in feed intake of gilts. The corresponding decreases for barrows and boars were approximately 4% and 8%, respectively. Diet-sex differences in average daily gain or feed-gain were not significant.

Newell and Bowland (1972) found significant diet-sex interactions when they compared the effects of two dietary regimens on boars, gilts, and barrows. One dietary program was a single 18% protein (approximately 0.8% lysine) diet fed from 10 kg to 90 kg body weight. The second dietary program involved a 16% protein diet (approximately 0.65% lysine) fed to 50 kg body weight followed by a 13% diet (approximately 0.45% lysine) fed to 90 kg body weight. Feeding the low-protein diets had a much greater effect on boars than on barrows or gilts. The average daily gain of boars was reduced by 14%, while the growth rate of gilts was reduced by only 7%, and barrows were unaffected.

Yen et al. (1986) evaluated the responses of Landrace × (Landrace × Large White) boars, barrows, and gilts to various levels of lysine (Table 25.2). Eight

Table 25.1 Effect of Diet Nutrient Density on Performance of Yorkshire and Lacombe Boars, Barrows, and Gilts from 20 to 89 kg Body Weight

	High-Nutrient Density Diet			*Medium-Nutrient Density Diet*		
Breed/Trait	*Boar*	*Barrow*	*Gilt*	*Boar*	*Barrow*	*Gilt*
Lacombe						
ADG (g)	799^{a}	804^{a}	736^{b}	814	811	793
ADFI (g)	2160^{a}	2399^{b}	2108^{a}	2358^{x}	$2485^{x,y}$	2519^{y}
F/G	2.72	3.02	2.92	2.96	3.10	3.13
Yorkshire						
ADG (g)	$660^{a,b}$	668^{a}	662^{b}	658^{x}	674^{x}	601^{y}
ADFI (g)	1788^{a}	2047^{b}	$1820^{a,b}$	1837^{x}	2101^{y}	1824^{x}
F/G	2.65^{a}	3.06^{b}	$2.90^{a,b}$	2.80^{x}	3.27^{y}	$3.17^{x,y}$

Abbreviations: ADG, average daily gain; ADFI, average daily feed intake; F/G, feed-gain.

[a,b,x,y] Within each diet, sex-type means without common superscripts differ ($P < .05$).

(Data from Castell and Strain 1985.)

Table 25.2 Effects of Dietary Lysine Concentration on Performance and Backfat Thickness of Boars, Barrows, and Gilts (50 to 90 kg Live Weight)

	ADG (g)[a]			*Feed/Gain*[b]			*Average Backfat (mm)*[c]		
Lysine (g/kg)	*Boars*	*Barrows*	*Gilts*	*Boars*	*Barrows*	*Gilts*	*Boars*	*Barrows*	*Gilts*
5.6	753	763	732	3.31	3.40	3.36	26.8	29.8	27.2
6.2	825	797	787	3.07	3.17	3.21	25.0	27.3	26.1
7.3	876	808	822	2.84	3.13	3.04	25.3	26.4	26.1
8.3	916	832	867	2.76	3.06	2.96	22.8	27.1	25.7
9.3	955	808	867	2.60	3.19	2.88	21.8	27.4	24.3
10.3	959	820	883	2.57	3.11	2.89	21.8	26.5	24.6
11.4	952	816	860	2.54	3.14	2.98	21.9	26.6	25.2
12.4	963	819	868	2.58	3.16	2.91	23.2	27.8	22.4
Overall[d]	900	808	836	2.76	3.16	3.02	23.6	27.3	25.2

Abbreviation: ADG, average daily gain.

[a] SE = 29.4.

[b] SE = 0.11.

[c] SE = 1.38; lysine × sex $P < .05$.

[d] SE for ADG = 10.4, feed/gain = 0.04, backfat = 0.49.

(Data from Yen et al. 1968.)

levels of lysine ranging from 0.75% to 1.45% of the diet were fed from 25 to 55 kg body weight. From 55 to 90 kg, the eight levels of lysine ranged from 0.56% to 1.24%.

During the growing period (25 to 55 kg body weight), there were no performance differences among the sex groups and no diet-sex interactions. From 55 to 90 kg body weight, boars gained approximately 11% faster than barrows and 8% faster than gilts. Feed intakes were similar, so feed efficiency was also superior for boars. Again, there were no statistically significant sex-diet interactions. However, the largest differences in growth among sexes occurred with the higher levels of lysine and protein. Over the entire range of lysine levels, there was a definite trend for boars and gilts to show a greater response than barrows to increases in dietary protein. For boars and gilts, the average growth rate across all lysine levels was about 20% and 14% greater, respectively, than observed at the lowest lysine level. Watkins et al. (1977) compared barrows and gilts from several breeds and crosses fed diets with different levels of protein. Diet-sex interactions were not statistically significant. However, the investigators cited trends that they interpreted to indicate that pigs varying in lean growth rate responded differently to changes in dietary protein level.

Carcass Composition

Differences in leanness among sex groups could provide a foundation for differences in nutritional requirements. Siers (1975) found Yorkshire gilts and boars to have significantly larger loin eye areas and higher ham and loin percentages than barrows. Bereskin and Steele (1986) compared Duroc, Yorkshire, and Duroc × Yorkshire boars and gilts. In this study, boars had approximately 6% less backfat than did gilts, but gilts had about 5% larger loin eye areas. Similar differences have been reported by others (Cleveland 1982; Bereskin 1983). Watkins et al. (1977), in their studies of barrows and gilts from several breeds, found gilts had approximately 13% less backfat and a higher (59.2% versus 57.0%) yield of lean cuts than did barrows. Mahan and Gerber (1985) reported similar relationships.

Do these differences in carcass composition cause differences in nutrient requirements? Yen et al. (1986) evaluated Landrace × (Landrace × Large White) boars, gilts, and barrows fed various levels of lysine. Differences among the sex groups were similar to those discussed earlier. Boars had approximately 6% less backfat than gilts and 14% less than barrows. The loin eye area of gilts was slightly (3%) greater than that of boars and 14% larger than that of barrows. Statistically, there was a significant diet-sex interaction for backfat thickness (Table 25.2). Generally, the backfat thickness of barrows did not decrease when the dietary lysine level was raised above 0.62%. In contrast, minimum levels of backfat were not achieved in boars and gilts until the dietary lysine level was raised to at least 0.83%. A similar differential response in barrows versus gilts and boars was observed when the proportion of lean in the ham was measured.

Watkins et al. (1977) measured the lean growth response of barrows and gilts as percent lean cuts. They fed diets containing from 12% to 18% protein. In five experiments, they reported a consistent trend for gilts to have a higher protein requirement than barrows.

There is some evidence to suggest that breed differences exist in the response of sex groups to changes in dietary protein or lysine levels. Castell and Strain (1985) saw no differences in backfat depth between Lacombe gilts or barrows when a medium-nutrient diet was fed. In Yorkshires fed the same diet (Table 25.3), gilts had 16% less backfat than barrows. When a high-nutrient diet was fed, the backfat depth of Lacombe barrows was 12% greater than that of gilts. Yorkshire barrows had 15% greater backfat thickness than gilts when the high-density diet was fed.

BREEDS AND LINES

Differences in performance and carcass composition among breeds and genetic lines of pigs have been reported. Watkins et al. (1977) found that Hampshire barrows and gilts grew approximately 14% slower than Durocs and Yorkshires. Hampshires had approximately 28% less backfat and a higher percentage (4%) of lean cuts. Bereskin and Steele (1986) reported that purebred Yorkshire boars and gilts gained approximately 10% faster than Durocs. Yorkshires had about 12% more backfat and 12% less loin eye area than did Durocs. The investigators observed an interesting breed-sex interaction for growth rate. Duroc boars and gilts grew at similar rates while Yorkshire boars grew 8% faster than gilts. Compared with their Duroc counterparts, Yorkshire boars grew approximately 16% faster. The advantage for Yorkshire gilts versus Duroc gilts was only 4%. Schneider et al. (1982) reported breed-sex interactions for backfat. The advantage for gilts versus barrows was much greater with Yorkshires than with Hampshires. The examples cited represent sound evidence for genetic differences in performance capabilities and carcass merit. However, the samples are very small segments of the total population within each breed. Also, the genetic variation within each breed is substantial. Consequently, it seems inappropriate to use the data to characterize the entire breed population.

Table 25.3 Effect of Diet Nutrient Density on Backfat Thickness of Yorkshire and Lacombe Boars, Barrows, and Gilts from 20 to 89 kg Body Weight

	Average Backfat Depth (cm)			
	Lacombe		*Yorkshire*	
Sex	*HND*[a]	*MND*[b]	*HND*[a]	*MND*[b]
Boar	2.94[c]	3.06[x]	3.24[c]	2.89[x]
Barrow	3.63[e]	3.52[y]	3.91[d]	3.66[y]
Gilt	3.24[d]	3.43[y]	3.40[c]	3.08[x]

Abbreviations: HND, high-nutrient density diet; MND, medium-nutrient density diet.

[a] HND calculated to contain 12.48 MJ/kg metabolizable energy and 0.82% lysine.

[b] MND calculated to contain 11.71 MJ/kg metabolizable energy and 0.76% lysine.

[c,d,e,x,y] Within each diet and breed, sex-type means without common superscripts differ ($P < .05$).

(Data from Castell and Strain 1985.)

Do genetic differences in performance and carcass potential reflect similar differences in nutrient requirements? Nutrient requirement differences among breeds have not been well established. However, several studies discussed later in this chapter indicate that the genetic capability of the pig for lean tissue growth does determine amino acid requirements. Bereskin et al. (1976) reported a significant diet-line interaction for feed conversion. In this study, increasing the dietary protein level from 12% to 16% in pigs selected for low fat improved feed/gain by 18%. The same diet change in the control line of pigs improved feed/gain by only 8%.

Davey (1976) evaluated the effect of protein or lysine level on the performance of Duroc and Yorkshire pigs selected for high or low fatness. Pigs fed diets with high levels of lysine (0.59% or 0.69%) grew 40% faster than those fed lower levels (0.40% or 0.48%). However, when the response within line was evaluated, there was a strong trend for the genetically lean pigs to increase growth more rapidly than genetically fat pigs. When the higher levels of lysine were fed to lean pigs, growth rate increased by 63% as compared with a 28% increase for genetically fat pigs. The differential in response was somewhat greater in the early part of the growth period (80 to 140 days). Lean pigs increased growth by 30% when fed the higher lysine levels. The genetically fat pigs grew only 12% faster when fed diets with the higher levels of lysine. Overall, the lean pigs fed the lower lysine levels produced only 20% more lean tissue than the fat pigs fed the lower levels of lysine. However, when the diets with higher lysine were fed, the lean pigs produced 44% more lean tissue than the fat pigs.

Pond et al. (1980) evaluated the effects of early protein deficiency of lean or obese swine. When a 12% protein diet was fed from 4 weeks of age to 12 weeks, obese pigs actually ate 63% more feed and grew 150% faster than lean pigs. When an 18% protein diet was fed during this early growing period, the feed consumption and growth rate of lean pigs and obese pigs were similar. From 30 kg to 90 kg body weight, there were marked diet-line interactions. Lean pigs grew 33% faster and required 20% less feed per gain than obese pigs. Lean pigs fed the inadequate protein level during the early growing period grew 20% slower than their counterparts that had received an adequate diet. With the obese pigs, feeding the protein-deficient growing diet depressed growth rate in the finishing period by only 9%.

Etherton et al. (1982) evaluated the effects of restriction of total nutrient intake to 65% of ad libitum in two breeds of swine differing in propensities for obesity. Nutrient restriction lowered growth rate in both breeds. However, nutrient restriction decreased growth in obese pigs by 40%, whereas the reduction was 56% in the lean breed. Nutrient restriction did not alter lean tissue development of the obese pigs but it did reduce it by 50% in genetically lean pigs.

Skeletal Development

Skeletal soundness is a primary concern of commercial and purebred swine producers. A predominant concern is that boars may require higher levels of calcium and phosphorus fortification than gilts and barrows for normal development. This concern is perpetuated by the relatively high incidence of soundness problems encountered in boars from performance testing environments. While it may seem logical that differences exist among sex groups, little supportive data exist from controlled studies. Crenshaw et al. (1981) compared the growth and skeletal development of boars, gilts, and barrows fed either 0.4% and 0.4% or 0.8% and 0.8% calcium and phosphorus. Bone ash and bone strength increased with increased calcium and phosphorus fortification for all sex groups. Bone from boars had lower strength than that of the other sex groups regardless of the level of calcium and phosphorus fed.

Nimmo et al. (1980) compared the performance of boars from two genetic lines fed two levels of calcium and phosphorus (0.65% Ca and 0.50% P versus 1.3% Ca and 1.0% P). Higher fortification increased the bone strength and bone ash of both breeds. In a second experiment, the investigators evaluated the performance of 180 Duroc boars fed various levels of calcium and phosphorus. The calcium and phosphorus levels fed were (%): 0.65 and 0.50, 0.975 and 0.75, 1.3 and 1.0. No differences in performance or feet and leg scores were observed.

Reproduction

Kornegay et al. (1985) reported a cooperative study evaluating the effect of elevated dietary calcium and phosphorus during growth and development on subsequent reproductive performance. The study involved 586 farrowings at five experiment stations. The levels of calcium-phosphorus fed were either 100% or 150% of the National Research Council's recommended allowances (1979). Dietary treatments were started at 3 to 6 weeks of age. Growth rate, feed intake, and feed/gain were unaffected by dietary treatment. Elevated dietary calcium and phosphorus during growth and development had no effect on subsequent reproductive performance or longevity.

Reproductive functions influence the bone calcium and phosphorus status of females. Maxson and Mahan (1986) observed consistently lower (2% to 5%) levels of bone ash in actively reproductive sows versus their nongravid counterparts (Table 25.4). Sows that reared larger litters (11 to 12 pigs) suffered greater bone demineralization than those rearing 6 to 7 pigs. The strength of the metatarsal, metacarpal, and rib bones of sows after their second parity was 30% to 40% lower than that of control females that had never been bred.

From the information discussed above, it would seem logical that genetic differences in reproductive productivity would be associated with different nutrient requirements. Despite the demand for additional calcium and phosphorus with larger litter size, Maxson and Mahan (1986) observed no changes in bone ash, bone strength, or litter performance as calcium and phosphorus increased from 0.65% and 0.50% to 1.17% and 0.90%. Experiments with longer lactation periods (Mahan and Fetter 1982) have indicated that higher supplementation of calcium and phosphorus may be of value. In this experiment, sows were carried through three parities. The levels of calcium and phosphorus fed were 0.65% and 0.50%, 0.80% and 0.60%, and 0.90% and 0.70%. The lactation period was 28 days. Bone mineralization expressed as percent ash was maintained in sows fed 0.90%/0.70% Ca-P but not at lower Ca-P levels.

More research is needed to determine whether genetic differences in reproductive capabilities dictate different levels of calcium and phosphorus in the diet. It is critical

Table 25.4 Effect of Production State on Percent Bone Ash

	Production State			
		Litter Size (No.)		
Item	*Nongravid*	*6–7*	*11–12*	*SE*
No. of Sows	7	68	64	
Bone ash (%)[a]				
Femur[b]	64.4	63.2	62.9	0.14
Humerus[b]	64.6	63.3	63.4	0.14
Metatarsal[b]	63.7	62.5	62.7	0.11
Metacarpal[b]	63.0	62.2	62.3	0.11
Vertebra[b,c]	59.7	57.9	57.3	0.23
Rib[d]	60.8	59.4	57.9	0.14

[a] Expressed as a percentage of dried, fat-free bone.
[b] Nongravid versus litter size response ($P < .01$).
[c] Litter size response ($P < .10$).
[d] Litter size response ($P < .01$).
(Data from Maxson and Mahan 1986.)

that there is a clear understanding of what the expected level of lactation feed intake is before diets are formulated. Some field observations indicate that breeds or lines of swine with higher reproductive capacities also tend to have lower ad libitum feed intakes during lactation. Such a situation would markedly affect the proper formulation of the diet.

Micronutrients

Differences in micronutrient requirements among breeds or lines of pigs have not been well documented. It would not be surprising for such differences to exist. For the most part, the cost of providing extra fortification as insurance against deficiency is relatively small. Consequently, for most micronutrients, the economic incentive is insufficient to support the in-depth experiments needed to assess the genetic-nutrition interactions.

There is some evidence in the literature to support the hypotheses that genetic influences on micronutrient requirements exist. Stowe and Miller (1985) evaluated the offspring of boars and gilts selected to be hyposelenemic or hyperselenemic. Offspring reflected the selenium (Se) status of their parents. The increase in serum Se due to 0.3 mg/kg supplemental dietary Se was greater among the hyposelenemic pigs than among the hyperselenemic pigs. Further research is needed to fully determine the genetic-nutrition implications of this observation.

Liptrap et al. (1970) examined sex differences in the zinc requirement of developing swine in two experiments. Differences in pig performance, serum alkaline phosphatase, and the incidence of parakeratosis indicated that boars and gilts have higher zinc requirements than barrows.

Dietary choline supplementation has been shown to improve reproductive performance (NCR-42 1976). In the NCR-42 cooperative study, the incidence of spraddle-legged pigs tended to be lower in the group receiving supplemental choline. However, the investigators noted that the spraddle leg condition was primarily confined to one breed at one station. It is not possible to determine if this observation is in fact a reflection of a true breed-diet interaction. More research is needed to define the scope and economic significance of genetic-nutrition interactions. A better understanding of the basic biological systems involved and the role of specific nutrients in those systems should help identify potential interactions. Cooperative research efforts involving nutritionists, physiologists, and geneticists will be critical to progress in this area.

REFERENCES

Bereskin, B. 1983. *J. Anim. Sci.* 57:867.
Bereskin, B., and N.C. Steele. 1986. *J. Anim. Sci.* 62:918.
Bereskin, B., R.J. Davey, and W.H. Petters. 1976. *J. Anim. Sci.* 43:1977.
Castell, A.G., and J.H. Strain. 1985. *Can. J. Anim. Sci.* 65:185.
Castell, A.G., R.L. Clipleff, and R.M. McKay. 1985. *Can. J. Anim. Sci.* 65:821.
Cleveland, E.R., P.J. Cunningham, and E.R. Peo. 1982. *J. Anim. Sci.* 54:719.
Crenshaw, T.D., et al. 1981. *J. Anim. Sci.* 52:1319.
Davey, R.J. 1976. *J. Anim. Sci.* 43:598.
Etherton, T.D., et al. 1982. *J. Nutr.* 112:2314.
Grummer, R.H. 1975. *Proceedings of the Symposium on the Effect of Genetic Variance On Nutritional Requirements of Animals.* pp. 113–123. Washington, DC: National Academy of Sciences.
Hertzer, H.O., and R.H. Miller. 1972. *J. Anim. Sci.* 35:730.
Kennedy, B.W. 1984. *J. Anim. Sci.* 59:338.
Kornegay, E.T., et al. 1985. *J. Anim. Sci.* 61:1460.
Liptrap, D.O., et al. 1970. *J. Anim. Sci.* 30:736.
Mahan, D.C., and A.W. Fetter. 1982. *J. Anim. Sci.* 54:285.
Mahan, D.C., and D.B. Gerber. 1985. *Nutr. Rep. Int.* 31:1015.
Maxson, P.F., and D.C. Mahan. 1986. *J. Anim. Sci.* 63:1163.
NCR-42 Committee on Swine Nutrition. 1976. *J. Anim. Sci.* 42:1211.
Newell, J.A., and J.P. Bowland. 1972. *Can. J. Anim. Sci.* 52:543.
Nimmo, R.D., et al. 1980. *J. Anim. Sci.* 51:112.
NRC. 1979. *Nutrient Requirements of Domestic Animals.* No. 2 *of Nutrient Requirements of Swine.* 8th ed. Washington, DC: National Academy of Sciences—National Research Council.
Pond, W.G., J.T. Yen, and R.V. Lindvall. 1980. *J. Nutr.* 110:2506.
Schneider, J.F., L.L. Christian, and D.L. Kuhlers. 1982. *J. Anim. Sci.* 54:728.
Siers, D.G. 1975. *J. Anim. Sci.* 41:522.
Skitsko, P.J., and J.P. Bowland. 1970. *Can. J. Anim. Sci.* 50:160.
Stowe, H.D., and E.R. Miller. 1985. *J. Anim. Sci.* 60:200.
Watkins, L.E., L.A. Swiger, and D.C. Mahan. 1977. *J. Anim. Sci.* 45:24.
Yen, H.T., D.J.A. Cole, and D. Lewis. 1986. *Anim. Prod.* 43:155.

Chapter 26

Mycotoxins in Swine Feeds

D.M. Forsyth

Mycotoxins are an insidious danger in feedstuffs. Their presence may go undetected, causing loss of production in livestock that goes unrecognized. Or, they may on occasion cause acute and fatal toxicities by their presence in large quantities in feedstuffs bearing little evidence of damage, as in the event that led to the discovery of aflatoxin (Goldblatt 1969). Mycotoxins cannot be presumed present in feedstuffs on the basis of presence of the causative mold, since toxins are only formed under certain conditions. Neither can feeds be presumed to be free of mycotoxins if no mold organisms are found; molds may have been present earlier, leaving behind their toxic legacy.

Mycotoxins are metabolites of filamentous fungi (Eumycetes), commonly referred to as molds, that are toxic to humans or animals. They are a diverse group of compounds, produced by a wide range of organisms, and they have markedly varied toxic effects. With improved detection and identification technology, the number of mycotoxins that has been identified has increased dramatically. It is fortunate then, that despite the ubiquitous nature of molds, only a few mycotoxins cause most of the problems in the feed supply for Midwestern United State swine producers. The mycotoxins presenting the greatest problems in swine feeds are aflatoxins and the metabolites from *Fusarium* species, with occasional incidences of other toxicities.

Besides the specific mycotoxins, there is concern for the nutritive quality of feeds that have been acted on by molds. In fact, when mycotoxins are not produced, molds may degrade, enhance, or leave unchanged the nutritive value of feeds.

Signs of molds leading to suspicion of mycotoxins vary from the obvious presence of fungal growth, through apparent damage to kernels of grain, to little or no visible evidence. Mycotoxin presence may be detected by biological effects on animals or by analysis for known offending substances. More specific signs and procedures are discussed under individual mycotoxins.

Although our immediate concern is for toxic effects in livestock, the ultimate consumption of food-producing animals by humans makes of paramount importance ensuring that the food supply remains wholesome. This is especially important with regard to aflatoxins, which are potent carcinogens. Procedures have been developed for removing or inactivating mycotoxins in feeds, but the best procedures for ensuring safe feeds are prevention of mycotoxin formation by good agronomic practices and proper preservation and storage of feeds.

AFLATOXIN

Aflatoxin is the mycotoxin of greatest concern due to its extreme toxicity and carcinogenicity. It has been responsible for the death of a large number of livestock and its cancer-causing properties are a risk to both humans and animals. Its recognition after losses of large numbers of turkey poults in England in 1960 has been reviewed by Heathcote and Hibbert (1978) and Moreau and Moss (1979).

Aflatoxin is the name given to a group of toxic metabolites from *Aspergillus flavus* and *Aspergillus parasiticus*. These organisms infect plant tissues, especially when they are stressed by drought or damaged by insects. *Aspergillus* spp. thrive under poor storage conditions (Smith and Moss 1985). *A. flavus* is a common inhabitant of soil and *A. parasiticus* is an insect pathogen. They especially present problems in peanuts, corn, and cottonseed meal. *A. flavus* can grow at temperatures of 6 °C to 54 °C, but prefers temperatures near 30 °C. The temperature, humidity, and other conditions conducive to production of aflatoxins have been reviewed (Diener and Davis 1969; Diener 1976; Moreau and Moss 1979).

The aflatoxins are a group of closely related compounds containing a methoxydihydrofuranocoumarin moiety. The predominant and most toxic form (to most species) is aflatoxin B_1. Aflatoxins B_1 and B_2 (fluorescing blue) and G_1 and G_2 (fluorescing green) were discovered first. Hydroxyaflatoxins (M_1 and M_2 [discovered in milk], B_{2a}, G_{2a}, GM_1, GM_2, B_3, R_0, P_1, and Q_1), dihydroxyaflatoxins (M_{2a} and GM_{2a}), and aflatoxin derivatives (0-alkyl aflatoxins, RB_{2a}, D_1, and D_2) are additional forms (Heathcote and Hibbert 1978).

Animals vary in their sensitivity to acute doses of aflatoxin according to species age, and sex. Ducklings, young pigs, calves, trout, and rabbits are highly sensitive, whereas rats, mice, sheep, and goats are quite resistant. Older animals are more resistant than younger ones, and females are more resistant than intact males (Heathcote and Hibbert 1978).

Signs of acute aflatoxicosis in swine include reduced body weight gain, depression, hemoconcentration, and liver damage. There is icterus, with a yellow swollen liver, mesenteric edema, and serous atrophy of fat. Microscopically, the liver shows fatty change, bile ductule cell proliferation and hypertrophy of ducts, lymphatic dilation, swollen or shrunken hepatic cell nuclei (depending on stage), and some pyknotic cells (Sysk et al. 1968; Cysewski et al. 1968). The median lethal dose (LD_{50}) for aflatoxin B_1 for the duckling, dog, rabbit, and trout is about 0.5 mg/kg, for the male rat it is 5 to 7 mg/kg, for the female rat it is 7 to 18 mg/kg, and for the pig it is 0.6 to 0.8 mg/kg (Butler 1969; Edds 1979a). Young pigs are more sensitive to both acute and chronic aflatoxicosis than are older pigs, although problems with exposure during gestation or through suckling are rare.

Acute toxicity is not often seen, especially with current concerns about and monitoring methods for aflatoxins. Chronic toxicosis from low-level ingestion of aflatoxin is much more common and results in serious economic loss from decreased animal performance. In pigs, anorexia and loss of weight were reported when the dose of aflatoxin was greater than 167 to 334 μg/kg body weight; levels above 83 μg/kg body weight were necessary to induce subacute toxicosis within 3 weeks (Sisk et al. 1968). Hintz et al. (1967a, 1967b) reported that 450 ppb of aflatoxin B_1 in the feed allowed normal growth and reproduction, but higher levels (615 ppb) depressed growth, although others have reported growth depression from slightly lower concentrations (Edds 1979a,b). Loss of appetite accompanies the decreased growth rate. The level of other nutrients in the diet influences the toxicity of aflatoxins and may help to explain some of the differences found. Feeding a high selenium level (2.5 mg/kg of feed) (Davila et al. 1983) protected against aflatoxin toxicity. Feeding additional thiamin and folic acid have been protective in rats (Bhavanishankar et al. 1986). Hemorrhaging, with prolonged clotting time, is a prevalent symptom of aflatoxicosis, and administration of vitamin K is an effective counter measure. Vitamin K supplementation may also improve weight gains during recovery from aflatoxicosis (Edds 1979b). Other aflatoxin-nutrition interactions have been reviewed by Newberne and Gross (1977) and Hamilton (1977).

Aflatoxin is a liver toxin, and damage in the liver occurs in all species. In chronic toxicity, the liver lesions may be slight and subtle on gross inspection. Prolonged exposure brings about disorganization of the lobular pattern, fibrosis, and the other changes that are also associated with acute toxicity.

Aflatoxin increases susceptibility to infection by interfering with immunity. Immunizations administered while animals are ingesting aflatoxins are not as successful as are those administered to animals not exposed to aflatoxins (Cysewski et al. 1978).

Aflatoxins are highly carcinogenic and cause liver tumors in swine as in other species. There may be a substantial time period between ingestion of aflatoxin and tumor development, but Carnaghan and Crawford (1964) reported that all pigs that survived acute aflatoxicosis subsequently developed hepatic carcinomas.

Analysis

Grain containing *A. flavus* examined under short wave ultraviolet light fluoresces with a characteristic bright greenish yellow fluorescence, and this has been used in grain elevators as a presumptive test for aflatoxin (Shotwell and Hesseltine 1981). It does not show the presence of aflatoxin, but only that *A. flavus* is, or was, present. Confirmation of aflatoxin by direct assay is necessary. Unfortunately, other substances also flouresce and can be confused during the initial screen, especially by those with little training.

For any mycotoxin analysis, the importance of proper sampling techniques cannot be overstated. Only a very small proportion of a feedstuff may be contaminated and the sample must be representative of the whole to be meaningful. The problem is especially great with large particles or seeds (e.g., corn or peanuts).

Typical procedures involved in analysis include sampling, preparation (grinding, mixing, subsampling), extraction, clean up (separation of interfering substances), detection and quantification, and confirmation of the identity of the compound (Davis et al. 1980).

Many analytical procedures have been used. Animal assays have been reviewed by Legator (1969). The standard methods of chemical analysis usually involve column chromatography, thin-layer chromatography, liquid chromatography, or some combination (AOAC 1984). Minicolumn methods have been developed to simplify and speed the analysis (AOAC 1984). Improvements in cleanup and detection have been offered (Kamimura et al. 1985) and will continue to be made. More recently, radioimmunoassay (RIA) and enzyme-linked immunosorbent assay (ELISA) methods have been developed (Chu 1984; Chu et al. 1987; El-Nakib et al. 1981; Ram et al. 1986). These methods are simple, rapid, and sensitive. The ELISA technique has provided the basis for a semiquantitative test kit that can be used in the field.

Detoxification of Feed

Prevention of formation of toxins by good harvesting and storage methods should be practiced to avoid contamination. Methods of detoxification have been developed, however, and they can be used when avoidance is impossible. Chemical methods that have been effective include solvent extraction and formaldehyde, methylamine, sodium hydroxide, calcium hydroxide, hydrogen peroxide, ozone, perchloric acid, methanol, or ammonia additions (Goldblatt and Dollear 1976; Moreau and Moss 1979; Edds 1979a). Although it damages protein quality, heat treatment (Hale and Wilson 1979) and ammoniation (Jensen et al. 1977) are probably the most practical methods. Recently, the use of hydrated sodium calcium aluminosilicate to adsorb aflatoxin, decreasing its absorption from the gastrointestinal tract and improving animal performance, has been reported (Phillips 1987).

The use of decontamination methods for grain in commercial channels is regulated. In 1988, a severe drought combined with hot weather increased the incidence of aflatoxin in corn in the Midwestern United States. The normal action level of 20 ppb was continued for corn destined for use by humans, immature animals, or dairy cattle, increased to 100 ppb for breeding cattle and swine or mature poultry, and increased to 200 ppb for finishing swine and to 300 ppb for finishing cattle. Blending of corn for animal feed was allowed under certain conditions, but ammoniation of corn shipped into interstate commerce was not allowed. This example illustrates that regulations are subject to change, and one must consult appropriate regulatory officials concerning any particular aflatoxin incidence.

TOXIC METABOLITES FROM FUSARIUM SPECIES

The toxic metabolites produced by several organisms of the *Fusarium* genus are of special importance to those dealing with swine, swine being more sensitive than other farm animals to their effects. Estrogenic activity from zearalenone, and feed refusal and emetic activity from trichothecenes are the most troublesome problems. These principles often exist together (Mirocha et al. 1976, 1979a,b). The variety of corn influences the susceptibility to infection (Atlin et al. 1983; Hurt et al. 1984; Hunter et al. 1986).

Complicating the understanding of the subject by nonspecialists is the fact that not only are many species, strains within species, and special stages of the organisms cited as causative agents of fusariotoxins, but also taxonomists have not always agreed on nomenclature and classification; consequently, different names have been used to describe essentially the same thing. *"Fusarium graminearum,"* *"Fusarium roseum,"* and *"Gibberella zeae"* have been used synomymously. The term *"Fusarium roseum"* was used to combine over 50 species, varieties, and forms into one species, but this scheme has now fallen into disuse. *"Gibberella zeae"* refers to the perfect (sexually reproductive) stage of *F. graminearum.* A manual for identification of *Fusarium* species (Nelson et al. 1983) has been published, and the complicated present state of *Fusarium* taxonomy has been reviewed extensively and explained by Joffe (1986). A comprehensive compilation of literature about fungal species, mycotoxins produced, and their effects in animals has been prepared by Marasas et al. (1984).

Zearalenone

Zearalenone and related compounds are produced by several species of *Fusarium* and have estrogenic activity that interferes with reproduction in swine and other animals. Moldy feeds may produce signs of estrus (swollen, reddened vulva) in immature gilts and interfere with the estrous cycle in cycling gilts. Zearalenone was isolated from *G. zeae* and the signs of mycotoxicosis in animals reproduced by Stob et al. (1962). The structure of zearalenone was determined by Urry et al. (1965) to be a resorcylic acid lactone. Christensen et al. (1965) isolated a uterotrophic metabolite and named it F2, which was the same as zearalenone. Both names are still used occasionally.

Zearalenone is different than other mycotoxins in that it exhibits estrogenic activity but it is not acutely toxic. A derivative has been used commercially to enhance weight gain in ruminants (Baldwin et al. 1983). The LD_{50} of zearalenone is too high to be practically meaningful, and death associated with zearalenone is most often caused by secondary infection from prolapse of the vagina.

Signs of Toxicity

Zearalenone has been extensively reviewed (Mirocha et al. 1971; Mirocha et al 1977; Christensen 1979; Haschek and Haliburton 1986; Joffe 1986). Its signs of toxicity are those of hyperestrogenism, involving primarily the reproductive tract and mammary gland. In natural cases of mycotoxicosis involving zearalenone, the effects due to zearalenone may be complicated by or confused with effects of other mycotoxins that are produced by the same organism and are commonly present together, such as T-2 toxin, deoxynivalenol, and diacetoxyscirpenol. Therefore, reports that attribute toxic effects to zearalenone from studies of feeding molded feeds should be interpreted with caution. In field cases of toxicity, the clinical picture may seldom be due to zearalenone alone, and, for example, feed intake may be decreased from trichothecene contamination. Zearalenone is often considered to be a mycotoxin produced under storage conditions, although it is also found in the field. Seasons that are cool and wet at silking of corn are conducive to infection with *G. zeae,* and conditions of high moisture (>25%) and low temperature (15 °C) promote zearalenone production (Eugenio et al. 1970; Tuite et al. 1974; Christensen 1979). These conditions are often prevalent in stored ear corn, but zearalenone is less likely to be produced in shelled corn because *Fusarium* organisms do not compete well with other organisms of decay thriving in these conditions (Christensen 1979).

Swine are particularly sensitive to zearalenone. In the prepuberal gilt, the vulva and uterus become swollen and edematous, and vaginal and/or anal prolapse may occur. The ovaries may partially atrophy. Histologically, there is ductal proliferation of the mammary glands and of all cell layers of the uterus, along with metaplasia of epithelium of the cervix and vagina (Kurtz et al. 1969). Abortion does not appear to be caused by zearalenone alone, but it can result from other toxins present. Zearalenone at high levels (60 or 90 ppm in the feed) interferes with embryonic development (Long and Diekman 1984). Lower concentrations (4 to 9 ppm) interfere with conception and cause pseudopregnancy (Etienne and Jemmali 1982; Young and King 1986a). Pregnancy was prevented in sows consuming 1 mg zearalenone/kg body weight on days 7 to 10 postmating, whereas consumption at other time periods allowed normal development of fetuses (Long and Diekman 1986). The mechanism involved may be through differences in the uterine environment of zearalenone-treated sows, although neither blastocyst migration nor intrauterine content of prostaglandin $F_{2\alpha}$, estradiol-17β, or progesterone were altered (Long et al. 1988). Reduced litter size, increased numbers of stillbirths, and increased neonatal mortality have been associated with zearalenone consumption by sows that remained pregnant (Miller et al. 1973; Sharma et al. 1974; Young et al. 1982).

Zearalenone, despite being uniquely different in chemical structure from estrogen, interacts directly with the estrogen receptors and evokes many of the biological and biochemical responses of estradiol (Kiang et al. 1978; Katzenellenbogen et al. 1979).

Zearalenone affects sexual development of young boars. Male reproductive tracts tended to be smaller when pigs were fed or dosed with high levels (500 to 600 ppm or 5 to 15 mg/kg body weight) of zearalenone (Christensen et al. 1972; Farnworth and Trenholm 1983). Feeding 40 ppm zearalenone for 4 weeks (at age 14 weeks) reduced subsequent libido scores (Berger et al. 1981). Prolonged feeding of low levels (0 to 9 ppm) of zearalenone did not affect libido, but it tended to reduce semen volume, total motile sperm, and percent sperm motility (Young and King 1986b).

Analysis

Biological assays were the first means of analysis for zearalenone, and they are still of value (MacDougald et al. 1987). Today, the most common analytical methods involve thin-layer chromatography (AOAC 1984; Swanson et al. 1984), liquid chromatography (Cohen and Lapointe 1980; Bagneris et al. 1986), gas chromatography, and combined gas chromatography-mass spectrometry (Mirocha et al. 1974). More recently, the immunological methods (RIA and ELISA) have been developed to improve the speed and reduce the cost of analysis (Chu 1984; Thouvenot and Morfin 1983; Liu et al. 1985).

Detoxification of Feed

Methods used to detoxify contaminated feeds are generally the same as those used for aflatoxin. Density segregation was successful in reducing zearalenone, aflatoxin, and deoxynivalenol (Huff and Hagler 1985). High temperature, aqueous ammonia, and hydrogen peroxide destroyed zearalenone, but these processes are unlikely to be adapted widely for feeds (Christensen 1979). Feeding alfalfa (15% or 25%) decreased the uterine enlargement in swine caused by zearalenone (James and Smith 1982). A unique means of dealing with zearalenone toxicity in pigs by immunization was proposed by Pestka et al. (1985); its efficacy has not yet been reported.

Trichothecenes

The trichothecenes, especially deoxynivalenol ([DON] or vomitoxin), are primarily responsible for the extraordinarily strong feed refusal response and occasional emetic response by pigs to grain infected with *Fusarium* spp. Approximately 50 naturally occurring trichothecene compounds have been isolated under laboratory conditions, the majority from *Fusarium* species but some from other fungi (NRC 1983; Joffe 1986). They are closely related sesquiterpenoids characterized as 12,13-expoxythrichothecenes. Primarily T-2 toxin, diacetoxyscirpenol, nivalenol, and DON (Joffe 1986), and perhaps a few others have been isolated from animal feeds associated with human and animal toxicosis.

Fusarium ear rot and stalk rot are present in corn to some degree every year, but occasionally are so prevalent as to affect a majority of the corn crop in a state. The same organisms affect barley and wheat, causing scabbed grain and producing mycotoxins (Pollman et al. 1985). In corn, problems are greatest when weather conditions are cool and wet at silking (Tuite et al. 1974). Corn that has been damaged by the fungus, commonly called "Gib corn" after *G. zeae,* may cause emesis in swine, if consumed, or almost total feed refusal. Curtin and Tuite (1966) suggested, from studies of extracts, that separate compounds might be involved in refusal and emesis. Yoshizawa and Morooka (1973) isolated DON, named after the known toxin nivalenol. In the same year, Vesonder et al. (1973) isolated an emetic factor and gave it the trivial name vomitoxin. This compound was later shown to also cause feed refusal (Vesonder et al. 1976) and both terms for the same compound (DON, vomitoxin) are still used.

Forsyth et al. (1977) added DON to feed and compared feed refusal to naturally infected corn. They concluded that DON failed to explain all of the feed refusal response. An additional trichothecene, 15-acetyl deoxynivalenol (a DON precursor), was later identified and might account for some of the response (Abbas et al. 1986; Pestka et al. 1987). Foster et al. (1986) have recently shown that DON alone does not account for all of the toxic effects seen in swine. Additional toxins and their metabolites are still being discovered (Gelderblom et al. 1988), and many occur simultaneously in infected feedstuffs.

Signs of Toxicity

DON causes feed refusal and emesis in swine. Toxicosis may occur, therefore, with no other signs than that of inanition (Pollman et al. 1985; Chavez and Rheaume 1986; Young et al. 1983; Lun et al. 1985). Feed intake of younger pigs is more affected than that of older pigs (Forsyth 1974). Feed containing more than 1 ppm of DON will cause at least partial feed refusal (Young et al. 1983).

DON-contaminated wheat diets did not appear to have deleterious effects on gilts or their progeny (Friend et al. 1982, 1986a), or on sexual development in boars or gilts (Friend et al. 1986b). Castrated males had lower weight gains than females, but the results were confounded by the presence of zearalenone (Cote et al. 1985).

Immunosuppression and hematological and histological changes due to trichothecenes are seen in laboratory animals (Joffe 1986) and, although seldom reported for swine given feed containing DON, could result from co-contamination with T-2 toxin, diacetoxyscirpenol, or other toxins. In natural cases of moldy feed intoxication, a number of toxins may be present, and the results of toxicity may vary according to complex interactions of synergistic, additive, or antagonistic nature, altering the clinical signs (Huff et al. 1988).

Analysis

The first indication of DON-containing feed may be by feed refusal by swine. Indeed, offering suspected feed to a few pigs is a rapid and practical screening technique. Rats are also affected, although they are less sensitive than swine, and can be used in screening assays (Forsyth 1974; DeUriarte et al. 1976). Other biological assay methods for the detection of trichothecenes have been described by Ueno (1983).

Before corn kernels are ground, infection by *Fusarium* organisms can be determined by observation by a trained plant pathologist. Chemical assay for the mycotoxins is usually by chromatography. Screening methods for trichothecenes using gas chromatography (Kuroda et al. 1979; Rood et al. 1988), thin-layer chromatography (Steyn 1981; Trucksess et al. 1986, 1987; Eppley et al. 1986), thin-layer chromatography with gas chromatography using flame ionization, electron capture, or mass spectrometric detection (Scott 1982; Ware et al. 1984), and nuclear magnetic resonance (Cox and Cole 1983; Blackwell et al. 1984) have been described. For more rapid analysis and larger numbers of samples RIA (Xu et al. 1986) and ELISA methods for trichothecenes have been developed (Chu 1984). Absorption by a hydrated sodium calcium aluminosilicate has been reported for analysis of several mycotoxins and for detoxification of aflatoxin (Phillips 1987).

Because mycotoxins are rarely distributed evenly throughout feedstuffs, proper sampling is essential. Guidelines to achieve accurate sampling have been described by Davis et al. (1980).

Detoxification of Feed

Efforts to improve acceptability of corn infected with *Fusarium* toxins by adding propionic acid, ammonium hydroxide, molasses (Tuite et al. 1974), vinegar, zinc (Forsyth 1974), copper (Fritschen et al. 1983), heating, or screening (J.R. Foster, personal communication) have not been successful. The trichothecenes are water-soluble, however, and can be removed by soaking and washing (Forsyth 1974; Forsyth et al. 1976; DeUriarte et al. 1976). The process can be hastened by use of NaOH together wtih washing (Forsyth 1974). The nutritional value of the corn is unimpaired after removal of the toxin, as shown by equivalent growth in a 92-day feeding trial of controls and pigs fed decontaminated corn that would not initially support growth (Forsyth et al. 1976). Other chemical and enzymatic methods of decontamination have been discussed for trichothecenes (NRC 1983), and benefits from treatment with sodium bisulfite have been demonstrated for DON (Young 1954; Young et al. 1987). The use of mold inhibitors, common in poultry feeds, is not as prevalent in low-moisture swine feeds, and it will not affect mycotoxins that are already present.

Pigs are particularly sensitive to ''Gib corn'' and may completely refuse feed in which 5% of the corn kernels are damaged (Tuite et al. 1974). Most other livestock, including beef cattle, dairy cattle, sheep, and chickens, are less sensitive to DON, so it is often recommended that DON-affected feed should be diverted to them and uncontaminated grain should be used for swine. There is not universal agreement on this point; for example, Hulan and Proudfoot (1982) found no effect in poultry, whereas Hamilton et al. (1981) reported that hens fed DON ate less feed than did hens fed control diets. It should be noted that T-2 toxin and diacetoxyscirpenol are toxic to cattle and could be present in DON-containing grain (see Joffe 1986).

OTHER MYCOTOXINS

The list of other mycotoxins is long (over 200 have been discovered), but fortunately reports of their causing mycotoxicosis in swine are rare or absent. A few that are potentially toxic are discussed briefly here.

Trichothecenes Besides DON

T-2 toxin, diacetoxyscirpenol (DAS), and fusarenon-x are nearly an order of magnitude more toxic than DON. DAS has been diagnosed as causing hemorrhagic bowel syndrome in swine in Minnesota. T-2 toxin has caused emesis and diarrhea in swine. T-2 toxin does not cause abortion when consumed, but it can lead to infertility (Mirocha 1979).

Ochratoxins

Ochratoxin, a metabolite of several *Aspergillus* spp. and *Penicillium* spp., is a nephrotoxin that has been reported to cause feed refusal in swine fed diets containing grain sorghum that had 5 mg of ochratoxin/kg (Harvey et al. 1987).

The fungi that produce ochratoxins are common in soil, plants, insects, and stored grain. Pigs clear ochratoxin slowly, and it has been considered to be a serious food-chain residue problem (Cheeke and Shull 1985).

Citrinin

Another nephrotoxin produced by species of *Penicillium* and *Aspergillus,* especially *Penicillium viridicatum,* is citrinin. Signs of toxicosis are similar to those of ochratoxin A; nephropathy with tubular necrosis and associated signs. Field cases are often complicated by both citrinin and ochratoxin contamination (Carlton and Tuite 1986).

Rubratoxins

Two toxins (rubratoxin A and B) are produced by *Penicillium rubrum* and *Penicillium purpurogenum.* They can produce liver and kidney degeneration and hemorrhages. The fungi have been isolated in cases in which mycotoxicosis was suspected, but involvement of the toxins has not been proved (Peden et al. 1986).

Cyclopiazonic Acid

Cyclopiazonic acid (CPA) is produced by a number of species of fungi and is toxic to swine and other species, involving primarily the liver, kidneys, and digestive system. Anorexia and diarrhea are signs (Peden et al. 1986).

Penicillic Acid

Two species of *Penicillium* (*P. cyclopium* Westl. and *P. puberulum* Bainier) are very common on grain and produce penicillic acid. Other species also produce this toxin. Penicillic acid is toxic to mice with an LD_{50} of 110 mg/kg body weight subcutaneously. It has antidiuretic activity and acts on the heart and is suspected of being carcinogenic. Its toxicity to swine is unknown (Moreau and Moss 1974).

REFERENCES

Abbas, H.K., C.J. Mirocha, and J. Tuite. 1986. *Appl. Environ. Microbiol.* 51:841.

AOAC. 1984. *Official Methods of Analysis.* 14th ed. Arlington, VA: Association of Official Analytical Chemists.

Atlin, G.N., et al. 1983. *Can. J. Plant Sci.* 63:847.
Bagneris, R.W., J.A. Gaul, and G.M. Ware. 1986. *J. Assoc. Off. Anal. Chem.* 69:894.
Baldwin, R.S., R.D. Williams, and M.K. Terry. 1983. *Regul. Toxicol. Pharmacol.* 3:9.
Berger, T., et al. 1981. *J. Anim. Sci.* 53:1559.
Bhavanishankar, T.N., T. Shantha, and R.P. Ramesh. 1986. *Nutr. Rep. Int.* 33:603.
Blackwell, B.A., R. Greenhalgh, and A.D. Bain. 1984. *J. Agric. Food Chem.* 32:1078.
Butler, W.H. 1969. In: *Aflatoxin*. Goldblatt, L.A. (Ed.). pp. 223–236. New York: Academic Press.
Carlton, W.W., and J. Tuite. 1986. In: *Diagnosis of Mycotoxicosis*. Dordrecht: Martinus Nijhoff.
Carnaghan, R.B.A., and M. Crawford. 1964. *Br. Vet J.* 120:201.
Chavez, E.R., and J.A. Rheaume. 1986. *Can. J. Anim. Sci.* 66:277.
Cheeke, P.R., and L.R. Shull. 1985. *Natural Toxicants in Feeds and Poisonous Plants*. Westport, CT: AVI Publishing Co.
Christensen, C.M. 1979. In: *Conference on Mycotoxins in Animal Feeds and Grains Related to Human Health*. pp. 1–79. Rockville, MD: Food and Drug Administration.
Christensen, C.M., G.H. Nelson, and C.J. Mirocha. 1965. *Appl. Microbiol.* 13:653.
Christensen, C.M., et al. 1972. *Appl. Microbiol.* 23:202.
Chu, F.S. 1984. *J. Food Protection* 47:562.
Chu, F.S., et al. 1987. *J. Assoc. Off. Anal. Chem.* 70:854.
Cohen, H., and M.R. Lapointe. 1980. *J. Assoc. Off. Anal. Chem.* 63:642.
Cote, L.M., et al. 1985. *J. Anim. Sci.* 61:942.
Cox, R.H., and R.J. Cole. 1983. In: *Trichothecenes, Chemical, Biological and Toxicological Aspects*. Ueno, Y. (Ed.). pp. 39–46. Amsterdam: Elsevier.
Curtin, T.M., and J. Tuite. 1966. *Life Sci.* 5:1937.
Cysewski, S.J., et al. 1968. *Am. J. Vet. Res.* 12:1577.
Cysewski, S.J., et al. 1978. *Am. J. Vet. Res.* 39:445.
Davilla, J.C., et al. 1983. *Am. J. Vet. Res.* 44:1877.
Davis, W.D., et al. 1980. *J. Assoc. Off. Anal. Chem.* 63:95.
DeUriarte, L.A., D.M. Forsyth, and J. Tuite. 1976. *J. Anim. Sci.* 42:1196.
Diener, U.L. 1976. *Proc. Am. Phytopath. Soc.* 3:126.
Diener, U.L., and N.D. Davis. 1969. In: *Aflatoxin*. Goldblatt, L.A. (Ed.). New York: Academic Press.
Edds, G.T. 1979a. In: *Conference on Mycotoxins in Animal Feeds and Grains Related To Animal Health*. pp. 80–155. Rockville, MD: Food and Drug Administration.
Edds, G.T., 1979b. In: *Interactions of Mycotoxins in Animal Production*. pp. 67–76. Washington, DC: National Academy of Sciences.
El-Nakib, O., J.J. Pestka, and F.S. Chu. 1981. *J. Assoc. Off. Anal. Chem.* 64:1077.
Eppley, R.M., et al. 1986. *J. Assoc. Off. Anal. Chem.* 69:37.
Etienne, M., and M. Jemmali. 1982. *J. Anim. Sci.* 55:1.
Farnworth, E.R., and H.L. Trenholm. 1983. *Can. J. Anim. Sci.* 63:967.
Forsyth, D.M., 1974. *J. Anim. Sci.* 39:1092.
Forsyth, D.M., L.A. DeUriarte, and J. Tuite. 1976. *J. Anim. Sci.* 42:1202.
Forsyth, D.M., et al. 1977. *Appl. Environ. Microbiol.* 34:547.
Foster, B.C., et al. 1986. *Can. J. Anim. Sci.* 66:1149.
Friend, D.W., et al. 1982. *Can. J. Anim. Sci.* 62:1211.
Friend, D.W., et al. 1986a. *Can. J. Anim. Sci.* 66:229.
Friend, D.W., et al. 1986b. *Can. J. Anim. Sci.* 66:765.
Fritschen, R.D., et al. 1983. *J. Anim. Sci.* 57:239 (Abstr.).
Gelderblom, W.C.A., et al. 1988. *Appl. Environ. Microbiol.* 54:1806.
Goldblatt, L.A. 1969. *Aflatoxin*. New York: Academic Press.
Goldblatt, L.A., and F.G. Dollear. 1976. In: *Mycotoxins in Human and Animal Health, Proceedings of a Conference*. Rodericks, J.V., C.W. Hesseltine, and M.A. Mehlman (Eds.). Park Forest, IL: Pathotox Publishing, Inc.
Hale, O.M., and D.M. Wilson. 1979. *J. Anim. Sci.* 48:1394 (Abstr.).
Hamilton, P.B. 1977. *Fed. Am. Soc. Exp. Biol.* 36:1899.

Hamilton, R.M.G., B.K. Thomson, and H.L. Trenholm. 1981. *Poult. Sci.* 60:1665 (Abstr.).
Hart, L.P., E. Gendloff, and E.C. Rossman. 1984. *Plant Dis.* 68:296–298.
Harvey, R.B., et al. 1987. *J. Am. Vet. Med. Assoc.* 190:673.
Haschek, W.M., and J.C. Haliburton. 1986. In: *Diagnosis of Mycotoxicoses.* Richard, J.L. and J.R. Thurston (Eds.). Dordrecht, The Netherlands: Martinus Nijhoff.
Heathcote, J.G., and J.R. Hibbert. 1978. *Aflatoxins: Chemical and Biological Aspects.* Amsterdam: Elsevier.
Hintz, H.F., et al. 1967a. *Proc. Soc. Exp. Biol. Med.* 124:266.
Hintz, H.F., et al. 1967b. *Proc. Soc. Exp. Biol. Med.* 126:146.
Huff, W.E., and W.M. Hagler, Jr. 1985. *J. Food. Prot.* 48:416.
Huff, W.E., et al. 1988. *J. Anim. Sci.* 66:2351.
Hulan, H.W., and F.C. Proudfoot. 1982. *Poult. Sci.* 61:1653.
Hunter, R.B., G.N. Atlin, and J.F. Muldoon. 1986. *Can. J. Plant Sci.* 66:291.
James, L.J., and T.K. Smith. 1982. *J. Anim. Sci.* 55:110.
Jensen, A.H., et al. 1977. *J. Anim. Sci.* 45:8–12.
Joffe, A.Z. 1986. *Fusarium Species: Their Biology and Toxicology.* New York: John Wiley and Sons.
Kamimura, H., et al. 1985. *J. Assoc. Off. Anal. Chem.* 68:458.
Katzenellenbogen, B.S., J.A. Katzenellenbogen, and D. Mordecai. 1979. *Endocrinology* 105:33.
Kiang, D.T., et al. 1978. *Cancer Res.* 38:3611.
Kuroda, H., et al. 1979. *J. Food Hyg. Soc.* Jpn 20:137.
Kurtz, H.J., et al. 1969. *Am. J. Vet. Res.* 30:551.
Legator, M.S. 1969. In: *Aflatoxin.* Goldblatt, L.A. (Ed.). New York: Academic Press.
Liu, M., et al. 1985. *Appl. Environ. Microbiol.* 50:332.
Long, G.G., and M.A. Diekman. 1984. *J. Anim. Sci.* 59:1662.
Long, G.G., and M.A. Diekman. 1986. *Am. J. Vet. Res.* 47:184.
Long, G.G., M.A. Diekman, and A.B. Scheidt. 1988. *J. Anim. Sci.* 66:452.
Lun, A.K., L.G. Young, and J.H. Lumsden. 1985. *J. Anim. Sci.* 61:1178.
MacDougald, O.A., et al. 1987. *Research Report from the Michigan State University Agricultural Experiment Station.* (Sept.) p. 165.
Marasas, W.F.O., P.E. Nelson, and T.A. Toussoun. 1984. *Toxigenic* Fusarium *Species, Identity and Mycotoxicology.* University Park, PA: The Pennsylvania State University Press.
Miller, J.K., A. Hacking, and V.J. Gross. 1973. *Vet. Rec.* 93:955.
Mirocha, C.J. 1979. In: *Conference on Mycotoxins in Animal Feeds and Grains Related to Animal Health.* Rockville, MD: Food and Drug Administration.
Mirocha, C.J., C.M. Christensen, and G.H. Nelson. 1971. In: *Microbial Toxins.* Vol. 7. Kadis, S., A. Ciegler, and S.J. Ajl (Eds.). New York: Academic Press.
Mirocha, C.J., S.V. Pathre, and C.M. Christensen. 1977. In: *Mycotoxins in Human and Animal Health.* Rodricks, J.V., C.W. Hesseltine, and M.A. Hehlman (Eds.). pp. 345–364. Forest Park South, IL: Pathotox Publishers, Inc.
Mirocha, C.J., B. Schauerhamer, and S.V. Pathre. 1974. *J. Assoc. Off. Anal. Chem.* 57:1104.
Mirocha, C.J., et al. 1976. *Appl. Environ. Microbiol.* 32:553.
Mirocha, C.J., et al. 1979a. *Appl. Environ. Microbiol.* 38:557.
Mirocha, C.J., et al. 1979b. *Appl. Environ. Microbiol.* 38:749.
Moreau, C., and M. Moss. 1979. *Moulds, Toxins and Food.* Chichester, England: John Wiley and Sons.
Nelson, P.E., T.A. Toussoun, and W.F.O. Marasas. 1983. *Fusarium species: An Illustrated Manual For Identification.* University Park, PA: The Pennsylvania State University Press.
Newberne, P.M., and R.L. Gross. 1977. In: *Mycotoxins in Human and Animal Health, Proceedings of a Conference.* Roderick, J.V., C.W. Hesseltine, and M.A. Mehlman (Eds.). Park Forest, IL: Pathotox Publishing, Inc.
NRC. 1983. *Protection Against Trichothecene Mycotoxins.* Washington, DC: National Academy Press.

Peden, W.M., J.L. Richard, and J.R. Thurston. 1986. In: *Diagnosis of Mycotoxicosis*. Dordrecht, The Netherlands: Martinus Nijhoff.
Pestka, J.J., et al. 1985. *J. Food Prot.* 48:953.
Phillips, T.D. 1987. In: *Recent Developments in the Study of Mycotoxins, Proceedings of a Symposium*. Cleveland, OH: Kaiser Aluminum & Chemical Corp.
Pollman, D.S., et al. *J. Anim. Sci.* 60:239.
Ram, B.P., et al. 1986. *J. Assoc. Off. Anal. Chem.* 69:904.
Rood, H.D., Jr., W.B. Buck, and S.P. Swanson. 1988. *J. Assoc. Off. Anal. Chem.* 71:493.
Scott, P.M. 1982. *J. Assoc. Off. Anal. Chem.* 65:876.
Sharma, V.D., R.F. Wilson, and C.E. Williams. 1974. *J. Anim. Sci.* 38:598.
Shotwell, O.L., and C.W. Hesseltine. 1981. *Cereal Chem.* 58:124.
Smith, J.E., and M.O. Moss. 1985. *Mycotoxins: Formation, Analysis and Significance*. Chichester, England: John Wiley and Sons.
Steyn, P.S. 1981. *Pure Appl. Chem.* 53:891.
Stob, M., et al. 1962. *Nature* 196:1318.
Swanson, S.S., et al. 1984. *J. Assoc. Off. Anal. Chem.* 67:580.
Sysk, D.B., W.W. Carlton, and T.M. Curtin. 1968. *Am. J. Vet. Res.* 29:1591.
Thouvenot, D.R., and R.F. Morfin. 1983. *Appl. Environ. Microbiol.* 45:16.
Trucksess, M.W., M.T. Flood, and S.W. Page. 1986. *J. Assoc. Off. Anal. Chem.* 69:35.
Trucksess, M.W., et al. 1987. *J. Agric. Food Chem.* 35:445.
Tuite, J.G., et al. 1974. *Cereal Sci. Today* 19:238.
Ueno, Y. 1983. In: *Trichothecenes, Chemical, Biological and Toxicological Aspects*. Ueno, Y. (Ed.). pp. 125–133. Amsterdam: Elsevier.
Urry, W.H., et al. 1966. *Tetrahedron Lett.* 27:3109.
Vesonder, R.F., A. Ciegler, and A.H. Jensen. 1973. *Appl. Microbiol.* 26:1008.
Vesonder, R.F., et al. 1976. *Appl. Environ. Microbiol.* 31:280.
Ware, G.M., et al. 1984. *J. Assoc. Off. Anal. Chem.* 67:731.
Xu, Y.C., G.S. Zhang, and F.S. Chu. 1986. *J. Assoc. Off. Anal. Chem.* 69:967.
Yoshizawa, T., and N. Morooka. 1973. *Agric. Biol. Chem.* 37:2933.
Young, J.C. 1986. *J. Agric. Food Chem.* 34:465.
Young, L.G., and G.J. King. 1986a. *J. Anim. Sci.* 63:1191.
Young, L.G., and G.J. King. 1986b. *J. Anim. Sci.* 63:1197.
Young, L.G., et al. 1982. *J. Anim. Sci.* 54:976.
Young, L.G., et al. 1983. *J. Anim. Sci.* 57:655.
Young, J.C., et al. 1987. *J. Agric. Food Chem.* 35:259.

Chapter 27

Intestinal Bacteria and Their Influence on Swine Nutrition

S.V. Radecki and M.T. Yokoyama

The gastrointestinal tract of the pig is an ideal environment for the establishment of a diverse bacterial population. Essential criteria for maintaining a stable indigenous population are met in this ecosystem. Substrates for the bacteria to ferment are continuously provided by ingested feeds, by the sloughing of mucopolysaccharides and epithelial cells from the intestinal wall, by secretions into the lumen, and by the recycling of bacterial cells. Fermentation metabolites are removed from the lumen through absorption and metabolism, or by passing through the intestinal tract and being voided along with undegraded residues. Numerous mesophilic bacteria are able to proliferate in this isothermic ecosystem. Mucous-coated epithelial tissue provides a surface for attachment and colonization.

Research has made clear that the indigenous bacteria play a significant role in the health and nutrition of the pig. Through their interactions with each other and with the pig, the indigenous bacteria can either prevent or suppress pathogenic bacteria from colonizing the intestinal tract. Although not completely understood, the significance of their effects on nutrition may be either beneficial or detrimental to the pig. This chapter reviews the current knowledge of the indigenous bacteria population in the gastrointestinal tract of the pig and its impact on nutrition.

ESTABLISHMENT OF THE INDIGENOUS POPULATION

At birth, the gastrointestinal tract of the young pig is germ free. Within hours after exposure to the environment, a large microbial population rapidly develops in the tract. Initially, *Escherichia coli* and species of *Streptococcus* and *Clostridium* proliferate to produce high numbers in the feces of the newborn, with a slower development of lactobacilli. Within the first weeks of life, the normal progression of change in the population is for a decrease in the predominance of *E. coli* along the entire gastrointestinal tract, concomitant with a colonization of a predominant facultatively anaerobic population in the proximal intestine (e.g., *Lactobacillus* and *Streptococcus* species) and a diverse, strictly anaerobic population in the distal intestine (e.g., *Bacteroides, Eubacterium, Bifidobacterium, Propionibacterium, Fusobacterium, Clostridium* species) (Ducluzeau 1985). The major factor responsible for this marked change is probably the initiation of suckling. Physiological and environmental factors may also have an important role in stabilizing the intestinal microflora and establishing an indigenous population. The relatively high pH of the newborn pig's stomach, due to the insufficient secretion of HCl, allows environmental bacteria to rapidly inoculate the intestinal tract. This high stomach pH permits bacteria to pass through the intestinal tract, colonizing different sections. However, as the pig suckles and the stomach pH decreases due to lactic acid production, only acid-tolerant bacteria are able to persist and proliferate in the proximal intestine (Smith and Jones 1963). Maternal milk possesses some bacteriostatic properties that can suppress *E. coli* (Nagy et al. 1979; Chidlow and Porter 1979), which may promote a more rapid stabilization of the indigenous population. Liquid milk replacers appear to decrease the *Lactobacillus* species and increase the *E. coli* and strictly anaerobic bacteria in the proximal small intestine (Ducluzeau 1985). Environmental factors, such as temperature (Tenk and Szabo 1979; Shimizu and Terashima 1982) and unsanitary rearing conditions, can delay the establishment of the indigenous bacterial population. Once the indigenous population has been successfully established, few qualitative changes in the population occur, even at weaning, when the young pig is exposed to solid food (Ducluzeau 1985). Some subdominant indigenous bacteria colonize the intestinal tract only after weaning.

DISTRIBUTION AND TYPES OF BACTERIA

Bacteria are distributed throughout the gastrointestinal tract of the pig. The anatomy and physiology of different sites along the gastrointestinal tract have a profound influence on where the major indigenous populations colonize, and also the diversity of the bacterial species (Savage 1977). Factors that influence the localization and diversity of indigenous bacterial populations include passage rate of the ingesta, pH, temperature, redox potential, osmolality, endogenous secretions, enzyme activities, anaerobiosis, and dry matter content of the ingesta. Sites along the gastrointestinal tract where more stasis and slower passage of the ingesta occur (e.g., stomach, cecum) will support a larger and more diverse population. At sites where the passage rate of ingesta is rapid (e.g., small intestine), bacteria that have faster growth rates and adhere to the intestinal wall have a clear advantage for colonization.

Numerous rod-shaped and coccal bacteria adhere to the esophageal tissue of the young pig. The rod-shaped bacteria most likely belong to the genus *Lactobacillus*. Segmented filamentous bacteria resembling *Alysiella* species have been observed in the esophagus of the pig (Tannock et al. 1987). This bacterium has previously been shown to inhabit the oral cavity of the pig (Kuhn 1981). In the stomach, a fairly large population of bacteria exists. Many of the facultatively anaerobic bacteria present in the stomach are probably transient, either passed down from regions of the mouth and esophagus or ingested with the feed and water. An indigenous bacterial population colonizes the keratinized epithelium of nonsecreting areas of the stomach (Kawai and Suegara 1977). On the squamous epithelium of the pars esophagea region of the suckling pig stomach, species frequently isolated include *Lactobacillus fermentum, Lactobacillus salivarius,* and *Streptococcus salivarius.* Early-weaned pigs have a higher prevalence of *Lactobacillus acidophilus* and *Streptococcus bovis* in their stomach (Fuller et al. 1978). *Lactobacillus* organisms and yeasts also colonize the columnar epithelium of the stomach (Tannock and Smith 1970). The occurrence of *Clostridium* organisms, *Veillonella* organisms, coliforms, and other unidentified species have been reported in the stomach (Decuypere et al. 1973; Dubos et al. 1965; Tannock and Smith 1970).

The transition from the environment of the stomach to that of the small intestine is drastic. The rapid passage of ingesta through the small intestine results in a fermentation rate that is lower than in any other section of the tract (Friend et al. 1964; Argenzio and Southworth 1974). This is especially true of the proximal small intestine. Bacteria isolated from the small intestine include those of the *Lactobacillus, Streptococcus,* and *Bifidobacterium* genera and coliforms, with yeasts isolated from the lower small intestine (Savage 1977). As in the stomach, many bacteria found in the small intestine are facultatively anaerobic and appear to be transient. Bacterial numbers and fermentation rates increase in the ileum (Vervaeke et al. 1979).

The cecum of the pig harbors a large and diverse bacterial population because of its large volume and stasis of substantial ingesta. The concentrations of bacteria from cecal ingesta are estimated to be 2.37×10^{10}/g and bacteria adhered to the cecal wall number $2.67 \times 10^{7}/cm^{2}$ of tissue surface area (Allison et al. 1979). The bacteria found in the cecum are predominantly strictly anaerobic species. Characterization of cecal isolates indicate that *Bacteroides ruminicola* and *Selenomonas ruminantium* account for 35% and 21% of the isolates, respectively. Other gram-negative bacteria isolated include *Butyrivibrio fibrisolvens* (6%) and *Bacteroides uniformis* (3%). Predominant gram-positive isolates include *L. acidophilus* (7.6%), *Peptostreptococcus productus* (3%), and *Eubacterium aerofaciens* (2.5%) (Robinson et al. 1981).

Like the cecum, the large intestine of the pig also supports a large and diverse bacterial population. Passage of undigested residues is slow in this region of the tract, and consequently, there are substantial amounts of substrates available for fermentation. The concentration of bacteria from colonic contents is estimated to be 13.3×10^{10}/g (Russell 1979) and bacteria adhered to the colon wall number $5.7 \times 10^{7}/cm^{2}$ of tissue surface area (Robinson et al. 1984). The predominant bacteria in the large intestine are strictly anaerobic, but many facultatively anaerobic bacteria are also present. The diverse population is predominantly gram-positive, consisting of *Streptococcus, Lactobacillus, Eubacterium,* and *Clostridium* species. Gram-negative bacteria include *Bacteroides, Acetovibrio, Selenomonas, Fusobacterium,* and *Escherichia* species. Cellulolytic bacteria, similar to those isolated from the rumen, such as *Bacteroides succinogenes* and *Ruminococcus flavefaciens* are found in the large intestine (Varel 1987), as well as a xylanolytic bacteria, resembling *Bacteroides ruminicola* (Terada et al. 1976; Varel et al. 1987). *Treponema succinifaciens,* a spirochete, has also been isolated from the pig colon (Cwyk and Canale-Parola 1979).

FERMENTATION OF DIETARY COMPONENTS

Carbohydrates

Fermentation of carbohydrates in the intestinal tract of the pig leads to the production of a number of low molecular weight organic acids. These are primarily acetic, propionic, butyric, and lactic acid (Argenzio and Southworth 1974; Imoto and Namioka 1978; Vervaeke et al. 1979; Kennelly et al. 1981). Other metabolites are also produced (e.g., succinate, ethanol, formate, H_2), but are quickly utilized in the fermentation activities of other bacteria. Glucose, primarily from the breakdown of starch and cellulose, is the major energy substrate for fermentation. The biochemical pathway involved in hexose metabolism for most anaerobes is the Embden-Myerhoff-Parnas pathway. Carbohydrate fermentation occurs along the entire gastrointestinal tract, but the highest activity is found in the stomach, cecum, and colon, where an accumulation of fermentable substrates occur. The proportion of lactic acid relative to the total organic acids produced varies from 5% to 10% in the upper tract to 1% to 2% in the lower tract (Argenzio and Southworth 1974). Lactic acid is found in high concentration in the stomach of young pigs receiving a milk-based diet (Ratcliffe 1985). Production of lactic acid from glucose represents an energy loss for the pig, which does not convert this acid into adenosine triphosphate (ATP) as efficiently as it does glucose. However, lactic acid may play an important role in lowering the pH of the stomach, which potentially protects the suckling pig from invasive, acid-sensitive, pathogenic bacteria.

The site and magnitude of organic acid production in the gastrointestinal tract is dependent on the type of diet fed and the level of intake. These factors influence the amount of substrate available for fermentation by the bacteria. Highly digestible feeds promote an upper tract fermentation, while more indigestible feeds (e.g., fiber) promote the fermentation in the lower tract. Diurnal fluctuations in volatile fatty acid (VFA) concentrations occur along the gastrointestinal tract with time after feeding, corresponding to the passage rate of ingesta (Argenzio and Southworth 1974). As carbohydrate intake increases, VFA concentration increases in the feces of pigs (Imoto and Namioka 1978). The relative proportions of the major VFA differ only slightly from the stomach to the rectum. Acetate, on a molar percent basis, makes up approximately 50% of the major VFA produced. Propionate is second in predominance at nearly 40%, while butyrate fluctuates around 10%.

However, in the small intestine, major shifts occur in VFA production rates, with the acetate percent rising to nearly 90% of the total and propionate falling to less than 10%, on a molar percent basis (Argenzio and Southworth 1974). Substantial fiber degradation and fermentation occurs in the lower intestinal tract and is influenced by such factors as the age of the pig, the fiber source, the amount of processing, and the adaptation of the bacterial population. As the pig matures, the ability of the intestinal bacteria to degrade cellulose increases (Varel and Pond 1985). With fiber constituting up to 15% of the daily feed intake, there is little change in VFA production in the lower intestinal tract (Kennelly et al. 1981). With high-fiber diets (e.g., 50% and 80% dehydrated alfalfa meal), the total number of bacteria does not change, but there is an increase in the number and activity of fibrolytic species (Varel 1987; Varel et al. 1987). If the digestibility of a fibrous feed increases, acetic acid production increases (Imoto and Namioka 1978).

Organic acids are readily absorbed primarily from the cecum and colon (Argenzio and Southworth 1974) and can be metabolized by the pig as a source of energy. Organic acids can provide up to 30% of the energy required for maintenance in the growing pig (Friend et al. 1964; Farrell and Johnson 1970; Imoto and Namioka 1978; Kim et al. 1978; Rerat et al. 1987), while in the gestating sow this value rises to 40% or more (Ratcliffe 1985). In the colon, the availability of carbohydrate substrates is probably the most limiting factor for fermentation. Nitrogenous substrates are much more available. Other sources of energy may be derived from endogenous secretions and recycled bacterial cells.

Proteins

Metabolism of nitrogenous compounds by intestinal bacteria results in the production of peptides, amino acids, ammonia, amines, branched-chain fatty acids, phenolics, and other metabolites. These compounds may be used in the resynthesis of bacterial protein and other cellular components, but many cannot be further utilized by either the bacteria or the pig. Degradation of nitrogenous compounds reduces their availability to the pig, but it is debatable if intestinal bacteria are actually in direct competition with the digestive process or only scavenging nitrogenous compounds that are inefficiently absorbed. Excess protein in the diet will result in higher levels of nitrogenous bacterial metabolites, presumably due to an increase in nitrogen availability in the intestinal tract. Other sources of nitrogen for the bacteria include sloughing mucosal cells and urea secreted into the lumen. In the stomach and small intestine, bacteria probably degrade proteins to peptides and amino acids, making a small but significant contribution to protein digestion (Zebrowska 1981). Further bacterial degradation of these peptides and amino acids to ammonia, amines, and hydrogen sulfide occurs in the ileum. Nitrogenous compounds, such as urea, are also hydrolyzed to ammonia in the upper intestinal tract (Dierick et al. 1986). The ureolytic bacteria that hydrolyze urea to ammonia appear to be the streptococci (Varel et al. 1987). In the small intestine, the ammonia production is about equally divided between urea hydrolysis and amino acid deamination. However, in the cecum and large intestine, most of the ammonia arises from the deamination of amino acids. In rats, high concentrations of ammonia increase cell turnover rate, increase the susceptibility of the host to viral and bacterial infections, and decrease the response of the immune system (Visek 1978). A similar effect in the intestine of the pig could also depress growth performance. Ammonia utilization by intestinal bacteria may be beneficial in preventing the recycling of ammonia through the pig. Studies indicate that most of the bacteria isolated from the colon prefer ammonia as a nitrogen source (Takahashi et al. 1980). Furthermore, some of the ammonia that is absorbed from the large intestine may be used by the pig for the synthesis of nonessential amino acids. This process becomes more important when the pig is consuming a low-nitrogen diet (Mason 1984). The ability of the pig to use amino acids derived from bacterial protein synthesized from urea in the colon has been demonstrated (Niiyama 1979). However, this amino acid contribution to the requirements of the pig is regarded as minor. A strain of *B. ruminicola,* isolated from the pig colon, has been shown to contain a high content of lysine, which could be of benefit to the pig (Takahashi et al. 1980). Bacterial deamination and decarboxylation of amino acids can also lead to the production of amines in the gastrointestinal tract. Decarboxylation of lysine by *E. coli* and other bacteria result in the production of cadaverine (Yen et al. 1979). Other amino acids, including aspartic, glutamic, arginine, histidine, alanine, and tryptophan, are also degraded by intestinal bacteria to their corresponding amines. Many of these amines are either toxic or pharmacologically active (Draser and Hill 1974) and may adversely affect the pig.

Bacterial degradation of tyrosine and tryptophan in the intestinal tract results in the production of several volatile phenolic and aromatic metabolites. Phenol, 4-methylphenol (*p*-cresol), 4-ethylphenol, phenylpropionic acid, indole, and 3-methylindole (skatole) are detected in the intestinal contents and feces of the pigs (Spoelstra 1977, 1978; Yoshihara 1979). *p*-Cresol is the predominant volatile phenolic metabolite excreted in the urine of weanling pigs (Yokoyama et al. 1982). A *Lactobacillus* has been isolated from pig feces, which produces *p*-cresol (Ward et al. 1987). Besides contributing to the malodor of swine feces (Spoelstra 1977; Hartung and Rokicki 1984), these bacterial metabolites cannot be used by the pig and are potentially toxic (Yokoyama and Carlson 1979).

Lipids

Little is known about the role of the intestinal bacteria on lipid digestion and utilization by the pig. Oleic acid is extensively hydrogenated to stearic acid by the intestinal bacteria of growing pigs (Freeman et al. 1968). When the long-chain fatty acids in the gastrointestinal tract of germ-free and conventional pigs fed the same diet were compared, stearic acid levels in the lower intestinal tract of germ-free pigs were low, as compared with high levels in conventionally raised pigs (Carlson and Bayley 1968). This difference in stearic acid levels was attributed to the bacterial hydrogenation of C18 unsaturated fatty acids. Hydrogenation of C18 unsaturated fatty acids occurs primarily in the cecum and colon (Salmon-Legagneur and Friend 1971). Fatty acids with odd numbers of carbon, such as pentadecanoic and heptadecanoic acids, are also synthesized by bacteria in the lower intestine of the pig (Bayley and Lewis 1965). The bacteria responsible for the hydrogenation of unsaturated fatty acids in the lower intestine of the pig have not been identified, but presumably are similar to species that have been described in the rumen. Dietary antibiotic supplementation will depress the bacterial hydrogenation of C18 unsaturated fatty acids in the large intestine of pigs (Mason and Just 1976). The role of bacterial hydrogenation of fatty acids in the lower intestine of the pig is unknown. Since fat absorption occurs in the small intestine, it is questionable if this process has much of an influence on body fat composition. However, if the hydrogenation of unsaturated fatty acids is serving as an electron sink, it could be important in the fermentative interactions between bacteria in the cecum and colon.

Intestinal bacteria can influence lipid absorption by the degradation of bile acids, which are necessary for the efficient absorption of lipids. Intestinal bacteria, especially *Lactobacillus* and *Eubacterium* species, will deconjugate and dehydroxylate primary bile acids (e.g., hyocholic and chenodeoxycholic) to secondary bile acids (e.g, hyodeoxycholic and lithocholic). These modifications influence lipid absorption by altering the turnover rate and recycling of bile acids. The antimicrobial carbadox has been shown to increase plasma chenodeoxycholic acid concentrations and fecal excretion rates of primary bile acids in young pigs (Tracy et al. 1986). Along with faster and more efficient weight gains, pigs fed carbadox show a decrease in the amount of lithocholic acid recycled in bile and a decrease in hyodeoxycholic acid concentrations in plasma. This sugests an inhibition of bacterial bile acid degradation in the intestinal tract by carbadox (Tracy and Jensen 1987). As mentioned above, the degradation of the primary bile acids by intestinal bacteria also leads to the production of lithocholic acid, which can be toxic to the pig. The secondary bile acids may be further metabolized by the intestinal bacteria or by hepatic enzymes to form tertiary bile acids, which are also potentially toxic (Gilliland and Speck 1977).

Minerals and Vitamins

Intestinal bacteria may influence the availability of minerals by actively sequestering or modifying them, and thus influence their uptake from the intestinal tract. Iron is sequestered by certain bacteria (Weinberg 1984), and some substances (e.g., citrate, siderophores) synthesized and excreted by intestinal bacteria act as chelating agents (Neilands 1981). Bacterial reductive reactions can change the valency state of elements, which could affect their chemical properties and absorption. Metabolism of certain elements by bacteria may be harmful to the pig. For instance, the reduction of sulfate to hydrogen sulfide (Gottschalk and Andreesen 1979) and the transformation of inorganic mercury to methylmercury (Rowland et al. 1977).

B-complex vitamins and vitamin K are synthesized by the indigenous bacteria in the intestinal tract of the pig (March 1979). However, this synthesis is probably not sufficient to meet the demands of the rapidly growing pig. Furthermore, since the small intestine is the primary site of vitamin absorption, and synthesis of vitamins occurs distally to these sites, the importance of this synthesis is further diminished.

CONCLUSIONS

The indigenous bacterial population in the gastrointestinal tract plays an integral role in the health and nutrition of the pig. Changes in the diet of the pig will alter the fermentation activities of the intestinal bacteria, which are in a continuous state of flux. Also, activities of bacteria localized in one particular site may have an impact on bacterial populations in other sites. The interaction between different bacterial populations would probably be most prominent between adjacent sites. Passage of indigenous and transient bacteria from upper regions to lower regions of the tract, the translocation of fermentation metabolites and intermediates, growth factors, and partially degraded substrates are means by which a bacterial population may influence more distal populations. Changes in the diet, level of intake, and antibiotic supplementation may affect the type of interactions that occur.

REFERENCES

Allison, M.J., et al. 1979. *Appl. Environ. Microbiol.* 37:1142.
Argenzio, R.A., and M. Southworth. 1974. *Am. J. Physiol.* 228:454.
Bayley, H.S., and D. Lewis. 1965. *J. Agric. Sci. (Camb).* 64:367–372.
Carlson, W.E., and H.S. Bayley. 1968. *Can. J. Anim. Sci.* 48:315.
Chidlow, J.W., and P. Porter. 1979. *Vet. Res.* 104:496.
Cwyk, W.M., and E. Canale-Parola. 1979. *Arch. Microbiol.* 122:231.
Decuypere, J., H.K. Henderickx, and I. Vervaeke. 1973. *Bakteriol. Parasitenkd. Infektionskr. Hyg. Abt. 1 Orig.* 223:348.
Dierick, N.A., et al. 1986. *Livestock Prod. Sci.* 14:161.
Draser, B.S., and M.J. Hill (Eds.). 1974. *Human Intestinal Flora.* p. 23. London, England: Academic Press.
Dubos, R., et al. 1965. *J. Exp. Med.* 122:67.
Ducluzeau, R. 1985. *Pig News Inform.* 6:415.
Farrell, D.J., and K.A. Johnson. 1970. *Anim. Prod.* 14:209.
Freeman, C.P., D.W. Holmes, and E.F. Annison. 1968. *Br. J. Nutr.* 22:651–660.
Friend, D.W., J.W.G. Nicholson, and H.M. Cunningham. 1964. *Can. J. Anim. Sci.* 44:303.
Fuller, R., P.A. Barrow, and B.E. Brooker. 1978. *Appl. Environ. Microbiol.* 35:582.
Gilliland, S.E., and M.L. Speck. 1977. *Appl. Environ. Microbiol.* 33:15.
Gottschalk, G., and J.R. Andreesen. 1979. *Microbiol. Biochem.* 21:85.
Hartung, J., and E. Rokicki. 1984. *Bakteriol. Parasitenkd. Infektionskr. Hyg. Abt. 1 Orig. Reihe B* 179:431.
Imoto, S., and S. Namioka. 1978. *J. Anim. Sci.* 47:467.
Kawai, Y., and N. Suegara. 1977. *Am. J. Clin. Nutr.* 30:1777.
Kennelly, J.J., F.X. Aherne, and W.C. Sauer. 1981. *Can. J. Anim. Sci.* 61:349.
Kim, K., et al. 1978. *J. Anim. Sci.* 46:1658.
Kuhn, D.A. 1981. *The Prokaryotes.* Vol. 1. p. 390. New York: Springer-Verlag.
March, B.E. 1979. *J. Anim. Sci.* 49:857.
Mason, V.C. 1984. *Proc. Nutr. Sci.* 43:45.
Mason, V.C., and A. Just. 1976. *Z. Tierphysiol. Tiernahr. Futtermittelkd.* 36:301–310.
Nagy, L.K., B.S. Bhogal, and T. Mackenzie. 1979. *Res. Vet. Sci.* 27:289.
Neilands, J.B. 1981. *Ann. Rev. Biochem.* 50:715.
Niiyama, M., et al. 1979. *Am. J. Vet. Res.* 40:716.
Ratcliffe, B. 1985. *Proceedings of the 3rd International Seminar on Digestive Physiology in the Pig.* Just, A., H. Jorgensen, and J.A. Ferdandex (Eds.). *Beretnina fra Statens Husdyrbrugsforsoa* 580:245.
Rerat, A., et al. 1987. *J. Anim. Sci.* 64:448.
Robinson, I.M., M.J. Allison, and J.A. Bucklin. 1981. *Appl. Environ. Microbiol.* 41:950.
Robinson, I.M., et al. 1984. *Appl. Environ. Microbiol.* 48:964.

Rowland, I., M. Daview, and P. Grasso. 1977. *Arch. Environ. Health* Jan.-Feb., p. 24.
Russell, E.G. 1979. *Appl. Environ. Microbiol.* 37:187.
Salmon-Legagneur, E., and D.W. Friend. 1971. *Ann. Biol. Anim. Biochim. Biophys.* 11:312–314.
Savage, D.C. 1977. *Ann. Rev. Microbiol.* 31:107.
Shimizu, M., and T. Terashima. 1982. *Microbiol. Immunol.* 26:467.
Smith, H.W., and J.E.T. Jones. 1963. *J. Pathol. Bacteriol.* 86:387.
Spoelstra, S.F. 1977. *J. Sci. Food Agric.* 28:415.
Spoelstra, S.F. 1978. *Appl. Environ. Microbiol.* 36:631.
Takahashi, M., Y. Benno, and T. Mitsuoka. 1980. *Appl. Environ. Microbiol.* 39:30.
Tannock, G., R.B. Blumershine, and R. Archibald. 1987. *FEMS Microbiol. Ecol.* 45:199–203.
Tannock, G.W., and J.M.B. Smith. 1970. *J. Comp. Pathol.* 80:359.
Tenk, I., and L. Szabo. 1979. *Magy. Allatorv. Lapga* 34:253.
Terada, A., K. Uchida, and T. Mitsuoka. 1976. *Z. Bakt. Hyg. I. Abt. Orig. A* 234:362.
Tracy, J.D., and A.H. Jensen. 1987. *J. Anim. Sci.* 65:1013–1018.
Tracy, J.D., et al. 1986. *J. Anim. Sci.* 62:997–1004.
Varel, V.H. 1987. *J. Anim. Sci.* 65:488.
Varel, V.H., and W.G. Pond. 1985. *Appl. Environ. Microbiol.* 49:858.
Varel, V.H., I.M. Robinson, and W.G. Pond. 1987. *Appl. Environ. Microbiol.* 53:2009.
Vervaeke, I.J., et al. 1979. *J. Anim. Sci.* 49:846.
Visek, W.J. 1978. *J. Anim. Sci.* 46:1447.
Ward, L.A., et al. 1987. *Appl. Environ. Microbiol.* 53:189.
Weinberg, E.D. 1984. *Physiol. Rev.* 64:65.
Yen, J.T., T.L. Veum, and K. Lauxen. 1979. *J. Anim. Sci.* 49(Suppl. 1):257.
Yokoyama, M.T., and J.R. Carlson. 1979. *Am. J. Clin. Nutr.* 32:173.
Yokoyama, M.T., et al. 1982. *Am. J. Clin. Nutr.* 35:1417.
Yoshihara, I. 1979. *Agric. Biol. Chem.* 43:1985.
Zebrowska, T. 1981. *Nutrition in Health and Disease and International Development. Symposia from XXI International Congress of Nutrition.* p. 909. New York: Alan R. Liss, Inc.

PART V

Applied Feeding of Swine

Chapter 28

Major Feedstuffs Used in Swine Diets

R.W. Seerley

The main objective of this chapter is to discuss briefly important feed formulation information relative to the major energy, protein, calcium, and phosphorus feedstuffs for swine. Many by-products for swine diets will not be discussed in detail. A more complete review of feedstuff evaluation has been provided by Pond and Maner (1984) and in other chapters in this book. Average composition of feedstuffs is presented in Table 28.1. The values provide a general guide for feed formulation, but analyses of specific feedstuffs to be used in the diet are recommended.

Plant genetic and environmental factors will influence the value of feedstuffs. Examples are cultivar used, soil quality, ground moisture, date of planting and harvesting, geographic location, test weight, foreign material, processing for storage and feeding, fungus, molds, and many other factors. These will not be discussed for each feedstuff, but each factor may affect the nutritive value of the feedstuff. The more extreme variations will be mentioned with certain feedstuffs. Some variations are well documented by research, but other discussion will be from observations and general knowledge.

Discussions on grain test weight and fineness of grinding feedstuffs will be general and lack some specific information that could be helpful to ration formulators and feed processors. Lower test weights are generally associated with lower quality due to less energy, more fiber, and more foreign material. Poorer performance can be expected with cereals of lower test weight, since more fiber and less energy results in poorer feed conversion. Rate of gain may not be adversely affected until poor palatability limits feed intake.

Table 28.1 Average Composition of Feedstuffs

			%							
	DM(%)	*ME (kcal/kg)*	*CP*	*EE*	*CF*	*Ca*	*P*	*K*	*Cl*	*Mg*
Alfalfa meal	92	2250	17.1	2.8	23.5	1.40	0.23	2.40	0.46	0.26
Barley	89	2900	10.5	2.0	6.0	0.05	0.36	0.50	0.15	0.12
Blood meal (flash-dried)	89	1950	80.0	1.0	1.0	0.29	0.24	0.90	0.27	0.22
Corn, yellow dent	88	3300	8.5	3.6	2.2	0.05	0.25	0.30	0.04	0.13
Corn, high-lysine	90	3434	10.1	4.3	3.3	0.03	0.20	0.35	—	0.13
Cottonseed meal, mech.	92	2500	41.0	4.0	12.0	0.17	1.00	1.20	0.04	0.40
Cottonseed meal, solv.	91	2450	41.0	1.1	12.1	0.16	1.00	1.25	0.03	0.40
Feather meal	92	2225	84.0	2.7	1.6	0.25	0.70	0.30	0.27	0.21
Fish meal, anchovy	91	2450	65.0	5.0	1.0	4.00	2.50	0.90	0.30	0.25
Fish meal, herring	92	2500	72.0	9.5	1.0	2.10	1.10	1.40	0.90	0.18
Fish meal, menhaden	92	2250	61.0	9.7	0.7	5.10	2.90	0.72	0.55	0.15
Linseed meal, mech.	90	2500	33.0	4.0	9.0	0.41	0.80	1.20	0.04	0.58
Linseed meal, solv.	90	2300	33.5	1.0	9.3	0.37	0.77	1.38	0.04	0.60
Meat and bone meal, 50%	92	2400	50.6	10.0	2.6	9.50	4.80	1.35	0.74	1.10
Meat meal, 55%	92	2500	55.0	8.0	2.6	8.00	3.90	0.60	1.27	0.28
Milk, whole dried	96	—	25.5	26.7	0.1	0.90	0.71	1.10	0.88	0.09
Milk, skimmed dried	92	3400	33.5	0.6	0.1	1.25	1.00	1.60	0.90	0.11
Oats	89	2675	11.4	4.2	10.6	0.10	0.35	0.38	0.10	0.15
Oat groats	91	3400	16.0	5.7	2.6	0.07	0.43	0.34	—	0.09

	%		mg/kg				
	Na	*S*	*Cu*	*Fe*	*Mn*	*Se*	*Zn*
Alfalfa meal	0.08	0.21	8.5	310.0	30.0	0.50	18.0
Barley	0.02	0.14	7.6	50.0	16.0	0.10	15.0
Blood meal (flash-dried)	0.32	0.33	10.0	3700.0	5.3	NA	NA
Corn, yellow dent	0.02	0.10	3.5	33.0	4.5	0.05	10.5
Corn, high-lysine	—	0.10	—	—	—	—	—
Cottonseed meal, mech.	0.04	0.40	18.0	150.0	22.0	0.90	60.0
Cottonseed meal, solv.	0.04	0.25	18.0	110.0	20.8	0.35	63.0
Feather meal	0.65	1.40	7.0	80.0	12.0	0.90	70.0
Fish meal, anchovy	0.90	0.55	9.1	220.0	9.5	1.40	103.0
Fish meal, herring	0.70	0.60	5.0	85.0	4.0	1.95	125.0
Fish meal, menhaden	0.40	0.45	11.0	440.0	35.0	2.10	150.0
Linseed meal, mech.	0.11	0.38	26.2	180.0	39.0	0.80	33.0
Linseed meal, solv.	0.14	0.39	26.0	310.0	37.8	0.80	NA
Meat and bone meal, 50%	0.72	0.26	1.7	600.0	13.5	0.26	90.0
Meat meal, 55%	1.40	0.50	10.0	450.0	10.0	0.45	85.0
Milk, whole dried	0.38	0.31	1.0	9.5	NA	NA	22.0
Milk, skimmed dried	0.50	0.32	1.1	9.5	2.1	0.12	38.0
Oats	0.06	0.21	5.9	71.0	38.0	0.30	NA
Oat groats	0.05	0.20	6.3	40.0	28.0	NA	NA

Table 28.1 (continued)

	mg/kg									
	Biotin	*Choline*	*Folacin*	*Niacin*	*Pantothenic*	*Pyridoxine*	*Riboflavin*	*Thiamin*	*Vitamin B_{12}*	*Vitamin E (IU/kg)*
Alfalfa meal	0.30	1370	4.4	40.0	29.0	6.5	15.0	3.40	0.004	115.0
Barley	0.15	980	0.5	50.0	7.4	3.0	1.3	4.00	—	36.0
Blood meal (flash-dried)	0.80	750	0.8	31.0	1.1	4.4	1.5	0.44	0.440	—
Corn, yellow dent	0.10	500	0.3	25.0	6.0	7.0	1.1	3.50	—	23.0
Corn, high-lysine	—	518	—	19.0	4.7	NA	1.1	—	—	—
Cottonseed meal, mech.	0.60	2750	2.5	3.0	8.0	5.3	4.5	7.00	—	15.0
Cottonseed meal, solv.	0.55	2925	2.6	4.0	7.5	3.0	4.0	3.5	—	15.0
Feather meal	0.04	890	0.2	20.0	9.0	4.5	2.1	0.1	0.080	—
Fish meal, anchovy	0.20	5100	0.2	135.0	20.1	4.0	7.5	0.1	0.500	6.0
Fish meal, herring	0.20	5250	0.5	140.0	21.9	4.0	9.5	0.1	0.550	17.0
Fish meal, menhaden	0.16	3075	1.0	55.0	8.8	4.0	4.8	0.2	0.150	7.0
Linseed meal, mech.	0.33	1700	2.8	37.0	16.0	NA	4.0	2.6	—	8.0
Linseed meal, solv.	NA	1500	1.3	31.0	16.0	NA	3.0	6.5	—	6.0
Meat and bone meal, 50%	0.12	2000	0.5	48.0	4.1	12.8	4.5	0.2	0.100	0.9
Meat meal, 55%	0.13	2200	0.5	60.0	6.0	NA	5.4	0.2	0.09	1.0
Milk, whole dried	0.38	NA	NA	7.9	23.0	NA	18.0	3.8	NA	NA
Milk, skimmed dried	0.33	1300	0.61	12.0	36.0	NA	21.0	3.5	—	—
Oats	0.30	1050	0.4	16.0	15.0	1.0	1.5	6.3	—	20.0
Oat groats	0.20	1230	0.3	15.0	11.0	NA	1.3	6.8	—	15.0

	%					
	Arginine	Cystine	Histidine	Isoleucine	Leucine	Lysine
Alfalfa meal	0.77	0.20	0.33	0.80	1.30	0.70
Barley	0.50	0.25	0.24	0.45	0.80	0.40
Blood meal (flash-dried)	2.50	1.40	3.50	0.90	10.00	7.00
Corn, yellow dent	0.50	0.20	0.20	0.37	1.10	0.24
Corn, high-lysine	0.66	0.20	0.35	0.35	0.99	0.42
Cottonseed meal, mech.	4.30	0.60	1.00	1.60	2.50	1.60
Cottonseed meal, solv.	4.60	0.60	1.10	1.33	2.40	1.75
Feather meal	5.30	4.00	0.55	3.35	6.00	1.60
Fish meal, anchovy	3.40	0.60	1.50	3.00	5.00	5.00
Fish meal, herring	5.00	0.70	1.70	3.10	5.10	5.70
Fish meal, menhaden	3.50	0.60	1.45	2.85	5.00	4.70
Linseed meal, mech.	2.60	0.60	0.60	1.70	1.90	1.10
Linseed meal, solv.	2.70	0.60	0.70	1.70	2.00	1.10
Meat and bone meal, 50%	3.50	0.30	1.00	1.60	3.20	2.60
Meat meal, 55%	3.70	0.70	1.10	1.80	3.30	3.00
Milk, whole dried	0.90	0.40	0.72	1.33	2.56	2.25
Milk, skimmed dried	1.10	0.40	0.80	2.10	3.30	2.50
Oats	0.80	0.20	0.18	0.50	0.90	0.40
Oat groats	0.80	0.25	0.25	0.50	1.00	0.50

Table 28.1 (continued)

	(%)					
	Methionine	*Phenylalanine*	*Threonine*	*Tryptophan*	*Tyrosine*	*Valine*
Alfalfa meal	0.27	0.90	0.70	0.35	0.60	0.90
Barley	0.18	0.60	0.40	0.15	0.30	0.60
Blood meal (flash-dried)	1.00	5.50	3.80	1.00	2.00	6.00
Corn, yellow dent	0.17	0.45	0.35	0.08	0.40	0.40
Corn, high-lysine	0.17	0.43	0.37	0.11	0.40	0.50
Cottonseed meal, mech.	0.60	2.20	1.40	0.55	1.10	2.00
Cottonseed meal, solv.	0.50	2.20	1.30	0.50	1.00	1.85
Feather meal	0.45	4.00	3.50	0.50	2.25	6.50
Fish meal, anchovy	1.90	2.50	2.70	0.75	2.20	3.40
Fish meal, herring	2.10	2.60	2.90	0.80	2.20	4.50
Fish meal, menhaden	1.80	2.30	2.40	0.70	1.95	3.20
Linseed meal, mech.	0.50	1.40	1.10	0.50	0.96	1.50
Linseed meal, solv.	0.50	1.50	1.20	0.50	1.10	1.65
Meat and bone meal, 50%	0.65	1.70	1.60	0.27	0.80	2.30
Meat meal, 55%	0.75	1.80	1.75	0.35	1.80	2.60
Milk, whole dried	0.60	1.33	1.00	0.40	1.33	1.74
Milk, skimmed dried	0.90	1.60	1.60	0.45	1.10	2.30
Oats	0.20	0.60	0.35	0.16	0.50	0.60
Oat groats	0.20	0.65	0.50	0.18	0.60	0.70

			%							
	DM(%)	*ME (kcal/kg)*	*CP*	*EE*	*CF*	*Ca*	*P*	*K*	*Cl*	*Mg*
Peas	90	3200	22.5	1.1	6.0	0.14	0.35	1.00	0.06	NA
Peanut meal, mech.	90	3300	46.0	6.0	7.0	0.18	0.55	1.15	0.03	0.30
Peanut meal, solv.	91	3000	47.5	1.4	8.0	0.25	0.65	1.20	NA	0.20
Poultry by-product meal	93	2800	58.0	13.5	2.4	3.80	2.20	1.10	NA	0.20
Rice, bran	91	2200	13.0	0.6	11.5	0.10	1.60	1.50	0.07	0.95
Rice, rough grain	89	2400	8.0	1.7	10.0	0.04	0.26	0.32	0.08	0.12
Rice, polishings	90	3000	12.1	11.0	4.0	0.05	1.30	1.10	0.11	0.70
Rye, grain	89	2710	12.5	1.8	2.8	0.06	0.30	0.45	NA	0.12
Safflower meal, mech.	91	2430	20.0	6.5	32.2	0.24	0.65	0.72	NA	0.33
Safflower meal, solv.	91	2430	23.4	1.0	30.6	0.34	0.84	0.76	NA	0.35
Sesame meal	93	2560	42.0	7.0	6.3	2.00	1.30	1.30	0.06	0.50
Shrimp meal	90	2108	39.9	3.9	14.1	9.73	1.84	0.83	1.04	0.54
Sorghum, grain	89	3230	8.9	2.8	2.3	0.03	0.28	0.32	0.09	0.25
Soybeans, whole cooked	90	3540	38.0	18.0	5.0	0.25	0.58	1.70	0.03	0.21
Soybean meal, mech., 42%	90	2990	42.5	4.0	6.3	0.25	0.60	1.75	0.07	0.25
Soybean meal solv., 44%	89	2850	44.5	0.8	7.0	0.25	0.63	2.00	0.04	0.27
Soybean meal, dehulled solv. 49%	90	3300	48.5	1.0	3.4	0.25	0.60	2.00	0.04	0.27
Sunflower meal	93	2600	42.0	2.5	12.5	0.40	1.00	1.00	0.10	0.75
Wheat, bran	89	2300	15.0	4.0	10.0	0.12	1.20	1.20	0.06	0.53
Wheat, shorts	89	2900	16.8	4.2	8.2	0.10	0.75	0.90	0.07	0.25

Table 28.1 (continued)

	%		mg/kg				
	Na	*S*	*Cu*	*Fe*	*Mn*	*Se*	*Zn*
Peas	0.04	NA	NA	50.0	NA	NA	30.0
Peanut meal, mech.	0.21	0.27	15.0	156.0	25.0	0.30	21.0
Peanut meal, solv.	0.10	0.30	15.0	142.0	27.0	—	30.0
Poultry by-product meal	0.10	—	NA	NA	30.0	NA	NA
Rice, bran	0.10	0.18	13.0	190.0	140.0	NA	30.0
Rice, rough grain	0.05	0.05	3.0	40.0	18.0	NA	17.0
Rice, polishings	0.10	0.17	3.0	160.0	12.0	—	26.0
Rye, grain	0.02	0.15	7.8	100.0	67.0	NA	31.0
Safflower meal, mech.	0.05	—	10.0	475.0	18.0	NA	40.0
Safflower meal, solv.	0.05	0.13	10.0	500.0	17.8	NA	39.8
Sesame meal	0.04	NA	NA	NA	48.0	NA	NA
Shrimp meal	1.57	—	—	105.0	30.0	—	28.0
Sorghum, grain	0.01	0.10	14.0	40.0	13.0	—	15.0
Soybeans, whole cooked	0.03	0.21	15.0	80.0	30.0	0.10	40.0
Soybean meal, mech., 42%	0.04	0.33	18.0	150.0	31.0	0.10	60.0
Soybeam meal solv., 44%	0.04	0.43	36.0	120.0	28.0	0.10	60.0
Soybean meal, dehulled solv. 49%	0.04	0.43	36.0	120.0	27.5	0.10	60.0
Sunflower meal	0.20	NA	3.5	33.0	22.0	—	—
Wheat, bran	0.05	0.22	10.5	170.0	100.0	0.70	95.0
Wheat, shorts	0.07	0.23	12.0	100.0	115.0	0.70	105.0

	mg/kg									
	Biotin	Choline	Folacin	Niacin	Pantothenic	Pyridoxine	Riboflavin	Thiamin	Vitamin B_{12}	Vitamin E (IU/kg)
Peas	0.20	640	0.4	17.0	5.0	NA	0.80	2.0	—	NA
Peanut meal, mech.	0.35	1800	0.7	170.0	46.0	NA	8.00	6.5	—	2.0
Peanut meal, solv.	0.35	1950	0.7	170.0	47.0	NA	10.0	6.0	NA	3.0
Poultry by-product meal	NA	6000	NA	40.0	10.0	NA	10.0	NA	30.0	2.1
Rice, bran	0.42	1200	NA	300.0	22.0	NA	2.6	22.4	—	60.0
Rice, rough grain	0.08	1000	0.4	33.0	10.0	NA	1.0	2.8	—	13.5
Rice, polishings	0.60	1240	—	510.0	47.0	—	1.8	20.0	—	90.0
Rye, grain	0.60	NA	0.6	16.0	9.0	NA	1.5	4.0	—	15.0
Safflower meal, mech.	1.40	800	0.4	86.0	4.0	NA	18.0	NA	—	1.0
Safflower meal, solv.	1.40	800	0.5	85.8	4.0	NA	18.0	NA	—	0.8
Sesame meal	—	1600	—	30.0	6.0	NA	3.5	2.8	—	—
Shrimp meal	—	—	—	—	—	—	—	—	—	—
Sorghum, grain	0.10	670	0.2	41.0	12.0	3.2	1.1	4.0	—	10.0
Soybeans, whole cooked	0.29	2420	3.5	22.0	15.6	NA	2.6	6.6	—	—
Soybean meal, mech., 42%	0.32	2650	0.5	36.0	14.0	NA	4.0	1.7	—	6.6
Soybean meal solv., 44%	0.32	2700	0.5	60.0	13.5	NA	3.0	1.7	—	3.0
Soybean meal, dehulled solv. 49%	0.32	2800	0.7	21.0	14.0	NA	2.9	1.7	—	3.0
Sunflower meal	—	2900	—	220.0	10.0	NA	3.1	—	—	11.0
Wheat, bran	0.10	980	1.8	320.0	30.0	NA	3.1	7.0	—	11.0
Wheat, shorts	NA	930	1.5	100.0	18.0	NA	2.0	20.0	—	30.0

Table 28.1 (continued)

	%					
	Arginine	*Cystine*	*Histidine*	*Isoleucine*	*Leucine*	*Lysine*
Peas	1.50	0.30	0.65	1.10	1.80	1.40
Peanut meal, mech.	5.00	0.70	1.10	1.70	3.20	1.50
Peanut meal, solv.	4.60	0.75	1.00	1.80	2.70	1.77
Poultry by-product meal	3.80	1.00	1.50	2.35	4.20	2.60
Rice, bran	0.72	0.10	0.23	0.46	0.70	0.49
Rice, rough grain	0.50	0.10	0.20	0.30	0.60	0.25
Rice, polishings	0.60	0.10	0.20	0.35	1.00	0.50
Rye, grain	0.50	0.20	0.27	0.50	0.70	0.40
Safflower meal, mech.	1.25	0.50	0.45	0.30	1.10	0.70
Safflower meal, solv.	1.95	0.35	0.50	0.28	1.20	0.70
Sesame meal	4.50	0.60	1.10	2.10	3.30	1.30
Shrimp meal	25.20	0.59	0.96	1.68	2.68	2.17
Sorghum, grain	0.40	0.20	0.25	0.50	1.40	0.25
Soybeans, whole cooked	2.80	0.55	1.00	2.10	2.80	2.40
Soybean meal, mech., 42%	3.10	0.60	1.10	2.70	3.70	2.70
Soybean meal solv., 44%	3.30	0.70	1.10	2.40	3.40	2.90
Soybean meal, dehulled solv. 49%	3.70	0.70	1.30	2.50	3.80	3.20
Sunflower meal	3.40	0.70	1.20	2.20	3.60	1.70
Wheat, bran	1.00	0.30	0.30	0.60	0.09	0.60
Wheat, shorts	1.10	0.30	0.40	0.60	1.10	0.75

	%					
	Methionine	*Phenylalanine*	*Threonine*	*Tryptophan*	*Tyrosine*	*Valine*
Peas	0.25	1.25	0.90	0.20	—	1.25
Peanut meal, mech.	0.40	2.50	1.25	0.45	—	2.10
Peanut meal, solv.	0.40	2.10	1.20	0.50	1.50	1.90
Poultry by-product meal	1.10	1.80	2.00	0.50	NA	2.70
Rice, bran	0.23	0.44	0.43	0.10	0.69	0.69
Rice, rough grain	0.10	0.35	0.25	0.10	0.40	0.50
Rice, polishings	0.20	0.40	0.35	0.13	NA	0.70
Rye, grain	0.20	0.60	0.40	0.12	0.25	0.60
Safflower meal, mech.	0.40	1.00	0.50	0.30	NA	1.00
Safflower meal, solv.	0.33	1.00	0.50	0.25	NA	1.00
Sesame meal	1.35	2.25	1.70	0.80	1.90	2.40
Shrimp meal	0.82	1.59	1.42	0.36	1.33	1.83
Sorghum, grain	0.10	0.50	0.30	0.10	0.40	0.50
Soybeans, whole cooked	0.50	2.00	1.60	0.52	NA	2.00
Soybean meal, mech., 42%	0.60	2.10	1.70	0.65	NA	2.20
Soybean meal solv., 44%	0.60	2.20	1.70	0.65	1.30	2.30
Soybean meal, dehulled solv. 49%	0.70	2.40	2.00	0.60	1.70	2.65
Sunflower meal	1.50	2.30	1.70	0.60	1.20	2.50
Wheat, bran	0.20	0.55	0.45	0.30	0.40	0.70
Wheat, shorts	0.20	0.70	0.60	0.20	0.50	0.80

Table 28.1 (continued)

	DM(%)	ME (kcal/kg)	%							
			CP	EE	CF	Ca	P	K	Cl	Mg
Wheat, middlings	89	2900	17.0	3.5	7.0	0.15	0.90	0.60	0.03	0.30
Wheat, hard	88	3210	13.5	1.9	2.5	0.05	0.40	0.50	0.05	0.11
Wheat, soft	88	3400	10.5	1.7	2.5	0.05	0.30	0.40	0.08	0.10
Whey, dried	93	3150	13.0	0.7	0.2	0.90	0.79	1.15	NA	0.13

	%		mg/kg				
	Na	S	Cu	Fe	Mn	Se	Zn
Wheat, middlings	0.60	0.16	4.4	40.0	43.0	0.80	64.0
Wheat, hard	0.05	0.12	10.0	50.0	62.0	0.06	14.0
Wheat, soft	0.06	0.11	9.7	40.0	51.0	0.06	14.0
Whey, dried	2.00	1.04	43.0	150.0	5.0	0.06	NA

	mg/kg									
	Biotin	Choline	Folacin	Niacin	Pantothenic	Pyridoxine	Riboflavin	Thiamin	Vitamin B_{12}	Vitamin E (IU/kg)
Wheat, middlings	0.10	1100	0.60	53.0	13.0	NA	2.0	20.0	—	57.0
Wheat, hard	0.10	800	0.40	56.0	13.5	NA	1.4	4.5	—	15.0
Wheat, soft	0.10	800	0.30	50.0	12.0	NA	1.2	4.5	—	15.0
Whey, dried	0.35	1980	0.90	11.0	46.0	NA	28.0	4.0	0.010	0.2

	%					
	Arginine	Cystine	Histidine	Isoleucine	Leucine	Lysine
Wheat, middlings	1.00	0.20	0.40	0.65	1.10	0.65
Wheat, hard	0.60	0.30	0.20	0.60	1.00	0.40
Wheat, soft	0.40	0.20	0.20	0.40	0.60	0.30
Whey, dried	0.35	0.30	0.20	0.80	1.20	1.00

	%					
	Methionine	*Phenylalanine*	*Threonine*	*Tryptophan*	*Tyrosine*	*Valine*
Wheat, middlings	0.15	0.60	0.50	0.20	0.40	0.70
Wheat, hard	0.20	0.70	0.35	0.17	0.50	0.60
Wheat, soft	0.15	0.50	0.30	0.12	0.35	0.40
Whey, dried	0.20	0.35	0.80	0.20	0.25	0.70

Abbreviations: CP, crude protein; EE, ether extract; CF, crude fiber; Mech., mechanical; solv., solvent.

CEREALS AND CARBOHYDRATE BY-PRODUCTS

Corn

The high-yielding hybrid varieties of corn are most commonly fed to swine. Corn is an excellent source of energy, is low in fiber, and makes a palatable diet when supplemented with adequate protein, minerals, and vitamins. Its quality is excellent when harvested and stored under appropriate conditions, including proper drying to 10% to 12% moisture and freedom from foreign material and molds. Corn is graded from 1 to 5, based largely on moisture content, damaged kernels, foreign material, condition, and mold appearance. Additional drying of good grain can improve the grade by lowering the corn to acceptable moisture content. Protein concentration is normally about 8.5%; lysine and tryptophan, respectively, are the first and second most limiting amino acids in corn-soybean meal diets, while the third- and fourth-limiting amino acids appear to be threonine and isoleucine, respectively (Grosbach et al. 1980). Approximately one half of the protein is zein (Mertz 1963), which is low in solubility and difficult to digest. Grinding the kernel breaks the hull and cell walls to yield nutrients more available for digestion. Other protein, largely in the germ, is more soluble and digestible than zein. Yellow and white corn are comparable in energy, protein, and minerals, but yellow corn has more carotene than white corn.

Number-2 grade corn is frequently used as a standard against which to compare other grains, and it will be so used in this chapter. Most other grains, except wheat, have a lower energy concentration than corn.

Corn should be ground medium to medium-fine for swine. Fine grinding will improve digestion and feed conversion, but the fine grinding may decrease palatability of the diet and has been associated with a higher incidence of gastric ulcers in growing-finishing pigs (See Chapter 22).

Shelled corn may be stored in high-moisture form (approximately 35% moisture) and can be fed free-choice along with an appropriate complete supplement. Care must be taken to balance the complete supplement and corn intake for efficient and economical production. When feeding high-moisture corn, feeders must be cleaned frequently to prevent accumulation of moldy feed.

Dried ear corn can be fed to older pigs and sows. Some small, low-investment operations utilize this form of feeding to maintain lower costs for harvesting, storing, and feed preparation.

High-Lysine Corn

Researchers (Mertz et al. 1964) at Purdue University discovered that opaque-2 kernels contained up to twice as much of the most limiting amino acid, lysine, and more of the second most limiting amino acid, tryptophan, than regular corn. Another genetic line called floury-2 corn is also higher than regular corn in lysine concentration. The advantage of these cultivars of corn is that less protein from other sources is needed to balance swine diets. One kilogram of opaque-2 corn is approximately equal to

1148 g of corn and 227 g of 44% soybean meal for crude protein and lysine concentration. Performance of swine fed properly formulated diets using either regular or high-lysine corn is similar. The disadvantage of high-lysine corn is that it has a powdery endosperm, which increases dustiness. The dust can be decreased by coarser grinding or by adding 2% or more fat to diets.

Wheat

The value of wheat in swine diets depends on its nutrient content and fineness of grind. Wheat is equal to corn in energy content but contains more crude protein and lysine. A unit of 96.6% corn and 3.4% soybean meal (44%) is equal in lysine content to one unit of wheat in swine diets. All wheat diets should be formulated on an amino acid basis, since lysine is the most limiting amino acid and it will be deficient in diets formulated on a protein basis.

The extensive use of high-quality wheat in human foods causes more low-quality wheat to be available for livestock. Low test weight wheat has a higher percentage of fiber and lower energy density than high test weight wheat. Wheat testing 695 g/L (54 lb/bu) contains about 3080 kcal metabolizable energy (ME)/kg, whereas 775 g/L (60 lb/bu) wheat averages 3300 kcal ME/kg. Hines and Pollmann (1982) reported 6% to 8% poorer feed conversions with 658 and 567 g/L wheat versus 760 g/L wheat.

Coarse grinding or rolling wheat is more suitable for older pigs. Recent research (Thompson and Hale 1985; Seerley et al. 1988) indicates a 9% increase in gains and 6% improved feed conversion by feeding finishing pigs coarse versus finely ground wheat diets. The recommended geometric mean diameter of wheat particles is 0.85 mm or larger for nursery and growing pigs up to 55 kg body weight and 1.80 mm or larger, provided each kernel is broken, for finishing pigs (Seerley et al. 1988).

Desirable grinding of wheat is more difficult than with corn. Screens with small holes in hammer mills cause every kernel to be broken, but the blades tend to disintegrate kernels to a fine powdery condition. Larger screen openings permit the small wheat kernels to pass through whole, which lowers the digestibility of the diet. Roller mills are being used successfully to break kernels and yet maintain a coarse grind.

Wheat can be used as the entire grain source in swine diets. However, some producers prefer corn-based or corn-wheat mixed diets. Wheat diets tend to cause bridging in feeders, wet feeder cups, occasionally poor performance, and hard-to-clean pens. Digestive disturbances also have been reported. Coarsely ground wheat prevents most of these problems, and mixing wheat with corn helps also.

Grain Sorghum

Grain sorghum, often referred to as milo, is used extensively as a cereal grain in swine and poultry diets. The plant is more suitable to harsh weather conditions such as high temperature and less consistent moisture than is corn. Grain sorghum is generally higher in crude protein than corn and equal to or slightly lower in energy content; however, there are more extremes in nutrient content and palatability. Therefore, a protein analysis prior to formulation of diets prevents some serious errors in dietary protein content. Crude protein content averages 8.9%, but can vary from 7% to 13%. The growing conditions such as ground moisture and soil conditions greatly affect the protein content. More than a 20% difference in ME density from twelve varieties has been reported (Nelson et al. 1975). The hybrid yellow endosperm varieties are more palatable to swine than the darker brown sorghums. The higher tannin content of the brown varieties may have production advantages in some regions, but these varieties are less palatable and the protein is less well utilized than the yellow varieties. Lysine is the most limiting amino acid in sorghum-soy diets. Higher lysine hybrids have been developed and are becoming available. Proper grinding of grain sorghum is important because of the hard seed coat. Whole kernels are not completely masticated by pigs and pass through the intestinal tract undigested. Hammer mills should break all of the kernels without producing a fine, dusty feed. Although grain sorghum is higher in crude protein than corn, an equal substitution should be used unless the protein concentration is known. Grain sorghum can be the only grain source for all ages of swine.

Oats

Oats may be fed in limited quantities in swine diets. High-quality oats are nutritionally equal to corn when fed to sows and older pigs, provided oats make up not more than one third of the diet. Higher levels can be fed, but performance will decrease because oats contain more fiber and only 80% of the ME density of corn. Oats provide a good source of bulk in sow diets because of its high fiber content (10.6%). Higher levels of oats can be used in finishing pig diets by pelleting to improve feed intake. Proper grinding is critical for best utilization. A fine grind is necessary to prevent sorting by pigs fed on self feeders and full-fed lactating sows. Feeders must be cleaned frequently of wet oat hulls. Coarse grinding of oats may be preferred in gestation diets to add bulk and to limit energy intake. The feeding of oats is less suitable during high temperatures because oats have a higher heat increment, lower energy content, and consequently, lower energy intake.

Oat Groats

The hull is removed from oats and the kernel is rolled to form what is commonly called rolled oats, which may be used for human consumption. Oat groats is a highly palatable, high-quality feedstuff, but it is too expensive for extensive use in swine diets. High digestibility makes oat groats a desirable ingredient in pig starter diets. Protein content averages 16% and permits the replacement of corn and some soybean meal in the diet. This protein and energy source is very suitable for baby pigs.

Barley

Barley is lower in energy and higher in fiber and protein content than corn. Crude protein content may range between 9% and 13%. Some varieties have been developed for the distillery industry and are lower in protein (10%). The high test weight, high-quality barley is used in the brewing industry, while lower-quality barley is available for animal feed. Highest-weight barley has 85% of the energy density of corn. Barley averages 6.0% fiber due to the hull surrounding the seed. Thus, grinding is important for maximum utilization. Barley is more suitable in sow and older pig diets than in young pig diets, and it has less value during hot weather because the higher fiber and higher heat increment tend to decrease feed intake. Using barley as 50% or less of the grain with available and economical corn seems to be better than attempting to use all-barley fortified diets.

Triticale

The hybrid cross between wheat and rye (triticale) has been studied and improved in recent years. The use of many varieties and crosses to improve yield and grain quality as well as adoption to local conditions has caused rather extensive variation in the nutrient composition. The principal interest is the higher lysine content and amino acid balance. When using triticale in diets it is important to know the variety and local evaluation of nutrient content. There are reports of potential ergot contamination and low palatability. An average value would be misleading when crude protein can range between 12% and 19% and lysine between 2.5% and 5.0% of the protein content.

Rye

This cereal grain is used mainly for human consumption, but it may be fed to swine at low levels because of poor palatability. Rye is generally limited to not more than 10% of pig diets when other grains are available. Gains will not be adversely affected by replacing up to 50% of the corn in swine diets with rye, but feed efficiency is decreased with levels of 25% replacement of corn (Hale et al. 1967). Another reason for limiting its use is the risk of ergot toxicity, which is caused by a fungus in rye. Pigs can tolerate a low level of ergot, but abortions may occur in gestating sows. Rye grain has about 12.5% crude protein and has a feeding value of 70% of that of corn because of its lower energy value.

Rice

The production of rice for human food is increasing because of improved cultivars and production techniques. Rice that does not meet the quality standards for humans is a good feed ingredient for swine diets. The rice hull (bran) can be separated from the kernel and then be fed for different purposes. While the grain has a feeding value nearly equal to corn (Noland 1960), the kernel with bran has lower energy and is about 85% of the value of corn. Rice is more suitable for sow gestation diets due to its bulk and laxative effect (See Chapter 36).

Cereal By-Products

The processing of cereal grains for human food and other products leaves many valuable residues that can be fed to animals. These feedstuffs provide nutrients for swine diets as an economical means of utilizing a low-quality product for conversion to a high-quality protein (pork) for the human diet.

Feeding these products requires skill in formulating diets for specific animals. The feedstuff may vary in nutrient content from time to time and between cereal processors. Using these products without proper analysis can result in improper feed formulation and poor animal performance. For more information on feeding cereal by-products to swine, see Chapter 36.

Citrus Pulp

The citrus industry has a large quantity of citrus by-products available for the livestock industry. The primary uses in the swine industry are for specialty feeding such as brood sow diets. Other uses center in local areas of processing for finishing pigs. Baird et al. (1974) showed that dried citrus pulp in growing pig diets as 10%, 20%, or 40% had a corn replacement value of 97%, 95%, and 82%, respectively. Growth rate was depressed more than feed conversion, thus nutrient balance was a greater problem than a lack of energy. Digestible energy is about 95% of the value of corn. The dried citrus pulp used at the Georgia Station contained 6% crude protein, 17.9% crude fiber, 2.4% ether extract, and 3194 kcal ME/kg. Dried citrus pulp is an effective laxative at a level of 10% in sow diets.

Molasses and Sugar

Sugar by-products are available and used when cereals are limiting. The prevailing data on sugar (Brooks 1972) illustrate improved growth and feed conversion with diets that contain sugar and properly supplemented nutrients. Sugar can be used effectively in sow diets also.

Cane molasses is a good energy source as well. Molasses is more laxative and tends to cause a loose stool in growing pigs, thus an upper level in diets is about 20%. The laxative effect is quite beneficial in some sow diets, and it is used for the laxative purpose as well as to support good feed intake. Molasses as 5% to 10% of the diet is effective in masking undesirable odor and taste in feeds.

SILAGES

Most silages are made from the whole corn plant or a number of different sorghum varieties. Silage made from corn or grain sorghum is a good feed source for brood sows and can be used to supplement rations during periods of low feedstuff availability. Corn silage can be used in gestation diets at 5 kg/d with 0.5 to 0.7 kg of protein supplement, minerals free choice, and additional energy during the last month of pregnancy. Alfalfa silage has also produced favorable performance in gestating sows. There is little information on the use of silages in lactating sow diets, but it is assumed that silages are too low in ME to be useful in meeting the great energy requirements of lactation. Corn silage and grass-legume silage have produced reproductive performance comparable to that of corn-soybean meal rations. The protein of grass-legume silage is 55% to 60% digestible, but energy is the limiting factor.

With proper supplementation, feed costs can be substantially reduced using either corn or grass-legume silage. Corn silage should be harvested at the proper maturation stage so that optimal nutrient quality and palatability are achieved. It is essential with most silages that a good protein supplement fortified with minerals and vitamins be added to balance deficiencies of the silages. Good-quality silage is an effective replacement for pasture and is most useful on farms where silage is fed to cattle.

FAT AND OIL PRODUCTS

The relative value of fat and oil sources has not been researched in swine diets to the extent to permit a fair evaluation of each source. The value of fats and oils in swine diets is reviewed in Chapter 8. Fats and oils are classified by the American Feed Control Officials and standards are given for each classification. The classes are well defined, yet the trade continues to use other terms (i.e., yellow grease or tallow), and sections of the country may use the same term, but refer to two different fat sources. The official terms in Section 33 are 33.1, animal fat; 33.2, vegetable fat, or oil; 33.3, hydrolyzed fat, or oil, feed grade; 33.4, the product consisting of methyl, ethyl, or other nonglyceride ester of fatty acids derived from animal and/or vegetable fats; 33.5, fat product, feed grade; 33.6, corn endosperm oil; 33.7, vegetable oil refinery lipid, feed grade; 33.8, corn syrup insolubles, feed grade.

When considering a feedstuff, quality, safety, and energy level are of primary interest. Standards in the three areas as shown are generally available for each fat source.

Quality Moisture
Impurities
Unsaponifiables
Total fatty acids
Free fatty acids
Color

Safety	Residues
	Stability
	Gossypol
Energy	Fat structure
	Uniformity

Moisture in fats accelerates the deterioration of equipment, may increase rancidity, and provides no energy. Impurities are often carcass particles, soil, or polyethylene. These decrease the fat quality and can clog screens and increase handling problems. Unsaponifiables include compounds such as hydrocarbons, sterols, pigments, and fatty alcohols, which can present problems in nutrition. Total fatty acids includes both free fatty acids and triglycerides, which is glycerol with fatty acids attached. The fatty acids contain more energy than glycerol, thus the ratio is a measure of energy density.

Free fatty acids is an important measure to understand. Hydrolyzed fat is largely free fatty acids. Other fat is mostly triglycerides, and high free-fatty-acid content may indicate oxidation or breakdown and potential rancidity. An antioxidant should be used to prevent the oxidation of the fat.

Color naturally ranges from white of beef tallow to dark brown of reprocessed fat, poultry fat, or acidulated soap-stock. Color has little effect on nutritional value, yet the color should be accurate for the product.

Residues such as pesticides or harmful products that could get into the food chain must be avoided. They can cause ill effects in the animals, as does gossypol toxicity from cottonseed oil.

Stability of fats must be maintained or the feed will deteriorate. Fats are prone to breakdown by oxidation to form peroxides, unstable compounds, and rancidity. The breakdown is prevented by the use of antioxidant additives. If these are not added and oxidation occurs, vitamin E and other antioxidant-type nutrients are destroyed. A vitamin E deficiency may occur. A peroxide value of 5.0 mEq of peroxide/kg or lower is an indication of little or no rancidity. The active oxygen method (AOM) test is a peroxide value after 20 hours of bubbling air through the sample, which tests the ability of the fat to resist oxidation. The test provides a general indication of potential rancidity.

Fat structure is important in nutrition. Although linoleic acid may be the only essential fatty acid for swine, others are very important in metabolism. Linoleic acid can be converted to linolenic and longer-chained fatty acids. The number of carbons (chain length) and saturated (no double bonds) to unsaturated (one to four double bonds) ratio are considered in nutrition. Most fats used in livestock feeding are long-chained with fatty acids of fourteen to twenty carbon molecules. Fat sources are different in their ratio of fatty acids (Table 28.2). The saturated to unsaturated ratio (S:U) affects the melting point and energy value of the fat as well as the fatty acid composition in the liver, fat, meat, and milk. These are important considerations for baby pig survival, feeding baby pigs, and carcass composition of market hogs. The iodine value and titer test are methods of estimating S:U ratio.

Table 28.2 Estimated Percentage of Major Fatty Acids with Iodine Number and Unsaturated:Saturated Ratio in Some Fat Sources[a]

Item	*Carbons: Double Bonds*	*Coconut*	*Beef Fat*	*Palm*	*Lard*	*Poultry*	*Peanut*	*Cotton-seed*	*Soybean*	*Corn*	*Safflower*
Iodine value		10	45	50	60	85	90	105	130	130	140
U:S ratio		0.1	0.9	1.1	1.5	2.5	5.3	2.9	6.1	7.0	8.1
Fatty acid											
Saturated											
Caprylic	8:0	7									
Capric	10:0	7									
Lauric	12:0	48									
Myristic	14:0	15	2	2	2	1					
Palmitic	16:0	9	26	42	25	21	12	23	12	10	8
Stearic	18:0	2	22	4	10	6	3	2	2	2	3
Unsaturated											
Palmitoleic	16:1	6	2		2	7					
Oleic	18:1		42	43	45	39	50	19	28	26	14
Linoleic	18:2	1	3	9	11	23	30	54	50	56	75
Linolenic	18:3								7	2	

[a]The total does not equal 100% because some fatty acids are omitted.

PLANT PROTEIN PRODUCTS

Soybean Meal

Soybean meal is the most widely used high-quality source of supplemental protein in the United States. Soybean meal is a ground by-product of the oil extraction process from whole soybeans. Oil is extracted by either the expeller, hydraulic, or solvent process with all yielding meal of about the same nutrient value. However, the fat content will be lower (2% to 4%) with the solvent process due to efficient extraction of oil. Soybean meal must be heat treated to inactivate a trypsin inhibitor and hemaglutenins in raw soybeans and to ensure good protein quality. Inadequate temperature fails to destroy the inhibitors and will result in poor performance of young pigs. Since sows can tolerate the inhibitors, very little or no cooking is required. Unextracted soybeans have been used successfully in sow diets (Crenshaw and Danielson 1985). The most limiting amino acid in corn-soybean meal diets, lysine, is one of the most heat-labile nutrients. Because margin of error is minimal, proper and careful heating is important. Baby pigs are most sensitive to poor-quality soybean meal.

Soybean meal contains 41% to 50% protein, depending on the amount of hull present and the oil extraction process used. The meal is well balanced for all amino acids except lysine and methionine. Soybean meal is also low in minerals and vitamins, especially calcium, phosphorus, carotene, and vitamin D.

Soybean meal and corn make an excellent combination for all ages of swine provided these are mixed in proportions that yield a balance of amino acids. The mixture must be supplemented with vitamins and minerals. Since dehulled soybean meal is lower in fiber and more palatable, it is recommended for prestarter and starter diets. Forty-one percent and 44% soybean meal may be substituted in growing-finishing diets if cost-effective. Soybean meal is too palatable and costly to feed free-choice with grain.

Soybean meal nutrient content and quality are quite consistent within processing plants. However, higher levels of calcium have been reported where $CaCO_3$ is added at low levels to improve flowability of the meal. A periodical analysis for calcium is worth the expense.

Soybeans

The primary interest in feeding whole soybeans has been to utilize home-grown beans. However, raw soybeans contain inhibitors that limit protein digestion. Several methods exist and numerous types of equipment are on the market to cook or extrude whole soybeans. Using the whole soybean is an acceptable feeding practice, but the benefits and economics of using it should be evaluated before changing from the use of soybean meal (see Chapter 35).

When properly cooked, soybeans contain about 3% crude protein and may be used to replace soybean meal in grower-finishing and breeding herd diets. Brood sows may be fed raw soybeans as a protein supplement in an otherwise balanced diet during gestation and slightly more during lactation (Crenshaw and Danielson 1986).

An advantage to using the whole bean is the higher energy (3540 kcal/kg) and oil (18%) content. However, the higher-fat diet may cause softer carcasses. Protein should be increased to prevent fatter carcasses and thereby minimize the effect of higher polyunsaturated fat in carcasses.

Cottonseed Meal

Cottonseed meal ranks second to soybean meal in annual production, with most of the U.S. production being used in cattle feeds. It is a good source of protein in swine diets when its limitations are taken into consideration. The protein content of cottonseed meal may vary from 36% to 41%, depending primarily on the amount of residual hulls present. Processors normally screen out the residual hulls and are able to make a meal with a desired protein content, usually 36% or higher.

Cottonseed meal is very low in lysine, high in fiber, and deficient in calcium, vitamin D, and carotene. It is high in phosphorus, but the phosphorus has very low bioavailability. The seeds of the cotton plant contain a natural pigment known as gossypol, which is toxic to pigs. Gossypol in the diet should be kept at a minimum and should not be higher than 0.01% of the total diet.

The development of glandless cotton varieties offers the potential for the increased production of cottonseed meal. The seed is virtually void of free gossypol. Although limited data exist on the use of glandless cottonseed meal in swine diets, the reports indicate that the digestibility of amino acids is superior to those of glanded cottonseed meals and equivalent to those of soybean meal. Cottonseed meal is normally limited to 5% in corn-based diets for pigs (Pork Industry Handbook [PIH] 3). The maximum effective level depends on variables such as variety, processing procedures, digestibility, adequate lysine in the diet, and class of pig. The highest level would be in finishing and sow diets.

Linseed Meal

Linseed meal is a by-product of oil extraction from flax seed and averages about 35% protein, but lysine content is low (1.2%). Linseed meal contains from 0.5% to 3.5% fat, depending on which oil extraction process is used. Linseed meal contains more fiber (9%) than some other sources of plant protein.

In experiments, younger pigs did not utilize linseed meal as well as finishing pigs. This indicates that linseed meal should be fed to young pigs at the lowest level and at higher levels for older pigs. Linseed meal is used to best advantage at a level of up to 50% of the protein sources in a balanced diet. The sources of protein should be rich in lysine.

Linseed meal is a good addition to sow diets, before and after farrowing, due to its laxative properties, but excessive amounts (>200 g/day) may cause diarrhea in weanling pigs. Linseed meal is a more satisfactory protein source for wheat- or barley-based diets than for corn-based diets.

Peanut Meal

Peanut meal is a by-product of oil extraction from dehulled peanut kernels. Protein content is 41% to 50%, and fat content is 4.5% to 8.0%. Because of the fat content, peanut meal tends to become rancid if stored more than 5 to 6 weeks in summer and 8 to 12 weeks in winter.

Peanut meal is low in methionine and tryptophan and is very low in lysine. It is also low in calcium, carotene, and vitamin D. Since peanut meal is so low in lysine it should be fed in combination with high-lysine feedstuffs such as soybean meal or flash-dried blood meal (Ilori et al. 1984). Peanut meal is very palatable and should not be fed free-choice.

Peanuts and peanut meal are sometimes affected by the mold *Aspergillus flavus*, which produces a toxin, aflatoxin B. Aflatoxins cause loss of appetite, reduced growth rate, and reduced level of vitamin A; if the aflatoxin level is high, death results. Therefore, peanuts and peanut meal should test negative for aflatoxin before they are used (see Chapter 26).

Sesame Meal

Sesame is regarded as one of the oldest cultivated oil seed crops. Despite this fact, very little sesame is grown in the United States. China and India are the major producers of sesame, providing over 40% of the world's production. Sesame meal may be produced by various processing methods with the entire seed used to produce the meal. Solvent extraction produces a meal that is higher in protein and lower in fat than meals prepared by the screw press or hydraulic methods. Sesame meals normally contain 38% to 48% crude protein, 7.0% to 11.0% fat, and 5.0% to 7.0% fiber. Sesame meal is a poor source of lysine but an excellent source of methionine and tryptophan. When sesame meal is used as a protein supplement for diets based on cereal grains, it should not be used as the sole source of supplemental protein. It should be blended with other supplemental protein sources such as soybean meal, flash-dried blood meal, and fish meal, which are good sources of lysine. Sesame meal may replace up to 10% of the soybean meal in corn-soybean meal diets in growing-finishing and sow diets.

Safflower Meal

Safflower seeds are composed of approximately 40% hull and 36% to 40% oil. Once the oil is removed, the protein content of this product is normally between 18% and 22%. This product contains approximately 60% hulls, thereby limiting the energy concentration and utilization of this meal by swine. Many methods have been used in an effort to reduce the hull content of safflower meal. Removal of the hull has resulted in a product that is composed of about 15% fiber and 40% protein. The protein of safflower meal is low in lysine and methionine.

In growing-finishing swine diets, decorticated safflower meal may be used to supply a small portion (5% to 10%) of the supplemental protein and should be combined with other lysine-rich protein concentrates.

Sunflower Meal

Production of sunflower seed in the United States has increased significantly over the last 20 years. The composition of the oil meal varies according to the composition of the seed, the method of extraction, and whether or not the seeds are dehulled. Expeller-processed meals contain less crude protein and more fiber and fat than meals produced by solvent extraction (41%, 13%, and 7.6% versus 47%, 11.0%, and 2.9%, respectively). Solvent-extracted meals are higher in lysine than those produced by a screw press. The meal is low in lysine, but rich in methionine content. Its use should be limited to one third of the protein source, and it should be mixed with richer sources of lysine.

Alfalfa Meal

Alfalfa meal is an excellent source of many nutrients such as high quality protein, B vitamins (riboflavin, pantothenic acid, and niacin), vitamin D, carotene, and calcium. A level of 25% to 30% fiber limits the amount of alfalfa meal that can be used in baby pig and growing-finishing diets. Alfalfa meal is most favorably used when high grain prices occur. In this case, alfalfa may be added at very high levels in gestation diets. Growing-finishing pigs can be fed from 2.5% to 10% alfalfa meal, but performance may be lowered at higher levels. Higher levels may be used with added fat to provide more energy and decrease dust. It has been shown that growing pigs preferred an alfalfa-free diet versus diets containing 10% or more alfalfa. Levels to use are dictated by other feedstuffs present and nutritional requirements. Using alfalfa meal in the gestation ration is usually most beneficial, but its use is optional.

Coconut Meal

Coconut meal, frequently called copra meal, is the by-product of oil extraction from the endosperm of coconuts. The meal contains about 21% crude protein, 10% fiber, and 6% ether extract. It is a richer source of phosphorus than calcium, and ash is relatively high, which is an indication that other minerals are present. Lysine as a percent of crude protein is low, and the digestibility of protein can be quite variable and frequently is low.

Feed intake has been shown to decrease as dietary content of coconut meal is increased, then rate of gain is depressed and feed requirement for gain increases. The quantity of coconut meal should be limited to 10% to 20% or less in swine if maximum performance is expected. The meal is less desirable than soybean meal because of lower palatibility, lower quality protein, and poorer digestibility.

Canola Meal (Rapeseed Meal)

Canola meal is a by-product of extracting oil from rapeseeds. The new term, canola, is preferred for the newer varieties of rapeseed with low glucosinolate content. Canola meal averages 38% crude protein, 11% fiber, and 4% ether extract. The protein is about 80% digestible and the limiting amino acids are similar to soybean meal on a protein basis. The feeding value is estimated to be 75% to 80% of that of 44% soybean meal. The suggested levels in all swine diets is up to 15% of the diet. There are anti-nutritional compounds in canola meal that limit levels in swine diets. The older cultivars may have eight times the glucosinolate content of the newer ones. The glucosinolates decrease feed intake and performance and cause enlarged thyroid gland and lower levels of circulating thyroid hormones (T_3 and T_4). Tannins and sinapine (the ester of 4-hydroxy3,5-dimethoxy-cinnamic acid) decrease palatability of diets. The use of canola meal in livestock and poultry diets has been reviewed by Baidoo and Aherne (1985).

ANIMAL PROTEIN PRODUCTS

The by-products of animal slaughtering can be made into excellent protein feedstuffs. The balance of amino acids is good and minerals and vitamins are generally higher than in plant sources. Performance of growing-finishing pigs fed diets with higher levels of meat meals may be equal to corn-soybean meal type diets, but some reports suggest that performance may be poorer when high levels of meat by-products are used. Those reports do not provide an explanation for the decrease in performance. Perhaps the heating process used caused nutrient loss, or nutrient content and balance were not as anticipated. Proper heating is important in order to maintain good palatability and not destroy amino acids and other nutrients. The nutrient content can vary more than soybean meal because the ratio of by-products may vary.

The meat meals are good sources of calcium and phosphorus, but because of the high levels, they must be limited in swine diets to avoid excessive calcium and phosphorus. A safe amount in pig diets is 5%, but more may be used in sow and boar diets.

Meat Meal

Meat meal is the rendered product from mammal tissues exclusive of blood, hair, hoof, horn, hide trimmings, manure, stomach, and rumen contents. The meal is mostly waste meat trimmings and organs. Average composition is 55% crude protein, 8.0% calcium, and 3.9% phosphorus. Meat meal is different from tankage in that no blood is added; furthermore, tankage has less calcium and phosphorus than meat and bone meal. When phosphorus content is over 4.0%, the product is termed meat and bone meal. The high mineral content is a limiting factor to the level of use in diets.

Meat and Bone Meal

Meat and bone meal usually contains around 50% protein, 9.5% calcium, and 4.8% phosphorus. Palatability of meat and bone meal is moderate to good. Quality depends largely on dilution with bone and tendinous tissues and on method and temperature of processing. Research has shown that the quality of these protein sources is lower than fish or soybean meal.

Leibholz (1979) found that meat and bone meal samples contained 42% to 54% crude protein, 2.38% to 3.39% lysine, 0.2% to 0.5% tryptophan, 8% to 15% calcium, and 4.4% to 6.0% phosphorus. A diet containing meat and bone meal is lower in tryptophan and ME than that of corn-soybean meal diets. Rate of gain and feed intake may decrease as increasing levels of meat and bone meal are added to the diet. Meat and bone meal may be used to replace up to one third of the soybean meal in a corn-soybean meal diet without adversely affecting rate of gain, feed efficiency, or carcass quality.

Blood Meal

Blood meal is a high-protein source with 80% to 85% crude protein on a dry matter basis. It may contain as much as 7.0% lysine but is low in isoleucine. Drying methods may lower the palatability, digestibility of protein, and availability of amino acids. Blood meal should be used in combination with other protein sources. Blood meal should be limited to 6% to 8% of swine diets. Feed intake and rate of gain were adversely affected at higher levels.

Poultry By-product Meal

The meal consists of the ground rendered clean parts of the carcass of slaughtered poultry, such as necks, feet, undeveloped eggs, and intestine, exclusive of feathers. It contains 58% crude protein and 13% fat, has good amino acid balance, and provides minerals and vitamins. Poultry by-product meal can replace some soybean meal and is an excellent source of protein for swine.

Fish Meal

Fish meals are high in protein (50% to 75%) and amino acids. The protein is of good quality and is highly digestible. Most mineral elements, particularly calcium and phosphorus and B vitamins, are moderate to high when compared with other protein sources. Saltwater species of fish commonly used for fish meal include menhaden, anchovy, herring, red fish, tuna, salmon, and white fish.

Quality of the fish meal will affect the feeding value. Processing factors such as partial decomposition before processing, overheating, molding, and excess oil may affect quality. Nutrient value will decrease when there is a higher amount of bone and head present than meat of the fish. The addition of up to 15% fish meal to the diet has increased performance in young pigs. Possible explanations for performance responses to fish meal include improved utilization of amino acids (absorption in the small intestine), better amino acid balance, underestimation of energy, and favorable action on intestinal microflora.

Shrimp Meal

Shrimp meal is made from the head and hull of whole shrimp. It must first be ground and then dried for commercial use. Salt content of the meal should never exceed 7%. The nutrient quality of the meal will depend on how much of the whole shrimp is present. Shrimp meal may contain 38% to 42% crude protein, 9.0% calcium, and 1.8% phosphorus. Metabolizable energy for swine is considerably lower than that of other protein sources. Shrimp meal is relatively equivalent to tankage in feeding value.

Dried Milk

Dried milk products include both dried whole milk and dried skim milk. Dried whole milk is the residue left after the drying of milk. The only difference between dried whole milk and dried skim milk is that in skim milk most of the fat and fat-soluble vitamins have been removed so that the other nutrients are increased proportionately. Whole milk is one of the highest quality feedstuffs that can be fed to pigs, and the only nutrients that are likely to be deficient in a diet composed mainly of dried whole milk are iron, copper, and vitamin D. In a diet containing a large portion of dried skim milk, a deficiency of the other fat-soluble vitamins could also occur.

Both dried whole milk and dried skim milk are highly palatable and are good sources of protein, vitamins, and minerals. It appears that lactase is produced in adequate amounts in older animals so that lactose is not a problem. Therefore, both dried whole milk and skim milk can be fed to all ages of swine, and their usage should be determined primarily on economic considerations.

Dried Whey

Dried whey is a by-product of cheese manufacturing and a kilogram contains about the same amount of nutrients as 14 kg of liquid whey. Dried whey is rich in riboflavin and

Table 28.3 Biological Availability of Phosphorus in Plant-Origin Feedstuffs

	Total Phosphorus (%)	*Availability*[a] *(%)*	*Available Phosphorus (%)*
Corn	0.28	11	0.03
Corn, high-moisture	0.30	59	0.18
Corn, pelleted	0.30	12	0.04
Barley	0.34	31	0.11
Oats	0.35	23	0.08
Wheat	0.39	51	0.20
Wheat middlings	0.96	34	0.33
Wheat bran	1.21	35	0.42
Soybean meal, dehulled	0.66	20	0.13
Soybean meal	0.59	38	0.22
Cottonseed meal	1.12	0	0.00

[a]Monosodium phosphate used as the standard and considered to be 100% available.
(Reprinted, by permission, from Cromwell 1982.)

pantothenic acid but may be low in vitamins A and D. It should contain at least 65% lactose and is normally composed of 13% to 17% of high-quality crude protein.

Dried whey can be fed to all ages of swine. Lactase, the enzyme required to break down lactose into its simple sugars, may not be produced in adequate amounts in older pigs. Dried whey is primarily added to the diets of young, early-weaned pigs. While levels of 10% to 30% whey are commonly used in diets, some research has indicated that dietary levels of 30% to 45% dried whey can be added to diet without depressing performance.

Quality of dried whey can vary dramatically. Overheating is a common problem and browning occurs; high-quality whey is normally a white powder.

Feather Meal

Feather meal is a by-product of dried and ground feathers from poultry processing plants. It contains about 84% crude protein, but only 2% ether extract; it is richer in calcium than phosphorus. Feather meal has < 2% lysine (2.6% of crude protein) and is relatively low in methionine. Feather meal should be used in swine diets on the basis of amino acids rather than crude protein content. The meal should be used in limited (5%) amounts for optimal performance; and it serves best in finishing and sow diets. The digestibility of the keratinous proteins is improved by steam heating or hydrolyzing in HCl.

CALCIUM AND PHOSPHORUS SOURCES

Cereals and plant protein sources are deficient in calcium and phosphorus for swine of all ages. A wide range of calcium and phosphorus feedstuffs is available, but good

Table 28.4 Availability of Calcium in Calcium Supplements for Swine

Calcium Source	*Availability of Calcium (%)*[a]
Calcitic limestone	
Fine	97
Medium	101
Coarse	95
Gypsum	104
Ground oyster shell	97
Marble	79
Dolomitic limestone	65

[a]Calcium carbonate precipitate was used as the standard and was considered 100% available.

(Reprinted, by permission, from Cromwell 1982.)

Table 28.5 Availability of Phosphorus in Phosphorus Supplements for Swine

Phosphorus Source	*Availability of Phosphorus (%)*
Monosodium phosphate	100
Monocalcium phosphate	100
Dicalcium phosphate	98
Steamed bone meal	95
Diammonium phosphate	95
Defluorinated phosphate	92
Curacao Island phosphate	69
Soft rock phosphate	34

(Reprinted, by permission, from Hays 1976.)

sources of these nutrients should be included in swine diets. The swine requirements should be based on available calcium and phosphorus. The available calcium and phosphorus can be calculated by estimating the percentage available from the total amounts.

The contribution of calcium by cereals and plant proteins to diets is almost insignificant, but cereals provide up to one half of the phosphorus in some diets. Part of the phosphorus is organically bound largely as phytate (Nelson et al. 1968) and chelates, and it is only partially utilized by monogastric animals. Cromwell (1982) reviewed calcium and phosphorus and presented data shown in Tables 28.3, 28.4, and 28.5.

REFERENCES

ASAE. 1974. *Agricultural Engineering Yearbook.* p. 381. American Society of the Agricultural Engineering Technology Committee.

Baidoo, S.K., and F.X. Aherne. 1985. *Agric. Forestry Bull.* 8:21.
Baird, D.M., R.J. Allison, and E.K. Heaton. 1974. *J. Anim. Sci.* 38:545.
Benevenga, N.J., J.K. Steinman, and T.D. Crenshaw. 1986. *Proceedings of the Georgia Nutrition Conference* p. 13. Athens: University of Georgia.
Brooks, C.C. 1972. *J. Anim. Sci.* 34:217.
Crenshaw, M.A., and D.M. Danielson. 1986. *J. Anim. Sci.* 60:163.
Cromwell, G.L. 1982. *Proceedings of the 1982 Georgia Nutrition Conference.* p. 129.
Grosbach, D.A., et al. 1980. *J. Anim. Sci.* 51(Suppl. 1):199.
Hale, O.M., J.C. Johnson, Jr., and B.L. Southwell. 1967. University of Georgia Agricultural Experiment Station Research Bulletin. p. 14. Athens, GA: University of Georgia.
Hays, V.W. 1976. *Phosphorus in Swine Nutrition.* Des Moines, IA: National Feed Ingredient Assoc.
Hines, R.H., and D.S. Pollmann. 1982. *Kansas State University Agricultural Experiment Station Report 422.* Manhattan: Kansas State University.
Holden, P., L. Frobish, and J. Pettigrew. 1984. *Nutrition.* Vol. 3 of *Pork Industry Handbook.*
Ilori, J.O., et al. 1984. *J. Anim. Sci.* 59:394.
Leibholz, J. 1979. *Anim. Feed Sci. Tech.* 4:53.
Mertz, E.T. 1963. *Corn Industry Research Conference.* Washington, DC, American Seed Trade Association.
Mertz, E.T., L.S. Bates, and O.E. Nelson. 1964. *Science* 145:279.
Nelson, T.S., et al. 1975. *Poult. Sci.* 54:1620.
Noland, P.R. 1960. *Arkansas Farm Res.* 9:30.
Pond, W.G., and J.H. Maner. 1984. *Swine Production and Nutrition.* Westport, CT: AVI Publishing Co.
Seerley, R.W., W.L. Vandergrift, and O.M. Hale. 1988. *J. Anim. Sci.* 66:2484.
Thompson, L.M., and O.M. Hale. 1985. *Swine Day Report.* p. 41. Athens, GA: University of Georgia.

Chapter 29

Feeding Neonatal Pigs

T.L. Veum

WEANING AT ONE DAY OF AGE

The term *neonatal* is defined as newly born but it also refers to the first 4 weeks of life.* Due to the rapid changes that occur in the development of the digestive system of the baby pig, this chapter focuses on the rearing of piglets weaned at 1 day of age. An earlier review on the nutrition of early-weaned piglets is available (Jones 1972).

Advantages of artificial rearing include the following:

1. Saving entire litters when extensive lactation failure occurs such that cross-fostering is not possible.
2. Saving piglets from large litters as an option to cross-fostering when the sow cannot nurse them all, especially the smaller piglets that often get pushed away and therefore starve (Lecce 1971).
3. Reducing neonatal death losses that occur from environmental causes. Death losses of pigs between birth and weaning range between 13% and 25% of all pigs born alive, with most of these losses occurring during the first 3 to 4 days postfarrowing and declining thereafter to weaning (Kernkamp 1965; Fahmy and Bernard 1971; Nielsen et al. 1974; Gastonbury 1977). Low birth weight is an important factor contributing to piglet mortality, with the most predominant causes of death being sow overlay and piglet starvation. Diseases have a minor contribution to death losses (Sharpe 1966; Leman et al. 1972; Nielsen et al. 1974; Gastonbury 1977).

   In contrast to the high death losses incurred with natural rearing, artificial rearing of piglets removed from the sow at 1 day of age has been accomplished with death losses below 5% (Veum and Bowman 1973; Lecce 1969, 1975; Sherry et al. 1978a,b; Mateo and Veum 1980a,b; Lauxen and Veum 1982).
4. Increasing the litters per sow per year through early rebreeding is a potential advantage, but currently it is not an advantage because of the delayed and erratic return to estrus and the smaller litter size that results from weaning piglets at a few

**Dorland's Illustrated Medical Dictionary.* 23rd ed. W.B. Saunders Co.

days of age (Moody and Speer 1971; Pay 1973; Svajgr et al. 1974; Walker and Eddie 1974). However, early weaning may have economic value in a farrowing system utilizing only gilts, in which the piglets are weaned and reared artificially after nursing colostrum and the dams are shipped to slaughter.

5. Improving feed efficiency by feeding the piglets directly, rather than indirectly via the sow.
6. Utilizing the neonatal piglet as a model for human infant nutrition research due to the biological and physiological similarities of pigs and humans (Book and Bustad 1974; Tumbleson 1986; Miller and Ullrey 1987).

Disadvantages of artificial rearing include the following:

1. The lower fertility rate of sows whose piglets are weaned at 1 day of age as compared with 2 to 3 weeks of age. This disadvantage in itself is of sufficient economic importance to prevent the widespread use of artificial rearing except for saving piglets as described above.
2. The high level of management and extra labor required to successfully operate an artificial rearing unit (Van der Hyde 1972).
3. The initial economic investment in a rearing facility, caging, and feeding equipment for piglets 1 to 2 days old.
4. The antibodies present in sow's milk that are capable of neutralizing the enterotoxigenic effects of *Escherichia coli* organisms (Svendsen and Larson 1977) as well as other enteric pathogens (Bourne 1973; Wilson 1974; Yabiki et al. 1977) are not utilized. Thus, piglets removed from the sow for artificial rearing, despite having received an adequate amount of colostrum, are deprived of this continuous source of specific milk immunoglobulins.

Environmental Requirements

Piglets weaned at 1 day of age require a warm, dry, draft-free environment. Artificial rearing units usually house piglets individually in some type of caging with wire or slatted flooring for waste removal. Individual caging is preferred to allow precise feeding and observation of each piglet and to prevent undesirable social behaviors such as ear and navel sucking (Van der Hyde 1972) due to the strong nursing instinct that exists at birth.

The perinatal and postnatal environmental requirements of piglets have been reviewed by Curtis (1970, 1974) and Pond and Houpt (1978). The lower critical temperature of the perinatal piglet is around 34 °C (Bianca and Blaxter 1961; Mount 1963a). The perinatal pig has little thermal insulation or pelage. Thus, when the effective environmental temperature falls to 34 °C, the piglet must raise its heat production rate above the minimum or suffer a reduction in body temperature. Piglet thermostability improves rapidly during its first 2 days of life (Curtis et al. 1967).

The ambient temperature preferred by piglets housed singly the first day of life is around 32 °C (Mount 1963b). The preferred temperature drops to 29 °C or 30 °C by

1 day of age and remains so throughout the neonatal period for piglets housed singly or in groups of five. In addition to air temperature, other environmental factors such as air flow (draft), humidity, flooring, and group size must be considered (Curtis 1970). For example, moving single newborn piglets from a concrete floor to a wooden box containing 10 cm of straw at 10 °C had the same thermal effect as raising the ambient temperature to 18 °C (Stephens 1971).

Passive Immunity and Nutrient Requirements

It is essential that the newborn pig consume colostrum at birth to activate the gluconeogenic hormone glucagon (Pegorier et al. 1981; Kasser et al. 1982; Spence et al. 1985) and to obtain adequate passive immunity (Brown et al. 1961; Lecce 1972; Bourne 1973) prior to removal for artificial rearing in practical, sanitary systems with minimal exposure to pathogens. The piglets do not need a prolonged period of nursing; 1 to 2 hours of good nursing may be adequate (Coalson and Lecce 1973a) and is best achieved by farrowing in such a manner that all the piglets are placed with the sow simultaneously for the first nursing. However, piglets that are reared in unsanitary conditions and/or exposed to disease organisms may benefit from a longer nursing of colostrum before removal for artificial rearing (Coalson and Lecce 1973b). The small intestine has a reduced capacity to absorb antibodies (macromolecules) by 1 to 1.5 days of age in piglets reared naturally or artificially (Speer et al. 1959; Asplund et al. 1962; Lecce and Coalson 1964; Lecce 1973), although closure was delayed considerably by subjecting the piglets to starvation at birth (Lecce and Morgan 1962). Colostrum-deprived piglets can be reared in sterile incubators (Coalson et al. 1973), sanitary isolation units (Lecce 1969), or nonsterile environments provided the piglets are administered porcine immunoglobulins (Scoot et al. 1972; McCallum et al. 1977).

The National Research Council (NRC) (1988) has published the minimum nutrient requirements (no allowance provided as a margin of safety) for baby pigs weighing from 1 to 5 kg live weight. Diets for pigs of this age are expected to contain a substantial amount (25% to 75%) of milk products.

Development of the Digestive Enzyme System

The growth of the digestive organs and changes in weight during the neonatal period have been described (Walker 1959b; Corring et al. 1978; Aumaitre and Corring 1978), including changes in pH (Walker 1959b), dry matter flow, and retention times as affected by milk and soybean proteins (Braude et al. 1970b; Wilson and Leibholz 1981b). In general, the digestive enzymes produced by the exocrine pancreas hydrolyze a major fraction of the ingested food in contrast to that hydrolyzed by the intestinal enzymes (Corring 1977). Changes do occur with age, however, with pancreatic protease representing 70% to 80% of the total activity up to 6 weeks of age, declining to 50% thereafter (Shields et al. 1980). The pancreatic contribution to amylase activity is reversed, contributing 30% at birth, then increasing to 70% by 4 weeks of age.

Similar changes occur in the digestive enzyme activities of weaned versus unweaned piglets from birth through 8 weeks of age for most enzymes (Hartman et al. 1961). Neither age at weaning (2 versus 4 weeks) nor feeding method (paste form versus dry meal) influence enzyme development or pig performance to 10 weeks of age (Shields et al. 1980). Digestive enzyme activity may be limiting the first week after weaning due to the change in diet (Lindemann et al. 1986).

The development of the digestive enzyme system in neonatal piglets has been reviewed (Aumaitre 1972; Pond and Houpt 1978). A brief review of pancreatic and intestinal mucosa enzyme activities and total enzyme production is presented here.

Pancreatic Enzymes

Fresh pancreatic tissue weight increases rapidly during the neonatal period in piglets nursing sows. From birth to 4 weeks of age, pancreatic growth occurs by hyperplasia, and after 4 weeks by hyperplasia and hypertrophy (Corring et al. 1978). The pancreas also adapts readily to changes in diet with corresponding changes in digestive enzyme production (Corring 1977). This adaptation requires 5 to 7 days in pigs. For example, pancreatic juice volume was doubled and the pancreatic activities of amylase, protease, and lipase increased fivefold in piglets fed soybean protein as compared with milk protein from 3 to 7 weeks of age (Pekas et al. 1966). Evidence indicates that pancreatic enzyme production is more important in the digestion of soybean protein than milk protein (Pekas et al. 1964).

The pancreatic enzymes lipase, amylase, chymotrypsin, and trypsin are present at birth (Kitts et al. 1956; Hartman et al. 1961; Corring et al. 1978). Enzymatic development varies according to the enzyme considered. Pancreatic lipase activities are high at birth and increase slightly with age (Kitts et al. 1956; Aumaitre 1972), although Hartman et al. found that weaning at 1 week of age caused a marked reduction in tributyrinase activity levels, which did not return to nonweaned pig levels until 6 or 7 weeks of age (Hartman et al. 1961). The specific pancreatic activities (per milligram of protein) for the proteolytic enzymes chymotrypsin and trypsin declined from birth to 2 or 3 weeks of age, respectively, before increasing up to 6 or 8 weeks of age, respectively (Corring et al. 1978), in the 8-week experiment. Piglets weaned at 2 weeks of age had higher pancreatic protease activities at 10 weeks of age than did piglets weaned at 4 weeks of age (Shields et al. 1980). Pancreatic amylase activity is very low at birth and increases rapidly with age (Kitts et al. 1956; Walker 1959a; Hartman et al. 1961). Piglets fed diets containing wheat were found to have higher pancreatic amylase activities than piglets fed diets containing lactose (Leibholz 1982b).

Intestinal Enzymes

Of the disaccharidases, only mucosal lactase activities are high at birth (Walker 1959a; Hartman et al. 1961; Dahlqvist 1961; Manners and Stevens 1972), reaching a maximum at 1 week before declining to 6 weeks (Ekstrom et al. 1975) or to 8 weeks of age (Aumaitre and Corring 1978; Kidder and Manners 1980). However, piglets fed diets containing approximately 52% lactose maintained higher intestinal mucosa activity levels of lactase than did piglets fed diets containing wheat (Leibholz 1982b).

Maltase activity, which is low in intestinal mucosa at birth (Bailey et al. 1956; Hartman et al. 1961; Dahlqvist 1961) increases gradually from birth to 8 weeks of age (Aumaitre and Corring 1978), and it is higher in piglets fed diets containing wheat as compared with lactose (Leibholz 1982b). Maltose was readily digested by 2- to 5-day-old piglets (Cunningham and Brisson 1957b). Sucrase activity was not found at birth by Dahlqvist (1961), Hartman et al. (1961), or Aumaitre and Corring (1978), although activity was present by 1 week of age (Manners and Stevens 1972). Intestinal sucrase levels increase rapidly with age (Dahlqvist 1961), reaching appreciable levels by 2 weeks of age (Bailey et al. 1956). The activities of all the intestinal disaccharidases were found to be low in the duodenum. Sucrase activity first appeared in the jejunum and ileum at 1 week and in the duodenum at 6 weeks (Aumaitre and Corring 1978). Considerable fluctuation in activity for all the mucosal enzymes along the intestinal tract has been documented (Stevens and Kidder 1972). Weaning at 3 weeks of age resulted in a rapid drop in lactase activity, with sucrase activity declining temporarily before recovering (Hampton and Kidder 1986).

Mucosal amylase activities are low at birth and increase with age (Kitts et al. 1956; Walker 1959a; Hartman et al. 1961), although the increase in activity is not as dramatic as in pancreatic tissue (Leibholz 1982b). Mucosal amylase activities were found to be similar from the proximate to the distal end of the small intestine (Kidder and Manners 1980; Shields et al. 1980; Leibholz 1982b).

Protein Sources and Utilization

The utilization of soybean and milk proteins by neonatal pigs reared artificially has been reviewed (Veum et al. 1986). Soybean proteins were found to be inferior to milk proteins for piglet growth (Schneider and Sarett 1969; Pond et al. 1971b; Newport 1980; Wilson and Leibholz 1981; Leibholz 1982). Soy flour was less acceptable to piglets 10 days old than was milk protein (Bayley and Holmes 1972). The type of milk protein also influenced neonatal pig performance, as dried skim milk was superior to skim milk hydrolysate and sodium caseinate plus sweet dried whey (Pettigrew et al. 1977a,b).

About 50% of the dried skim milk protein could be replaced with soybean meal for piglets reared artificially starting at 1 or 2 days of age (Sherry et al. 1978a; Zamora and Veum 1978; Zamora et al. 1979). These piglets were fed by machine every 90 minutes (sixteen feedings daily in slurry form), which may have improved their performance as compared with piglets in earlier trials that were fed diets containing 50% soybean meal protein three to five times daily. The level of soybean meal protein in the diet could be increased with increasing age, indicating rapid adaptation of the digestive system (Zamora and Veum 1979), as previously suggested by Sherry et al. (1978a). About one half of the dried skim milk protein could be replaced by an isolated soy protein without impairing neonatal pig performance, although complete replacement with a soy isolate resulted in scours, reduced growth, and a high death loss (Newport 1980). A soy concentrate depressed piglet performance even more than the soy isolate (Newport and Keal 1982).

Dried skim milk tended to produce greater piglet performance than did casein, while both milk proteins were clearly superior to isolated soy protein as evaluated by piglet performance, nutrient digestibilities, and nitrogen retention (Mateo and Veum 1980c; Leibholz 1982a,b). Other studies have found casein to be superior to isolated soy protein (Maner et al. 1961; Pond et al. 1971b), with the protein quality of isolated soy protein plus methionine being about 85% as compared with that of milk proteins for baby pigs (Schneider and Sarett 1969; Wilson and Leibholz 1981a). Pond et al. (1971a) concluded that the inferior performance of piglets fed isolated soy protein as compared with casein was not due to an insufficiency of the pancreatic enzymes chymotrypsin, trypsin, amylase, or lipase, but to some other contributing factor(s). Casein also produces a faster postprandial decrease in gastric content pH and a slower rate of passage through the small intestine than isolated soy protein (Maner et al. 1961). The buffering action of isolated soy protein delays the activation of pepsinogen in the stomach, which reduces the efficiency of protein digestion. Additional studies have compared milk and soy proteins with regard to digesta retention times, pH, and nitrogen digestibilities over the entire tract, and amino acid digestibilities and nitrogen retention from the small intestine in pigs between 7 and 35 days of age (Wilson and Leibholz 1981b,c,d,e).

Based on amino acid profile, chicken egg albumen should be an excellent source of protein for neonatal pigs (Cotterill et al. 1977). However, casein produced greater growth and nitrogen (N) balance than spray-dried egg albumen (DA), DA supplemented with amino acids, or dry autoclaved DA, while wet autoclaved DA was similar to casein (Watkins and Veum 1986). Injecting the pigs fed DA or autoclaved DA with 100 μg biotin/day did not improve performance. Uncooked egg albumen was found to be an unsatisfactory protein source for neonatal pigs (Pettigrew and Harmon 1977). Furthermore, the avidin-biotin complex has been found to cause a biotin deficiency (Gyorgy and Ross 1941; Cunha et al. 1946). Egg albumen also contains trypsin and chymotrypsin inhibitors (Kassell 1970). While avidin and the protease inhibitors are inactivated by heating (Green 1970; Kassell 1970), the protein and lysine availabilities are easily reduced by heating (Kelly and Scott 1968; Hurrell and Carpenter 1976). Excessive heating of whole milk (88 °C for 30 minutes) prior to spray drying increased protein denaturation and reduced pig performance as compared with heating to a lower temperature (66 °C) and drying immediately (Braude et al. 1971).

Fish protein concentrate was equal to casein in supporting neonatal pig performance when diet consumption and growth of all the pigs was low (Pond et al. 1971b). However, with high dietary intakes, the performance of piglets fed diets containing dried skim milk protein or 50% dried skim milk protein and 50% fish protein concentrate (plus dried whey) were similar, while total replacement of the dried skim milk with fish protein concentrate plus dried whey greatly reduced piglet performance (Newport 1979). Further research indicated a linear decline in piglet performance with each increase in a functional fish protein concentrate (plus dried whey) as a replacement for dried skim milk (Newport and Keal 1983). Fish meal produced piglet performance similar to that of isolated soy protein and soybean meal, while milk proteins were clearly superior (Leibholz 1982a).

Replacement of 50% of the dried skim milk protein with a single-cell (bacterial) protein did not reduce piglet performance, although higher dietary levels of the single-cell protein reduced performance (Newport and Keal 1980).

Carbohydrate Sources and Utilization

The utilization of carbohydrates by neonatal piglets has been reviewed (Veum and Mateo 1986). Artificially reared neonatal piglets utilized the monosaccharide glucose and the disaccharide lactose equally well starting at 1 day of age when the diets contained either isolated soy protein or casein as the protein source (Mateo and Veum 1980a,c), confirming earlier research with these sugars (Becker et al. 1954; Aherne et al. 1969). However, in rats, diets with lactose increased the biological value of the protein sources as compared with diets without lactose (Eggum 1973; Forsum 1975). The addition of lactose to an isolated soy protein diet improved the performance of pigs over 21 days of age (Sewell and West 1965).

Sucrose is utilized about as well as glucose by 1-week-old piglets (Mateo and Veum 1980b; Veum and Mateo 1981), but not by piglets less than 1 week of age (Becker et al. 1954; Kidder et al. 1963a; Aherne et al. 1969) because the newborns do not produce adequate amounts of intestinal sucrase (Johnson 1949). Piglets reared artificially and fed diets containing sucrose adapted physiologically by increasing intestinal production of sucrase as compared with piglets nursing sows (Manners and Stevens 1972).

Piglets fed diets containing cornstarch do not grow well as a result of a lower diet consumption, even though starch digestibility was not reduced (Cunningham and Brisson 1957a; Cunningham 1959; Mateo and Veum 1980; Veum and Mateo 1981). Diet consumption and growth was also low for neonatal piglets fed diets containing wheat starch as compared with lactose, while apparent digestibilities were similar (Leibholz 1982b). Piglets weaned at 2 weeks of age and fed a cereal-based diet adjusted physiologically, as evidenced by a greater total amylase activity (primarily due to greater pancreatic activity) as compared with piglets weaned at an older age (Shields et al. 1980). The baby pig is not able to utilize xylose (Wise et al. 1954) or fructose (Johnson 1949; Becker et al. 1954), although fructose utilization improves with age (Kidder et al. 1963b; Steele et al. 1971).

Fat Sources and Utilization

Sow's milk contains 30% to 40% fat on a dry matter basis (deMann and Bowland 1963), which emphasizes the importance of adequate levels of digestive lipase. The growth of piglets from 3 to 24 days of age was improved when corn oil or coconut oil was included in the diet (Veum et al. 1974). Piglets from 3 to 5 or 6 weeks of age can utilize fat calories from corn oil (Allee et al. 1971) or corn oil and peanut oil (Cline et al. 1977) as efficiently as carbohydrate calories. However, it is important that formulation methods be used to maintain a constant nutrient:calorie ratio when incorporating fat into the diet (Allee et al. 1971). Several reports suggested that young pigs (weaned at 2 to 3 weeks) did not utilize fat calories efficiently (Asplund et al. 1960; Eusebio et al. 1965; Frobish et al. 1969, 1970, 1971; Leibbrandt et al. 1975a,b), possibly due to inadequate intakes of other nutrients (e.g., lysine:calorie ratio). The protein:calorie ratio for neonatal pigs should be at least 67 mg protein/kcal of digestible energy when soybean meal and dried skim milk each provide 50% of the dietary protein (Sherry et al. 1978b).

Fatty-acid chain length (molecular weight) has a greater effect on fat digestibility than does degree of unsaturation, with short-chain fatty acids being more digestible than the longer-chain fatty acids (Lloyd and Crampton 1957; Lloyd et al. 1957; Leibbrandt et al. 1975b). An inverse relationship between melting point (unsaturation) and digestibility (Bayley and Lewis 1965; Hamilton and McDonald 1969) also exists for fats fed to neonatal pigs (Sherry et al. 1978b). Piglet digestibilities of corn oil and lard were considerably greater than those for tallow (Carlson and Bayley 1968).

The substitution of medium-chain triglycerides for soybean oil in the diet did not improve neonatal piglet performance or nitrogen retention (Newport et al. 1979). In a comparison of dietary fat sources, pig performance and apparent fat digestibilities indicated that soybean oil was equal to butterfat for pigs from 2 to 28 days of age, while butterfat was slightly superior to coconut oil and far superior to tallow (Braude and Newport 1973). From 2 to 7 days of age, however, butterfat was superior to all the fat sources. The digestion of oleic and linoleic acids was higher than that of palmitic and stearic acids (Braude et al. 1976).

Feeding Management

The majority of automated systems developed for artificial rearing use individual bowls or cups (Braude et al. 1969; Lecce 1969, 1975; Sherry 1978a), although McCallum et al. (1977) developed an automated nipple feeding system to reduce wastage. The frequency of cleaning feeding equipment can be reduced by adding formalin (a preservative) to the diet (Robertson et al. 1971; Menge and Frobish 1976), especially when the diets are refrigerated prior to feeding.

The liquid feeding systems provide diet continuously (Pettigrew and Harmon 1977; Pettigrew et al. 1977a,b), twice daily (Braude et al. 1970a), four times daily (Pond et al. 1961), every 90 minutes (Veum and Bowman 1973; Veum and Mateo 1986; Veum et al. 1986), or hourly (Braude et al. 1970a; Braude and Newport 1973). Piglets fed their daily ration in 24 portions (hourly) were less likely to develop diarrhea when challenged with enteropathogenic *Escherichia coli* and rotavirus than piglets consuming their daily ration in three meals (Lecce et al. 1983).

Braude et al. (1970a) found that piglets weaned at 2 days of age and fed either a cow's milk (12.5% total solids) diet or a reconstituted cow's milk diet (20% total solids) at high levels had faster growth rates than did piglets nursing sows. The artificially reared pigs in this study were housed in individual cages; feeding equipment was sterilized twice daily and the cages, twice weekly. Piglets weaned at 2 days of age and individually fed their diet in a liquid form consumed more dry matter and gained considerably more weight to 28 days than piglets kept in groups and fed the same diet in pelleted form from 7 to 28 days (Braude and Newport 1977).

Piglets weaned at 1 to 3 days of age and fed a liquid diet ad libitum with dried skim milk as the protein source gained in excess of 200 g/day (Pettigrew and Harmon 1977; Pettigrew et al. 1977a). Good growth has also been obtained with diets fed in mash or dry meal form for the purposes of measuring growth (Menge and Frobish 1972) and conducting mineral balance studies (Miller and Ullrey 1987). In the majority of experimental studies conducted with neonatal piglets, however, individual piglet growth was lower than that generally obtained by piglets nursing sows. This is primarily due to nutrient limitations in the experimental diets and/or restricted diet intake based on the feeding regimen utilized, such as equalizing nutrient intake across treatments in balance and bioavailability experiments (Veum and Mateo 1986; Watkins and Veum 1986).

Subsequent Performance

Most of the negative effects of nutritional deprivation on growth and development during the neonatal period appears to be reversible in the pig. Carcass traits were unaffected by early dietary treatments, and decreases in total muscle RNA and DNA that resulted from suboptimal neonatal nutrition were completely reversed by 6 months of age (Martin et al. 1974).

Neonatal piglets fed diets containing $\leq$25% milk protein as a percentage of the dietary protein had severely depressed postneonatal growth from 23 to 51 or 65 days of age as compared with piglets fed neonatal diets in which $\geq$45% of the protein was milk protein (Sherry et al. 1978a). However, in nutrition studies with neonatal piglets in which the diets contained $\geq$50% milk protein (as a percentage of the dietary protein), postneonatal pig performance was similar for all the pigs fed the same diet from 3 to 11 weeks of age (Zamora and Veum 1978, 1979; Zamora et al. 1979). Evaluation of various carbohydrate sources for neonatal pigs also indicated that the neonatal diet fed did not influence postneonatal pig performance from 3 to 9 weeks of age when all the pigs were fed the same diet (Mateo and Veum 1980a,b,c; Veum and Mateo 1981).

Piglets weaned at 2 days of age and reared artificially on a high-calorie liquid diet for 5 weeks, followed by dry feeding, reached slaughter weight earlier than control piglets weaned at 8 weeks of age (Horakova et al. 1971). Piglets reared artificially from 1.8 to 6.5 kg and fed a high-calorie liquid diet also reached 20 and 75 kg faster than piglets weaned at 6.5 kg (Campbell and Dunkin 1983). These results indicate that artificial rearing does not have a detrimental effect on subsequent performance when the nutritional and environmental requirements are optimized during the neonatal rearing period.

SUMMARY

Artificial rearing of neonatal piglets removed from the sow at 1 or 2 days of age is an effective way of avoiding piglet death as a result of starvation due to the sow's lactation failure or insufficient milk glands. The diets fed should contain at least 50% milk protein as a percentage of the dietary protein. Neonatal piglets utilize fat, glucose, lactose, and corn syrup calories effectively. The nutrition and management procedures for successful artificial rearing of neonatal piglets are well described. The main limitation to the practical use of artificial rearing systems in swine production, however, is the reduction in sow fertility associated with such early weaning. The neonatal pig is an excellent model for human infant nutrition research due to the biological and physiological similarities of the two species.

REFERENCES

Aherne, F., et al. 1969. *J. Anim. Sci.* 29:444.
Allee, G.L., D.H. Baker, and G.A. Leveille. 1971. *J. Nutr.* 101:1415.
Asplund, J.M., R.H. Grummer, and P.H. Phillips. 1960. *J. Anim. Sci.* 19:709.
Asplund, J.M., R.H. Grummer, and P.H. Phillips. 1962. *J. Anim. Sci.* 21:412.
Aumaitre, A. 1972. *Wld. Rev. Anim. Prod.* 8:54.
Aumaitre, A., and T. Corring. 1978. *Nutr. Metab.* 22:244.
Bailey, C.B., W.D. Kitts, and A.J. Wood. 1956. *Can. J. Agric. Sci.* 36:51.
Bayley, H.S., and J.H.G. Jones. 1972. *J. Anim. Sci.* 35:1101 (Abstr.)
Bayley, H.S., and D. Lewis. 1965. *J. Agric. Sci.* 64:373.
Becker, D.E., et al. 1954. *Science* 120:345.
Bianca, W., and K.L. Blaxter. 1961. *Proc. VIIIth Int. Congr. Anim. Prod.* p. 113. Stuttgart: E. Ulmer.
Book, S.A., and L.K. Bustad. 1974. *J. Anim. Sci.* 38:997.
Bourne, F.J. 1973. *Proc. Nutr. Soc.* 32:205.
Braude, R., and M.J. Newport. 1973. *Br. J. Nutr.* 29:447.
Braude, R., and M.J. Newport. 1977. *Anim. Prod.* 24:271.
Braude, R., H.D. Keal, and M.J. Newport. 1976. *Br. J. Nutr.* 35:253.
Braude, R., K.G. Mitchell, and S.F. Suffolk. 1969. *J. Inst. Anim. Tech.* 20:43.
Braude, R., et al. 1970a. *Br. J. Nutr.* 24:501.
Braude, R., M.J. Newport, and J.W.G. Porter. 1970b. *Br. J. Nutr.* 24:827.
Braude, R., M.J. Newport, and J.W.G. Porter. 1971. *Br. J. Nutr.* 25:113.
Brown, H., et al. 1961. *J. Anim. Sci.* 20:323.
Campbell, R.G., and A.C. Dunkin. 1983. *Anim. Prod.* 36:425.
Carlson, W.E., and H.S. Bayley. 1968. *Can. J. Anim. Sci.* 48:315.
Cline, T.R., et al. 1977. *J. Anim. Sci.* 44:72.
Coalson, J.A., and J.G. Lecce. 1973a. *J. Anim. Sci.* 36:381.
Coalson, J.A., and J.G. Lecce. 1973b. *J. Anim. Sci.* 36:1114.
Coalson, J.A., et al. 1973. *J. Anim. Sci.* 36:259.
Corring, T. 1977. *Wld. Rev. Nutr. Diet.* 27:132–144.
Corring, T., A. Aumaitre, and G. Durane. 1978. *Nutr. Metab.* 22:231.
Cotterill, O.J., J. Glauert, and G.W. Froning. 1977. *Poult. Sci.* 57:439.
Cunha, T.J., D.C. Lindley, and M.E. Ensminger. 1946. *J. Anim. Sci.* 5:219.
Cunningham, H.M. 1959. *J. Anim. Sci.* 18:964.
Cunningham, H.M., and G.J. Brisson. 1957a. *J. Anim. Sci.* 16:370.
Cunningham, H.M., and G.J. Brisson. 1957b. *J. Anim. Sci.* 16:574.
Curtis, S.E. 1970. *J. Anim. Sci.* 31:576.
Curtis, S.E. 1974. *J. Anim. Sci.* 38:1031.
Curtis, S.E., C.J. Heidenreich, and R.B. Harrington. 1967. *Am. J. Vet. Res.* 28:1887.
Dahlqvist, A. 1961. *Nature* 190:31.
deMan, J.M., and J.P. Bowland. 1963. *J. Dairy Res.* 30:339.
Eggum, B.O. 1973. *Experimental Technique for Rats. A Study of Certain Factors Influencing*

Protein Utilization in Rats and Pigs. p. 120. Copenhagen: National Institute of Animal Science.
Ekstrom, K.E., et al. 1975. *J. Nutr.* 105:1032.
Eusebio, J.A., et al. 1965. *J. Anim. Sci.* 24:1001.
Fahmy, M.H., and C. Bernard. 1971. *Can. J. Anim. Sci.* 51:351.
Forsum, E. 1975. *Nutr. Rep. Int.* 11:419.
Frobish, L.T., et al. 1969. *J. Anim. Sci.* 29:320.
Frobish, L.T., et al. 1970. *J. Anim. Sci.* 30:197.
Frobish, L.T., et al. 1971. *J. Anim. Sci.* 33:385.
Gastonbury, J.R.W. 1977. *Aust. Vet. J.* 53:315.
Green, N.M. 1970. *Methods in Enzymology.* Vol. XVIIIA. pp. 414–417. New York: Academic Press.
Gyorgy, P., and C.S. Ross. 1941. *Science* 93:477.
Hamilton, R.M.G., and B.E. McDonald. 1969. *J. Nutr.* 97:33.
Hampton, D.J., and D.E. Kidder. 1986. *Res. Vet. Sci.* 40:24.
Hartman, P.A., et al. 1961. *J. Anim. Sci.* 20:114.
Horakova, U., A. Holub, and J. Zezula. 1971. *Acta. Vet. Brno.* 40(Suppl. 2):29.
Hurrell, R.F., and K.J. Carpenter. 1976. *Br. J. Nutr.* 35:383.
Johnson, S.R. 1949. *Fed. Proc.* 8:387.
Jones, A.A. 1972. *Proc. Br. Soc. Anim. Prod.* Vol. 1. pp. 19–32.
Kassell, B. 1970. *Methods in Enzymology. Vol. XIX.* pp. 890–906. New York: Academic Press.
Kasser, T.R., J.H. Gahagan, and R.J. Martin. 1982. *J. Anim. Sci.* 55:1351.
Kelly, M., and H.M. Scott. 1968. *Poult. Sci.* 47:850.
Kernkamp, H.C.H. 1965. *J. Am. Vet. Med. Assoc.* 146:337.
Kidder, D.E., and M.J. Manners. 1980. *Br. J. Nutr.* 43:141–153.
Kidder, D.E., M.J. Manners, and M.R. McCrea. 1963a. *Res. Vet. Sci.* 4:131.
Kidder, D.E., et al. 1963b. *Res. Vet. Sci.* 4:145.
Kitts, W.D., C.B. Bailey, and A.J. Wood. 1956. *Can. J. Agric. Sci.* 36:45.
Lauxen, R.C., and T.L. Veum. 1982. *Nutr. Rep. Int.* 26:415.
Lecce, J.G. 1969. *J. Anim. Sci.* 28:27.
Lecce, J.G. 1971. *J. Anim. Sci.* 33:47.
Lecce, J.G. 1972. *World Rev. Anim. Prod.* 8:45.
Lecce, J.G. 1973. *J. Nutr.* 103:751.
Lecce, J.G. 1975. *J. Anim. Sci.* 41:659.
Lecce, J.G., and D.O. Morgan. 1962. *J. Nutr.* 78:263.
Lecce, J.G., et al. 1983. *J. Clin. Microbiol.* 17:689.
Leibbrandt, V.D., et al. 1975a. *J. Anim. Sci.* 40:1070.
Leibbrandt, V.D., et al. 1975b. *J. Anim. Sci.* 40:1081.
Leibholz, J. 1982a. *Anim. Prod.* 34:9.
Leibholz, J. 1982b. *Anim. Prod.* 35:199.
Leman, A.D., et al. 1972. *J. Am. Vet. Med. Assoc.* 161:1248.
Lindemann, M.D., et al. 1986. *J. Anim. Sci.* 62:1298.
Lloyd, L.E., and E.W. Crampton. 1957. *J. Anim. Sci.* 16:377.
Lloyd, L.E., E.W. Crampton, and V.G. MacKay. 1957. *J. Anim. Sci.* 16:383.
Maner, J.H., W.G. Pond, and J.K. Loosli. 1961. *J. Anim. Sci.* 20:614.
Maner, J.H., et al. 1962. *J. Anim. Sci.* 21:49.
Manners, M.J., and J.A. Stevens. 1972. *Br. J. Nutr.* 28:113.
Martin, R.J., et al. 1974. *J. Anim. Sci.* 39:521.
Mateo, J.P., and T.L. Veum. 1980a. *Anim. Prod.* 30:407.
Mateo, J.P., and T.L. Veum. 1980b. *Nutr. Rep. Int.* 22:419.
Mateo, J.P., and T.L. Veum. 1980c. *J. Anim. Sci.* 50:869.
McCallum, I.M., J.I. Elliot, and B.D. Owen. 1977. *Can. J. Anim. Sci.* 57:151.
McCallum, I.M., B.D. Owen, and M.J. Farmer. 1977. *Can. J. Anim. Sci.* 57:489.
Menge, H., and L.T. Frobish. 1972. *J. Anim. Sci.* 42:99.

Miller, E.R., and D.E. Ullrey. 1987. *Ann. Rev. Nutr.* 7:361.
Moody, N.W., and V.C. Speer. 1971. *J. Anim. Sci.* 23:510.
Mount, L.E. 1963a. *Fed. Proc.* 22:818.
Mount, L.E. 1963b. *Nature* 199:1212.
Newport, M.J. 1979. *Br. J. Nutr.* 41:103.
Newport, M.J. 1980. *Br. J. Nutr.* 44:171.
Newport, M.J., and H.D. Keal. 1980. *Br. J. Nutr.* 44:161.
Newport, M.J., and H.D. Keal. 1982. *Br. J. Nutr.* 48:89.
Newport, M.J., and H.D. Keal. 1983. *Br. J. Nutr.* 49:43.
Newport, J.M., J.E. Story, and B. Tuckley. 1979. *Br. J. Nutr.* 41:85.
Nielsen, N.C., et al. 1974. *Nord. Vet. Med.* 26:137.
NRC. 1988. *Nutrient Requirements of Swine.* Washington, DC: National Academy of Sciences.
Pay, M.G. 1973. *Vet. Rec.* 92:255.
Pegorier, J.P., et al. 1981. *J. Dev. Physiol.* 3:203.
Pekas, J.C., V.W. Hays, and A. Thompson. 1964. *J. Nutr.* 82:277.
Pekas, J.C., A.M. Thompson, and V.W. Hays. 1966. *J. Anim. Sci.* 25:113.
Pettigrew, J.E., and B.G. Harmon. 1977. *J. Anim. Sci.* 44:374.
Pettigrew, J.E., et al. 1977a. *J. Anim. Sci.* 45:261.
Pettigrew, J.E., et al. 1977b. *J. Anim. Sci.* 44:383.
Pond, W.G., and K.A. Houpt. 1978. *The Biology of the Pig.* Ithaca, NY: Cornell University Press.
Pond, W.G., et al. 1961. *J. Anim. Sci.* 20:88.
Pond, W.G., et al. 1971a. *J. Anim. Sci.* 33:1270.
Pond, W.G., et al. 1971b. *J. Anim. Sci.* 33:587.
Robertson, V.A.W., et al. 1971. *Res. Vet. Sci.* 12:59.
Schneider, D.L., and H.P. Sarett. 1969. *J. Nutr.* 98:279.
Scoot, A., B.D. Owens, and J.L. Agar. 1972. *J. Anim. Sci.* 35:1201.
Sewell, R.F., and J.P. West. 1965. *J. Anim. Sci.* 24:239.
Sharpe, H.B.A. 1966. *Br. Vet. J.* 122:99.
Sherry, M.P., M.K. Schmidt, and T.L. Veum. 1978a. *J. Anim. Sci.* 46:1250.
Sherry, M.P., M.K. Schmidt, and T.L. Veum. 1978b. *J. Anim. Sci.* 46:1259.
Shields, R.G., Jr., K.E. Ekstrom, and D.C. Mahan. 1980. *J. Anim. Sci.* 50:257.
Spence, C.A., et al. 1985. *J. Anim. Sci.* 60:1280.
Steele, N.C., et al. 1971. *J. Anim. Sci.* 33:983.
Stephens, D.B. 1971. *Anim. Prod.* 13:303.
Stevens, J.A., and D.E. Kidder. 1972. *Br. J. Nutr.* 28:129.
Svajgr, A.J., et al. 1974. *J. Anim. Sci.* 38:100.
Svendsen, J., and J.L. Larsen. 1977. *Nord. Vet. Med.* 29:533.
Tumbleson, M.E. (Ed.). 1986. *Swine in Biomedical Research.* Vols. 1 through 3. New York: Plenum Press.
Van der Hyde, H. 1972. *Proc. Br. Soc. Anim. Prod.* 1:33–36.
Veum, T.L., and G.L. Bowman. 1973. *J. Anim. Sci.* 37:67.
Veum, T.L., and J.P. Mateo. 1981. *J. Anim. Sci.* 53:1027.
Veum, T.L., and J.P. Mateo. 1986. *Swine in Biomedical Research.* Vol. 2. pp. 735–743. New York: Plenum Press.
Veum, T.L., R.G. Zamora, and M.P. Sherry. 1986. *Swine in Biomedical Research.* Vol. 2. pp. 1113–1124. New York: Plenum Press.
Veum, T.L., et al. 1974. *J. Anim. Sci.* 39:984 (Abstr.)
Walker, D.M. 1959a. *J. Agric. Sci. (Camb.)* 52:357–363.
Walker, D.M. 1959b. *J. Agric. Sci.* 52:352.
Walker, N., and S.M. Eddie. 1974. *Anim. Prod.* 18:153.
Watkins, K.L., and T.L. Veum. 1986. *Swine in Biomedical Research.* Vol. 2. pp. 1125–1135. New York: Plenum Press.
Wilson, R.H., and J. Leibholz. 1981a. *Br. J. Nutr.* 45:301.

Wilson, R.H., and J. Leibholz. 1981b. *Br. J. Nutr.* 45:321.
Wilson, R.H., and J. Leibholz. 1981c. *Br. J. Nutr.* 45:337.
Wilson, R.H., and J. Leibholz. 1981d. *Br. J. Nutr.* 45:347.
Wilson, R.H., and J. Leibholz. 1981e. *Br. J. Nutr.* 45:359.
Wise, M.B., et al. 1954. *J. Anim. Sci.* 13:365.
Yabiki, T., M. Kashiwazaki, and S. Namioka. 1974. *Am. J. Vet. Res.* 35:1483.
Zamora, R.G., and T.L. Veum. 1978. *Nutr. Rep. Int.* 18:495.
Zamora, R.G., and T.L. Veum. 1979. *Nutr. Rep. Int.* 19:49.
Zamora, R.G., M.K. Schmidt, and T.L. Veum. 1979. *Philippine Agric.* 62:191.

Chapter 30

Feeding Pigs Weaned at Three to Four Weeks of Age

T.R. Cline

There has been a continuing trend in the swine industry over the past 30 to 40 years to wean pigs at a younger age. Years ago it was not uncommon for pigs to "wean" themselves from their mothers after they were consuming large quantities of dry feed and the sow's milk production declined to virtually nothing. This may have occurred when the pigs were 10 to 12 weeks of age. As swine production gradually moved toward more intensive systems, the weaning age declined because sow productivity (litters per year, pigs weaned per sow per year, etc.) could be increased. Today, most swine producers wean pigs from their dams at 3 to 4 weeks of age. Weaning at this age places a great deal of attention on nursery management, nutrition, and feeding.

NURSERY CONSIDERATIONS

Proper sanitation, temperature control, and ventilation are the keys to successful operation of a pig nursery. If the building is clean (relatively free of disease-causing organisms), warm (or hot, depending on the age of the pig), draft-free, and reasonably dry, the newly weaned pig will have an opportunity to grow rapidly when provided with a nutritious starter diet. For detailed information on swine nursery units, the reader is urged to read Pork Industry Handbook fact sheets on "Swine Nursery Units" (Driggers and Jensen 1980) and "Management and Nutrition of the Newly Weaned Pig" (Aherne et al. 1987).

NUTRIENT REQUIREMENTS

Qualitatively, the nutrient requirements of the early-weaned pig are the same as those of growing-finishing pigs, but when expressed as a percentage of the diet, they are higher than for older pigs. All young pigs require energy, amino acids, fatty acids, minerals, vitamins, and water.

Energy

The National Research Council publication on nutrient requirements of swine (NRC 1988) indicates that diets fed to pigs weighing 10 to 20 kg should contain 3500 kcal digestible energy (DE)/kg. This value is not a true requirement but rather the level of energy in a corn-soybean meal diet. NcNutt and Ewan (1984) estimate that the metabolizable energy (ME) requirement of the 4-week-old weaned pig is 115 kcal $\times$ d^{-1} $(kg^{.75})^{-1}$. Generally speaking, higher-density diets (e.g., those containing supplemental fat) will support a faster rate of gain and will improve feed conversion whereas lower-energy diets such as barley-based diets will have a poorer feed conversion. It is important to keep in mind that as the energy density of the diet is increased for the nursery-age pig, other nutrients, particularly amino acids, need to be increased concomitantly. For an in-depth discussion of energy utilization and theoretical aspects of energy requirements, the reader is referred to Chapter 7 and the ARC publication, *The Nutrient Requirements of Pigs* (ARC 1981).

Amino Acids

Even though the pig needs ten indispensable amino acids (see Table 30.1 for exact level), only three or four seem to have practical concern. Virtually all cereal-based diets are first-limiting in lysine. Threonine, tryptophan, and/or methionine may be limiting in some instances, but if the lysine requirement is met, the others will usually be adequate, particularly when intact proteins are used as the only source of amino acids. When synthetic lysine is substituted for intact proteins in the diet, one or more of the amino acids listed above may become limiting. Refer to Chapter 9 for basic information about amino acids.

Fatty Acids

Even though evidence is limiting, linoleic acid should be considered an essential or indispensable fatty acid. The requirement is small and is supplied by natural ingredients. Plant oils contain relatively large amounts of linoleic acid whereas animal fats contain smaller but significant quantities (see Chapter 8).

Minerals

The National Research Council (NRC) (1988) lists requirements (Table 30.1) for twelve minerals. If others are required (e.g., chromium and fluoride), they are needed in such trace amounts that all practical starter diets would contain adequate levels.

Practical starter diets need to be supplemented with calcium, phosphorus, sodium, chloride, iron, zinc, copper, selenium, iodine and manganese. Dicalcium phosphate, ground limestone, and salt are routinely used as macromineral (calcium, phosphorus, sodium, chlorine) sources. The safest and usually the most economical way to add trace minerals is to use a high-quality commercial base mix or a trace mineral premix.

Vitamins

The NRC (1988) lists minimum requirements for thirteen vitamins. Of these, A, D, E, K, riboflavin, niacin, pantothenic acid, and B_{12} are routinely added to diets of nursery-age pigs. Choline, thiamin, biotin, and ascorbic acid are added to several commercially available starter feeds, but their need is not well documented.

Variable results have been obtained when ascorbic acid has been added to pig starter diets. Yen and Pond (1981) obtained a growth response to 330 mg/kg feed, but when the work was repeated (Yen and Pond 1984, 1987), no benefit was evident. Mahan and Saif (1983) reported a trend toward performance improvement by feeding or injecting ascorbic acid, but blood clearance studies indicated that even large doses were completely cleared by 4 hours postinjection. Kornegay et al. (1986) also reported that ascorbic acid is of no benefit in either warm or cold nursery facilities.

Russett et al. (1979a,b) have shown that starter pigs do require choline and that this requirement does not exceed 330 ppm. Practical corn-soybean meal starter diets contain adequate choline (NCR-42 Committee 1980). Methionine-choline interactions have been studied, but the results are not clear-cut. Russett et al. (1979a) did not find a significant interaction even though the pigs did respond to choline. Lovett et al. (1986) report that there is an interaction, but the pigs in their experiment did not respond to either methionine or choline when added individually.

Water

The requirement for water has not been quantitated as for other nutrients, but it is equal to the pig's water loss and the quantity used for weight gain. Water consumption is related to dry matter intake and early-weaned pigs consume more in relative terms than do older pigs, possibly as much as 7 parts water to 1 part feed (ARC 1981). Ad libitum access to clean, fresh water at all times is recommended (see Chapter 18).

DIGESTIVE PHYSIOLOGY

This subject is discussed at length earlier in the book (Chapter 3), but it should be kept in mind that there are changes in the digestive capabilities of the pig that occur rapidly from birth through the first 6 to 8 weeks. The newly weaned pig is apparently much better equipped to digest milk nutrients than nutrients from other sources, particularly plant materials. This is certainly true for sugars and proteins. It is apparent that pigs adapt to diets composed primarily of plant material within relatively short periods of

Table 30.1 Nutrient Requirements of Swine Allowed Feed Ad Libitum (90% dry matter)

	Swine Live Weight (kg)				
Intake and Performance Levels	*1–5*	*5–10*	*10–20*	*20–50*	*50–110*
Expected weight gain (g/day)	200	250	450	700	820
Expected feed intake (g/day)	250	460	950	1900	3110
Expected efficiency (gain/feed)	0.800	0.543	0.474	0.368	0.264
Expected efficiency (feed/gain)	1.25	1.84	2.11	2.71	3.79
Digestible energy intake (kcal/day)	850	1560	3230	6460	10570
Metabolizable energy intake (kcal/day)	805	1490	3090	6200	10185
Energy concentration (kcal ME/kg diet)	3220	3240	3250	3260	3275
Protein (%)	24	20	18	15	13
	Requirement (% or amount/kg diet)[a]				
Nutrient					
Indispensable amino acids (%)					
Arginine	0.60	0.50	0.40	0.25	0.10
Histidine	0.36	0.31	0.25	0.22	0.18
Isoleucine	0.76	0.65	0.53	0.46	0.38
Leucine	1.00	0.85	0.70	0.60	0.50
Lysine	1.40	1.15	0.95	0.75	0.60
Methione + cystine	0.68	0.58	0.48	0.41	0.34
Phenylalanine + tyrosine	1.10	0.94	0.77	0.66	0.55
Threonine	0.80	0.68	0.56	0.48	0.40
Tryptophan	0.20	0.17	0.14	0.12	0.10
Valine	0.80	0.68	0.56	0.48	0.40
Linoleic acid (%)	0.1	0.1	0.1	0.1	0.1

Mineral elements					
Calcium (%)	0.90	0.80	0.70	0.60	0.50
Phosphorus, total (%)	0.70	0.65	0.60	0.50	0.40
Phosphorus, available (%)	0.55	0.40	0.32	0.23	0.15
Sodium (%)	0.10	0.10	0.10	0.10	0.10
Chlorine (%)	0.08	0.08	0.08	0.08	0.08
Magnesium (%)	0.04	0.04	0.04	0.04	0.04
Potassium (%)	0.30	0.28	0.26	0.23	0.17
Copper (mg)	6.0	6.0	5.0	4.0	3.0
Iodine (mg)	0.14	0.14	0.14	0.14	0.14
Iron (mg)	100	100	80	60	40
Manganese (mg)	4.0	4.0	3.0	2.0	2.0
Selenium (mg)	0.30	0.30	0.25	0.15	0.10
Zinc (mg)	100	100	80	60	50
Vitamins					
Vitamin A (IU)	2200	2200	1750	1300	1300
Vitamin D (IU)	220	220	200	150	150
Vitamin E (IU)	16	16	11	11	11
Vitamin K (menadione) (mg)	0.5	0.5	0.5	0.5	0.5
Biotin (mg)	0.08	0.05	0.05	0.05	0.05
Choline (g)	0.6	0.5	0.4	0.3	0.3
Folacin (mg)	0.3	0.3	0.3	0.3	0.3
Niacin, available (mg)	20.0	15.0	12.5	10.0	7.0
Pantothenic acid (mg)	12.0	10.0	9.0	8.0	7.0
Riboflavin (mg)	4.0	3.5	3.0	2.5	2.0
Thiamin (mg)	1.5	1.0	1.0	1.0	1.0
Vitamin B_6 (mg)	2.0	1.5	1.5	1.0	1.0
Vitamin B_{12} (μg)	20.0	17.5	15.0	10.0	5.0

NOTE: The requirements listed are based upon the principles and assumptions described in the text of this publication [NRC 1988]. Knowledge of nutritional constraints and limitations is important for the proper use of this table.

[a] These requirements are based upon the following types of pigs and diets: 1- to 5-kg pigs, a diet that includes 25% to 75% milk products; 5- to 10-kg pigs, a corn-soybean meal diet that includes 5% to 25% milk products; 10- to 110-kg pigs, a corn-soybean meal diet. In the corn-soybean meal diet, the corn contains 8.5% protein; the soybean meal contains 44%.

Reprinted, by permission, from NRC 1988.

time, since the postweaning lag period does not continue more than a week or two. Many of the differences in performance of pigs fed various nutrient sources (to be discussed in detail below) are no doubt due to the pig's digestive capabilities.

SIMPLE VERSUS COMPLEX DIETS

As used in this chapter, the term *simple diet* refers to a cereal and soybean meal diet fortified with vitamins and minerals and usually medicated. Complex diets, by default, contain ingredients other than those listed above. Ingredients commonly used include dried skim milk, dried whey, whey protein concentrate, casein, fish meal, soy flour, oat meal, sugar, fats and oils, and other feed additives. Complex diets are also fortified with vitamins and minerals and are medicated.

Fats, Oils, and Energy

Contrary to early published studies, it has now been established that pigs weaned at 3 to 4 weeks of age do utilize fat efficiently, although the results obtained in pig starter trials are not in complete agreement. Cline et al. (1977) showed that young pigs could utilize corn oil and peanut oil calories as well as glucose or lactose calories. Lawrence and Maxwell (1983) observed that coconut oil promoted more rapid growth in baby pigs than did either corn oil or lard. An interesting fact in this work was that inclusion of fat in the starter diet actually decreased weight gain during the first 2 weeks of the trial. Recent work by Forsyth and Cline (1986) tended to confirm this. Added oil showed no benefit until 4 weeks after weaning. It is possible that in both of these cases, the fat utilization data were confounded with a protein and/or lysine deficiency.

The response in gain of pigs fed added fat seems to be variable, but an improvement in feed conversion is usually noted. Atteh and Leeson (1983) indicated that neither 5% nor 10% added fat (an animal-vegetable blend) increased gain, but feed conversion was improved by the addition of 10% of fat. Gore et al. (1986) did not obtain a gain response when 5% of soybean oil was added to weanling pig diets, but an improvement in feed efficiency was noted and nursery dust was reduced by 45%.

The variability in performance response may depend on the energy level in the basal diet and/or the protein level in the diet. McConnell et al. (1982) determined that gain of the early-weaned pig was maximized at a level of 3520 kcal ME/kg diet. Feed conversion was improved at greater ME densities than 3520 kcal/kg, but gain was not improved further.

Data defining protein needs at different energy levels can be misleading due to the fact that protein levels, as stated, may not reflect levels of limiting amino acids, but several investigators have studied the so-called protein × energy interaction. Menge and Frobish (1976) suggest that the protein requirement of pigs fed corn-soybean meal-milk product diets is between 20% and 24% when the calorie:protein ratio (kcal:g) is 15 to 18. Campbell (1977) has suggested that the protein requirement to maximize carcass nitrogen is 23% when pigs are fed high-energy wheat-soybean meal-meat meal diets. It has been shown that protein level does not affect the maintenance energy requirement (Campbell and Dundin 1983), but there is no question that there is an interaction between energy used for gain and protein level (McCracken et al. 1980; Zang et al. 1986). Given the ME intake, one can calculate both fat and protein gain in the young pig (McCracken 1980).

Processing can affect energy (oil) availability in feedstuffs. Adams and Jensen (1984) have shown that the digestibility of fat extracted from soybeans or sunflower seeds is 90%, whereas the digestibility of the oil in intact seeds is only 75%. Mechanical pressure generated by certain processing methods such as pelleting or extrusion increases availability of oil in whole seeds (e.g., soybeans, presumably by rupturing the fat cells). The availability of the oil in these products is equal to that of extracted oil.

In summary, the addition of fats or oils to pig starter diets that are properly formulated usually increases rate of weight gain after the first 2 weeks and almost always improves feed efficiency. Furthermore, the resultant decrease of dust in the nursery is probably beneficial. The economics of fat additions may vary considerably.

Milk and Other Animal Products

Adding milk products to a cereal-soybean meal diet usually will improve rate of gain and feed conversion of weanling pigs. Casein, dried whey, and dried skim milk have all shown beneficial effects. Both Rodriguez and Young (1981) and Graham et al. (1981) have reported that dried whey, buttermilk, or dried skim milk will increase performance of weanling pigs. Armstrong and Clawson (1980) obtained a response from the inclusion of 30% of dried whey in the diet of 3- to 4-week-old pigs, and whey protein concentrate has also been shown to be beneficial in pig starter diets (Cinq-Mars et al. 1986).

Generally speaking, adding milk products to a cereal-soybean meal diet improves the digestibility and/or utilization of both energy and protein or amino acids. This has been adequately demonstrated by Wilson and Leibholz (1981a,b,c,d), Walker and Maxwell (1986a,b), and Owsley et al. (1986). The reasons for digestibility differences are not entirely clear (also see Digestive Physiology section of this chapter), but Decuypere et al. (1981a,b) suggest that solubility of the protein plays a role. They found that nitrogen digestibility was higher in soluble materials but that some soluble soy flours may actually be less digestible because they do not clot or coagulate in the stomach as does casein.

Growth and feed conversion responses are often obtained from including other animal products that, as stated previously, are probably more highly digestible to the newly weaned pig. Newport and Keal (1983) improved early-weaned pig performance by adding fish meal alone or in combination with dried skim milk.

Other Plant Proteins

Decuypere et al. (1981a,b) have published research indicating that certain soy flours support increased gains as compared with soybean meal in early-weaned pigs, but as stated above, some soy flours are actually detrimental due supposedly to their solubility characteristics that lead to a very rapid rate of passage. Generally, other oilseed meals are well utilized by starter pigs if proper amino acid levels are maintained. An exception to this may be canola meal. McIntosh et al. (1986) have recently shown that, contrary to their work with growing-finishing pigs, as the amount of canola meal in the starter diet increases, daily feed intake and gain decrease linearly. Raw legume seed products containing trypsin inhibitors will also be poorly utilized.

Flavor Enhancers

Little recent research has been published in the scientific literature concerning the use of flavors or sweeteners. Research by Kornegay et al. (1979) indicates that feed flavors have little value in weanling pig diets, but the type or quality of the basal diet may affect results obtained. Baidoo et al. (1986) have shown that the use of some commercially available flavor products enhanced feed intake and subsequent performance of young pigs fed canola meal diets, and the response was greater as the dietary level of canola meal increased. There was no effect of flavor product on consumption of soybean-meal–based diets.

Given a choice of diets containing sugar or other sweeteners, early-weaned pigs will consume more of a ''sweet'' diet. When not given a choice, the pigs usually consume equal quantities of either diet.

Unidentified Growth Factors

One can find articles in the popular press and in advertisements about unidentified growth factors (UGF), but nothing appears in recent scientific literature to substantiate the many claims. It is the author's opinion that exotic feed ingredients need not be fed to 3- to 4-week-old pigs as a source of UGF. That is not to say that all essential nutrients have necessarily been discovered, but if other organic or inorganic compounds are found to be required, the minute amount needed will probably be present in the natural ingredients of either simple or complex diets.

Summary

More reports have been published dealing with the subject of simple versus complex starter diets in recent years than other studies combined. Although the economics may be questioned at times, the biology of the benefits derived from using complex starter diets for pigs weaned at 3 to 4 weeks of age is very convincing.

NUTRITIONAL DIARRHEA

As is the case with many research areas, conflicting data have been published concerning the effect of nutrition on piglet diarrhea. Ethridge et al. (1984a,b) showed that incidence and severity of diarrhea increases as diet digestibility decreases and that the inclusion of oat groats and casein in the diet prevented diarrhea. Small numbers of pigs were involved in their experiments. Using an intestinal loop technique, Armstrong and Cline (1976) found evidence that oats may have some protective effect against fluid accumulation in the gut, but other carbohydrate sources or protein level were without effect. They also showed that neither protein level nor oats in the diet had any effect on *Escherichia coli* numbers in the intestine (Armstrong and Cline 1977).

The inclusion of oats in practical diets has not been beneficial in terms of gain, feed conversion, or diarrhea incidence (Rivera et al. 1978; Kornegay et al. 1981). Feeding a complex diet did not prevent diarrhea (Ball and Aherne 1982), but restricting intake of feed did. Limiting the time that the pig had access to the feeder caused more diarrhea than when pigs were ad libitum fed.

Pouteaux et al. (1982) indicated that pigs fed milk, soybean, or pea proteins performed at the same level and had identical diarrhea scores. Lecce et al. (1985) made an interesting observation that a high level of protein supported a faster rate of gain of pigs infected with rotavirus. Even though all pigs had diarrhea, those fed 26% protein gained faster than those fed 11% protein. Also, those fed cow's milk gained faster than those fed soy flour.

Feeding of immunoglobulins may have some protective effect against *E. coli* diarrhea. Kennelly et al. (1979) observed that pigs drenched with pathogenic *E. coli* gained faster and had less scours if they were fed immunoglobulins. There was no difference in performance of control and immunoglobulin-fed pigs if they were not drenched with the pathogenic bacteria.

It appears that sanitation, temperature and humidity control, and proper ventilation in concert with good nutrition are the keys to the control of diarrhea in early-weaned pigs.

FEED ADDITIVES

Antibiotics and Copper

Antibiotics are usually efficacious in starter diets if they are going to be effective in any phase of the life cycle. Several recent reports indicate that antimicrobials are effective growth promoters in young pigs and that combinations of antimicrobials are often the most efficacious.

Blair and Shires (1981) reported that both salinomycin and carbadox improved gain and feed:gain ratio in starter diets. Patterson (1984) showed that carbadox and sulphadimidine gave additive responses in terms of gain. Stahly et al. (1980) and Roof and Mahan (1982) have shown that the growth response associated with high-level copper feeding is also additive with the response obtained with antibiotics. Yen et al. (1976) demonstrated that carbadox increased nitrogen digestibility in young pigs. Roof and Mahan (1982) also suggested that carbadox increased nitrogen retention in pigs weaned at 4 weeks of age, and Campbell (1982) has reported that carbadox "spared" dietary protein or gave a greater response in low-protein diets.

Other combinations that have been used extensively for a number of years, such as chlortetracycline-sulfamethazine-penicillin and tylosin-sulfamethazine, continue to be effective in the diet of early-weaned pigs. There is some question as to the value of penicillin in the former combination. Bridge et al. (1982) indicate that the growth-promoting activity of tetracycline-sulfa-penicillin is not due to the penicillin. When penicillin was omitted from the mixture, pigs performed the same as positive controls, but when either tetracycline or sulfa was omitted, gain was decreased by 12%.

It is generally assumed that one reason antibiotics and other chemotherapeutics are more efficacious in the early-weaned pig is because of the "stress" caused by weaning. This may indeed be true, but all stresses do not increase the response to antimicrobials. The NCR-89 Committee on Swine Management (1984) has shown that space restriction does not enhance the efficacy of antibiotics in nursery pigs.

As stated previously, the nursery-age pig virtually always responds in terms of gain and feed conversion to antibiotics. It would be a rare instance where this would not be true. The use of these feed additives is also almost always economical, which may or may not be the case in other phases of the life cycle. The reader is urged to read Chapter 17 for an in-depth discussion about antimicrobials.

Organic Acids

With increased research and knowledge concerning digestive development and the possible lack of hydrochloric acid production in the young pig (see Chapter 3), there has been great interest in studying the possible efficacy of organic acids in the diet of early-weaned pigs. Conflicting data have been published. For example, Falkowski and Aherne (1984) indicated neither fumaric nor citric acids improved gain but both improved feed conversion, while Giesting and Easter (1985) reported that fumarate, citrate, and propionate all increase gain. Radecki et al. (1988) found that fumarate improved both gain and feed conversion for the first week postweaning, but citrate additions to the diet were without effect. Henry et al. (1985) noted a response in gain from citrate, but not fumarate, and in a prefence trial they found that pigs preferred an acid-free diet. Edmonds et al. (1985) also reported that citrate and fumarate improved feed conversion. Furthermore, Burnell et al. (1988) indicated that feeding 1% citric acid does decrease the pH of intestinal content of pigs and also improves performance, particularly in simple corn-soybean meal diets.

It appears that organic acids usually will improve feed conversion and, depending on diet composition, may increase rate of gain. Prices may change dramatically, but current economics do not warrant the use of organic acids in starter diets.

Probiotics

Even though several reports appear in the popular press and in *Field Day* reports concerning the efficacy of probiotics, few articles appear in the scientific literature. Pollman et al. (1980) found that the use of a *Lactobacillus acidophilus* culture was of no benefit in pig starter diets. Recently, Lessard and Brisson (1987) indicated that the inclusion of a *Lactobacillus* fermentation product in the diet of pigs weaned at 4 weeks of age increased rate of gain slightly; also of interest was the fact that IgG levels were increased in the pigs at 7 weeks of age. IgA levels were not affected. The inconsistent response obtained from the use of probiotics in starter diets may be due to the presence or absence of colonization of the organisms in the small intestine. If the bacteria do not colonize in the small intestine, a beneficial response is unlikely; if colonization takes place, the gut environment may be "improved" and increased performance may result. Methodology to assure colonization is not available.

SUMMARY

Since sow productivity can be increased by weaning at an early age (3 to 4 weeks), nursery pig nutrition has received added attention in recent years. Current trends in the industry point toward the use of high-energy, complex diets. These diets are composed of high levels of animal (milk) products and fat. Since they are relatively expensive, they are used for only limited feeding periods before a transition is made to simpler cereal-soybean meal–based diets. Almost all of these diets contain one or more antibiotics (medicated) and many also contain copper sulfate. Other feed additives find variable use.

REFERENCES

Adams, K.C., and A.H. Jensen. 1984. *J. Anim. Sci.* 59:1557–1566.
Aherne, F.X., M.G. Hogberg, and H.W. Jones. 1987. *Pork Industry Handbook Fact Sheet PIH-111.* West Lafayette, IN: Purdue University Cooperative Extension Service.
ARC. 1981. *The Nutrient Requirements of Pigs.* Farnham Royal, England: Commonwealth Agricultural Bureaux.
Armstrong, W.D., and A.J. Clawson. 1980. *J. Anim. Sci.* 50:377–384.
Armstrong, W.D., and T.R. Cline. 1976. *J. Anim. Sci.* 42:592–598.
Armstrong, W.D., and T.R. Cline. 1977. *J. Anim. Sci.* 45:1042–1050.
Atteh, J.O., and S. Leeson. 1983. *Can. J. Anim. Sci.* 63:699–705.
Baidoo, S.K., M.K. McIntosh, and F.X. Aherne. 1986. *Can. J. Anim. Sci.* 66:1039–1049.
Ball, R.O., and F.X. Aherne. 1982. *Can. J. Anim. Sci.* 62:907–914.
Blair, R., and A. Shires. 1981. *Can. J. Anim. Sci.* 61:961–964.
Bridge, R., B. Owen, and R.M. Beames. 1982. *Can. J. Anim. Sci.* 62:967–970.
Burnell, T.W., G.L. Cromwell, and T.S. Stahly. 1988. *J. Anim. Sci.* 66:1100–1108.
Campbell, R.G. 1977. *Anim. Prod.* 24:69–76.
Campbell, R.G. 1982. *Anim. Prod.* 34:111–114.
Campbell, R.G., and A.C. Dunkin. 1983. *Anim. Prod.* 36:185–192.
Cinq-Mars, D., et al. 1986. *J. Anim. Sci.* 62:145–150.
Cline, T.R., et al. 1977. *J. Anim. Sci.* 44:72–77.
Decuypere, J.A., P. Knockaert, and H.K. Hendericks. 1981a. *J. Anim. Sci.* 53:1297–1308.
Decuypere, J.A., A. Meeusen, and H.K. Hendricks. 1981b. *J. Anim. Sci.* 53:1011–1018.
Driggers, L.B., and A. Jensen. 1980. *Pork Industry Handbook Fact Sheet PIH-70.* West Lafayette, IN: Purdue University Cooperative Extension Service.
Edmonds, M.S., OA. Izquierdo, and D.H. Baker. 1985. *J. Anim. Sci.* 60:462–469.

Etheridge, R.D., R.W. Seerly, and T.L. Huber. 1984a. *J. Anim. Sci.* 58:1403–1411.
Etheridge, R.D., R.W. Seerly, and R.D. Wyatt. 1984b. *J. Anim. Sci.* 58:1396–1402.
Falkowski, J.F., and F.X. Aherne. 1984. *J. Anim. Sci.* 58:935–938.
Forsyth, D.M., and T.R. Cline. 1986. Unpublished data.
Giesting, D.W., and R.A. Easter. 1985. *J. Anim. Sci.* 60:1288–1294.
Gore, A.M., E.T. Kornegay, and H.P. Veit. 1986. *J. Anim. Sci.* 62:1–7.
Graham, P.L., D.C. Mahan, and R.G. Shields, Jr. 1981. *J. Anim. Sci.* 53:299–307.
Henry, R.W., D.W. Pickard, and P.E. Hughes. 1985. *Anim. Prod.* 40:505–509.
Kennelly, J.J., R.O. Ball, and F.X. Aherne. 1979. *Can. J. Anim. Sci.* 59:693–698.
Kornegay, E.T., et al. 1986. *J. Anim. Sci.* 63:484–491.
Kornegay, E.T., H.R. Thomas, and K.L. Bryant. 1981. *J. Anim. Sci.* 53:130–137.
Kornegay, E.T., S.E. Tinsely, and K.L. Bryant. 1979. *J. Anim. Sci.* 48:999–1006.
Lawrence, N.J., and C.V. Maxwell. 1983. *J. Anim. Sci.* 57:936–942.
Lecce, J.G., et al. 1985. *J. Anim. Sci.* 61:1043–1048.
Lessard, M., and G.J. Brisson. 1987. *Can. J. Anim. Sci.* 67:509–516.
Lovett, T.D., et al. 1986. *J. Anim. Sci.* 63:467–471.
Mahan, D.C., and L.J. Saif. 1983. *J. Anim. Sci.* 56:631–639.
McConnell, J.C., et al. 1982. *J. Anim. Sci.* 55:841–847.
McCracken, K.J. 1980. *Br. J. Nutr.* 43:305–320.
McCracken, K.J., S.M. Eddie, and W.G. Stevenson. 1980. *Br. J. Nutr.* 43:289–305.
McIntosh, M.K, et al. 1986. *Can. J. Anim. Sci.* 66:1051:1056.
McNutt, S.D., and R.C. Ewan. 1984. *J. Anim. Sci.* 59:738–745.
Menge, H., and L.T. Frobish. 1976. *J. Anim. Sci.* 43:1019–1023.
MCR-42 Committee on Swine Nutrition. 1980. *J. Anim. Sci.* 50:99–102.
NCR-89 Committee on Confinement Management of Swine. 1984. *J. Anim. Sci.* 58:801–804.
Newport, M.J., and H.D. Keal. 1983. *Anim. Prod.* 37:395–400.
NRC. 1988. *Nutrient Requirements of Swine.* 9th ed. Washington, DC: National Academy of Sciences-National Research Council.
Owsley, W.F., et al. 1986. *J. Anim. Sci.* 63:492–496.
Patterson, D.C. 1984. *Anim. Prod.* 38:487–493.
Pollmann, D.S., D.M. Danielson, and E.R. Peo, Jr. 1980. *J. Anim. Sci.* 51:638–644.
Pouteaux, V.A., G.I. Christison, and C.S. Rhodes. 1982. *Can. J. Anim. Sci.* 62:1199–1209.
Radecki, S.V., M.R. Juhl, and E.R. Miller. 1988. *J. Anim. Sci.* 66:2598–2605.
Rivera, E.R., et al. 1978. *J. Anim. Sci.* 46:1685–1693.
Rodriquez, J.P., and L.G. Young. 1981. *J. Anim. Sci.* 53:683–692.
Roof, M.D., and D.C. Mahan. 1982. *J. Anim. Sci.* 55:1109–1117.
Russett, J.C., et al. 1979a. *J. Anim. Sci.* 49:708–714.
Russett, J.C., et al. 1979b. *J. Anim. Sci.* 48:1366–1373.
Walker, W.R., et al. 1986a. *J. Anim. Sci.* 63:505–512.
Walker, W.R., et al. 1986b. *J. Anim. Sci.* 63:513–524.
Wilson, R.H., and J. Leibholz. 1981a. *Br. J. Nutr.* 45:301–320.
Wilson, R.H., and J. Leibholz. 1981b. *Br. J. Nutr.* 45:321–336.
Wilson, R.H., and J. Leibholz. 1981c. *Br. J. Nutr. 45:337#346.*
Wilson, R.H., and J. Leibholz. 1981d. Br. J. Nutr. 45:347–358.
Yen, J.T., and W.G. Pond. 1981. *J. Anim. Sci.* 53:1292–1296.
Yen, J.T., and W.G. Pond. 1984. *J. Anim. Sci.* 58:132–137.
Yen, J.T., and W.G. Pond. 1987. *J. Anim. Sci.* 64:1672–1681.
Yen, J.T., et al. 1976. *J. Anim. Sci.* 42:375–380.
Zhang, Y., I.G. Partridge, and K.G. Mitchell. 1986. *Anim. Prod.* 42:389–395.

Chapter 31

Feeding Growing-Finishing Pigs

L.F. Tribble

The growing-finishing period is considered to cover the weight range from about 20 to 100 kg. Once it reaches 20 kg in good health, the most critical periods of the market pig's life have passed. However, the growing-finishing pig still responds to good nutrition, environment, and disease prevention.

Pigs are adaptable to a wide variety of environments as indicated by the fact that they are produced throughout the world. In the United States, many are produced successfully in outside lots or pastures, but the majority of pigs are produced in larger units that use some type of confinement (Van Arsdall and Nelson 1984). The major advantage for the production of swine in confinement is the reduction in labor requirements. One person can produce more pork in the large confinement operations than in less intense systems. Furthermore, the confinement buildings buffer the environment, thus maintaining a more uniform environment throughout the year. This provides more comfortable surroundings for the pig, which results in increased productivity, especially in feed efficiency. Seymour et al. (1968) found the optimum temperature to be near 20 °C, with reduced performance occurring at 6 °C to 7 °C and 26 °C to 32 °C. Feed efficiency is reduced at the lower temperatures (Seymour et al. 1964; Wahlstrom et al. 1971). Verstegen et al. (1982) found that feed requirements were increased by 25 to 39 g/day for growing-finishing pigs for each degree Celsius below the lower critical temperature. The feed contained 3 kcal metabolizable energy (ME)/g. The thermo-neutral zone for the pig is from 15 °C to 29 °C, depending on size, level of feed intake, and wind velocity (Heitman et al. 1958; Holmes and Close 1977).

There is an interaction between energy density of the diet and environmental temperature. High-energy diets are more efficiently utilized at high temperatures than are low-energy diets, but at low temperatures the difference in efficiency is minimal between high- and low-energy diets (Coffey et al. 1982; Noblet et al. 1985; Stahly et al. 1981). Feed intake is reduced at high temperatures, but if energy density is high, a higher level of energy intake may be maintained. Rate of gain will decline, but efficiency will be maintained until extremely high temperatures are reached. At low temperatures, feed intake is increased, rate of gain is maintained, but feed efficiency declines. A point may be reached for both hot and cold temperatures where the pig cannot maintain homeostasis and production declines. The pig responds to a suitable environment, and management procedures should be employed to provide a comfortable environment for the pig during the growing-finishing period.

The nutrient requirements of the growing-finishing pig have been fairly well determined and are reported by the National Research Council (NRC) (1979, 1988). These requirements refer to minimum requirements and apply best to a corn-soybean meal diet, fed ad libitum in a thermoneutral comfort zone.

A specific energy requirement has not been determined for growing-finishing pigs. Suggested diet energy density is about 3400 kcal digestible energy (DE)/kg for pigs from 20 to 110 kg, which is the energy density of a corn-soybean meal grower diet (NRC 1988). Seerley et al. (1978) found that a diet containing more than 3300 kcal ME/kg did not increase average daily gains of growing-finishing pigs. They stated that additional calories are not likely to enhance growth rate. Pigs tend to eat to meet their energy requirement, and the data of Seerley et al. (1978) would indicate that diets that are more energy dense than 3300 kcal ME/kg would not be expected to improve gains. However, the more energy dense the diet, the less feed would be required per unit of gain. Energy (kcal) required per unit of gain would remain about the same (Baird et al. 1970). Pigs can efficiently utilize diets composed of all of the grains even though they vary in diet density. The comparative feeding values of these grains may be based on their density of DE or ME.

Protein requirements as listed by the NRC (1988) are 15% and 13% for pigs weighing 20 to 50 and 50 to 100 kg, respectively. These values would be satisfactory for diets composed of corn or sorghum and soybean meal. Higher or lower levels of protein would be required with different combinations of grains and supplemental protein sources. The protein content would be determined by the amino acid densities of the feed ingredients. The major concern would be the combination that would furnish a satisfactory level of lysine.

Lysine requirements (NRC 1988) are 0.75% and 0.60% for pigs weighing 20 to 50 and 50 to 110 kg, respectively. Easter and Baker (1980) showed that pigs fed corn-soybean meal diets containing 14%, 11.5%, and 11% protein and supplemental lysine to pigs weighing 23 to 45, 45 to 75, and 75 to 93 kg, respectively, performed equal to those fed diets containing 16%, 13%, and 12% protein. They also demonstrated that the lysine requirements declined 0.02% for each 1% decrease in diet protein density. Satisfactory growth was obtained at 11.3% protein on a corn-soybean meal diet when 50% of the protein came from soybean meal (Smith et al. 1967). A diet concentration of 12.8% protein was required for maximum feed efficiency, and carcass leanness improved up to 14.3% diet protein, which indicates that the requirement depends on the criterion used. Actually, the requirement for the pig is not for protein but for indispensable amino acids. Most of the amino acid requirements have been determined for the young pig and interpolated for the growing-finishing pig. For example, the threonine requirement is 3.1% of the protein in the diet for the pig from 10 to 110 kg (NRC 1988). Brown et al. (1973) determined the lysine requirement of the finishing pig to be 0.48% for maximum daily gain and 0.62% for maximum gain per feed. The latter value would be near the 0.60% lysine requirement established by the NRC (1988). Using nitrogen retention as the criterion, Brown et al. (1974) determined the isoleucine requirement for finishing pigs to be 0.31% of the diet and the tryptophan requirement to be 0.059% of the diet. They also determined that the sulfur amino acid requirement was not greater than 0.17% of the diet, which is considerably lower than the NRC (1988) value of 0.4%.

Research continues on minerals to more precisely define the requirements of the modern meat-type pig. A salt level of 0.25% of the diet appears adequate to meet the requirements for sodium and chlorine (NRC 1988; Hagsten et al. 1976). NRC (1988) requirements for calcium and phosphorus appear to be adequate for rate and efficiency of gain (Thomas and Kornegay 1981). Maximum bone mineralization requires slightly higher levels of calcium and phosphorus. Magnesium and potassium would appear to be adequate in practical diets for growing-finishing swine. The trace elements copper, iodine, iron, manganese, selenium, and zinc are usually added to practical growing-finishing pig diets, although proof of the need for all of them is lacking. The copper requirement is 3 to 4 ppm (NRC 1988), and most practical diets would contain adequate copper. Interest in much higher levels of copper (up to 250 ppm) for its antibiotic-like growth effect was stimulated by Barber et al. (1955). It is well recognized that the area around the Great Lakes is deficient in iodine. Feeds produced in other areas of the country should be adequate. Cromwell et al. (1975) determined the iodine requirement to be between 0.086 and 0.132 ppm, which is slightly lower than the 0.14 ppm cited by the NRC (1988). The iron requirements should be met by practical diets of NRC-recommended levels. The manganese requirement of 2 ppm (NRC 1988) is probably met by practical diets but often is supplemented as insurance against a possible deficiency. Selenium has been found to be deficient over a rather wide geographical area. The United States Food and Drug Administration (FDA) approved the supplementation of 0.1 ppm selenium to all swine diets in 1974 and raised to 0.3 ppm selenium supplementation of all swine diets in 1982. Groce et al. (1971) observed classical selenium and vitamin E deficiency lesions in pigs fed practical diets containing 0.04 ppm selenium. No pathological lesions were found in pigs fed supplemental levels of 0.1 or 0.5 ppm selenium. No benefit in average daily gain and feed efficiency was obtained from supplementing a practical diet containing 0.08 ppm of selenium with 0.1 ppm selenium (Wilkinson et al. 1977). The importance of supplementing practical diets with zinc was established when Tucker and Salmon (1955) reported that supplemental zinc cured parakeratosis in swine. The NRC (1988) stated zinc requirement levels of 50 to 60 ppm, but levels of 100 ppm are frequently used in practical diets. The level of calcium and phytate in the diet have been shown to interfere with the availability of zinc (Church and Pond 1988).

All of the fat-soluble vitamins are supplemented to practical diets for growing-finishing swine. Vitamins A and D are usually supplemented at more than twice the NRC (1988) minimum requirement levels. The NRC (1988) levels are best estimates of minimum requirements of pigs fed corn-soybean meal or sorghum-soybean meal diets. Vitamin E functions together with the mineral selenium, although each has specific requirements. Ullrey (1981) stated that with supplemental levels of 0.1 ppm selenium, the vitamin E requirement is between 10 and 20 IU/kg. A level of 0.5 mg/kg of menadione equivalent of vitamin K is listed by the NRC (1988) and is usually supplemented at that level in all swine diets.

Among the B vitamins, thiamin, pyridoxine, biotin, and folacin are present in adequate levels in practical swine diets. The remaining B vitamins are supplemented at or in excess of NRC (1988) requirements. An example of the level of vitamin supplementation is shown in Table 31.1 at Texas Tech University as compared to NRC (1988) listed minimum requirements.

ANTIBIOTICS AND HIGH LEVELS OF COPPER

Antibiotics, chemical compounds with antibiotic activity, and high levels of copper are added to growing-finishing swine diets for growth promotion and improvement of feed efficiency. Antibacterials have been fed to growing-finishing swine at growth-promoting levels of <50 g/ton for over 35 years. Hays and Muir (1979) stated that summaries confirm that antibiotics continue to be effective in improving rate and efficiency of gain. However, antibiotic-resistant strains have developed, and there is concern about possible human health hazards, animal health hazards, and effectiveness in animals (Solomons 1978). Langlois et al. (1978) reported data comparing antibiotic resistance in a herd in which antibiotics had not been fed for 42 months as compared with a herd fed antibiotics continuously. They found that the herd continuously fed antibiotics had a higher level of resistant organisms than the herd without antibiotics. However, the resistance persisted in the herd not fed antibiotics and indications are that once resistance is established, a long time period is required before appreciable reduction in resistance is noted. Great Britain has limited the use of antibiotics to a therapeutic

Table 31.1 Vitamin Supplementation of Diets of Growing-Finishing Swine[a]

Vitamin	Unit of Measure	Growing Swine		Finishing Swine	
		NRC[b]	*TTU*[c]	*NRC*[b]	*TTU*[c]
A	IU	1300	4400	1300	3300
D	IU	150	440	150	330
E	IU	11	11	11	8.25
K (menadione equivalent	mg	0.5	4.4	0.5	3.3
Riboflavin	mg	2.5	4.4	2.0	3.3
Niacin	mg	10	22	7	16.5
Pantothenic acid	mg	8	18	7	13.5
Choline	mg	300	382	300	286.5
Cyanocobalamin	μg	10	22	5	16.5

Abbreviation: TTU, Texas Tech University.

[a] Figures represent units per kilogram of diet.

[b] Estimated minimum dietary requirements.

[c] Levels supplemented to corn-soybean meal or sorghum-soybean meal diets.

(Data from NRC 1988.)

basis. Braude (1978), in evaluating the situation in Great Britain, stated that there is no evidence that the restrictions imposed have improved the human disease situation. The feeding of growth-promoting levels of antibiotics appears to be safe and effective. A number of antibacterial agents are available, and a list of approved levels of usage may be found in the *Feed Additive Compendium* (1990).

High levels of copper (100 to 250 ppm) have been used as a growth-promoting substance for several years. The first report by Barber et al. (1955) was followed by considerable research in the United States. Copper is an effective substitute for antibiotics or may be fed in combinations with antibiotics (Cromwell et al. 1981). See Chapter 17 for additional information.

COMPARISON OF BARROWS AND GILTS

Barrows consistently gain faster and eat more feed than do gilts (Newell and Bowland 1972; Shields and Mahan 1980; Siers 1975; Wagner et al. 1963; Young et al. 1968). Efficiency of gain tends to favor the gilts. Barrows tend to be fatter than gilts. Since the gilt is leaner, does she require more protein in the diet? The general answer is that gilts do, but the magnitude is probably not large (Bayley and Summers 1968; Fuller 1984; Newell and Bowland 1972; Wallace 1968). However, Shields and Mahan (1980) and Wagner et al. (1963) failed to show a sex response to different levels of protein between barrows and gilts. Perhaps gilts are more efficient in the utilization of protein than are barrows. Since barrows gain faster, there may be an advantage to splitting the sexes for more uniform marketing. The difference in protein requirement may not justify splitting the sexes. For more information on differences between barrows and gilts, see Chapter 25.

EFFECT OF NUTRITION ON CARCASS COMPOSITION

The composition of the carcass in swine is primarily determined by genetics. Nutrition can only develop the pig up to the genetic potential of the animal. Any essential nutrient may affect the carcass composition through its effect on growth. The major nutrients involved in body composition are energy and protein (amino acids) and energy:protein ratio.

Reducing energy intake by limited feeding (Tribble et al. 1956) or by diluting the energy with fiber (Boenker 1961) will reduce the fat deposition and increase the yield of lean. Both methods reduce the rate of gain, and added fiber increases feed intake and feed per gain. The effect of limited feeding on efficiency is not consistent. Tribble et al. (1956) reported more efficient gains, while Wallace (1968) found less efficient gains from limited feeding. The effect on the composition of the carcass of adding fat to the diet to increase energy density of the diet is also not consistent. Since the pig tends to eat to meet its energy requirement, adding fat does not always result in increased energy intake. Tribble et al. (1977) added 4% and 8% of tallow to a sorghum-soybean meal diet and obtained no increase in gain or fat in the carcass. The

Table 31.2 Sample Diets for Growing-Finishing Pigs[a]

	Growing Pigs			Finishing Pigs		
Ingredient	*1*	2	*3*	*4*	*5*	*6*
Corn	79.4			84.55		
Sorghum		75.9			81.75	
Barley			82.3			88.75
Soybean meal	17.5	14.1	7.4	13	10.6	4.5
Cottonseed meal		7.0			5.3	
Canola meal			7.4			4.5
Salt	0.3	0.3	0.3	0.3	0.3	0.3
Dicalcium phosphate	0.9	0.7	0.6	0.5	0.3	0.2
Calcium carbonate	0.9	1.0	1.0	0.9	1.0	1.0
Vitamin-trace mineral[b]	1.0	1.0	1.0	0.75	0.75	0.75

[a]Calculated to meet the requirements for lysine, calcium, and phosphorus according to NRC 1979.

[b]Contained the following units per kilogram of premix: Vitamin A, 440,000 IU; vitamin D, 44,000 IU; vitamin E, 1100 IU; vitamin K, 440 mg; riboflavin, 440 mg; niacin, 2200 mg; pantothenic acid, 1800 mg; choline, 38,200 mg; cyanobalamin, 2200 μg; copper, 550 mg; iodine, 75 mg; manganese, 2750 mg; iron, 5000 mg; and zinc, 10,000 mg.

average daily intake of energy was similar among the various diets. Wagner et al. (1963) obtained increased fatness from adding 10% of fat to the diet.

Adequate protein is required to allow for development of muscle to the genetic potential of the animal. A deficient protein diet results in a fatter pig with more backfat and more intramuscular fat (Seymour et al. 1964; Kornegay et al. 1973; Wallace 1968). Feeding protein in excess of the requirement (25%) resulted in reduced backfat and increased lean cuts, but daily gain was also reduced (Newell and Bowland 1972). Low protein with high-energy–dense diets are especially bad for carcass composition. The high energy reduces feed intake, which further reduces the intake of protein, which results in a fatter carcass. Increasing protein in the presence of added fat to narrow the calorie:protein ratio results in normal body composition and intramuscular fat (Wagner et al. 1963).

The chemical composition of the fat deposited is directly related to the chemical composition of the fat consumed (Ellis and Isbell 1926; Vestal and Shrewsbury 1944). The feeding of highly unsaturated fats such as soybean or peanut oil will result in soft oily carcasses.

Examples of diets using feedstuffs most commonly available in various parts of the United States are shown in Table 31.2. Corn and sorghum may be substituted for each other on a unit weight basis, since they are similar in lysine content. The example using cottonseed meal and canola meal are included as a partial substitute for soybean meal, since these feedstuffs may be available in some areas. Other combinations that supply adequate available amino acids, especially lysine, may be used, such as the combination of peanut meal and flash-dried blood meal (Ilorie et al. 1984).

REFERENCES

Baird, D.M., H.C. McCampbell, and J.R. Allison. 1970. *J. Anim. Sci.* 31:518.
Barber, R.S., et al. 1955. *J. Nutr.* 9:378.
Bayley, H.S., and J.D. Summers. 1968. *Can. J. Anim. Sci.* 48:181.
Boenker, D.E. 1961. "The Evaluation of Calorie Protein Ratios in Swine Nutrition," Ph.D. thesis. University of Missouri, Columbia.
Braude, R. 1978. *J. Anim. Sci.* 46:1425.
Brown, H.D., B.G. Harmon, and A.H. Jensen. 1973. *J. Anim. Sci.* 37:708.
Brown, H.W., B.G. Harmon, and A.H. Jensen. 1974. *J. Anim. Sci.* 38:59.
Church, D.C., and W.G. Pond. 1988. *Basic Animal Nutrition and Feeding.* 3rd ed. New York: John Wiley and Sons.
Clawson, A.J., et al. 1962. *J. Anim. Sci.* 21:62.
Coffey, M.T., et al. 1982. *J. Anim. Sci.* 54:95.
Cromwell, G.L., D.T.H. Sihombing, and V.W. Hays. 1975. *J. Anim. Sci.* 41:813.
Cromwell, G.L., T.S. Stahly, and W.D. Williams. 1981. *Feedstuffs.* November 2, p. 30.
Easter, R.A., and D.H. Baker. 1980. *J. Anim. Sci.* 50:467.
Ellis, N.R., and H.S. Isbell. 1926. *J. Biol. Chem.* 69:219.
Feed Additive Compendium. 1990. Chicago: Miller Publishing Co.
Fuller, M.F. 1985. Sex differences in nutrition and growth of pigs. In: *Recent Developments in Swine Nutrition.* Cole, D.J.A., and W. Haresign (Eds.). pp. 177–189. London: Butterworth.
Groce, A.W., et al. 1971. *J. Anim. Sci.* 32:905.
Hale, O.M., J.C. Johnson, Jr., and E.P. Warren. 1968. *J. Anim. Sci.* 27:1577.
Hays, V.W., and W.M. Muir. 1979. *Can. J. Anim. Sci.* 59:447.
Heitman, H., Jr., C.F. Kelly, and T.E. Bond. 1958. *J. Anim. Sci.* 17:62.
Holmes, C.W., and W.H. Close. 1977. "The influence of climate variables on energy metabolism and associated aspects of productivity in the pig." In: *Nutrition and the Climatic Environment.* Haresign, W., H. Swan, and D. Lewis (Eds.). pp. 51–73. London: Butterworth.
Ilorie, J.O., et al. 1984. *J. Anim. Sci.* 59:394.
Kornegay, E.T., H.R. Thomas, and J.H. Carter. 1973. *J. Anim. Sci.* 36:79.
Langlois, B.E., G.L. Cromwell, and V.W. Hays. 1978. *J. Anim. Sci.* 46:1383.
Newell, J.A., and J.P. Bowland. 1972. *Can. J. Anim. Sci.* 52:543.
Noblet, J., J. LeDividich, and T. Bikawa. 1985. *J. Anim. Sci.* 61:452.
NRC. 1979. *Nutrient Requirements of Swine.* 8th ed. Washington, DC: National Academy of Sciences.
NRC. 1988. *Nutrient Requirements of Swine.* 9th ed. Washington, DC: National Academy of Sciences.
Seerley, R.W., M.C. McDaniel, and H.C. McCampbell. 1978. *J. Anim. Sci.* 47:427.
Seymour, E.W., V.C. Speer, and V.W. Hays. 1968. *J. Anim. Sci.* 27:389.
Seymour, E.W., et al. 1964. *J. Anim. Sci.* 23:375.
Shields, R.G., Jr., and D.C. Mahan. 1980. *J. Anim. Sci.* 51:1340.
Siers, D.G. 1975. *J. Anim. Sci.* 41:522.
Smith, J., Jr., A.J. Clawson, and E.R. Barrick. 1967. *J. Anim. Sci.* 26:752.
Solomons, I.A. 1978. *J. Anim. Sci.* 46:1360.
Stahly, T.S., and G.L. Cromwell. 1979. *J. Anim. Sci.* 49:1478.
Stahly, T.S., G.L. Cromwell, and M.P. Aviotti. 1979. *J. Anim. Sci.* 49:1242.
Stahly, T.S., G.L. Cromwell, and J.R. Overfield. 1981. *J. Anim. Sci.* 53:1269.
Tribble, L.F., et al. 1956. Missouri Agricultural Experiment Station Research Bulletin 609.
Tribble, L.F., et al. 1979. *J. Anim. Sci.* 48:541.
Tucker, H.F., and W.D. Salmon. 1955. *Proc. Soc. Exp. Biol. Med.* 88:613.
Ullrey, D.E. 1981. *J. Anim. Sci.* 53:1039.
Van Arsdall, R.N., and K.E. Nelson. 1984. *USDA Agriculture Economic Report No. 511.* Washington, DC: United States Department of Agriculture.

Verstegen, M.W.A., H.A. Bandsma, and G. Mateman. 1982. *J. Anim. Sci.* 55:88.
Vestal, C.M., and C.L. Shrewsbury. 1935. *Indiana Agricultural Experiment Station Bulletin, 400.* Lafayette, IN.
Wagner, G.R., et al. 1963. *J. Anim. Sci.* 22:202.
Wahlstrom, R.C., J.F. Fredrickson, and G.W. Libal. 1971. *J. Anim. Sci.* 32:1138.
Wallace, H.D. 1968. In: *The Pork Industry.* p. 77. D.G. Topel, (Ed.). Ames, IA: Iowa State University Press.
Wilkinson, J.E., et al. 1977. *J. Anim. Sci.* 44:229.
Young, L.G., et al. 1968. *Can. J. Anim. Sci.* 48:71.

Chapter 32

Feeding Developing Gilts and Boars

R.C. Wahlstrom

Maximum reproductive efficiency is a necessity for swine operations to be successful. The performance of replacement gilts and boars has a profound influence on the total efficiency of the breeding herd. Developing gilts must be provided with the nutrition, environment, and management conditions necessary for the female to attain puberty, express estrus, mate, and conceive at a relatively early age (7 to 9 months). Likewise, boars must be developed to reach early puberty with adequate sexual aggressiveness and have the ability to mate readily and produce high conception rates. Factors that are important in developing gilts and boars for maximum production in the breeding herd are discussed in this chapter.

SELECTION AND MANAGEMENT OF DEVELOPING GILTS

Selection of Gilts

Gilt selection should start at birth by identifying gilts born in large litters of uniform size that were farrowed without difficulty. Litters should be free from hernias, cryptorchids, and other abnormalities. Ear notching two to three times as many gilts as will be needed for replacements will allow for additional selection at weaning, prebreeding, and breeding. Birth dates, litter size, identification, and breed composition should be recorded. It is important to know the breed composition in order to maintain a crossbreeding program in proper rotation.

At weaning, reject gilts from sows that have not shown above-average milking ability. Examine underlines and reject individuals with inverted or necrotic nipples. Twelve to fourteen evenly spaced, developed teats are preferred. Final selection should be made at prebreeding when gilts weigh approximately 75 to 90 kg. Select 25% to

30% more gilts than needed for breeding. Base selection on growth rate, leanness (backfat), soundness, and normal-appearing external genitalia. Replacement gilts should be able to move freely with adequate bone to support further skeletal growth. Gilts with small, infantile vulvas should be culled.

Management for Development

Gilts from large litters will be more likely to express their genetic potential for litter size if they are reared in litter groups of six to eight from birth to weaning. This can be accomplished by cross-fostering male pigs to other sows whose gilts are not being selected as replacements.

Following weaning, replacement gilts should be fed and managed in a manner that will stimulate their growth and development to reach early puberty. Gilts will ovulate one to two more eggs on the second and subsequent estrus periods than on first estrus. Thus, gilts that express estrus at a younger age and are bred at the second or third estrus period will require less feed as well as less overhead maintenance costs without affecting reproductive performance.

Housing

Rearing gilts in enclosed confinement buildings delays the onset of puberty and increases the incidence of behavioral anestrus (Christenson and Ford 1979). The effect of confinement on delaying onset of puberty differs among breeds. Large White, Landrace, and crosses of these breeds are not affected to the extent of most other breeds (Christenson 1981). A practical solution used by some producers is to remove gilts from confinement before breeding age and house them in outside lots until they express first estrus.

Confinement-reared gilts should be grouped eight to twelve per pen and allowed 0.9 to 1.3 m^2/pig of pen floor space during the period from selection to breeding. Avoid overcrowding and large groups, as they may delay puberty.

Seasonal Effects

Research on the effect of season of birth of gilts on age at puberty has been inconclusive. This may not be unusual in that seasonal conditions can be quite variable from year to year and between different research stations. Recent evidence would indicate that gilts born in the summer or fall reach puberty earlier than those born in winter or spring (Christenson 1981). Primary seasonal effects are day length (light) and temperature.

Although studies on the effect of light on age at puberty have not been conclusive, most of the evidence seems to indicate an advantage of exposing gilts to prolonged light periods. Insufficient light exposure has been indicated as a possible cause of delayed puberty in gilts housed in confinement buildings that restrict response to light (Ntunde et al. 1979). However, Dufour and Bernard (1968) reported a slight decrease in age to puberty when gilts were raised in complete darkness. A possible mechanism for the effect of light on reproduction has been proposed by Hughes and Varley (1980).

High environmental temperatures, above 30 °C, have been shown to increase the incidence of anestrus, decrease ovulation rate and conception rate in cycling gilts, and decrease feed intake (Teague et al. 1968). Producers should increase the number of gilts exposed during the months of June through September in order to maintain a constant number of bred gilts.

Social Environment

Two methods of stimulating estrus in the prepuberal gilt are mixing and relocation of gilts, referred to as "transport phenomenon," and exposure of gilts to sexually mature boars. Mixing and relocating to a new environment has been shown to cause 15% to 30% of gilts to show estrus in 3 to 10 days. For maximum synchronization, the two methods should be combined.

Boar exposure may be by continuous fence line contact or daily exposure of a mature boar into the gilt pen. Exposure to boars before gilts reach 130 days of age may actually delay puberty. Likewise, the age at puberty is considerably increased if gilts are first introduced to a boar at 180 days or later. For maximum synchronization of first estrus, boar introduction should occur between 150 and 170 days (Brooks and Cole 1973; Hughes and Cole 1976). Rotating boars daily may result in an improvement of estrus synchronization as compared with exposure to a single boar (Brooks and Cole 1970).

SELECTION AND MANAGEMENT OF DEVELOPING BOARS

When selecting replacement boars at approximately 6 months of age, consider performance (growth rate and feed efficiency), backfat, soundness of feet and legs, sexual behavior and aggressiveness of the individual, as well as the source herd. The seedstock producer is responsible for providing boars with the genetic potential to produce fast-growing, efficient, healthy, sound pigs with desirable carcass traits. Selection between birth and weaning should eliminate those litters having inverted nipples, hernias, cryptorchids, or other genetic abnormalities or structural unsoundness.

Social contact is important in the development of normal sexual behavior in young boars. This interaction may be in groups of all male or mixed sex. Boars housed in groups reached puberty earlier and demonstrated greater sexual aggressiveness as compared with boars housed singly (Hemsworth et al. 1978; Thomas et al. 1979). Esbenshade et al. (1979) reported that confinement housing had little, if any, effect on growth, soundness, or sexual development of young boars. However, Thomas et al. (1979) found that boards housed in earth lots reached puberty earlier than those on concrete confinement. Young boars should not be exposed to environmental temperatures above 30 °C for 6 to 8 weeks prior to breeding. Temperatures above 30 °C can cause a reduction in fertility for a 2- to 6-week period following heat stress.

Commercial producers should purchase boars about 2 months before breeding, isolate them for 30 days, and then allow 30 days of fence line contact with nonpregnant females prior to breeding.

RELATIONSHIP OF NUTRITION DURING GROWTH AND REPRODUCTIVE DEVELOPMENT OF GILTS

Preweaning Nutrition

There is a paucity of information on the effect of preweaning nutrition on development of the breeding animal. It is difficult to assess nutritional and environmental effects during this period. It has been suggested by Revelle and Robison (1973) that physiological maturation of gilts in larger litters is delayed due to increased nutritional and/or sociological stress. Thus, females from large litters are unable to express their genetic superiority. These researchers also suggest that gilts from litters of six to twelve reach puberty at a younger age than gilts from larger litters.

Postweaning Nutrition

This section considers how nutrition during the two periods of rearing and preestrus (flushing) affect reproductive development. The effect of level of feed intake during rearing on age of puberty has been inconclusive. A high level of feeding was reported by some to result in a younger age at puberty (Haines et al. 1959; Zimmerman et al. 1960), while others reported a delay in sexual maturity due to increased feed intake (Self et al. 1955). The effects of energy, protein, and minerals will be discussed separately.

Energy Intake During Rearing

In a review, den Hartog and van Kampen (1980) cited fourteen publications reporting that food restriction delayed age at puberty, eight that found no effect, and five that reported a favorable effect of food restriction. Other factors contributing to differences in age at puberty are age at the beginning of the restricted energy regimen, breed, season of year, and degree of restriction imposed.

Table 32.1 presents data (Friend 1976; Friend et al. 1981) indicating that weight for age rather than age per se is the more important determinant of age at puberty, since gilts in the two experiments differed in average daily gain but were similar in body weight at puberty. The data also show that if daily energy level is reduced to 62% (experiment 1) or 54% (experiment 2) of ad libitum-fed gilts, age at puberty is increased.

Table 32.1 Effect of Energy Intake on Puberty

	Experiment 1[a]		*Experiment 2*[b]	
	Feeding Method		*Feeding Method*	
	Ad Libitum	*Restricted*	*Ad Libitum*	*Restricted*
Avg. daily feed (kg)	3.02[c]	1.08[d]	2.96[c]	1.60[d]
Avg. daily gain (kg)	0.95[c]	0.60[d]	0.69[c]	0.41[d]
Age at puberty (d)	173[c]	194[d]	159[e]	170[f]
Weight at puberty (kg)	101[e]	92[f]	97	92

[a] Data from Friend 1976.

[b] Data from Friend et al. 1981.

[c,d] Within each experiment, means in the same row without common superscripts differ ($P < .01$).

[e,f] Within each experiment, means in the same row without common superscripts differ ($P < .05$).

Table 32.2 Metabolizable Energy Intake and Puberty in Gilts

	ME (kcal/d)		*Age at Puberty (d)*		*Weight at Puberty (kg)*	
	Feeding Method		*Feeding Method*		*Feeding Method*	
No. of Trials	*Ad Libitum*	*Restricted*	*Ad Libitum*	*Restricted*	*Ad Libitum*	*Restricted*
9	8920	5530	201	217	91	74
6	8910	6010	212	201	94	74

(Data from Anderson and Melampy 1972.)

Other workers have suggested puberty in gilts is influenced less by body weight than age. Lodge and McPherson (1961) reported a difference of only 2 days in age of gilts that differed by 33 kg in body weight at puberty. A summary of fourteen experiments by Anderson and Melampy (1971) confirms a lower body weight at puberty in restricted gilts but an increased age at puberty in gilts only from experiments where metabolizable energy (ME) was reduced to an average of 62% of that of full-fed gilts (Table 32.2). More recently, it has been suggested that minimum threshold levels of age, live weight, and fatness may be necessary for the attainment of puberty (Kirkwood and Aherne 1985; Burnett and Walker 1988).

Difficulty in mating gilts reared on a high feeding level has been reported by Pomeroy (1960), who found excessively fat animals did not show normal estrus behavior. It was suggested that this may be due to estrogens secreted by the ovaries being dissolved in fat depots. Gilts with a greater backfat thickness were found to have lower conception rates (Hafez 1959).

Replacement gilts should be fed a high-energy ration ad libitum to time of selection at about 150 days of age (80 to 90 kg body weight). Energy intake can then be restricted without delaying puberty. Limit daily feed to about 2 kg of a 14% protein ration containing 6 Mcal of ME until 2 weeks before breeding. Small adjustments to this level of feeding may be necessary due to differences in environment, particularly temperature, and breed or type of animal.

Energy Intake Before Estrus

Increasing the energy level fed prior to estrus is referred to as "flushing." Flushing may be accomplished by increasing feed intake from about 2 to 3 or 3.5 kg daily or by increasing energy density of the diet. This practice has been shown to consistently increase the number of ovulations. It does not, however, consistently increase litter size. The optimum duration of a high-energy regimen is about 11 to 14 days before estrus or mating (Anderson and Melampy 1972).

Although high-energy diets fed before mating increase number of ovulations, the continuation of these diets after mating causes a higher embryonic death loss. Therefore, it is advisable to reduce feeding level to approximately 2 kg daily immediately after breeding.

Effect of Dietary Protein

Protein restriction during the rearing period increases age at puberty. Diets of 10% protein fed from 42 days of age (Cunningham et al. 1974) and from 103 days of age (Wahlstrom and Libal 1977) or 8% protein fed from 146 days of age (Jones and Maxwell 1974) delayed puberty by approximately 19, 25, and 10 days, respectively. Jones and Maxwell (1974) also reported that the number of corpora lutea decreased with a decreased level of dietary protein, but embryo survival was not affected. It is possible that diet concentrations of specific amino acids are more limiting for reproductive criteria than protein content per se. There is evidence that a severe imbalance in essential amino acids may delay the onset of puberty in gilts (Friend 1973). Zimmerman et al. (1967) replaced part of the supplemental protein in a fortified all-plant diet (corn-soybean meal) with protein of animal origin (meat and bone scraps). It was reported that there were no differences due to diet for age at puberty, ovulation rate, or embryo survival.

Calcium and Phosphorus

One of the major reasons for culling females from a breeding herd is structural unsoundness and feet and leg problems. Calcium and phosphorus are the two dietary nutrients most involved in bone development. National Research Council (1988) recommendations of calcium and phosphorus levels for growing-finishing swine to 100 kg do not support maximum bone development and strength in developing gilts (Kornegay and Thomas 1981; Thomas and Kornegay 1981). These researchers reported serum phosphorus and bone mineralization decreased when phosphorus was below NRC recommendations. However, stronger, denser bones were not related to increased structural soundness, and dietary calcium and phosphorus levels did not influence soundness scores (Kornegay and Thomas 1981; Kornegay et al. 1981a,b). A regional five-state study did not find any differences in reproductive performance or longevity of gilts developed on diets containing 100% or 150% of NRC-recommended levels of calcium and phosphorus (Kornegay et al. 1985). In contrast, Nimmo et al. (1981a,b) found that dietary levels of 0.65% calcium and 0.5% phosphorus from 21 days of age to 93 kg did not support maximum skeletal development and resulted in a high percentage (30%) of gilts having to be removed during the first gestation period because of the inability to stand. Gilts fed 0.975% calcium and 0.75% phosphorus during growth did not exhibit these symptoms.

Other Nutrients

Since maximum growth rate is desired in developing gilts, the requirements of growing-finishing swine have been considered adequate unless research has shown additional needs during the growth period for gilts entering the breeding herd. Except for calcium and phosphorus, as discussed previously, research has not shown a need for mineral or vitamin supplementation above NRC-recommended levels for developing gilts destined for the breeding herd.

Zinc deficiency symptoms including reduced gains, feed consumption, serum zinc concentration, and alkaline phosphatase activity, as well as the appearance of parakeratosis, were more severe in gilts than in barrows. Parakeratosis was not observed in barrows fed diets containing <30 ppm of zinc, while 26.7% of the gilts fed equivalent diets exhibited parakerotic lesions (Liptrap et al. 1970). Gilts can tolerate up to 5000 ppm of supplemental zinc from zinc oxide during growth and development. The high zinc level caused elevated serum alkaline phosphatase activity and serum zinc and lower serum copper (Hill and Miller 1983). The investigators did not report any effect on age at puberty or conception rate.

Selenium is deficient in feedstuffs produced in many areas of the United States. Supplementation must comply with regulations of the Food and Drug Administration. Levels of 5 ppm of selenium are considered toxic for swine. Dietary selenium of 10 ppm from 8 weeks of age to breeding lowered conception rate and increased the number of services per conception (Wahlstrom and Olson 1959).

Many feed additives have growth-promoting potential. They may be used during the early growth period at approved levels. It is not necessary or profitable to routinely feed antibiotics to developing gilts. However, the use of high levels of antibiotics approximately 10 days prebreeding to 10 days postbreeding may improve conception rate and litter size in some herds (Hays 1978).

FEEDING DEVELOPING BOARS

Boars should be developed to about 110 kg by feeding high-energy diets ad libitum in order to allow for meaningful rate of gain and backfat probe data for use in selection

Table 32.3 Nutrient Recommendations for Developing Gilts and Boars

	Live Weight (kg)							
	Gilts				*Boars*			
	10–20	*20–55*	*55–100*	*100-Breeding*	*10–20*	*20–55*	*55–100*	*120-Breeding*
ME (kcal/day)	[a]	[a]	[a]	6000	[a]	[a]	[a]	6000
Protein (%)	18	16	15	14	20	18	16	14
Lysine (%)	1.0	0.8	0.7	0.65	1.15	1.0	0.8	0.65
Tryptophan (%)	0.18	0.15	0.12	0.12	0.20	0.17	0.14	0.12
Threonine (%)	0.7	0.6	0.5	0.5	0.75	0.65	0.6	0.5
Methionine + cystine (%)	0.55	0.45	0.35	0.4	0.55	0.45	0.35	0.4
Calcium (%)	0.75	0.7	0.6	0.65	0.9	0.75	0.7	0.65
Phosphorus (%)	0.6	0.55	0.5	0.5	0.7	0.6	0.55	0.5
Salt (%)	0.25	0.25	0.25	0.5	0.25	0.25	0.25	0.5
Zinc (mg/kg)	100	75	50	75	100	75	50	75
Iron (mg/kg)	100	75	50	75	100	75	50	75
Manganese (mg/kg)	20	20	20	20	20	20	20	20
Copper (mg/kg)	7	6	5	6	7	6	5	6
Iodine (mg/kg)	0.15	0.15	0.15	0.15	0.15	0.15	0.15	0.15
Selenium (mg/kg)	0.3	0.15	0.1	0.1	0.3	0.15	0.1	0.1
Vitamin A (IU/kg)	4000	3000	2000	4000	4000	3000	2000	4000
Vitamin D (IU/kg)	400	300	200	400	400	300	200	400
Vitamin E (IU/kg)	20	18	15	20	20	18	15	20
Vitamin K (menadione) (mg/kg)	2	1.5	1	2	2	1.5	1	2
Riboflavin (mg/kg)	5	4	3	5	5	4	3	5
Niacin (mg/kg)	35	30	25	35	35	30	25	35
Pantothenic acid (mg/kg)	20	15	12	20	20	15	12	20
Choline (mg/kg)	500	400	300	500	500	400	300	500
Vitamin B_{12} (μg/kg)	20	15	10	20	20	15	10	20
Biotin (μg/kg)	100	50	50	100	100	50	50	100

[a] Self-fed a diet containing 3300 to 3600 kcal ME/kg.

programs. Energy intake can then be restricted by limiting feed intake to about 2 kg daily. Increasing the dietary fiber level to reduce energy content can also accomplish a restricted energy intake but at a higher feed level. Energy requirements are approximately 25% greater during extreme cold temperatures for boars exposed to outside lots in winter months.

The protein (amino acid) requirement of growing boars is greater than that of barrows or gilts. This is not unexpected, since boars gain faster than gilts and equal to (Newell and Bowland 1972; Knudson et al. 1985) or faster than (Siers 1975; Wood and Riley 1982) barrows and are also more efficient and have less backfat than do gilts and barrows (Siers 1975). Average daily gain and feed:gain ratio are maximized for growing boars fed corn-soybean meal diets at levels of 20% protein during the growing period of 24 to 55 kg followed by 18% protein from 55 to 100 kg (Tyler et al. 1983). A 14% to 15% protein diet is suggested for boars being limited-fed from 6 to 8 months of age. Developing boars require 0.15% to 0.25% more dietary lysine than barrows of similar weight (Williams et al. 1984). Requirements for other indispensable amino acids have not been established for developing boars.

Adequate dietary levels of calcium and phosphorus are necessary for maximum bone development because of rapid mineral deposition during early growth. Growing boars fed diets containing calcium and phosphorus levels of 125% to 200% of NRC (1979) suggested levels had heavier and stronger bones than boars fed 100% calcium and phosphorus levels (Nimmo et al. 1980; Kesel et al. 1983). The calcium:phosphorus ratio of the diet should be maintained at about 1.3:1, and the phosphorus level should be between 0.5% and 0.8% for optimum performance and bone development of growing boars. Specific nutrient recommendations for developing gilts and boars are presented in Table 32.3.

SUMMARY

Developing gilts and boars to be used in the breeding herd should be self-fed high-energy diets that promote optimal growth and development. This practice is necessary to obtain meaningful selection data on individual growth and backfat. Energy can be limited after weights of 80 to 90 kg in gilts and 100 to 110 kg in boars without affecting sexual maturity or future reproductive performance. Energy can be restricted by hand feeding approximately 2 kg of a 14% corn-soybean meal protein diet fortified to contain minerals and vitamins at levels suggested in Table 32.3. Animals housed in enclosed, environmentally controlled confinement require about 10% less feed than those reared outside. Feed intake should also be increased approximately 25% during extreme cold, such as may occur in December, January, and February in northern areas of the United States.

REFERENCES

Anderson, L.L., and R.M. Melampy. 1972. In: *Pig Production.* Cole, D.J.A. (Ed.). pp. 329–366. London: Butterworths.

Brooks, P.H., and D.J.A. Cole. 1970. *J. Reprod. Fertil.* 23:435.
Brooks, P.H., and D.J.A. Cole. 1973. *Anim. Prod.* 17:305.
Burnett, P.J., and N. Walker. 1988. *Anim. Prod.* 46:427.
Christenson, R.K. 1981. *J. Anim. Sci.* 52:821.
Christensen, R.K., and J.J. Ford. 1979. *J. Anim. Sci.* 49:743.
Cunningham, P.J., et al. 1974. *J. Anim. Sci.* 39:63.
den Hartog, L.A., and G.J.M. van Kempen. 1980. *Neth. J. Agric. Sci.* 28:211.
Dufour, J., and C. Bernard. 1968. *Can J. Anim. Sci.* 48:425.
Esbenshade, K.L., et al. 1979. *J. Anim. Sci.* 48:246.
Friend, D.W. 1973. *J. Anim. Sci.* 37:701.
Friend, D.W. 1976. *J. Anim. Sci.* 43:404.
Friend, D.W., G.W. Lodge, and J.I. Elliot. 1981. *J. Anim. Sci.* 53:118.
Hafez, E.S.E. 1959. *J. Anim. Sci.* 18:1178 (Abstr.).
Haines, C.E., A.C. Warnick, and H.D. Wallace. 1959. *J. Anim. Sci.* 18:347.
Hays, V.W. 1978. The role of antibiotics in efficient livestock production. In: *Nutrition and Drug Interrelations.* Hatch, J.N., and J.Coon (Eds.). pp. 545–576. New York: Academic Press.
Hemsworth, P.H., J.K. Findlay, and R.G. Beilharz. 1978. *Anim. Prod.* 27:201.
Hill, G.M., and E.R. Miller. 1983. *J. Anim. Sci.* 57:106.
Hughes, P.E., and D.J.A. Cole. 1976. *Anim. Prod.* 23:89.
Hughes, P.E., and M.A. Varley. 1980. *Reproduction in the Pig.* London: Butterworths.
Jones, R.D., and C.V. Maxwell. 1974. *J. Anim. Sci.* 39:1067.
Kesel, G.A., et al. 1983. *J. Anim. Sci.* 57:82.
Kirkwood, R.N., and F.X. Aherne. 1985. *J. Anim. Sci.* 60:1518.
Knudson, B.K., et al. 1985. *J. Anim. Sci.* 61:789.
Kornegay, E.T., and H.R. Thomas. 1981. *J. Anim. Sci.* 52:1049.
Kornegay, E.T., H.R. Thomas, and J.L. Baker. 1981a. *J. Anim. Sci.* 52:1070.
Kornegay, E.T., et al. 1981b. *J. Anim. Sci.* 52:1085.
Kornegay, E.T., et al. 1985. *J. Anim. Sci.* 61:1460.
Liptrap, D.O., et al. 1970. *J. Anim. Sci.* 30:736.
Lodge, G.A., and R.M. McPherson. 1961. *Anim. Prod.* 3:19.
National Research Council. 1988. *Nutrient Requirements of Swine.* 9th ed. Washington, DC: National Academy Press.
Newell, J.A., and J.P. Bowland. 1972. *Can. J. Anim. Sci.* 52:543.
Nimmo, R.D., et al. 1980. *J. Anim. Sci.* 51:100.
Nimmo, R.D., et al. 1981a. *J. Anim. Sci.* 52:1330.
Nimmo, R.D., et al. 1981b. *J. Anim. Sci.* 52:1343.
Ntunde, B.N., R.R. Hacker, and G.J. King. 1979. *J. Anim. Sci.* 48:401.
Pomeroy, R.W. 1960. *J. Agric. Sci.* 54:57.
Revelle, T.J., and O.W. Robison. 1973. *J. Anim. Sci.* 37:668.
Self, H.L., R.H. Grummer, and L.E. Casida. 1955. *J. Anim. Sci.* 14:573.
Siers, D.G. 1975. *J. Anim. Sci.* 41:522.
Teague, H.S., W.L. Roller, and A.P. Grifo, Jr. 1968. *J. Anim. Sci.* 27:408.
Thomas, H.R., et al. 1979. *Anim. Prod.* 28:231.
Thomas, H.R., and E.T. Kornegay. 1981. *J. Anim. Sci.* 52:1041.
Tyler, R.W., et al. 1983. *J. Anim. Sci.* 57:364.
Wahlstrom, R.C., and G.W. Libal. 1977. *J. Anim. Sci.* 45:94.
Wahlstrom, R.C., and O.E. Olson. 1959. *J. Anim. Sci.* 18:141.
Williams, W.D., et al. 1984. *J. Anim. Sci.* 58:657.
Wood, J.D., and J.E. Riley. 1982. *Anim. Prod.* 35:55.
Zimmerman, D.R., E.R. Peo, Jr., and D.B. Hudman. 1967. *J. Anim. Sci.* 26:514.
Zimmerman, D.R., et al. 1960. *J. Anim. Sci.* 19:687.

Chapter 33

Feeding Sows to Maximize Reproductive and Lactation Capabilities

G.W. Libal

Feeding the sow for maximum reproduction involves recognizing that the nutrient requirements are different during different stages of the sow's reproductive life. Nutrient levels may immediately affect the sow or may have an affect on subsequent production. Interpretation of research results as to nutrient requirements may lead to several different conclusions, depending on the response criteria chosen. Much of the research reported evaluated the sow's responses to nutrient levels or nutrition management over a relatively short portion of its reproductive life. Extremely valuable was the research that involved long-term or lifelong performance of the sow. Research summarized deals with energy, protein and amino acids, minerals, vitamins, and water, as well as interactions among the various nutrients. Utilization of various feedstuffs is also addressed. Conclusions as to the proper nutrient levels or the correct sow feeding management are not made. However, the literature has been reviewed and summarized to allow the readers to draw their own conclusions.

Measuring the effect of nutrition on the reproductive performance of swine is extremely difficult. The sow has the capability to cope with minor nutritional deficiencies. Positive or negative responses to nutrition are often very subtle and hard to measure. Individual animal variation in nutritional requirement or the degree of response to proper or deficient nutrient levels make real differences hard to detect. Many other environmental factors mask the sow's responses to nutrition. Interactions between nutrition and environment exist, but because they are sometimes not apparent, they are not always taken into consideration when drawing conclusions on sow nutrient requirements. Selection pressure for maternal traits and changing management systems can affect the requirements of the sow. The body of information about properly feeding sows is large. Much of the important information on basic concepts of sow nutrition is documented. However, there are still major voids in the information. While the effects of certain nutrient levels have been documented, the cause and effect mechanism often is not clear. Interactions between individual nutrients or between nutrient levels and certain environmental conditions and management practices have not been completely investigated. Contradictory or inconsistent results from research involving sows are present for many of the nutrients. Additive effects of responses obtained with addition of individual nutrients need additional investigation.

This chapter is an attempt to summarize the body of published information on feeding the sow for maximum reproductive performance. It is hoped that the reader will be able to sense the nutritional areas in which a consensus can be reached, the areas in which research results are too contradictory to draw conclusions, and the areas that have been ignored by researchers.

PROTEIN AND AMINO ACIDS

Gestation

The effect of restricted protein intake on growing-finishing pigs is well documented. Restricted protein intake of gilts during the prepuberal developmental stages has been investigated by Wahlstrom and Libal (1977), Cunningham et al. (1974), and Jones and Maxwell (1974). Reducing protein levels to 10% of the diet during the developmental period resulted in lower body weight at estrus and significantly older gilts at first estrus (Wahlstrom and Libal 1977; Cunningham et al. 1974). Jones and Maxwell (1974) reported the same trend when daily intake of crude protein was below 254 g/day (14% protein). They also reported an increase of number of corpora lutea at 30 days but no difference in embryo survival due to higher protein intake. Wahlstrom and Libal (1977) observed no differences in number of corpora lutea at 25 days or in number of pigs born live due to dietary protein levels prior to conception.

Severe protein restriction of the sow during gestation has been evaluated by Atinmo et al. (1974, 1976). Feeding a diet during gestation limited to 0.5% protein resulted in reduced brain and liver weights of newborn pigs. The pigs also had reduced serum albumin levels at birth and a lower RNA concentration of brain tissue at birth and slaughter. Growth rate of offspring of protein-restricted sows was significantly lower from 6 weeks until slaughter. Earlier research by Pond et al. (1968) produced no apparent effects on offspring for growth or carcass measurements. The investigators concluded that the dam was an effective buffer against protein deprivation. However, Hammell et al. (1976) reported an inconsistent but interesting learning response of offspring of protein-restricted sows. Pigs spent more time in a water maze and had higher avoidance scores when their dams had been fed a gestation protein level of 2% followed by 5% protein during lactation.

Reproductive performance as well as nitrogen balance of gravid gilts as related to gestation protein intake has been reported by Jones and Maxwell (1982) and Willis and Maxwell (1984). In those trials, as low as 146 or 119 g/day of protein supported reproductive performance (litter size and storage of nitrogen in reproductive tissue). However, muscle nitrogen retention was maximized at intake levels as high as 364 g/day of protein. These values agree favorably with those reported by Miller et al. (1969), who reported maximum nitrogen retention for sows with nitrogen intake between 285 and 345 g/day. Nitrogen retention is greater for gravid gilts than for nongravid gilts (Cuaron et al. 1983). These workers also found that accumulated third-day feeding compared with every-day feeding was detrimental to nitrogen retention, with the greatest urinary nitrogen excretion occurring during the second 24 hours after feeding.

Listed below are the amino acid requirements of the gravid sow as reported in the literature. Requirements are listed as reported by the researchers, either as a percentage of the diet or as grams per day or both. In most cases, the two reported values are linked together by the assumed feeding level of 1.8 kg/day.

Lysine	0.43%	7.8 g/day	Woerman and Speer (1976)
	0.47%		Corley et al. (1983)
	0.43%	7.7 g/day	Cuaron et al. (1984)
Tryptophan	0.084%	1.53 g/day	Meisinger and Speer (1979)
	0.09%		Corley et al. (1983)
	0.07%	1.4 g/day	Easter and Baker (1977)
Threonine	0.30%	5.4 g/day	Leonard and Speer (1983)
		6.83 g/day	Cuaron et al. (1984)
Methionine plus cystine	0.18%		Holden et al. (1971)
Isoleucine	0.25%		Speer et al. (1990)
Leucine	0.34%	6.8 g/day	Easter and Baker (1977)
Valine		5.9 g/day	Robles-Cabrera and Speer (1983)
Phenylalanine plus tyrosine	0.48%		Speet et al. (1990)
Phenylalanine	0.20%		Speer et al. (1990)
Arginine		0.0 g/day	Easter et al. (1974)

Lactation

Protein levels provided during lactation have been investigated by a number of research teams with the research approach varying from providing ad libitum consumption of feeds of different protein content to controlling level of feed consumption and thus daily level of crude protein. Protein level fed during gestation has been constant in some trials and has varied as a part of a protein sequence evaluation in others. The conclusion drawn as to appropriate lactation feeding level has differed somewhat, depending on the approach taken.

Baker et al. (1970b) demonstrated that the growth rates of pigs during a 21-day suckling period were reduced if an 8.7% protein diet had been fed throughout gestation even if a 16% protein lactation diet was provided during lactation. Providing a 16% protein diet during the first one third of gestation did not improve performance. However, when supplied during the last one third of gestation, pig performance was equal to that of pigs from sows receiving the high-protein diet throughout gestation. Both gilt and sow litters responded similarly. Hawton and Meade (1971) evaluated the effects of daily protein levels of 154, 250, and 341 g during gestation on offspring development. Pig gains to 21 days were greatest for the highest daily gestation protein level. Holden et al. (1968) evaluated gestation protein levels of 8%, 12%, 16%, and 20% fed at 1.82 kg over four parities. This allowed for daily protein levels ranging from 146 to 364 g. Crude protein content of sows' milk at 2 weeks and pig weights at weaning increased with increasing gestation protein levels. Number of pigs produced was not affected. The lower level of protein during gestation was satisfactory to support reproduction but not to support maximum pig gains. Lucas et al. (1969) reported that essential plasma amino acid levels increased during both gestation and lactation with the increasing daily gestation protein levels in the previous study.

Protein intake during lactation and its effects on milk composition and pig performance has been evaluated. Elliot et al. (1971) found that colostrum from sows fed 15% protein diets for 30 days prior to parturition and throughout a 35-day lactation was higher in protein and slightly higher in total solids and solids not fat than samples from sows receiving 5% or 10% protein. Milk samples at 7, 14, and 21 days of lactation did not reflect dietary treatments. Mahan et al. (1971a) also found that milk composition was not altered by dietary protein level during lactation. The only differences observed were increases in nonprotein nitrogen (NPN) and decreases in albumin as protein was reduced from 18% to either 14% or 10%. As dietary protein decreased, lower milk volume and quantity of milk constituents were observed. Sows receiving an opaque-2 corn diet (9.7% protein) responded similarly to those receiving the 10% protein diet.

Listed below are estimates of the amino acid requirements of the lactating sow as reported in the literature. Requirements are given as reported by the researcher, either as a percentage of the diet or in grams per day or both. In most cases, the assumption linking the two values together is feed consumption during lactation averaging 5.45 kg per day.

Lysine	0.60%	20.0 g/day	Boomgaardt et al. (1972)
	0.55%		Lewis and Speer (1973)
	0.50%		Lewis and Speer (1974a)
Tryptophan	0.12%	3.9 g/day	Lewis and Speer (1974b)
	0.091%		Lewis and Speer (1974a)
Threonine	0.42%	5.45 g/day	Lewis and Speer (1975)
Methionine plus cystine	0.23%		Ganguli et al. (1971)
Isoleucine	0.39%		Haught and Speer (1977)
Leucine	0.46%		Rousselow et al. (1979)
Valine	0.53%		Rousselow and Speer (1980)
Phenylalanine plus tyrosine	0.75%	41.2 g/day	Lellis and Speer (1985)
Phenylalanine	0.34%	18.7 g/day	Lellis and Speer (1987)

The effect of protein levels provided primiparous sows during both gestation and lactation was evaluated by several workers. DeGeeter et al. (1972, 1973) found that litter size and birth weights of pigs were similar for sows receiving 5% or 17% protein diets during gestation, although gestation weight gain was less for sows receiving the low-protein diet. A carry-over effect of low gestation protein was lower growth rate during lactation for pigs, including cross-fostered pigs nursing sows that had received low-protein diets during gestation. Survival rate was not affected except in the presence of enteritis, which claimed more pigs nursing sows that had received low-protein diets. Although both gestation and lactation protein levels affected performance of pigs during lactation, the effect of lactation protein level was more dramatic. A subsequent effect on weaned pig performance was also documented, with pigs from sows receiving low-protein during gestation gaining at a slower rate than pigs from sows receiving adequate protein. Similar protein levels were evaluated for first-litter gilts by Shields et al. (1985). It was found that litter weights were lower and sow mortality higher when 5% protein was fed as compared with 14% protein during gestation. Protein was catabolized during late gestation and fat reserves mobilized during lactation to a greater extent for sows fed the 5% protein gestation diet.

The NCR-42 Committee on Swine Nutrition (1978) reported that sows fed 9% protein tended to farrow fewer pigs, but that gestation protein level had little effect on pig weights or numbers at 14 days. It appeared that the response of 14-day weight to lactation protein level (12% versus 16%) was greater for pigs from sows receiving 9% protein during gestation than for pigs from sows receiving 15% protein. No advantage for 20% protein during lactation was observed. Mahan (1977, 1979) observed that sows fed either 8.5% or 9% protein diets gained less during gestation than sows fed 12% or 14% protein. Lactation weight gain was greater, although feed intake during lactation was not higher for the sows fed low protein during gestation. It appeared that milk production was suppressed initially for sows fed low protein. Weaning weights of pigs were affected negatively in one trial, but not in the other, by the low gestation protein levels for sows. The investigator concluded that either a 14%-14% or 14%-15% protein sequence for gestation and lactation was superior to a low protein (8.5% or 9%) followed by a higher protein level for lactation. A 12%-16% gestation and lactation protein sequence also produced satisfactory reproductive results. Mahan and Grifo (1975) found that the amino acid-protein requirement during lactation was higher if sows had been fed an 8.2% corn diet during gestation. Sow lactation feed consumption, sow weight gain, and pig weights at weaning responded to lactation protein levels increasing from 12% to 20%. Haye et al. (1981) reported that gestation-lactation protein sequences for sows of 14%-14%, 12%-14%, and 9%-18% all produced similar antibody response and serum immunoglobulin concentrations in their offspring.

ENERGY

The energy needs of the reproducing sow at various stages of production and life cycle may be the most studied and, yet, the least understood portion of nutrition management of swine. Depending on the criteria evaluated, several logical recommendations can be made for the sow's requirements. The sow has the ability to protect the developing fetus from energy limitation and the ability to transfer body stores of energy-rich nutrients to conceptus development and milk production. Thus, short-duration studies evaluating energy for the reproducing sow may lead to conclusions that do not take into consideration the long-term consequences for future production of that sow. Evaluation of the energy requirements of sows at one stage of production without regard for the energy supplied at other stages may lead to recommendations that are of little value when considering the entire life cycle of reproducing swine.

Prebreeding

The response of gilts to increased energy levels prior to breeding (flushing) is well documented. Edey et al. (1972) found that gilts fed a high plane of nutrition (ad libitum) from 170 days of age produced 2.5 more corpora lutea than gilts fed a low plane of nutrition (1.4 kg of feed/day). Cox et al. (1987) reported that an energy level of 9.96 Mcal of metabolizable energy (ME)/day resulted in 2.4 more corpora lutea than when 5.77 Mcal of ME/day was fed the last 11 days of the estrus cycle for 8- to 9-month-old gilts. Administration of insulin also increased estimates of ovulation rate by 2.4. Moore et al. (1973) reported that allowing gilts ad libitum consumption for 24 hours at the onset of estrus yielded no increase in ovulation rate. However, ad libitum consumption of feed for 14 days prior to estrus resulted in 1.9 additional corpora lutea. Effects of the higher energy and insulin administration appeared to be additive. Schultz et al. (1966) found that gilts receiving 3.6 kg of feed for one estrous cycle before breeding had three additional corpora lutea than gilts receiving 1.8 kg of feed. They also documented the detrimental effects of high energy during early pregnancy. Ray and McCarty (1965) demonstrated that temporary fasting of gilts for 24, 48, or 72 hours after mating had no detrimental effects on ovulation rate or embryo survival. No response to higher feed levels was observed by Ruiz et al. (1968) when the higher feeding level was maintained for the entire breeding period for gilts pen mated. Increased embryo mortality during the first 25 days postbreeding was found when the higher feeding level was maintained past breeding. Positive response to increasing energy prior to breeding has not been reported in the literature for mature sows or sows that are being rebred (Myers and Speer 1973). Tribble and Orr (1982) found that doubling the sow's feed from 1.8 to 3.6 kg from weaning to breeding did not shorten interval to estrus or improve reproductive performance. First-litter sows tended to more readily consume the higher feeding level, possibly indicating a higher energy requirement than second- and third-litter sows.

Knabe et al. (1986) found that depriving sows of feed for 48 hours immediately prior to weaning actually increased the weaning-to-breeding interval and adversely affected farrowing rates of primiparous sows. Allrich et al. (1979) reported that fasting sows for 2, 3, or 4 days after weaning had no effect on interval from weaning to estrus or on embryo survival. However, for sows weaned after a 30-day lactation, fasting reduced number of live pigs born. No beneficial aspects to fasting sows after weaning at 21 or 30 days of lactation were observed.

Gestation

Buitrago et al. (1974a) found that gilts were responsive in gestation weight gain to energy level fed during gestation (2.2, 5.1, and 8.0 Mcal of digestible energy [DE]). Weight change during lactation also reflected the gestation feeding levels, but in the opposite direction, with increasing weight loss occurring as a result of higher gestation energy levels. The only response in reproduction to varying energy levels was lighter birth weights for pigs fed the low-energy diet. Frobish et al. (1966) reported that feeding 10.8 Mcal of ME resulted in more net sow weight gain per reproductive cycle, but no change in reproductive performance as compared with sows receiving 5.4 Mcal. Frobish et al. (1973) evaluated energy levels for gilts over three reproducing cycles. Numbers and weights of pigs weaned were not different for sows receiving 3.0, 4.5, 6.0, or 7.5 Mcal of ME. However, birth weights of pigs reflected the sow's energy levels, and sow weight change was greater for sows receiving higher energy. The greatest increase in sow weight occurred between the 3.0- and 4.5-ME treatment groups. Fewer sows receiving 7.5 Mcal of ME completed three reproductive cycles than from groups receiving the lower energy levels. Similar results were reported by Libal and Wahlstrom (1977). A linear response in sow gestation gain to ME levels from 4.0 to 7.0 Mcal was observed. There was a tendency for sows gaining more during gestation to gain less or lose more weight during lactation. A linear decrease in number of live pigs born due to gestation energy level was observed. Although no difference in number of pigs weaned was found due to gestation energy level supplied, pig and litter weaning weights peaked for litters from sows receiving 6.0 Mcal of ME. Feeding 4.4 Mcal of ME resulted in lower gestation gains and lighter pigs at birth than when 7.3 Mcal of ME was provided to gilts in a study by Vermedahl et al. (1969). However, number of live pigs born and vigor of pigs was not affected. Hoppe (1990) evaluated gestation energy levels of 6.0 and 9.0 Mcal of ME for Large White × Landrace sows for four parities. The 6.0-ME level supported adequate gains and reproductive performance with less extreme changes in weight during gestation and lactation. Sow backfat was greater for sows receiving 9.0 Mcal of ME after one parity and remained greater over four parities. Body weight was the same between groups of sows, indicating that a change in body composition had resulted due to feeding regimen imposed.

It has been proposed that body condition may be the best indicator of adequacy of energy during gestation. However, Esbenshade et al. (1986) found that changes in sow body condition typically observed in commercial production units may be too subtle to have an effect on reproductive performance. Correlations between body condition and other criteria were low. Pond et al. (1983) reported that sows from genetically obese lines responded to gestation feeding levels of 2.0 Mcal of DE by gaining more weight and more fat than contemporary control or lean-line sows. They observed that all sows gained weight when fed 6.0 Mcal of DE during gestation. Using gravid sows in both normal and thin condition, de Lange et al. (1980) found that nitrogen and energy balances before parturition were not related to sow condition. After parturition, however, thin sows produced less energy in their milk than normal sows. Additional feed during lactation more adequately prevented protein loss from thin sows than normal-condition sows. Johnston et al. (1987) found that sow backfat at weaning was not related to days to first estrus after weaning for sows with a weaning-to-estrus interval < 10 days. However, when the interval was more than 10 days, backfat level was a factor.

The method or frequency of delivery of feed to the sow was evaluated by Michel et al. (1980). Feeding 1.9 kg of feed daily or feeding 5.7 kg of feed every third day resulted in sows losing similar weight during lactation and weaning litters similar in number and weight. Gilts gained less weight during gestation in both the first and second parity and also farrowed fewer live pigs in the first parity when fed every third day. Backfat changes (increase during gestation and decrease during lactation) were greater for sows fed daily.

Restriction of feed or nutrients during gestation has been evaluated by Pond et al. (1985, 1986) and Hard and Anderson (1982). Restriction of feed intake to one third of normal during the first two thirds of gestation resulted in reduced weight gain and fat accretion of offspring during young adulthood (Pond et al. 1985). Hard and Anderson (1982) observed that offspring of dams that had severe nutrient deprivation during the middle and last thirds of gestation exhibited no detrimental effects on reproduction and actually reached puberty at an earlier age. Pond et al. (1986) reported that feeding primiparous gilts one third of their energy requirement to day 84 or day 108 resulted in reduced fetal weight and no evidence of pregnancy anabolism. They also documented that the greater weight gain of pregnant animals compared with nonpregnant animals was attributable to increase in uterine and mammary tissue. Buitrago et al. (1974b) reported that severe restriction of energy of the dam during gestation resulted in a reduction of fat, glucose, and protein of the fetus.

Preparturition

It has been theorized that increasing energy during late gestation would better meet the energy demands of pregnancy, provide additional nutrient stores for milk production, and, depending on the energy source, increase the substrate or products needed by the newborn to survive during the first critical days after parturition. McNamara et al. (1985) found that fatty acid metabolism changes during the late stages of pregnancy redirect energy flow from maternal adipose tissue to mammary and fetal development. Thulin et al. (1989) reported that only trace amounts of free fatty acids cross the placental tissues during late gestation and their contribution to fetal energy supply and storage was limited. Ojamaa et al. (1980) found that severe restriction of energy from day 85 of gestation did not result in differences in litter size at parturition. However, feeding 0.45 kg of feed daily did result in no gestation sow gain and a tendency for a shorter gestation period and lighter pigs at birth as compared with sows fed 1.36 kg daily.

Liver and muscle glycogen concentrations were reduced as well. Pond et al. (1981) fed gravid sows double their allotted gestation energy level (6.0 versus 12.0 Mcal of DE) from day 100 of gestation until parturition. The additional energy was supplied by cornstarch. No changes were observed in birth or weaning weights or survival rate due to the additional energy. Results from a large cooperative study indicated that increasing gestation feeding levels by 1.36 kg from day 90 of gestation to parturition was advantageous in increasing numbers of pigs born alive and weaned and in increasing birth and weaning weights (Cromwell et al. 1989). Sows fed the additional levels of feed gained more weight during gestation and lost more weight during lactation, with more net gain to the end of lactation than sows receiving the lower feeding level. The differences observed were relatively small; but, because of the 1080 litters observed, were statistically documented. Boyd et al. (1978a) evaluated increasing ME levels from the control gestation level of 5.75 Mcal to 9.3 Mcal from day 100 of gestation to parturition with either tallow or cornstarch. Nonsignificant increases in survival rate were observed with the addition of tallow, particularly among pigs weighing <1.0 kg at birth. Fat content of colostrum, but not milk, was increased in sows receiving the diets supplemented with tallow. Addition of tallow to the lactation diet caused higher fat content of milk throughout the lactation period. Boyd et al. (1978b) also observed that tallow additions during late gestation resulted in higher piglet glucose concentrations at birth and at 6 and 24 hours after birth. Level of liver glycogen was also numerically, but not significantly, higher for pigs from dams receiving tallow as compared with those receiving cornstarch supplementation. Seerley et al. (1974) observed that feeding corn oil to sows from day 109 of gestation until parturition resulted in greater survival of pigs weighing <1.0 kg and higher linoleic acid and total fatty acid content of the liver and muscles of newborn pigs. Pigs from sows fed corn oil also had better thermostability than pigs from sows fed cornstarch. Seerley et al. (1978a) found that sows that had received animal fat from day 104 of gestation provided pigs with colostrum and milk that was higher in oleic acid and total lipids during the first 6 days of lactation as compared with sows receiving cornstarch. However, when pigs were fasted during the first 6 days after parturition, fat utilization by pigs from sows fed fat was relatively low. The addition of 15% lipid to the sow's diet in the form of casein-encapsulated white grease from day 109 of gestation through lactation resulted in increased piglet survival and weight gain (Cieslak et al. 1983). The greatest improvement in survival occurred for those pigs weighing from 700 to 1100 g at birth. Feeding either 10% fat or 23% high-fructose corn syrup from day 88 of gestation and through lactation (Coffey et al. 1987) resulted in no differences in pig numbers, weights, or survivability. However, fewer stillbirths and higher lipid content of milk as well as more total milk volume resulted from sows receiving fat. Seerley (1989) fed sows 5% solid fat from day 80 of gestation or 10% solid fat from day 100 of gestation and continued feeding the diets through lactation. Pigs from either group of sows had higher liver glycogen levels and also higher blood glucose levels at birth than pigs from sows not fed fat. However, survival rate was high for all groups of pigs and was not affected by the sow's nutritional treatment. Weaned pig gains were lower for pigs from sows fed diets containing fat.

Lactation

Energy intake requirement during lactation is affected by energy demands dependent on number of pigs nursing and by quantity of energy stored as body fat as well as the degree to which these body stores can be reduced without affecting subsequent performance. As stated earlier, voluntary feed intake during lactation can be influenced by level of energy intake during gestation and thus logically by levels of body stores of fat. Intake itself becomes the limiting factor in nutritionally managing the sow herd during lactation.

Feeding sows during lactation based on the number of pigs nursing has been investigated by Hitchcock et al. (1971) and Libal and Wahlstrom (1975). In both studies, a comparison was made between feeding 0.45 kg of feed per nursing pig and ad libitum feeding. In both trials (the former was 49 days long and the latter was 21 days long), feed intake was less and sow weight losses greater over the lactation period when the limited feeding regimen was imposed. However, no differences in numbers or weights of pigs were observed due to feed intake level. Pigs that received creep feed (in the former trial only) consumed significantly more feed if their dams were receiving restricted levels of lactation feed. The feeding level in these two trials (0.45 kg/pig) is below the estimated needs of the sow for each additional pig nursing (0.5 to 0.6 kg/pig) as estimated by Verstegen et al. (1985) with an energy balance trial. Stahly et al. (1979) evaluated the effects of gradually increasing sow feed levels over a 7-day period as compared with allowing ad libitum feed consumption. All sows received the lactation diet ad libitum after the initial week. Increasing the feeding levels by 0.9 kg/day from 0 on day 0 to 6.3 kg on day 7 resulted in less total feed consumption and more total weight loss for sows over the 21-day lactation. However, no differences in pig survival or weights due to lactation regimen were observed. Noblet and Etienne (1986) evaluated the effect of lactation energy levels of 14.2 and 10.4 Mcal of ME/day on milk production, milk composition, and litter performance. While total milk production was reduced, concentration of fat and nitrogen in the milk was increased from sows receiving the lower lactation energy level, leading to equal intake of energy by pigs of both sow groups. No difference in litter growth rate was observed.

Nelssen et al. (1985a) found that 12 or 14 Mcal of ME/day was adequate for maintaining sow weight, for postweaning estrus interval, and for litter performance to weaning. However, 10 Mcal was not sufficient energy for these criteria. In three trials, Reese et al. (1982a) documented that feeding 8 Mcal of ME/day during lactation resulted in greater sow weight loss, and fewer sows exhibiting estrus by day 7 postweaning (by day 70 in two trials) than when 16 Mcal was fed. In the one trial where an intermediate level of ME was provided, sows fed 12 Mcal of ME responded similarly to those receiving the higher energy level. In subsequent performance (Reese et al. 1982b), sows that had received the low-energy intake during lactation gained more weight, deposited more backfat, and farrowed lighter pigs in parity two. However, farrowing rate was not influenced by the previous lactation energy treatment. Lactation performance during the second lactation was largely a function of the immediate lactation feeding treatment (high or low energy) and not the previous lactation treatment. Again, estrus was delayed when 8 Mcal of ME/day was fed during lactation. Johnston et al. (1986) concluded that 12.5 Mcal of ME/day during lactation supported adequate rebreeding performance and reproductive performance equal to 16 Mcal of ME/day during lactation. Reese et al. (1984) reported that sows that lost more body fat during lactation when restricted in dietary energy (8 Mcal ME/day) had slower return to estrus than sows that lost less body fat, even when weight changes were similar. Failure to return to estrus could not be predicted by backfat levels. However, the group of sows that received 16 Mcal of ME/day had higher body fat and fewer individuals failing to return to estrus by day 14 of lactation. Armstrong et al. (1986) reported that a similar low-energy intake during lactation resulted in lower body condition of sows as compared with those fed approximately 12 Mcal of ME/day. However, no difference in return to estrus was observed between the two groups. Klaver et al. (1981) observed that thin sows produced less milk, energy, and protein than sows in adequate condition and that lactation feeding level had no effect on quantity or composition of milk. Energy utilized for milk production can be supplied directly from the feed, or energy can be mobilized from the sow's tissue stores. Bendemuhl et al. (1987, 1989) documented that energy and protein intake during lactation had an effect on sow body composition. Composition of weight lost during lactation was diet dependent. Sows fed diets deficient in protein but adequate in energy lost large amounts of protein from muscles and organs. Energy deficiency resulted in fat loss. Verstegen et al. (1985) have estimated that the sow's efficiency of milk production from feed is about 62%. Noblet and Etienne (1987) reported that utilization of energy for milk production from food is 72% and from body reserves is 88%. The overall efficiency of storing energy during pregnancy and its mobilization during lactation is approximately 68% to 71%.

There is evidence that the source of energy supplied during lactation may be as important as the amount of energy. Seerley et al. (1978b) found that colostrum of sows fed corn oil as an additional energy source from day 109 of gestation contained more calories and total lipids as well as linoleic acid than did colostrum of sows fed cornstarch. Fat utilization by the pigs was similar for offspring of both sow groups. Miller et al. (1971) reported that, as compared with an isocaloric diet without fat, the addition of 10% corn oil to lactation diets caused sows' colostrum and milk to be elevated in linoleic acid and that the fat stores of pigs consuming the milk reflected the fatty acid profile of the milk at 21 days of age. In contrast, Nelssen et al. (1985b) found that replacing cornstarch with tallow in lactation diets of primiparous sows was not beneficial when energy intake was equal. Coffey et al. (1982) observed that adding animal fat to prelactation diets or both prelactation and lactation diets increased milk yield at day 14 of lactation. Percent total lipids and vitamin A in the milk were increased by fat addition to the lactation diet. In a nutrient balance study, Lellis and Speer (1983) evaluated lactation diets containing energy from either dextrose or tallow. Efficiency of milk production was greater for sows receiving tallow. Addition of tallow led to higher milk fat as a percentage of dry matter, and sows gained more weight during lactation when fed the diet that included tallow.

Higher milk yield and greater sow weight losses were documented for sows fed fructose supplied by corn syrup than when an equivalent amount of carbohydrate was supplied as dextrose or when a corn-soybean diet was provided (White et al. 1984a).

That pigs displayed elevated plasma glucose and fructose and lower insulin increase after eating a diet containing fructose suggests that fructose spares glucose (White et al. 1984b).

The effects of adding fat to the diet of lactating sows on performance of their offspring to market weight have been evaluated. Friend (1974) found that feeding fat to sows for 5 days prior to farrowing resulted in more fat in the milk and higher levels of linoleic acid in the carcass fat of day-old pigs. This increase in linoleic acid persisted until market weight. No differences in performance of pigs to market weight or carcass merit due to lactation fat levels were observed. Stahly et al. (1981) reported that addition of 10% fat that was high in oleic or linoleic acid to lactation diets increased ME and fat content of milk as compared with milk from sows fed a low-fat diet. However, pig survival and pig gains to weaning were not changed. Subsequent performance included depressed feed intake and gains from weaning to 49 days of age, compensatory performance after 49 days of age, and a resulting equal performance from birth to market weight for offspring of sows fed fat.

Interactions of sources of energy or total energy intake with environmental conditions during lactation are also important. Cox et al. (1983) observed that supplementing lactation diets with fat in the summer months may be advantageous because of lower feed intake and longer weaning-to-estrus intervals. Shurson et al. (1986) reported the results of a study specifically designed to evaluate fat addition to sow's diets as related to seasonal differences and found that the interaction did not exist under conditions of the study. Interval to estrus was longer in the summer than the winter, and sows receiving fat in their diets tended to return to estrus more quickly. However, the response to fat was similar in both seasons. Sows receiving fat in their diets weaned heavier litters and individual pigs because of higher milk yields and higher fat concentration in their milk. Schoenherr et al. (1989b) found that the effects of heat stress on milk yield and litter weight are minimized by choice white grease addition to the diet. Fiber additions were detrimental to these same criteria. In a thermoneutral environment, milk yield was increased by addition of either fat or fiber in early lactation but not in late lactation. Heat exposure depressed feed intake (Schoenherr et al. 1989a) but did not alter digestibility of feed components. Dietary fiber additions depressed energy retention and apparent nitrogen digestibility. Dietary fat additions did not affect energy digestibility but increased nitrogen digestion and retention in both a thermoneutral and a hot environment.

Compounds that can be fed or administered in some other manner have been used in an attempt to alter the metabolism of the sow, increase the stores of desirable nutrients within the fetus, alter the metabolism of the newborn to enhance the chances of survival, or alter the nutrient content of the colostrum and milk of the sow. None is presently used, but some appear promising if economically feasible.

In an attempt to increase embryo survival, Schultz et al. (1966) fed orally active progesterone from 4 days postbreeding. Embryo survival was increased in the treated group. Feeding orally active progesterone (altrenogest) for 7 days after weaning did not result in a higher percentage of gilts exhibiting estrus in summer months (Stevenson et al. 1985), but it did result in a delay in estrus and an associated increased farrowing rate and larger litters from more of the treated sows.

The effect of chlorpropamide, an oral hypoglycemic compound, was evaluated for sows by Wachholz and Wahlstrom (1973). Feeding chlorpropamide caused increases in fetal blood glucose. Litter size and embryo survival were not affected. The effects of late gestation feeding of dichlorvos have been reported by Siers et al. (1976) and Young et al. (1979). In the former study, dichlorvos feeding from day 80 of gestation resulted in more live pigs at birth and heavier litters at all stages of growth. Lipid content of the colostrum was increased for sows receiving dichlorvos. In the latter study, sows receiving dichlorvos produced litters with an average of 0.5 more live pigs regardless of whether they were parasite-infected or parasite-free. Individual pig weight and litter weight were increased as a result of feeding dichlorvus. Bishop et al. (1985) reported that the addition of triamcinolone, a dietary glucocorticoid, to a diet that contained soybean oil for 9 days prepartum resulted in increased pig weights and increased fat content of colostrum. This glucocorticoid failed to increase energy reserves as measured by liver glycogen concentration of the newborn pig.

The effects of 1,3-butanediol, a synthetic carbohydrate with ketogenic properties, on pig metabolites and survival have been reported by Spence et al. (1985) and Stahly et al. (1986). In the former report, it was indicated that 1,3-butanediol or a mixture of acetate and lactate produced similar effects when fed to sows from day 90 of gestation. More total liver glycogen at birth and a trend for more plasma glucose after 24 hours and 36 hours of fasting were observed when compared with pigs from sows receiving cornstarch. However, sow plasma beta-hydroxybutyrate was higher and plasma glucose was lower for sows fed 1,3-butanediol. In the latter report, sows fed either lard or 1,3-butanediol weaned more pigs as a result of higher survival rate from birth to weaning as compared with sows receiving cornstarch. Improvement in survival was greater for pigs from sows fed the synthetic carbohydrate than for pigs from sows fed fat.

Use of exogenous growth hormone during the first 21 days of gestation has been evaluated by Kveragas et al. (1986). Sows administered porcine growth hormone injections exhibited higher plasma insulin and glucose levels, indicating an insulin resistance. Serum free fatty acids were elevated in sows fed a control diet but not in sows fed a diet containing both glucose and fat, and pigs from this group had higher serum glucose concentrations. Pigs receiving injections had more total body lipids and tended to have higher free-fatty-acid concentrations.

The effect of maternal diabetes on energy reserves of newborn pigs and on subsequent reproductive performance was reported by Ezekwe and Martin (1978), Ezekwe et al. (1984), and Ezekwe (1986). Maternal diabetic conditions were established with sows on day 80 of gestation by intravenous injections of alloxan in the first study and streptozotocin in the latter studies. Liver weight and total liver glycogen were increased for offspring of sows injected with alloxin. Serum glucose concentration increased and insulin concentration decreased when a high dose of streptozotocin (100 mg/kg) was administered. Pig liver glycogen and lipid content were increased. Maternal free-fatty-acid concentration also increased. Either alloxan or streptozotocin was effective in altering the nutrient supply to the newborn pig. No effects on the reproductive status or energy status of pigs produced in the next parity were observed. The residual effects of streptozotocin on the sow appear to be dose related. Evidence of continued diabetic condition as measured by maternal glucose and free-fatty-acid concentration was found for doses of 100 mg/kg but not for doses of 50 mg/kg.

Aherne and Speer (1974) reported that including thyroprotein at 220 mg/kg of lactation diet resulted in increased 21-day pig gains as a result of milk containing higher concentrations of dry matter, protein, and energy. Total milk production at various stages of lactation was numerically greater for sows fed thyroprotein, and those sows lost more weight and backfat and produced smaller litters at their subsequent farrowings. Giesemann et al. (1989) found that feeding thyroprotein for 2 days prior to weaning and for 14 days following weaning had no effect on postweaning return to estrus or interval to estrus. Sows fed thyroprotein did have elevated levels of T_3 and T_4.

MINERALS

Zinc

Hill et al. (1983a,b,c) evaluated zinc (Zn) levels ranging from 0 to 5000 ppm in diets of gravid gilts. Number and weight of pigs at parturition were not affected by dietary Zn level. However, higher numbers of abnormal pigs were farrowed by sows receiving no supplemental Zn. Sows fed 5000 ppm Zn exhibited a mild Zn toxicity with less body weight at the completion of two parities, higher incidence of osteochondrosis, lower hepatic iron (Fe) stores, higher renal copper (Cu) and Zn concentrations, and higher Zn and lower Cu concentrations in the aorta. There were also higher Zn and lower Cu concentrations in the serum. Colostrum contained less Cu and phosphorus (P) than did colostrum from sows receiving less supplemental Zn. Pigs produced by sows receiving 5000 ppm Zn had heavier organ weights, higher Fe and Zn stores, lower Cu stores, and higher liver calcium (Ca) and manganese (Mn) levels. P and Zn levels were higher in the kidney on day 1 than on day 21. The opposite effect was seen for pigs from sows receiving 0, 50, and 500 ppm Zn. Further evidence of the mild toxicity and the interrelationship of dietary Zn and other minerals was reported by Hill et al. (1983d). Feeding the sow 5000 ppm Zn induced a Cu deficiency in early-weaned offspring fed diets unsupplemented with Cu. Number and weight of pigs at parturition were not affected by dietary zinc level. However, higher numbers of abnormal pigs were farrowed by sows receiving no supplemental zinc. This work seems to agree with earlier findings by Hedges et al. (1976) that supported supplementation of a diet that contained 33 ppm Zn from natural feed ingredients. Although reproductive performance was not improved by 50 ppm Zn addition, Zn body stores of the offspring and their growth rate was increased.

Iron

The Fe requirement of sows during gestation and lactation has not been established. Spruill et al. (1971) found that supplementation of sow diets with 700 ppm resulted in a slight nonsignificant change in placental transfer of Fe as measured by blood parameters of the newborn offspring. Mammary transfer of Fe was unchanged. However, higher hemoglobin, hematocrit, and serum Fe were observed for pigs at 21 days of lactation. The investigators suggested that access to the sow's feces may explain the improvement in Fe status. Ducsay et al. (1984) demonstrated that injections of Fe-dextran through the middle of gestation produced higher levels of uteroferrin, which is involved with maternal-to-fetal transfer of Fe. However, the increase in placental transfer of Fe was small and probably of little value in prevention of anemia. Lillie and Frobish (1978) found no difference in sow or offspring hematology at parturition and 21 days postpartum when gestation and lactation diets were supplemented with 100 or 200 ppm Fe.

Copper

Lillie and Frobish (1978) evaluated dietary Cu additions to sow gestation and lactation diets at levels of 0, 15, 30, and 60 ppm. They found that 15 ppm Cu supported optimum sow hematology and that 60 ppm Cu supported highest birth and weaning weights of offspring. Lillie and Frobish (1978) and Ducsay (1986) both demonstrated that observed tissue and plasma levels of Cu are the result of an interrelationship between Cu and Fe.

Magnesium

Harmon et al. (1976) demonstrated that Mg levels of 400 and 150 ppm for gestation and lactation, respectively, resulted in negative Mg balance during lactation. Levels of 900 and 650 ppm for the two production periods were adequate for positive balance. The lower levels of Mg did support adequate numbers and weights of offspring as well as sow weight changes.

Selenium

Selenium (Se) is a mineral that is essential in very small amounts. It is a component of glutathione peroxidase, which has a role in protecting subcellular membranes against damage by detoxifying peroxides (Rotruck et al. 1973). Since vitamin E also protects against peroxide formation, the level of Se needed in the diet depends to a certain extent on the level of vitamin E provided. Results of controlled studies show the efficacy of additions of 0.1 ppm Se to gestation and lactation diets containing 0.03 and 0.05 ppm, respectively (Mahan et al. 1974, 1975). Serum Se levels of sows increased and colostrum and milk Se levels increased with 0.1 ppm Se addition. Serum Se was much higher for offspring of Se-supplemented sows, and deficiency symptoms, histopathic lesions, and mortality were delayed in pigs fed purified, vitamin E-free, Se-free diets. Wilkinson et al. (1977) reported that the addition of 0.1 ppm Se to a basal diet containing 0.1 ppm Se resulted in a decrease in the magnitude of decline in blood and serum

Se levels for sows 28 days postparturition. Mahan et al. (1977) reported that sow serum, milk, and tissue levels of Se reached near maximum levels with 0.1 ppm addition of Se, and little advantage was achieved by increasing the level to 0.5 ppm. Concentration of Se in the hair reflected the higher feeding level and was higher for gravid than for nongravid females. Piatkowski et al. (1979) reported that nonpregnant females would maintain higher liver Se levels over time than pregnant females, especially when fed unsupplemented diets.

Calcium and Phosphorus

Levels of dietary Ca and P during growth and development and gestation were evaluated by Nimmo et al. (1981a,b). Grower levels of 0.65% Ca and 0.50% P, and 13 g Ca followed by 10 g P daily during gestation were not adequate to meet Ca and P requirements of the gilt. Gain and feed per gain were not affected by the lower mineral levels, but bone characteristics were less desirable at slaughter weight than for gilts receiving 0.975% and 0.75% Ca and P, respectively. More gilts were removed from the low mineral group because of feet and leg problems. A greater Ca balance was obtained during lactation in gilts receiving the higher gestation Ca levels. Pig performance and sow weight changes were not affected by dietary Ca or P levels. Arthur et al. (1983) evaluated the effect of Ca and P levels in diets during growth on subsequent structural soundness of sows. Providing 150% rather than 100% of the NRC recommendation for Ca and P did not change the incidence or severity of feet and leg lesions. In a large regional study, no advantages as measured by sow attrition, pig production, or sow weights were observed for increasing grower Ca and P levels to 150% of the NRC-recommended levels (Kornegay et al. 1985). Kornegay et al. (1973) evaluated gestation and lactation Ca and P levels of 10.3 g, and 11.0 g versus 15.5 g and 15.0 g. A greater number of sows fed the higher Ca and P levels completed five parities. However, farrowing and weaning performance and sow serum and bone characteristics were not influenced by mineral levels. Kornegay and Kite (1983) found that 10 g of P in combination with 15 g of Ca was adequate to support normal farrowing performance, return to estrus, and rebreeding performance. Mahan and Fetter (1982) evaluated Ca-P levels of 0.65%-0.50%, 0.80%-0.60%, and 0.90%-0.70% for gestation and lactation over three parities. No differences in litter performance, milk mineral levels, or pig bone characteristics were observed due to sow Ca-P levels. However, sow bone ash values would indicate that the 0.90%-0.70% Ca-P level was most adequate over three parities. Maxson and Mahan (1986) evaluated the effect of P levels of 0.5%, 0.6%, 0.7%, 0.8%, and 0.9% for sows during lactation when the Ca:P ratio was constant at 1.3:1. No differences in sow or pig performance, milk composition, or sow bone characteristics were observed due to the different levels of P. Levels of P of 0.45%, 0.55%, and 0.65% during lactation were evaluated by Harmon et al. (1975). Levels of P during gestation were either 0.33% or 0.68%. The lower P levels did not influence pig numbers or weights, milk production or composition, or sow bone composition except for bone ash. The lower bone ash would suggest that 0.45% P may be inadequate for sows over multiple parities. Harmon et al. (1974) evaluated diets for gestation and lactation containing 0.31% or 0.52% P with P supplemented from different sources. A high incidence of posterior paralysis was observed among sows during the sixth to eighth week of lactation for sows receiving the low-P diet. Bone characteristics would indicate that dicalcium phosphate was a good supplemental source of P, Curacao phosphate was intermediate in availability, and that soft phosphate was a less available source of P. Ca levels of 0.3% and 0.7% during the last trimester of gestation were evaluated by Itoh et al. (1967). They found that less Ca was absorbed and less Ca was deposited in the fetuses of sows receiving the lower Ca level.

Salt

Dietary salt levels were evaluated in a regional study that included data from 1020 litters (Cromwell et al. 1989b). Salt levels were 0.5% and 0.25% in the first trial and 0.25% and 0.125% in the second trial. Daily intake was calculated to be 9.0 g, 4.5 g, and 2.25 g for sodium and 13.5 g, 6.75 g, and 3.37 g for chlorine during gestation for the three salt-treatment sow groups. In the first trial, feeding 0.25% salt resulted in lighter pigs at birth and a tendency for lighter pigs at weaning. While numbers of pigs born and weaned and sow weight changes during gestation and lactation were not affected by salt level, sows that received 0.5% salt during the first parity produced large litters in the second parity, while those sows that had received 0.25% salt had a decrease in litter size from the first to the second parity. In the second trial, reducing salt from 0.25% to 0.125% did not affect reproductive performance.

VITAMINS

Vitamin A

The absolute requirement for vitamin A by the sow during reproduction is difficult to establish due to extensive storage of vitamin A in the liver and constant plasma levels maintained with varied feeding levels of vitamin A or carotene. Heaney et al. (1959) found that gilts that had been depleted of vitamin A for 6 months did not respond to feeding levels of vitamin A in terms of their own health or reproduction. However, liver and plasma levels of vitamin A of the pigs and vitamin A content of colostrum and milk was much higher when 16 μg of supplemental vitamin A was fed as compared with 5 μg or 2.5 μg. This work was supported by that of Selke et al. (1967), who found that vitamin A levels from 0 to 23,510 IU/kg of feed resulted in no differences in reproduction or vitamin A status of the sows or pigs. However, colostrum and 14-day milk vitamin A levels were higher with the higher vitamin A feeding levels. Brief and Chew (1985) found that reproductive performance of gilts and performance of pigs receiving supplements of β-carotene and vitamin A were no different from the performance of gilts not receiving supplements. However, injecting gilts with β-carotene or vitamin A resulted in higher plasma β-carotene and vitamin A levels, less embryonic mortality, and heavier pigs at birth and weaning. These data would indicate an advantage of improved vitamin A status for the sow but would indicate that there are limitations of improvement that can be made by feeding vitamin A or its precursor. The study did demonstrate that β-carotene is effectively converted to vitamin A when fed but not when injected.

Vitamin D

Vitamin D requirements of the reproducing sow have not been clearly established. However, vitamin D status of the newborn pig is related to vitamin D status of the dam. Goff et al. (1984) demonstrated that the pig reflected the dam's status because of placental transfer of metabolites and mammary transfer of cholecalciferol itself.

Vitamin E

The level of vitamin E required for reproduction has not been clearly established. Young et al. (1977, 1978) demonstrated no relationship between level of Se or vitamin E fed during growth, development, and gestation and reproductive performance of gilts. However, death loss was higher for groups of growing and developing gilts receiving no supplemental vitamin E or Se. Serum and colostrum of sows and serum of offspring reflected the dietary levels of vitamin E. Vitamin E status of prenursing and postnursing newborn pigs would indicate that supplementation of the dam results in greater influence on offspring vitamin E status by mammary transfer than by placental transfer. Malm et al. (1976) showed that supplementation of gestation diets of sows resulted in severalfold increases in alpha-tocopherol levels in milk and colostrum. They also reported that serum tocopherol levels of offspring were higher than those of the dams when vitamin E was supplemented at 100 IU/kg of diet. Addition of lard, but not corn oil, to the gestation and lactation diets tended to promote higher serum and colostral tocopherol levels. No differences in reproductive performance were observed. Loudenslager et al. (1986) reported that addition of 50 IU/kg of vitamin E with 0.1 ppm Se to the sow gestation diet resulted in increased plasma and colostrum vitamin E levels and higher biological antioxidant status of the offspring throughout the nursing period.

Vitamin K

No requirement has been established for vitamin K for the breeding herd. The National Research Council (1988) lists the menadione requirement for breeding swine to be 0.5 mg/kg.

Folic Acid

Matte et al. (1984) demonstrated that maintaining high serum folate levels of sows from weaning through 60 days of gestation by injections led to significantly more pigs at parturition. Tremblay et al. (1986) found that feeding folic acid in the diet was as effective a method of maintaining serum folate levels as injecting folic acid. By measuring serum folate levels and relating folate levels obtained by feeding to levels obtained by injection, it was estimated that the folic acid requirement for the sow during gestation was approximately 4.3 ppm.

Additions of 1 ppm folic acid to gilts diets over three parities was effective in improving number of total and live pigs born by approximately one pig (Lindemann and Kornegay 1989). However, the advantage in number of pigs was largely lost by weaning at 28 days (0.31 pigs). There was a slight trend toward less breedings required per female farrowed for the supplemented group. Thaler et al.(1989) evaluated feeding levels of 1.65 and 6.62 ppm of supplemented folic acid to gilts over two parities. Feeding folic acid resulted in more total and live pigs born in parity one but not in parity two. In addition, sow weight loss and backfat thickness loss during lactation increased quadratically for sows fed folic acid. The response to folic acid appeared to be greater for the 1.65-ppm feeding level. Tremblay et al. (1989a) reported an increase in embryo survival during early gestation with dietary additions of 5 mg/kg of folic acid for sows that had high ovulation rates. Tremblay et al. (1989b) reported an interrelationship between serum folate levels and serum Zn levels. Both were elevated when 5 mg/kg of folic acid was added to the diets of sows during early gestation. Matte and Girard (1989) evaluated the effect of folic acid injections in sows during lactation. Serum folates increased throughout lactation for all sows but the increase was more pronounced for the sows that received folic acid injections. Milk folates and serum folates of the offspring reflected the sow's serum folate levels. No difference in pig growth parameters could be associated with folic acid levels.

Riboflavin

The riboflavin requirement of the gestating sow was estimated by Frank et al. (1984) by measuring reproductive performance and erythrocyte glutathione reductase activity. Riboflavin supplemented at 0.77 ppm resulted in abnormal gestation lengths (both long and short), lower litter weights and gestation gains, as well as more stillborn pigs. Mortality of pigs was higher when 1.77 ppm was fed than when sows received higher levels. The requirement was estimated to be between 3.2 and 3.3 mg/kg of diet or 6.4 to 6.6 mg/day. The riboflavin requirement during lactation based on glutathione reductase activity of offspring 24 days postfarrowing was 16.3 and 16.2 mg/day for sows and gilts, respectively (Frank et al. 1988). Enzymatic activity of offspring was directly related to sow feeding levels, indicating no protective mechanism by the sow against riboflavin deficiency of the pig.

Pantothenic Acid

Davey and Stevenson (1963) reported that the requirement for pantothenic acid was at least 12 mg/kg of feed for reproduction in swine. This conclusion was based on the fact that pig survival to weaning was reduced and evidence of incoordination of hind feet and "goose stepping" was observed when lower levels were fed. These findings are generally in agreement with those of Ullrey et al. (1955), who had established a requirement level of 12.5 mg/kg.

Pyridoxine

Ritchie et al. (1960) found no advantage to supplementing diets with normal levels of pyridoxine (1 mg/kg) fed to gilts and sows during gestation. However, Russell et al. (1985) found that the pyridoxine requirement of sexually mature gilts exceeded 2.1 mg/kg based on activity coefficients for erythrocyte glutamic-oxaloacetate transaminase and muscle enzyme activity. Easter et al. (1983) found an advantage in litter size at birth and weaning with the addition of 1 mg/kg to the gestation diet of gilts.

Vitamin B_{12}

Fredrick and Brison (1961) reported that supplementing sows with vitamin B_{12} at the rate of 400 μg/day helped maintain pregnancy and increased survivability of pigs in the first days after birth. The National Research Council (1988) lists the requirement for sows at 15 μg/kg of diet.

Vitamin C

No requirement for vitamin C in diets of reproducing swine has been established. Yen and Pond (1983) fed diets supplying up to 1 g of vitamin C daily from day 108 of gestation to 7 days postpartum and observed no advantage in reproduction or lactation performance.

Thiamin

No evidence of a requirement of thiamin for normal reproductive performance in swine is available. The National Research Council (1988) lists the requirement at 1 mg/kg of diet.

Niacin

No information on the niacin requirement of reproducing swine is available. The National Research Council (1988) lists the requirement for reproducing sows to be 10 mg/kg.

Choline

The need for choline in diets of reproducing swine is well documented, but the level of supplementation needed has not been clearly established. The most extensive trial was reported by the NCR-42 Committee on Swine Nutrition (1976). They reported that more total and live pigs were born, more pigs survived to 2 weeks, and fewer spraddle-legged pigs were observed when gestation and lactation diets were supplemented with 770 mg/kg of choline as compared with unsupplemented diets. Kornegay and Meacham (1973) reported more live pigs born during the fifth and sixth parities when 880 mg/kg of supplemental choline were administered, and Maxwell et al. (1987) reported an advantage in weaning weights when either 882 or 551 mg/kg supplemental choline was provided. Stockland and Blaylock (1974) found lower conception rates and farrowing rates with fewer pigs born and weaned from sows receiving unsupplemented diets as compared with those receiving either 412 or 824 mg/kg of supplemental choline. The lower level resulted in 1236 mg of total choline per kg of diet. Boyd et al. (1982) found no advantage to the addition of 770 mg/kg over 220 mg/kg of supplemental choline for litter performance with or without supplemental fat added to the farrowing diet. Seerley et al. (1981) reported no advantage to supplementing diets of sows with 550 mg/kg of choline and no interaction of choline level with fat additions to the sows' diets. The nonsupplemented diet contained 1110 mg/kg choline.

Biotin

The need for supplemental biotin in reproducing swine diets is not clear due to conflicting results in controlled research studies. Improvement of foot lesions in sows by supplementation with biotin in herds with a history of symptoms typical of those caused by a biotin deficiency has been reported by Brooks et al. (1977) and Penny et al. (1980). Improvement of reproductive performance has also been reported with biotin supplementation (Brooks et al. 1977). Misir and Blair (1986) reported that available biotin levels of 0.147 to 0.217 ppm were sufficient to correct lesions of an induced biotin deficiency in sows. Bryant et al. (1985a,b,c) reported fewer foot lesions on developing gilts receiving 0.22 ppm supplemental biotin than on those receiving no supplemental biotin. Farrowing and lactation performance was not influenced by the addition of 0.44 ppm biotin supplementation to gestation and lactation diets over four parities. However, weaning-to-estrus interval and conception rate improved with supplemental biotin. Foot lesions were improved over the four parities with supplemental biotin, but soundness scores were not different between groups. Hair scores and number of hairs per square centimeter were improved by supplementation with 0.44 ppm biotin. Microbiological assay revealed biotin levels in the unsupplemented diet to exceed 0.10 ppm. No differences in response were observed due to type of grain in the diet (corn or wheat). In contrast, Hamilton and Veum (1984) found no advantage to supplementing gestation and lactation diets with 0.55 ppm biotin over a 3-year study.

Culling rates, feet and leg soundness, interval to rebreeding, and incidence of dermatitis were similar between supplemented and unsupplemented sow groups. The only difference in pig production was larger litters weaned in the first parity by biotin-supplemented sows. The level of biotin in the control diet was determined to be 0.17 ppm.

WATER

Friend (1971) found that sows allowed ad libitum consumption of feed and water consumed water at the rate of 2.3 and 3.9 kg/kg of dry matter during gestation and lactation, respectively. Feed and water consumption both declined during gestation. Friend (1973) reported a similar relationship between feed consumption and water consumption with unbred gilts.

Patterson et al. (1979) evaluated the effect of added sodium sulfate in the water of sows from 30 days postbreeding through gestation and a 28-day lactation. Sodium sulfate levels of 3320 ppm and total dissolved solids of 5060 ppm had no effect on sow reproductive performance. Water consumption did increase during lactation for those sows receiving the high levels of sodium sulfate. Andres and Cline (1989) reported a similar study with mice. Sulfate levels up to 5000 ppm did not have a negative affect on size or weaning weight of the litter or on gestation or lactation weight gain of the dam.

Water deprivation of lactating sows as a management tool for terminating lactation was evaluated in a regional study (Knabe et al. 1986). Depriving sows of water for 48 hours immediately prior to weaning had no effect on percentage of sows bred, conception rates, or farrowing rates, nor did it have any effect on interval from weaning to estrus.

ANTIBIOTICS

Antibiotics have long been used in diets of breeding animals to improve reproductive efficiency. The value of chlortetracycline in diets of sows at breeding was documented by Messersmith et al. (1966). Feeding either 1 g or 0.5 g of chlortetracycline daily before breeding and through a 21- to 24-day breeding period resulted in significant improvement in farrowing rate. Feeding 1 g of chlortetracycline daily from weaning to 15 days postbreeding resulted in increased birth weights and a trend toward increased conception and farrowing rates of sows (Soma and Speer 1975). Ruiz et al. (1968) found that 1.25 g of a sulfa-antibiotic mixture fed daily for 1 week prior to and throughout a 21-day breeding period resulted in more pigs farrowed and weaned by gilts, but no improvement in farrowing rate. The inclusion of the same antibiotic mixture from weaning to 3 days postbreeding resulted in no improvement in ovulation rate, ova recovery rate, or fertility rate of sows slaughtered 3 days postbreeding (Hays et al. 1978). Myers and Speer (1973) reported a trend toward improvement of farrowing rate and number of pigs when sows were fed 1 g of chlortetracycline daily from weaning to breeding and throughout the gestation period.

The effect of antibiotics on reproductive performance was best documented in the University of Kentucky Princeton herd (Langlois et al. 1978). After 9 years of routine but not continuous use of chlortetracycline in the herd, no antibiotic was used for 3 years. During that period, a decline was recorded for conception rate, litter size at birth and weaning, and weaning weights as compared with the previous years. Litter size at birth and weaning was higher for another herd, which had continuous chlortetracycline feeding during the same 3-year period. On the positive side, antibiotic-resistant coliform numbers as well as total coliform numbers decreased in the antibiotic-free herd and increased in the herd that received antibiotics continuously.

Bane et al. (1988) reported that salinomycin was not effective in increasing reproductive performance of sows when fed for 14 days prior to parturition and through a subsequent gestation. Holzgraefe et al. (1986) reported that feeding lasalocid to sows from 35 days postbreeding to parturition resulted in more live pigs 14 days postpartum. Colostrum fat content was reduced by dietary lasalocid feeding. This change in colostrum fat level may be explained by the changes in products of fermentation as a result of lasalocid feeding (Holzgraefe et al. 1985a). Molar concentration of propionate was higher and of acetate was lower in the cecum of sows fed lasalocid. Mineral digestion and retention was affected by lasalocid intake but was dependent on type of diet fed (Holzgraefe et al. 1985b). For more information on antibiotics see Chapter 17.

MOLDS

Zearalenone is one of the toxins that may be produced by the mold *Fusarium,* which grows on corn in the field. It has been reported by Young et al. (1981) that weaned gilts fed 6 to 9 ppm zearalenone exhibited vaginal and uterine changes as well as red and swollen vulvas. Long and Diekman (1984) reported no effect on embryo development at 40 days postbreeding when gilts received diets with up to 30 ppm zearalenone. However, no fetuses were found in the uterus of gilts receiving 60 or 90 ppm zearalenone. The uterine tissue appeared to be stimulated by both estrogen and progesterone when 90 ppm was fed. Young et al. (1982) evaluated zearalenone in levels up to 4.8 ppm in gilts from first estrus through two parities. Reproductive performance seemed to decrease with increasing levels of zearalenone, even though all levels were quite low. Gilts nursing sows fed the highest levels exhibited heavier reproductive tract weight by 21 days. However, neither zearalenone nor its metabolites were found in sows' milk. Young et al. (1990) fed diets containing 0, 5, and 10 ppm zeralenone in diets of first and second parity sows from day 7 of lactation until day 40 after weaning. While 5 ppm had little effect, 10 ppm of zearalenone resulted in increased nonpregnant sows, decreased litter size, and longer weaning-to-estrus interval. For more information on molds and toxins see Chapter 26.

FEEDSTUFF UTILIZATION

Because of the ability of sows to reproduce with minor nutrient deficiencies and to utilize nutrients supplied from both body stores and feedstuffs, a wide variety of feedstuffs can be utilized in sows' diets. Only a few of them have been evaluated.

Hesby et al. (1970a,b) found that opaque-2 corn, fortified with minerals and vitamins, was satisfactory for sows during gestation. Normal corn fortified in the same manner did not support adequate reproductive performance. Baker et al. (1970a) found either fortified corn or fortified opaque-2 corn gestation diets satisfactory for first parity sows. However, feeding opaque-2 corn diets without additional protein was unsatisfactory for sows during lactation (Mahan et al. 1971a). Milk production was depressed with either an opaque-2 or a 10% protein normal corn diet. Mahan et al. (1971b) found that opaque-2 corn diets produced litter gains equal to those from first litter sows fed 12% or 14% protein diets and from second litter sows fed 10% protein diets. Negative nitrogen balance for sows fed opaque-2 corn or 10% protein diets during lactation was observed by Mahan et al. (1971c).

Young et al. (1973) reported that barley, supplemented with minerals and alfalfa hay, supported satisfactory reproductive performance. In the second parity, supplementation of barley diets with soybean meal led to heavier pig birth weights. In a subsequent trial (Young et al. 1976), it was observed that protein supplementation of barley diets resulted in heavier pigs at birth and greater pig survival.

Sows fed wheat shorts with a free-choice mineral supplement farrowed more pigs with lighter birth weights and returned to estrus more slowly than counterparts fed a corn-soybean meal diet (Young and King 1981). Digestible energy content of wheat shorts was estimated to be 2.93 kcal/kg.

Palmer et al. (1970) reported an increase in litter size at birth when 6% whole Menhaden fish meal was included in the all-plant diet of gestating sows. Gestation gain of sows and gilts was also increased. Baker et al. (1974a) noted no improvement in reproductive performance when 3% Menhaden fish meal was added.

Mung beans were evaluated as a protein source for gilts during gestation (Luce et al. 1989). Feeding mung beans at 89% or 61% of the protein supplement resulted in decreased litter size and weight. Crenshaw and Danielson (1985) found that raw soybeans could be effectively utilized in gestation diets for swine. With no negative effects, inclusion of raw soybeans resulted in increased pig weight and increased milk fat at 3 days. Kepler et al. (1982) reported that ground whole sunflowers could be included in gestation diets as a protein and energy source for sows at 25% of the diet with no adverse effects and at 50% of the diet with some feed refusal problems.

Haught et al. (1977) reported that reproductive performance of sows fed sorghum diets in which one half of the supplemental protein was supplied by cottonseed meal was similar to that of sows that had diets based on soybean meal.

By-products of the alcohol industry can be utilized effectively by gestating sows. All the supplemental protein added to a corn diet during gestation can come from brewer's dried grains (Wahlstrom and Libal 1976) or distillers dried grains with solubles (Thong et al. 1978) without adverse effects.

Results of balance studies (Van Dyke et al. 1986) indicate that screened swine waste solids can be utilized as an energy source for gestating gilts. However, this product contributes little as a protein source.

Kornegay (1981) reported that the digestibility of soybean hulls by sows was 69.4% for dry matter and 67.4% for crude protein. Based on performance trials with growing-finishing pigs, levels of 15% soybean hulls or more could be used in sow diets.

Baker et al. (1974b) reported that either 5% wheat bran or 5% dehydrated alfalfa meal could be added to sow lactation diets without adverse effects. Including 50% alfalfa in the gestation diets of sows had no adverse effects on sow or pig performance (Calvert et al. 1985; Pollman et al. 1981). Inclusion of 96.75% alfalfa hay gave satisfactory performance over three consecutive parities (Danielson and Noonan 1975), and including 95% alfalfa meal in gestation and lactation diets resulted in reduced pig weaning weight as the only negative reproductive performance (Calvert et al. 1985). Pollman et al. (1979) also reported that sows fed 97% sun-cured alfalfa or 66% tall wheatgrass gained less during gestation but exhibited similar reproductive performance to sows receiving a corn-soybean meal diet. Nuzback et al. (1984) found that sun-cured alfalfa was digested equally by the gestating sow if in the form of meal or pellets and that smaller particle size was utilized more efficiently by the sow.

REFERENCES

Aherne, F.X., and V.C. Speer. 1974. *J. Anim. Sci.* 38:310.
Allrich, R.D., et al. 1979. *J. Anim. Sci.* 48:359.
Andres, C.J., and T.R. Cline. 1989. *J. Anim. Sci.* 67:1313.
Antinmo, T., W.G. Pond, and R.H. Barnes. 1974. *J. Anim. Sci.* 39:703.
Antinmo, T., et al. 1976. *J. Anim. Sci.* 43:606.
Armstrong, J.D., J.H. Britt, and R.R. Kraeling. 1986. *J. Anim. Sci.* 63:1915.
Arthur, S.R., et al. 1983. *J. Anim. Sci.* 56:876.
Baker, D.H., B.G. Harmon, and A.H. Jensen. 1974b. *J. Anim. Sci.* 39:838.
Baker, D.H., et al. 1970a. *J. Anim. Sci.* 30:364.
Baker, D.H., et al. 1970b. *J. Anim. Sci.* 31:526.
Baker, D.H., et al. 1974a. *J. Anim. Sci.* 38:325.
Bane, D.P., R.F. Bevill, and W.F. Hall. 1988. *J. Anim. Sci.* 66:3094.
Bishop, T.C., T.S. Stahly, and G.L. Cromwell. 1985. *J. Anim. Sci.* 61:1467.
Boomgaardt, J., et al. 1972. *J. Anim. Sci.* 34:408.
Boyd, R.D., et al. 1978a. *J. Anim. Sci.* 47:874.
Boyd, R.D., et al. 1978b. *J. Anim. Sci.* 47:883.
Boyd, R.D., et al. 1982. *J. Anim. Sci.* 54:1.
Brendemuhl, J.H., A.J. Lewis, and E.R. Peo, Jr. 1987. *J. Anim. Sci.* 64:1060.
Brendemuhl, J.H., A.J. Lewis, and E.R. Peo, Jr. 1989. *J. Anim. Sci.* 67:1478.
Brief, S., and B.P. Chew. 1985. *J. Anim. Sci.* 60:998.
Brooks, P.H., D.A. Smith, and V.C.R. Irwin. 1977. *Vet. Rec.* 101:46.
Bryant, K.L., et al. 1985a. *J. Anim. Sci.* 60:136.
Bryant, K.L., et al. 1985b. *J. Anim. Sci.* 60:145.
Bryant, K.L., et al. 1985c. *J. Anim. Sci.* 60:154.
Buitraga, J.A., et al. 1974a. *J. Anim. Sci.* 39:47.
Buitraga, J.A., et al. 1974b. *J. Anim. Sci.* 38:766.
Calvert, C.C., N.C. Steele, and R.W. Rosebrough. 1985. *J. Anim. Sci.* 61:595.
Cieslak, D.G., V.D. Leibbrandt, and N.J. Benevenga. 1983. *J. Anim. Sci.* 57:954.
Coffey, M.T., R.W. Seerley, and J.W. Mabry. 1982. *J. Anim. Sci.* 55:1388.
Coffey, M.T., J.A. Yates, and G.E. Combs. 1987. *J. Anim. Sci.* 65:1249.
Corley, J.R., et al. 1983. *J. Anim. Sci.* 56:108.
Cox, N.M., et al. 1983. *J. Anim. Sci.* 56:21.
Cox, N.M., et al. 1987. *J. Anim. Sci.* 64:507.
Crenshaw, M.A., and D.M. Danielson. 1985. *J. Anim. Sci.* 60:163.
Cromwell, G.L., et al. 1989a. *J. Anim. Sci.* 67:3.

Cromwell, G.L., et al. 1989b. *J. Anim. Sci.* 67:374.
Cuaron, J.A., R.P. Chapple, and R.A. Easter. 1983. *J. Anim. Sci.* 56:96.
Cuaron, J.A., R.P. Chapple, and R.A. Easter. 1984. *J. Anim. Sci.* 58:631.
Cunningham, P.J., et al. 1974. *J. Anim. Sci.* 39:63.
Danielson, D.M., and J.J. Noonan. 1975. *J. Anim. Sci.* 41:94.
Davey, R.J., and J.W. Stevenson. 1963. *J. Anim. Sci.* 22:9.
DeGeeter, M.J., et al. 1972. *J. Anim. Sci.* 35:772.
DeGeeter, M.J., et al. 1973. *J. Anim. Sci.* 37:459.
de Lange, P.G.B., et al. 1980. *J. Anim. Sci.* 50:886.
Ducsay, C.A., et al. 1984. *J. Anim. Sci.* 59:1303.
Ducsay, C.A., et al. 1986. *J. Anim. Sci.* 62:706.
Easter, R.A., and D.H. Baker. 1977. *J. Anim. Sci.* 44:417.
Easter, R.A., R.S. Katz, and D.H. Baker. 1974. *J. Anim. Sci.* 39:1123.
Easter, R.A., et al. 1983. *Nutr. Rep. Int.* 28:945.
Edey, T.N., et al. 1972. *J. Anim. Sci.* 35:1223.
Elliott, R.F., et al. 1971. *J. Anim. Sci.* 32:1128.
Esbenshade, K.L., et al. 1986. *J. Anim. Sci.* 62:1187.
Ezekwe, M.O. 1986. *J. Anim. Sci.* 62:1005.
Ezekwe, M.O., and R.J. Martin. 1978. *J. Anim. Sci.* 47:1121.
Ezekwe, M.O., et al. 1984. *J. Anim. Sci.* 59:974.
Frank, G.R., J.M. Bahr, and R.A. Easter. 1984. *J. Anim. Sci.* 59:1567.
Frank, G.R., J.M. Bahr, and R.A. Easter. 1988. *J. Anim. Sci.* 66:47.
Fredrick, G.L., and G.J. Brisson. 1961. *Can. J. Anim. Sci.* 41:212.
Friend, D.W. 1971. *J. Anim. Sci.* 32:658.
Friend, D.W. 1973. *J. Anim. Sci.* 37:1137.
Friend, D.W. 1974. *J. Anim. Sci.* 39:1073.
Frobish, L.T., V.C. Speer, and V.W. Hays. 1966. *J. Anim. Sci.* 25:729.
Frobish, L.T., N.C. Steele, and R.J. Davey. 1973. *J. Anim. Sci.* 36:293.
Ganguli, M.C., et al. 1971. *J. Anim. Sci.* 33:394.
Giesemann, M.A., et al. 1989. *J. Anim. Sci.* 67:157.
Goff, J.P., R.L. Horst, and E.T. Littledike. 1984. *J. Nutr.* 114:163.
Hamilton, C.R., and T.L. Veum. 1984. *J. Anim. Sci.* 59:151.
Hammell, D.L., et al. 1976. *J. Anim. Sci.* 43:589.
Hard, D.L., and Anderson, L.L. 1982. *J. Anim. Sci.* 54:1227.
Harmon, B.G., et al. 1974. *J. Anim. Sci.* 39:1117.
Harmon, B.G., et al. 1975. *J. Anim. Sci.* 40:660.
Harmon, B.G., et al. 1976. *J. Anim. Sci.* 42:860.
Haught, D.G., and V.C. Speer. 1977. *J. Anim. Sci.* 44:595.
Haught, D.G., et al. 1977. *J. Anim. Sci.* 44:249.
Hawton, J.D., and R.J. Meade. 1971. *J. Anim. Sci.* 32:888.
Haye, S.N., E.T. Kornegay, and D.C. Mahan. 1981. *J. Anim. Sci.* 53:1262.
Hays, V.W., et al. 1978. *J. Anim. Sci.* 46:884.
Heaney, D.P., et al. 1959. *J. Anim. Sci.* 18:925.
Hedges, J.D., E.T. Kornegay, and H.R. Thomas. 1976. *J. Anim. Sci.* 43:453.
Hesby, J.H., et al. 1970a. *J. Anim. Sci.* 31:481.
Hesby, J.H., et al. 1970b. *J. Anim. Sci.* 31:474.
Hill, G.M., E.R. Miller, and P.K. Ku. 1983a. *J. Anim. Sci.* 57:123.
Hill, G.M., E.R. Miller, and H.D. Stowe. 1983b. *J. Anim. Sci.* 57:114.
Hill, G.M., et al. 1983c. *J. Anim. Sci.* 57:130.
Hill, G.M., et al. 1983d. *J. Nutr.* 113:867.
Hitchcock, J.P., et al. 1971. *J. Anim. Sci.* 33:30.
Holden, P.J., R.C. Ewan, and V.C. Speer. 1971. *J. Anim. Sci.* 32:900.
Holden, P.J., et al. 1968. *J. Anim. Sci.* 27:1587.
Holzgraefe, D.P., G.C. Fahey, Jr., and A.H. Jensen. 1985a. *J. Anim. Sci.* 60:1235.

Holzgraefe, D.P., et al. 1985b. *J. Anim. Sci.* 60:1247.
Holzgraefe, D.P., et al. 1986. *J. Anim. Sci.* 62:1145.
Hoppe, M.K., et al. 1990. *J. Anim. Sci.* 68:2235.
Itoh, H., et al. 1967. *J. Anim. Sci.* 26:335.
Johnson, L.J., et al. 1986. *J. Anim. Sci.* 63:804.
Johnson, L.J., et al. 1987. *J. Anim. Sci.* 64:36.
Jones, R.D., and C.V. Maxwell. 1974. *J. Anim. Sci.* 39:1067.
Jones, R.D., and C.V. Maxwell. 1982. *J. Anim. Sci.* 55:848.
Kepler, M., G.W. Libal, and R.C. Wahlstrom. 1982. *J. Anim. Sci.* 55:1082.
Klaver, J., et al. 1981. *J. Anim. Sci.* 52:1091.
Knabe, D.A., T.J. Prince, and D.E. Orr, Jr. 1986. *J. Anim. Sci.* 62:1.
Kornegay, E.T. 1981. *J. Anim. Sci.* 53:138.
Kornegay, E.T., and B. Kite. 1983. *J. Anim. Sci.* 57:1463.
Kornegay, E.T., and T.N. Meacham. 1973. *J. Anim. Sci.* 37:506.
Kornegay, E.T., H.R. Thomas, and T.N. Meacham. 1973. *J. Anim. Sci.* 37:493.
Kornegay, E.T., et al. 1985. *J. Anim. Sci.* 61:1460.
Kveragas, C.L., et al. 1986. *J. Anim. Sci.* 63:1877.
Langlois, B.E., G.L. Cromwell, and V.C. Hays. 1978. *J. Anim. Sci.* 46:1369.
Lellis, W.A., and V.C. Speer. 1983. *J. Anim. Sci.* 56:1334.
Lellis, W.A., and V.C. Speer. 1985. *J. Anim. Sci.* 61:1448.
Lellis, W.A., and V.C. Speer. 1987. *J. Anim. Sci.* 65:1006.
Leonard, R.P., and V.C. Speer. 1983. *J. Anim. Sci.* 56:1345.
Lewis, A.J., and V.C. Speer. 1973. *J. Anim. Sci.* 37:104.
Lewis, A.J., and V.C. Speer. 1974a. *J. Anim. Sci.* 38:785.
Lewis, A.J., and V.C. Speer. 1974b. *J. Anim. Sci.* 38:778.
Lewis, A.J., and V.C. Speer. 1975. *J. Anim. Sci.* 40:892.
Libal, G.W., and R.C. Wahlstrom. 1975. *J. Anim. Sci.* 41:1542.
Libal, G.W., and R.C. Wahlstrom. 1977. *J. Anim. Sci.* 45:286.
Lillie, R.J., and L.T. Frobish. 1978. *J. Anim. Sci.* 46:678.
Lindemann, M.D., and E.T. Kornegay. 1989. *J. Anim. Sci.* 67:459.
Long, G.G., and M.A. Diekman. 1984. *J. Anim. Sci.* 59:1662.
Loudenslager, M.J., et al. 1986. *J. Anim. Sci.* 63:1905.
Lucas, E.W., et al. 1969. *J. Anim. Sci.* 29:429.
Luce, W.G., et al. 1989. *J. Anim. Sci.* 67:329.
Mahan, D.C. 1977. *J. Anim. Sci.* 45:1061.
Mahan, D.C. 1979. *J. Anim. Sci.* 49:514.
Mahan, D.C., and A.W. Fetter. 1982. *J. Anim. Sci.* 54:285.
Mahan, D.C., and A.P. Grifo, Jr. 1975. *J. Anim. Sci.* 41:1362.
Mahan, D.C., D.E. Becker, and A.H. Jensen. 1971b. *J. Anim. Sci.* 32:470.
Mahan, D.C., D.E. Becker, and A.H. Jensen. 1971c. *J. Anim. Sci.* 32:476.
Mahan, D.C., A.L. Moxon, and J.H. Cline. 1975. *J. Anim. Sci.* 40:624.
Mahan, D.C., A.L. Moxon, and M. Hubbard. 1977. *J. Anim. Sci.* 45:738.
Mahan, D.C., et al. 1971a. *J. Anim. Sci.* 32:482.
Mahan, D.C., et al. 1974. *J. Anim. Sci.* 39:536.
Malm, A., et al. 1976. *J. Anim. Sci.* 42:393.
Matte, J.J., and C.L. Girard. 1989. *J. Anim. Sci.* 67:426.
Matte, J.J., C.L. Girard, and G.J. Brisson. 1984. *J. Anim. Sci.* 59:1020.
Maxson, P.F., and D.C. Mahan. 1986. *J. Anim. Sci.* 63:1163.
Maxwell, C.V., R.K. Johnson, and W.G. Luce. 1987. *J. Anim. Sci.* 64:1044.
McNamara, J.P., et al. 1985. *J. Anim. Sci.* 61:410.
Meisinger, D.J., and V.C. Speer. 1979. *J. Anim. Sci.* 48:559.
Messersmith, R.E., et al. 1966. *J. Anim. Sci.* 25:752.
Michel, E.J., et al. 1980. *J. Anim. Sci.* 50:93.
Miller, G.M., J.H. Conrad, and R.B. Harrington. 1971. *J. Anim. Sci.* 32:79.

Miller, G.M., et al. 1969. *J. Anim. Sci.* 28:204.
Misir, R., and R. Blair. 1986. *Res. Vet. Sci.* 40:212.
Moore, C.P., et al. 1973. *J. Anim. Sci.* 37:734.
Myers, D.J., and V.C. Speer. 1973. *J. Anim. Sci.* 36:1125.
National Research Council. 1988. *Nutrient Requirements of Swine.* 9th revised ed. Washington, DC: National Academy Press.
NCR-42 Committee on Swine Nutrition. 1976. *J. Anim. Sci.* 42:1211.
NCR-42 Committee on Swine Nutrition. 1978. *J. Anim. Sci.* 46:1673.
Nelssen, J.L., et al. 1985a. *J. Anim. Sci.* 61:1164.
Nelssen, J.L., et al. 1985b. *J. Anim. Sci.* 60:171.
Nimmo, R.D., et al. 1981a. *J. Anim. Sci.* 52:1343.
Nimmo, R.D., et al. 1981b. *J. Anim. Sci.* 52:1330.
Noblet, J., and M. Etienne. 1986. *J. Anim. Sci.* 63:1888.
Noblet, J., and M. Etienne. 1987. *J. Anim. Sci.* 64:774.
Nuzback, L.J., D.S. Pollmann, and K.C. Behnke. 1984. *J. Anim. Sci.* 58:378.
Ojamaa, K.M., J.I. Elliot, and T.G. Hartsock. 1980. *J. Anim. Sci.* 51:620.
Palmer, W.M., H.S. Teague, and A.P. Grifo, Jr. 1970. *J. Anim. Sci.* 31:535.
Patterson, D.W., et al. 1979. *J. Anim. Sci.* 49:664.
Penny, R.H.C., et al. 1980. *Vet. Rec.* 107:350.
Piatkowski, T.L., et al. 1979. *J. Anim. Sci.* 48:1357.
Pollmann, D.S., D.M. Danielson, and E.R. Peo, Jr. 1979. *J. Anim. Sci.* 48:1385.
Pollmann, D.S., et al. 1981. *J. Anim. Sci.* 51:294.
Pond, W.G., H.J. Mersmann, and J.T. Yen. 1985. *J. Nutr.* 115:179.
Pond, W.G., J.T. Yen, and L.H. Yen. 1986. *J. Anim. Sci.* 63:472.
Pond, W.G., et al. 1968. *J. Anim. Sci.* 27:1583.
Pond, W.G., et al. 1981. *J. Anim. Sci.* 52:535.
Pond, W.G., et al. 1983. *J. Nutr.* 113:436.
Ray, D.E., and J.W. McCarty. 1965. *J. Anim. Sci.* 24:660.
Reese, D.E., E.R. Peo, Jr., and A.J. Lewis. 1984. *J. Anim. Sci.* 58:1236.
Reese, D.E., et al. 1982a. *J. Anim. Sci.* 55:590.
Reese, D.E., et al. 1982b. *J. Anim. Sci.* 55:867.
Ritchie, H.D., et al. 1960. *J.Nutr.* 70:491.
Robles-Cabrera, A., and V.C. Speer. 1983. *J. Anim. Sci.* 57:1479.
Rotruck, J.T., et al. 1973. *Science* 179:588.
Rousselow, D.L., and V.C. Speer. 1980. *J. Anim. Sci.* 50:472.
Rousselow, D.L., V.C. Speer, and D.G. Haught. 1979. *J. Anim. Sci.* 49:498.
Ruiz, M.E., et al. 1968. *J. Anim. Sci.* 27:1602.
Russell, L.E., P.J. Bechtel, and R.A. Easter. 1985. *J. Nutr.* 115:1124.
Schoenherr, W.D., T.S. Stahly, and G.L. Cromwell. 1989a. *J. Anim. Sci.* 67Z:473.
Schoenherr, W.D., T.S. Stahly, and G.L. Cromwell. 1989b. *J. Anim. Sci.* 67:482.
Schultz, J.R., et al. 1966. *J. Anim. Sci.* 25:157.
Seerley, R.W. 1989. *J. Anim. Sci.* 67:1889.
Seerley, R.W., F.M. Griffith, and H.C. McCampbell. 1978a. *J. Anim. Sci.* 46:1009.
Seerley, R.W., J.S. Maxwell, and H.C. McCampbell. 1978b. *J. Anim. Sci.* 47:1114.
Seerley, R.W., R.A. Snyder, and H.C. McCampbell. 1981. *J. Anim. Sci.* 52:542.
Seerley, R.W., et al. 1974. *J. Anim. Sci.* 38:64.
Selke, MR., C.E. Barnhart, and C.H. Chaney. 1967. *J. Anim. Sci.* 26:759.
Shields, R.G., Jr., D.C. Mahan, and P.F. Maxson. 1985. *J. Anim. Sci.* 60:179.
Shurson, G.C., et al. 1986. *J. Anim. Sci.* 62:672.
Siers, D.G., et al. 1976. *J. Anim. Sci.* 42:381.
Soma, J.A., and V.C. Speer. 1975. *J. Anim. Sci.* 41:100.
Speer, V.C., et al. 1990. *J. Anim. Sci.* 68:2394.
Spence, C.A., et al. 1985. *J. Anim. Sci.* 60:1280.
Spruill, D.G., V.W. Hays, and G.L. Cromwell. 1971. *J. Anim. Sci.* 33:376.

Stahly, T.S., G.L. Cromwell, and H.J. Monegue. 1986. *J. Anim. Sci.* 63:1156.
Stahly, T.S., G.L. Cromwell, and W.S. Simpson. 1979. *J. Anim. Sci.* 49:50.
Stahly, T.S., G.L. Cromwell, and W.S. Simpson. 1981. *J. Anim. Sci.* 51:352.
Stevenson, J.S., D.L. Davis, and D.S. Pollmann. 1985. *J. Anim. Sci.* 61:480.
Stockland, W.L., and L.G. Blaylock. 1974. *J. Anim. Sci.* 39:1113.
Thaler, R.C., et al. 1989. *J. Anim. Sci.* 67:3360.
Thong, L.A., et al. 1978. *J. Anim. Sci.* 46:674.
Thulin, A.J., et al. 1989. *J. Anim. Sci.* 67:738.
Tremblay, G.F., et al. 1986. *J. Anim. Sci.* 63:1173.
Tremblay, G.F., et al. 1989a. *J. Anim. Sci.* 67:724.
Tremblay, G.F., et al. 1989b. *J. Anim. Sci.* 67:733.
Tribble, L.F., and D.E. Orr. 1982. *J. Anim. Sci.* 55:608.
Ullrey, D.E., et al. 1955. *J. Anim. Sci.* 57:401.
Van Dyke, N.J., T.J. Prince, and D.T. Hill. 1986. *J. Anim. Sci.* 63:1150.
Vermedahl, L.D., et al. 1969. *J. Anim. Sci.* 28:465.
Verstegen, M.W.A., J. Mesu, and G.J.M. van Kempen. 1985. *J. Anim. Sci.* 60:731.
Wachholz, D.E., and R.C. Wahlstrom. 1973. *J. Anim. Sci.* 37:131.
Wahlstrom, R.C., and G.W. Libal. 1976. *J. Anim. Sci.* 42:871.
Wahlstrom, R.C., and G.W. Libal. 1977. *J. Anim. Sci.* 45:94.
White, C.E., H.H. Head, and F.W. Bazer. 1984b. *J. Nutr.* 114:361.
White, C.E., et al. 1984a. *J. Anim. Sci.* 59:141.
Wilkinson, J.E., et al. 1977. *J. Anim. Sci.* 44:224.
Willis, G.M., and C.V. Maxwell. 1984. *J. Anim. Sci.* 58:647.
Woerman, R.L., and V.C. Speer. 1976. *J. Anim. Sci.* 42:114.
Yen, J.T., and W.G. Pond. 1983. *J. Anim. Sci.* 56:621.
Young, L.G., and G.L. King. 1981. *J. Anim. Sci.* 52:551.
Young, L.G., R.P. Forshaw, and G.C. Smith. 1973. *J. Anim. Sci.* 37:898.
Young, L.G., R.P. Forshaw, and G.C. Smith. 1976. *J. Anim. Sci.* 42:1182.
Young, L.G., H. Ping, and G.J. King. 1990. *J. Anim. Sci.* 68:15.
Young, L.G., et al. 1977. *J. Anim. Sci.* 45:1051.
Young, L.G., et al. 1978. *J. Anim. Sci.* 47:639.
Young, L.G., et al. 1981. *J. Anim. Sci.* 52:1312.
Young, L.G., et al. 1982. *J. Anim. Sci.* 54:976.
Young, R., Jr., D.K. Hass, and L.J. Brown. 1979. *J. Anim. Sci.* 48:45.

PART VI

Feeding Unique Feedstuffs to Swine

Chapter 34

Utilization of Liquid Whey in Feeding Swine

V.D. Leibbrandt and N.J. Benevenga

Liquid whey is the serum or watery part of milk that separates from the curd during cheese making. The liquid by-product can be dried and used as an ingredient in human and animal diets. When drying whey is impractical, cheese plants frequently dispose of liquid whey via conventional sewage processing plants. The high organic matter content of whey makes such disposal costly. Thus, liquid whey become available as a livestock feed.

Two liquid wheys are commonly available. Sweet whey is the effluent from whole milk following the manufacture of natural or rennet cheeses (Swiss, Munster, Cheddar, Monterey Jack, etc.) and processed cheese. Acid whey is produced from acid casein processing of skim milk during cottage, pot, or farmer cheese making. The pH of sweet whey varies from 5 to 7 while that of acid whey varies from 4 to 5. Acid whey also possesses a somewhat pungent odor (Gilles 1974).

NUTRIENT COMPOSITION

Approximately 10 kg of milk are used to produce 0.5 to 1 kg of cheese. The whey that remains is about 7% dry matter and contains about 90% of the lactose, 20% of the protein, 40% of the calcium, and 43% of the phosphorus originally in the milk. The nutrient composition of sweet and acid whey dry matter is shown in Table 34.1.

Lactose makes up a large portion of the whey dry matter, but the metabolizable energy (ME) content of liquid whey is low due to the low dry matter content in the by-product. Liquid whey is estimated to contain 230 kcal of ME/kg.

Table 34.2 shows the amino acid composition of sweet and acid whey. Generally, amino acid availability from milk and whey products is considered high. Feeding whey as a liquid reduces the chance that lysine will bind to carbohydrates by overheating during drying. Brown discolored liquid whey that appears to have been overheated should

Table 34.1 General Nutrient Composition of Whey Dry Matter

Nutrient	*Sweet Whey (%)*	*Acid Whey (%)*
Protein	13.0	11.7
Lactose	69.4	63.2
Fat	1.0	0.4
Ash	8.3	10.6
Calcium	0.9	2.4
Phosphorus	1.1	1.6

(Data from Glass and Hedrick 1977a,b.)

Table 34.2 Amino Acid Composition of Whey Proteins

	Sweet Whey		*Acid Whey*	
Amino Acid	*% of Liquid Whey*[a]	*% of Dry Whey*	*% of Liquid Whey*[a]	*% of Dry Whey*
Lysine	0.077	1.10	0.087	1.24
Histidine	0.018	0.25	0.020	0.28
Arginine	0.023	0.33	0.023	0.33
Tryptophan	0.021	0.30	0.020	0.29
Aspartic acid	0.090	1.28	0.086	1.23
Threonine	0.060	0.85	0.041	0.59
Serine	0.046	0.66	0.039	0.56
Glutamic acid	0.156	2.23	0.155	2.22
Proline	0.060	0.85	0.054	0.77
Glycine	0.017	0.24	0.014	0.20
Alanine	0.041	0.58	0.035	0.50
Cystine	0.020	0.28	0.018	0.26
Valine	0.051	0.73	0.044	0.63
Methionine	0.015	0.22	0.015	0.21
Isoleucine	0.052	0.74	0.046	0.66
Leucine	0.090	1.28	0.088	1.26
Tyrosine	0.024	0.34	0.026	0.37
Phenylalanine	0.030	0.43	0.031	0.44

[a]Based on liquid whey containing 7% dry matter.

(Data from Glass and Hedrick 1977a.)

be fed only as an energy source, since the availability of amino acids is questionable.

Whey derived from cow's milk contains three major protein fractions (Table 34.3). Lactalbumin, the largest fraction, contains alpha-lactalbumin, beta-lactoglobulin, and serum albumin subfractions. The lysine content of the alpha- and beta-subfractions (13.5% and 12.7%, respectively) is greater than the average for all proteins (8.8%) in sweet whey.

Table 34.3 Protein Fractions in Whey Dry Matter

Fraction	%
Lactalbumin	
Alpha lactalbumin	19.7
Beta lactoglobulin	43.7
Serum albumin	4.7
Proteose-peptone	18.9
Immunoglobulins	13.0
Total	100.0

(Data from Smith 1976.)

Acid whey contains slightly greater mineral content than does sweet whey. Mineral content can vary due to season, type of cheese produced, and geographical location. The phosphorus in whey may have greater nutritional value than that from plant sources, since it is not in the phytin phosphorus form.

The cheese produced and the addition of salt-laden press drippings influence the whey salt content. Natural cheeses like Cheddar, Colby, brick American, and Mozzarella are salted after whey drainage and before pressing. Whey collected during pressing can contain 10% sodium chloride and should not be fed to animals. Salt is added to cottage cheese after the creaming process, making salt addition to acid whey less likely (Modler 1985).

Salt toxicity when feeding whey is often a concern. Bohstedt and Grummer (1954) found finishing pigs could tolerate up to 2% sodium chloride in the diet without exhibiting salt toxicity symptoms when the animals could consume water ad libitum. Animals consuming whey as their only liquid source should not develop salt toxicity because liquid whey contains 93% to 94% water. If liquid whey is fed in restricted amounts, animals should have access to drinking water.

Vitamin content of milk and type of cheese produced influence the vitamins found in whey. Generally, fat-soluble vitamins are retained in the cheese and are at low levels in the whey. Most water-soluble vitamins remain in the whey during cheese production.

UTILIZATION

The high lactose content of whey solids makes the feedstuff attractive for use by weanling pigs because mucosal lactase activity of the small intestine relative to metabolic body size ($W^{.75}$) is greater for pigs from 2 to 4 weeks of age than for pigs 100 or 180 days old (Ekstrom et al. 1975b). Despite this fact, young pigs cannot consume as large a liquid volume as can grower-finisher pigs.

Feeding grower pigs a diet containing 40% dried whey can cause digestive upsets and diarrhea (Ekstrom et al. 1976) but Ekstrom et al. (1976a) found that this whey level did not affect performance. Grower pigs drinking liquid whey ad libitum consumed

25% to 50% (Cieslak et al. 1986) or 30% (Vignes 1976) of their daily dry matter intake from whey without decreasing their performance.

Feeding lactose-rich diets can increase lactase utilization by grower-finisher pigs. Pigs fed diets containing 40% dried whey exhibited higher total lactase activity in the small intestine than did control pigs (Ekstrom et al. 1975a). High lactose diets also increase the digestive capacity of the large intestine. Approximately 30% to 32% of the lactose in a 40% dried whey diet fed to 107-kg pigs appeared in the large intestine (Kim et al. 1978a), doubling the lactase activity of the cecal and colonic contents and increasing volatile fatty acid (VFA) production 1.5 to 2 fold (Kim et al. 1978b).

Liquid whey is frequently considered as an energy source but its greatest nutritional potential is as an amino acid source. Whey protein contains a greater portion of lysine and several other essential amino acids than does that from soybean or fish meal (Table 34.4) and is superior in quality to that from casein (Smith 1976).

Whey protein is a concentrated source of essential amino acids that are deficient in cereal grains (Al-Ani et al. 1972; Womack and Vaughan 1972; Chan et al 1976). Consequently, combining whey and corn should minimize the total protein needed to satisfy essential amino acid requirements for growing-finishing swine. Cieslak et al. (1986) calculated that 6.2 g of protein/kg body weight in the diet would meet the amino acid need of a 20-kg pig when 30% of the protein came from corn and 70% came from whey. Ten grams of protein per kilogram of body weight are required when using a corn-soybean meal amino acid spectrum as described by the National Research Council (NRC 1979).

A University of Wisconsin study (Cieslak 1979) showed that pigs consuming large volumes of liquid whey can meet their protein needs when liquid whey is the only liquid source and it is fed free-choice with vitamin- and mineral-fortified corn. The experimental treatments are described in Table 34.5. One treatment approximated a feeding

Table 34.4 Grams of Amino Acid per 100 Grams of Ingredient Protein

Amino Acid	*44% Soybean Meal*[a]	*Menhaden Fishmeal*[a]	*Sweet Whey*[b]	*Acid Whey*[b]
Lysine	6.6	7.7	8.8	10.3
Histidine	2.5	2.4	2.0	2.3
Arginine	7.3	6.1	2.6	2.8
Tryptophan	1.5	1.1	2.4	2.4
Threonine	3.9	4.1	6.8	4.9
Cystine	1.5	0.9	2.3	2.2
Valine	4.6	5.2	5.9	5.2
Methionine	1.2	2.9	1.8	1.8
Isoleucine	4.5	4.7	5.9	5.4
Leucine	7.7	7.3	10.9	10.5
Tyrosine	3.4	3.2	2.7	3.1
Phenylalanine	4.8	4.0	3.5	3.7

[a] Data from NRC 1988.

[b] Values from Glass and Hedrick 1977a.

Table 34.5 Description of Treatment

Treatment	*Protein Source*	*Liquid Source*	*Crude Protein % of Dry Matter*	*Crude Protein Intake (g/d)*	*Feeding Method*	*Method Used to Control Protein Level*
CS-18	Corn and soybean meal	Water	17.9	381	Mixture of corn, soybean meal, vitamins, and minerals with water free-choice	Fixed by formulation
CFC	Corn and soybean meal	Water	11.4	82	Mixture of corn, soybean meal, vitamins, and minerals with water free-choice	Adjusted weekly to crude protein concentration in dry matter consumed by pigs on the CW treatment
IFC	Corn and soybean meal	Water	15.1	236	Mixture of corn, soybean meal, vitamins, and minerals with water free-choice	Adjusted weekly to match protein intake by pigs fed CW
CW	Corn and whey	Whey	11.4	259	Mixture of corn, soybean meal, vitamins, and minerals with whey free-choice	Determined by relative intake of corn + vitamin + mineral mixture and liquid whey
CSW-15	Corn and soybean meal	Whey	15.2	318	Mixture of corn, soybean meal, vitamin and minerals with whey free-choice	Crude protein level of dry diet adjusted weekly so combined dry matter intake from corn-soy mixture and liquid whey fed free-choice was 15%
CSW-17	Corn and soybean meal	Whey	17.1	341	Mixture of corn, soybean meal, vitamins, and minerals with whey free-choice	Crude protein level of dry diet adjusted weekly so combined dry matter intake from corn-soy mixture and liquid whey fed free-choice was 17%

regime used in swine production (18% crude protein, vitamin, mineral fortified corn-soybean meal diet fed free choice with water [CS-18]). Three of the six treatments (corn-whey [CW]; corn-soybean-whey, 15% crude protein [CSW-15], and corn-soybean-whey, 17% crude protein [CSW-17]) evaluated the effects of different levels of supplemental protein when liquid cheddar cheese whey was fed free-choice with a dry corn-based diet. The crude protein level of the total dry matter consumed was maintained at 15% (CSW-15) and 17% (CSW-17) by adjusting levels of soybean meal. Protein intake of pigs fed the CW-diet depended on the amounts of corn and whey consumed.

Two additional treatments compared soybean meal and liquid whey as supplements to corn. In the intake floating control (IFC) treatment, the average crude protein intake of pigs fed a corn-soybean meal diet, was maintained at the same level as pigs fed the CW diet, allowing comparisons between protein sources when pigs consumed the same amount of crude protein.

A concentration floating control (CFC) treatment examined performance of pigs fed a corn-soybean meal diet containing the same percentage of crude protein as the CW diet. Soybean meal levels of CFC diet varied so the percentage of crude protein (dry matter basis) was similar to that of the CW diet. Although the protein concentration of the CFC diet was the same as the CW diet, pigs fed the CFC diet consumed less total protein.

Pigs fed the CW diet maintained a growth rate similar to that of pigs fed the CSW-15 or CS-18 diet (Figure 34.1). The body weights of pigs fed the CW and corn-soybean meal (CS-18) diets were similar, even though the dry matter consumed by pigs fed liquid whey contained 6% less crude protein (17.9% versus 11.9%). Pigs fed the CW diet also had greater rate of gain than pigs fed the corn-soybean meal CFC diet, which contained the same percentage protein. After 14 weeks, pigs fed the CW diet weighed an average of 92.7 kg, while pigs assigned to the CFC diet weighed only 30.5 kg. The reduced gain of pigs fed the IFC diet relative to pigs fed the same amount of protein from corn and whey also indicated that the protein in corn and whey contains amino acids required for growth.

The dry matter conversion efficiency of pigs fed liquid whey was similar to that of pigs fed the CS-18 diet (Table 34.6). While pigs fed the CSW-15, CSW-17, CW, and CS-18 diets had similar dry matter conversion efficiencies, pigs fed the CS-15 and CSW-17 diets gained more weight per unit of protein consumed than pigs fed the CS-18 diet. This increased efficiency of protein utilization also suggests that the corn-whey protein combination is superior to protein in the corn-soybean meal combination.

Feeding acid whey free-choice with corn, as was done with sweet whey, decreased whey intake and gains by grower-finisher pigs (Benevenga 1982, unpublished). Increasing the protein level of the dry ingredient mixture to 13% restored performance and caused pigs to consume 30% of their dry matter intake from liquid acid whey during the grower-finisher period. Barber et al. (1978) found that replacing 30% of a barley-based diet with either acid or sweet whey resulted in similar performance by pigs from 20 to 90 kg body weight, suggesting that the two whey types contained similar nutritive value. Benevenga (1984) varied the combination of corn and whey proteins in a baby pig slope-ratio assay and found that the protein quality of acid whey was

Regime	*Description*
CS-18	18% crude protein, corn-soybean meal weanling pig diet fortified with vitamins and minerals.
CSW-15	Corn-Soybean meal-whey diet in which crude protein constitutes 15% of the dry matter.
CSW-17	Same as CSW-15, except crude protein constitutes 17% of the dry matter.
CW	Ground, shelled corn fortified with vitamins and minerals and fed free-choice with whey.
IFC	Intake floating control in which crude protein intake of corn-soybean meal diet with water is maintained equal to that of CW regime.
CFC	Concentration floating control in which crude protein concentration of dry matter in corn-soybean meal diet with water is maintained similar to that of CW regime.

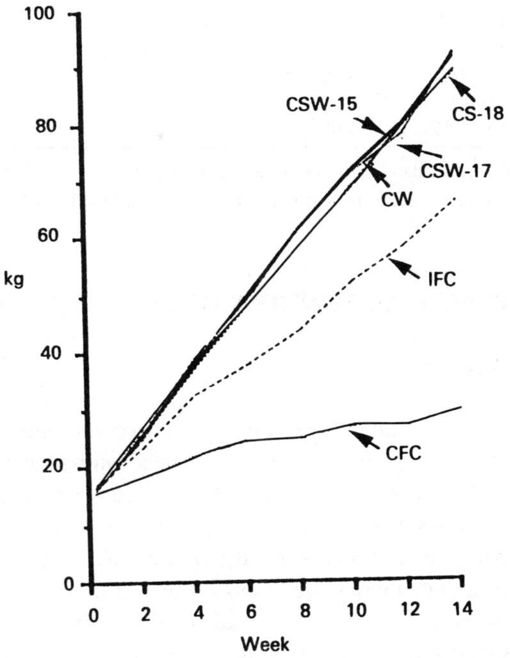

(Adapted, by permission, from Cieslak 1979.)

FIGURE 34.1 *Effect of whey dietary regimes on pig weight.*

inferior to that of sweet whey. A slope-ratio study involving acid whey from a different source showed acid and sweet whey protein qualities were similar. Whey source and processing may influence feeding value.

Condensed whey is produced by removing water from whey through evaporation or reverse osmosis. Concentrating whey is expensive and can cause lactose crystallization when the dry matter exceeds 25%. Feeding condensed whey free-choice with a corn-soybean meal diet and as the only liquid source was unsuccessful (Vignes 1976), but concentrated whey can be successfully fed to grower-finisher pigs if drinking water is provided. Hanrahan (1971) fed concentrated whey (16.6% to 19.7% solids) to pigs so whey provided 0%, 20%, 40%, or 60% of their dry matter intake. Pig performance was acceptable on all treatments but daily feed intake and daily gain from the 60% whey diet were lower than those from the control diet.

Table 34.6 Effect of Treatment on Performance and Carcass Characteristics

	CFC[a]	*IFC*[a]	*CS-18*	*CW*	*CSW-15*	*CSW-17*
Average daily gain (kg)	0.14	0.53	0.75	0.78	0.76	0.76
Average daily dry matter intake (kg)	0.70	1.72	2.12	2.19	2.11	1.99
Dry matter conversion	4.96	3.23	2.84	2.79	2.52	2.62
Average slaughter weight (kg)	—	—	98.2	99.1	96.8	99.1
Dressing %[b]	—	—	74.1	75.5	75.5	74.7
Length (cm)	—	—	79	78	79	78
Average backfat depth (cm)	—	—	3.5	4.0	3.7	3.6
Loin eye area (cm^2)	—	—	29.4	26.6	29.0	28.7

[a]Carcass data were not collected on pigs fed CFC and IFC diets.

[b]Means for CS-18 and CSW-17 were significantly different ($P < .05$) from those of CW and CSW-15 treatments.

PRACTICAL CONSIDERATIONS

Animals

Feeding liquid whey during the grower-finisher period is best because the potential feed savings is great and pigs can consume large volumes of liquid. Pigs should average 18 kg body weight before they are fed corn and whey free-choice. Weanling pigs may not consume sufficient whey volume to satisfy their amino acid needs and to make whey feeding economical (Modler 1985). Feeding liquid whey can cause a wet environment, increasing stress on young pigs. Limited field experience shows that liquid whey can replace up to half of the daily dry feed intake by gestating sows when the by-product replaces water as the liquid source (Muller 1979). Avoid feeding liquid whey during lactation because large liquid intakes prevent sows from consuming adequate energy. A wet environment caused by whey feeding can also jeopardize piglet survival.

Consumption

Grower-finisher pigs fed vitamin- and mineral-fortified grain free-choice with liquid whey should consume a minimum of 50% of their protein from whey. Results from a series of experiments at the University of Wisconsin show grower-finisher pigs consume 8 to 12 kg/pig/day and average 10 kg/pig/day of liquid sweet when whey is the only liquid source and it is fed free-choice with vitamin- and mineral-fortified ground corn. Daily liquid whey consumption increases until pigs reach about 60 kg and then remains constant or decreases slightly (Figure 34.2).

Holmes (1970) found that decreasing whey temperature from 40 °C to 20 °C significantly reduced whey consumption. Pigs housed in a 16 °C environment and fed whey

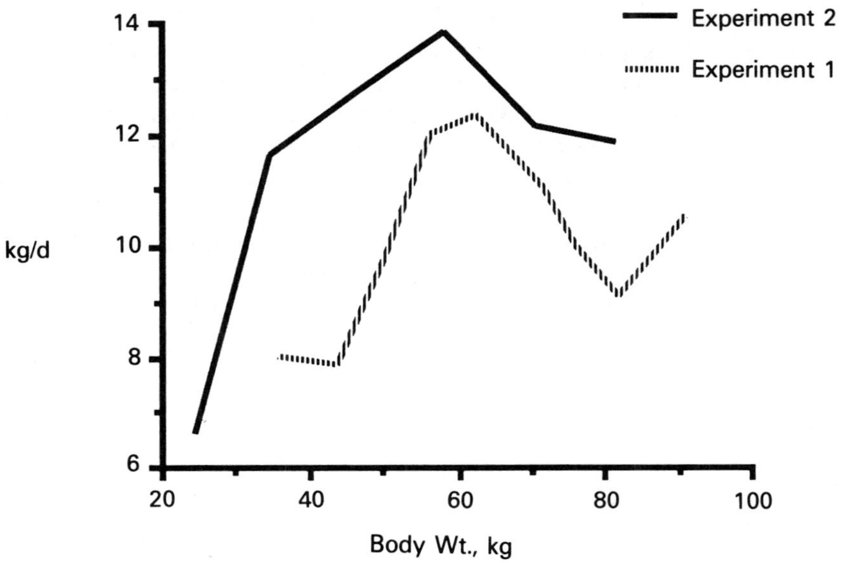

(Adapted, by permission, from Vignes et al. 1976.)

FIGURE 34.2 *Effect of body weight on voluntary liquid whey consumption, kg/d.*

at 15 °C grew slower and required more dry matter per kilogram of body weight than did pigs offered whey at 40 °C. Raising the environmental temperature to 22 °C diminished the adverse effects of feeding whey at 15 °C (Holmes 1971). Feeding cold whey to pigs in a cold environment could adversely affect performance due to the extra heat production required to warm the whey.

Storage Life

Between one third and one half of the nutritional value of liquid whey is lost during storage (Dunkin 1969; Fox and O'Conner 1969; Hanrahan 1969). Vignes (1976) found that fresh liquid Swiss cheese whey stored for 48 hours lost as much as 10% of the dry matter, 14% of the protein, and 37% of the lactose. The lactic acid produced during this period lowered pH by one unit. The low pH of acid whey prevents the growth of lactic acid-producing bacteria and extends storage life beyond that of sweet whey.

Pasteurization can decrease lactic acid production in liquid whey, but the by-product available for feeding is often unpasteurized. Additives to preserve liquid whey have not been cleared. Adding 0.1% of a 37% formaldehyde solution (formalin) to whey prior to storage at the cheese plant has been shown to maintain whey pH at 5.8 to 6.1 for 2 to 3 days. Untreated whey can reach a pH of 4 within 4 hours. Adding more than 0.15% formalin has been shown to reduce palatability.

Organic acids added to fresh whey lower the pH and inhibit bacterial growth. Formic acid added at 2% or propionic acid added at 0.2% levels effectively preserves whey but adversely affects palatability. Hydrogen peroxide added at 0.5 ml/L also preserves whey, but the cost exceeds that of formaldehyde (Modler 1985). Peters and Froseth (1983) found copper sulfate (1.3 g $CuSo_4 \cdot 5\ H_2O$/L) to be a preferred preservative over penicillin, propionic acid, or formalin. Feeding copper sulfate-preserved whey could cause excessive copper intakes when pigs consume large volumes of the liquid; therefore, the copper sulfate ($CuSO_4 \cdot 5\ H_2O$) level should not exceed 0.5 g/L.

Reduced storage temperature should extend the storage life of fresh whey. Peters and Froseth (1982) reported pH and dry matter content did not change when fresh whey was stored at 5 °C but that levels decreased dramatically when whey was stored at 22 °C and 35 °C.

Animal Health

Death loss among pigs fed liquid whey free-choice tends to increase. This is probably due to a damp environment and generally less sanitary conditions than with conventional feeding. These conditions can cause pig discomfort during cold weather and can increase water vapor that must be removed in environmentally regulated facilities. Death due to a hemorrhagic bowel syndrome and twisted gut has been observed, especially among pigs approaching slaughter weight. Overconsumption of whey following the delivery of fresh whey or after the whey supply has run out may increase the risk of intestinal disorders. Providing a continuous supply of fresh palatable whey will minimize this problem and minimize gastric upsets that may result during adaptation to the whey diet. Avoid frequent switching of liquid whey and dry diets.

Facility Modification and Durability

The lactic acid in whey will dissolve concrete and corrode metal. The continual contact with whey causes floors near troughs and drinkers to become rough and abrasive. The wet environment that frequently occurs can further deteriorate facilities.

Any operation using liquid whey will need a storage tank to hold enough volume to service the operation for 1 to 2 days if sweet whey is fed and up to 4 days if acid whey is used. Wood, fiberglass, or stainless steel tanks work best because they resist corrosion. Steel or galvanized coated tanks corrode quickly, and the acid of whey will dissolve iron oxide from rust, producing a flavor that makes whey unpalatable. Withdraw liquid from the side wall rather than the bottom of the tank to prevent whey particles from plugging distribution lines.

Modified nipple drinker watering systems are used when whey is fed as the only source of liquid. A pressure pump made of corrosion-resistant materials removes whey from the storage tank and pumps it to nipple drinkers in each pen via a plastic pipe. The filter between the drinker and the supply line is usually removed or modified to reduce plugging from whey particles. Provide at least two drinkers per 25 pigs. Place drinkers over the waste disposal system and space them at least 2 feet apart.

Whey can also be pumped into troughs extending the length of the pen with the whey level maintained by a float and valve arrangement. Defecation in the trough can be a problem if the trough is not covered. Troughs should be made of wood or lined with ceramic, plastic, or stainless steel.

Slurry or wet feeding systems have been used when liquid whey is not used as the sole source of supplemental protein. These systems combine liquid whey with dry feed ingredients and circulate the mixture throughout the facility via a supply line. A valve at each pen controls the flow of feed to the pen so that feed delivery can be adjusted when consumption is not consistent across pens. The operator using this system must anticipate animal needs and provide sufficient feed to maximize growth without causing feed wastage. This system does not allow animals to voluntarily select between whey and corn to balance their amino acid intake. The operator must also determine the proper dry matter level and whey-dry feed mixture to use.

Increased Waste Production

Grower-finisher pigs consuming liquid whey ad libitum will drink 50% to 100% more water than pigs fed a conventional diet (Vignes 1976), increasing the waste volume produced. Feeding liquid whey will increase the waste storage capacity needed or increase the frequency of emptying of existing storage capacity. Operations using solid waste handling may also experience difficulty handling the low dry matter waste that results from whey feeding.

Vitamin and Mineral Fortification

Vitamin-mineral premixes designed for use with conventional swine diets can be used to supplement cereal grains fed free-choice with liquid whey, but they do not account for the mineral balance and availability in liquid whey. The premix formula shown in Table 34.7 was developed (Crenshaw 1984) for use when liquid whey and grains are fed free-choice.

Economics

Feeding liquid whey provides the greatest economic advantage when it is fed free-choice with corn as the only supplemental protein. Table 34.8 shows the feed savings per pig at varying soybean meal prices and average daily liquid whey intakes. The feed savings must exceed the combined cost for whey transportation, facility modification, added waste handling, increased death loss, reduced facility life, and additional management before liquid whey feeding can be advantageous. A net economic benefit must occur most of the time despite fluctuating prices of protein supplements to justify switching from a conventional to a liquid whey feeding program.

Table 34.7 Base Mix to Fortify Corn for Feeding Free-Choice with Liquid Whey to Grower-Finisher Pigs[a]

Ingredient	*Level*[b]
Ground limestone (%)	41.0
Zinc carbonate (%)	0.64
Ferrous carbonate (%)	0.62
Cupric sulfate (25.4% Cu) (%)	0.08
Selenium mix[c]	0.10
Vitamin mix[d]	1.00
Carrier[e] (%)	56.56
	100.00

[a]Base mix added to corn at a rate of 2.5%.

[b]Levels are as a percentage or amount per kilogram of base mix.

[c]Provides 13 mg/kg of base mix.

[d]Provides the following per kilogram of base mix: vitamin A, 100,000 IU; vitamin D_3, 16,000 IU; vitamin K, 280 mg; niacin, 800 mg; vitamin B_{12}, 0.4 mg.

[e]Fine-ground corn containing 2% mineral oil for dust control.

Table 34.8 Feed Cost Savings When Liquid Whey and Corn Are Fed Free-Choice to Grower-Finisher Pigs

Soybean Meal Price			
$/Ton	*¢/lb*	*Feed Savings ($/Pig)*[a]	*Value of Savings (¢/gallon of Whey)*[b]
180	9	7.56	2.2
200	10	8.40	2.4
220	11	9.24	2.6
240	12	10.08	2.8
260	13	10.92	3.1
280	14	11.76	3.4
300	15	12.60	3.6
320	16	13.44	3.8
340	17	14.28	4.1
360	18	15.12	4.3

[a]Feed savings based on grower-finisher pigs gaining 77.3 kg while consuming a 14% crude protein diet containing 15% soybean meal, (44%). Average feed conversion = 3.3.

[b]Based on a 13.6-kg (3.5-gallon) average daily liquid whey intake for a 100-day period.

Liquid sweet whey can provide 25% to 30% of the dry matter when it is combined with a complete feed and fed as a gruel (Lachance et al. 1985). Such a program does not fully exploit the economic advantage of using liquid whey as the only supplemental protein. Feeding a complete liquid feed requires greater equipment expense than when liquid is delivered to pens via a watering system.

REFERENCES

Al-Ani, M.R. et al. 1972. *Nutr. Rep. Int.* 5:111.

Barber, R.S., et al. 1978. *Anim. Feed Sci. Technol.* 3:163.

Benevenga, N.J. 1984. *J. Anim. Sci.* 59(Suppl. 1):96.

Bohstedt, G., and R.H. Grummer. 1954. *J. Anim. Sci.* 13:933.

Chan, H.W., et al. 1976. *Nutr. Rep. Int.* 14:597.

Cieslak, D.G. 1979. Evaluation of whey protein as a supplement to corn using growing pigs and rats. M.S. thesis, University of Wisconsin, Madison, WI.

Cieslak, D.G., et al. 1986. *Anim. Feed Sci. Technol.* 14:171.

Crenshaw, T.D. 1984. Wisconsin Swine Facts and Analysis. Fact sheet SW 84-5, Department of Meat and Animal Science, University of Wisconsin, Madison.

Dunkin, A.C. 1969. *N.Z. J. Agric.* 118:22.

Ekstrom, K.E., et al. 1975a. *J. Nutr.* 105:851.

Ekstrom, K.E., et al. 1975b. *J. Nutr.* 105:1032.

Ekstrom, K.E., et al. 1976. *J. Anim. Sci.* 42:106.

Fox, D.F., and F. O'Conner. 1969. *Irish J. Agric. Res.* 8:271.

Gilles, M.T. 1974. *Whey Processing and Utilization.* Park Ridge, NJ: Noyes Data Corp.

Glass, L., and T.I. Hedrick. 1977a. *J. Dairy Sci.* 60:185.

Glass, L., and T.I. Hedrick. 1977b. *J. Dairy Sci.* 60:190.

Hanrahan, T.D. 1969. *Irish J. Agric. Res.* 8:271.

Hanrahan, T.D. 1971. *Irish J. Agric. Res.* 10:9.

Holmes, C.W. 1970. *Anim. Prod.* 12:485.

Holmes, C.W. 1971. *Anim. Prod.* 13:1.

Kim, K-I., et al. 1978a. *J. Anim. Sci.* 46:1658.

Kim, K-I., et al. 1978b. *J. Anim. Sci.* 46:1648.

Lachance, B., et al. 1985. *Proceedings of the Symposium on Swine Production. Counseil des Production Animales du Quebec.* Ottawa, Ontario: Research Program Service, Research Branch, Agriculture Canada.

Modler, H.W. 1985. *The Use of Whey as Animal Feed and Fertilizer.* Ottawa, Ontario: Food Research Institute, Agriculture Canada.

Muller, P.G. 1979. *Economic evaluation of feeding liquid whey to livestock. Part 2 Project Report: Whey utilization, nutritional aspects, feeding practices and systems, transportation cost, national benefits.* Ottawa, Ontario: Food Research Institute, Research Branch, Agriculture Canada.

NRC. 1979. *Nutrient Requirements of Swine.* 8th ed. Washington, DC: National Academy of Sciences.

NRC. 1988. *Nutrient Requirements of Swine.* 9th ed. Washington, DC: National Academy of Sciences.

Peters, D.N., and J.A. Froseth. 1982. *J. Anim. Sci.* 55(Suppl. 1):521.

Peters, D.N., and J.A. Froseth. 1983. *J. Anim. Sci.* 57(Suppl. 1):263.

Smith, G. 1976. *World Rev. Nutr. Diet.* 24:88.

Vignes, J.L. 1976. Utilization of fresh liquid whey or condensed whey (20% DM) by the growing-finishing pig. M.S. thesis, University of Wisconsin, Madison, WI.

Womack, M., and D.A. Vaughan. 1972. *J. Dairy Sci.* 55:1081.

Chapter 35

Raw and Processed Soybeans in Swine Diets

D.M. Danielson and J.D. Crenshaw

Many areas of the world have enjoyed and been dependent on the soybean *(Glycine max)* for nutritional needs for nearly 5000 years. Its origin and early history are unknown. It is generally accepted that the soybean is a native of eastern Asia. Nagata (1959, 1960) suggests that the species originated in the northern and central regions of China proper. It was considered one of the five sacred grains, that is, rice, soybean, wheat, barley and millet, essential to the existence of Chinese civilization (Morse 1950).

The first published acknowledgement of the soybean in the United States was by Mease (1804). In 1850, the United States Department of Agriculture (USDA) initiated research to study the use of the legume as forage, green manure, silage, or hay crop. It was not until 1940 that production of soybeans for beans surpassed the production for hay.

As the world need for large quantities of vegetable oil increased at the beginning of the twentieth century, so too did the importance of the soybean. The supply of soybean meal as a by-product increased rapidly during World War II because of the increased demand for edible vegetable oils. Simultaneously, the high price of livestock encouraged the feeding of supplemental protein feeds. As the oil industry grew, the nutritional value of soybean meal, a by-product of the oil extraction process, became widely recognized. Consequently, it has become the most important protein supplement in livestock and poultry feeds in the United States. The total increase in soybean production over the years has been spectacular in American agricultural history.

World recognition of soybean qualities, in addition to the knowledge that the climatic requirements for the soybean are about the same as that for corn, is producing a shift in geographic production areas. The United States once produced more than 75% of the total world soybean supply; by 1985, it produced only 58.9% (USDC 1988). The shift in production resulted from significant increases in soybean production in Brazil, Indonesia, Mexico, South Korea, Canada, Columbia, and several

European countries. This shift and the increase in total world production substantiates recognition of the nutritional qualities of soybeans.

NUTRITIONAL IMPORTANCE

Raw Soybeans (Full-Fat)

At the time soybean meal was becoming popular and well-recognized as an excellent protein supplement in livestock and poultry feeds, many producers attempted to utilize raw soybeans (unheated) in feeding systems. To their dismay, there was growth retardation and reduced efficiency in animal performance when raw soybeans replaced soybean meal as a feed protein supplement.

Research studies have indicated that raw soybeans contain factors that retard growth in swine (Robinson 1930; Jimenez et al, 1963; Hooks et al. 1965, 1967a,b; Combs et al. 1967; Sheppard et al. 1967; Young 1967, 1969; Combs and Wallace 1969; Jensen et al. 1970, 1971; Young et al. 1970; Hanke et al. 1972; Yen et al. 1974, 1977; Crenshaw and Danielson 1985b). Osborne and Mendel (1917) demonstrated that heating raw soybeans deactivated the antigrowth factors. Although several of the antigrowth factors (trypsin inhibitors, urease, and lipoxidase) can be deactivated by proper heat treatment, there are some antigens that are not easily deactivated.

The protein quality of the raw soybean (full-fat) is dependent on its amino acid balance (Table 35.1). When relating to the essential amino acids, methionine is the only amino acid considered to be marginal in this feedstuff. The amino acid profile of soybeans or soybean meal is complementary to the amino acid profile of most of the common grains (maize, barley, wheat, sorghum grain, or oats) used in swine feed.

Proximate composition of full-fat soybeans (Table 35.1) indicates the contribution that they afford when included as a supplement in livestock diets. The value of this feedstuff as an energy source is reflected by the 18% ether extract content.

The high fat content of the soybean allows for simple incorporation of fat into animal diets. In addition to increasing the energy density of a diet, the fat from the soybean reduces feed dustiness and subsequent dust accumulation in confinement buildings. Previous research by Chiba et al. (1985) reported that 5% fat reduced dust accumulation in swine confinement by approximately 50%. In typical swine diets formulated with raw or cooked soybeans, an additional 3% to 4% dietary fat is contributed by the soybeans. Suggested diets formulated with whole soybeans or soybean meal are presented in Table 35.2.

Until recently, soybeans in swine diets have been fed primarily in the form of soybean meal, or roasted or extruded beans. However, age of the animal may influence the extent to which antigrowth factors in raw soybeans affect performance. Jimenez et al. (1963), Doty (1965), Combs et al. (1967), Combs and Wallace (1969), Young (1970), Crenshaw and Danielson (1985b), and Danielson (1986) reported that young growing pigs fed uncooked soybeans gain slowly and inefficiently due to the inhibition of trypsin, the key proteolytic enzyme essential for effective protein digestion.

Table 35.1 Nutrient Composition of Whole Soybeans and Soybean Meal

		Soybean Meal	
	Whole Soybean	*Dehulled, Solvent Extracted*	*Solvent Extracted*
Dry matter (%)	90	90	90
ME (kcal/kg)	3625	3385	3220
Crude protein (%)	36.7	48.5	44
Ether extract (%)	18.8	0.9	1.1
Crude fiber (%)	5.2	3.4	7.3
Calcium (%)	0.26	0.26	0.30
Phosphorus (%)	0.61	0.64	0.65
Arginine (%)	2.54	3.67	3.20
Histidine (%)	0.87	1.20	1.12
Isoleucine (%)	1.60	2.13	2.00
Leucine (%)	2.64	3.63	3.37
Lysine (%)	2.25	3.12	2.90
Methionine (%)	0.46	0.71	0.52
Cystine (%)	0.55	0.70	0.66
Phenylalanine (%)	1.80	2.36	2.10
Tyrosine (%)	1.26	1.71	1.50
Threonine (%)	1.42	1.90	1.70
Tryptophan (%)	0.54	0.69	0.64
Valine (%)	1.62	2.47	2.02

(Adapted, by permission, from NRC 1988.)

The data in Table 35.3 (Danielson 1986) indicate that raw soybeans replacing soybean meal on an equal weight basis in starter diets significantly reduced average daily feed intake, average daily gain, and feed efficiency.

An experiment reported by Crenshaw and Danielson (1985b) indicates that replacing soybean meal with raw soybeans in growing-finishing diets either on equal weight basis or on an isonitrogenous basis reduces live-animal performance. As presented in Table 35.4, the initial weight and days on experiment dictate the degree of reduced performance.

Jensen et al. (1970) and Crenshaw and Danielson (1983) reported that gestating swine reproduced normally when fed diets containing raw soybeans as the sole source of supplemental protein in a complete diet. The success of this type of feeding regimen could relate to reproductive functions being protected by the dam, which buffers the fetus against nutritional discrepancies. In growth critera, this type of protection is not present.

Moser and Lewis (1981) summarized 25 trials in which pig survival was improved by 2.6% when the energy content of gestation diets was increased by the addition of animal fat or vegetable oil (energy).

Thus, theorizing that the inhibitors in raw soybeans are primarily growth related has prompted further studies utilizing raw soybeans as a source of protein and energy

Table 35.2 Suggested Swine Diets Using Whole Soybeans or Soybean Meal

	Weight Class (kg)									
Ingredient (%)	*5–20*		*20–50*		*50–100*		*Gestation (2–2.5 kg/d)*		*Lactation (Ad Libitum)*	
Corn	63.40	55.85	75.15	68.90	80.75	76.15	84.70	81.45	79.10	74.25
Soybean meal	32.70		21.70		16.05		10.75		16.40	
Whole soybeans		40.25[a]		28.00[a]		20.70[a]		13.90		21.15
Dicalcium phosphate	1.75	1.70	0.85	0.80	0.95	0.90	2.25	2.50	2.15	2.40
Limestone	0.85	0.90	1.00	1.00	0.95	0.95	1.00	0.85	1.05	0.90
Salt	0.30	0.30	0.30	0.30	0.30	0.30	0.30	0.30	0.30	0.30
Vit-AB-TM mix[b]	1.00	1.00	1.00	1.00	1.00	1.00	1.00	1.00	1.00	1.00
Calculated analysis										
Crude protein (%)	19.8	19.3	16	16	14	14	12	12	14	14
Lysine (%)	1.10	1.10	0.81	0.84	0.66	0.68	0.52	0.53	0.67	0.69
Calcium (%)	0.85	0.85	0.65	0.65	0.65	0.65	0.97	0.97	0.97	0.97
Phosphorus (%)	0.70	0.70	0.50	0.50	0.50	0.50	0.77	0.77	0.77	0.77
ME (kcal/kg)	3160	3252	3186	3259	3186	3239	3136	3171	3136	3191

[a] Cooked or extruded full-fat soybeans only. Raw soybeans not recommended.

[b] Vitamin-antibiotic-trace mineral mix.

Table 35.3 Performance of Pigs Fed Starter Diets (Pelleted and Nonpelleted) Supplemented with Raw Soybeans or Soybean Meal (42 d)

	Dietary Treatments			
	Nonpelleted		*Pelleted*	
Criteria	*SBM*	*RSB*	*SBM*	*RSB*
No. of pigs	20	20	20	20
Initial weight (kg)	7.5	7.8	7.6	7.6
Final weight (kg)	22.0	10.7	23.2	9.4
Avg. daily gain (kg)[a]	0.34	0.07	0.37	0.04
Avg. daily feed intake (kg)[a]	0.64	0.28	0.68	0.34
Feed conversion[a]	1.87	4.16	1.82	7.85

Abbreviations: SBM, soybean meal; RSB, raw soybeans.
[a]SBM versus RSB ($P < .01$).
(Data from Danielson 1986.)

in lactation as well as in gestation diets (Danielson and Crenshaw 1985; Matzat et al. 1985; Newman et al. 1987; Danielson 1986; Yen and Pond 1986). Based on the results of these studies, it seems feasible that raw soybeans can be successfully used as the supplemented protein in both gestation and lactation diets without affecting dam and litter performance.

The experiments conducted by Crenshaw and Danielson (1985c) and Danielson (1986) utilizing raw soybeans are presented in Table 35.5. Each of the two experiments recorded the performance over three consecutive reproduction cycles. In experiment 1, raw soybeans were utilized only during the gestation phase. In experiment 2, a third treatment was included, which utilized raw soybeans on an equal weight basis when replacing soybean meal. During gestation, all animals received 1.81 kg of their respective diets daily and all were ad libitum fed a soybean meal diet during lactation.

In the first experiment (Table 35.5), 88 of possible 90 litters were farrowed for each dietary treatment. Feeding raw soybeans (RSB) did not affect number of pigs born alive. For the three parities, live pigs at parturition and 21 days were as follows: soybean meal (SBM), 887 and 732, and RSB, 924 and 765, respectively. Birth weights and 21-day weights were as follows: SBM, 1.52 kg and 5.42 kg, and RSB, 1.59 kg and 5.41 kg, respectively. Birth weights of pigs from RSB dams were heavier, but weaning weights did not differ. Sow weight changes during gestation and lactation did not differ, although a slight reduction in average daily feed intake of dams fed RSB during lactation was observed.

In the second experiment (Table 35.5), there was a slight increase in the birth weight of pigs farrowed from dams fed RSB, but a smaller number of live pigs was farrowed. Survival at day 21 did not differ to any great extent; 21-day weights of pigs were heavier for the SBM litters. Gestation and lactation weight changes were the same for all treatments. Average daily feed intake during lactation was reduced for RSB dams. However, the fat content of the milk was higher when raw soybean diets were fed during gestation. The milk fat content remains higher throughout lactation when

Table 35.4 Performance of Growing Pigs Fed Diets Supplemented with Raw Soybeans

	Initial Weight Groups								
	Group A 23-kg Pigs			*Group B 45-kg Pigs*			*Group C 68-kg Pigs*		
Criterion[a]	*SBM*[b]	*EWB*[b]	*ISO*[b]	*SBM*	*EWB*	*ISO*	*SBM*	*EWB*	*ISO*
Days on study	98	98	98	56	56	56	28	28	28
Avg. initial wt. (kg)	24.5	25.0	24.3	46.3	46.2	46.2	69.3	69.5	69.5
Avg. final wt (kg)	96.7	60.8	60.8	95.2	75.3	78.2	92.5	86.2	85.2
Avg. daily gain (kg)	0.74[c]	0.37[d]	0.37[d]	0.88[c]	0.52[d]	0.57[d]	0.83[e]	0.60[f]	0.56[f]
Avg. feed intake (kg/d)	2.39[c]	1.66[d]	1.74[d]	3.13[e]	2.57[f]	2.65[f]	3.37[e]	3.02[f]	2.94[f]
Feed/gain	3.23[c]	4.47[d]	4.70[d]	3.56[c]	4.94[d]	4.65[d]	4.05[g]	5.03[h]	5.25[h]

Abbreviations: SBM, soybean meal; EWB, equal weight basis; ISO, isonitrogenous; avg., average; wt. weight.

[a] Values represent the average of four pens per treatment outcome group.

[b] Dietary treatment.

[c,d] Values in the same row within initial weight groups bearing different superscripts differ ($P < .001$).

[e,f] Values in the same row within initial weight groups bearing different superscripts differ ($P < .01$).

[g,h] Values in the same row within initial weight groups bearing different superscripts differ ($P < .05$).

(Data from Crenshaw and Danielson 1985b.)

Table 35.5 Effect of Raw Soybeans Fed During Gestation or Gestation through Lactation for Three Parities on Sow and Litter Performance

	Dietary Treatment				
	Experiment 1[a]		*Experiment 2*[b]		
Criteria	*SBM*	*RSB*	*SBM*	*ISO*	*EWB*
Litter performance					
Litters	88	88	56	52	58
Live pigs	10.08	10.50	9.86	9.71	8.97
Birth wt. (kg)	1.52	1.59	1.60	1.64	1.64
Pigs d 7	8.83	9.33	8.76	8.36	8.00
Wt. d 7 (kg)	2.64	2.66	2.85	2.82	2.83
Pigs d 14	8.49	8.92	8.20	8.02	7.67
Wt. d 14 (kg)	3.77	4.06	4.33	3.97	4.09
Pigs d 21	8.32	8.69	7.92	7.78	7.52
Wt. d 21 (kg)	5.42	5.41	5.81	5.00	5.20
Survival (%)	82.53	82.79	80.33	80.52	83.86
Sow wt. change (kg)					
Gestation	43	46	43	40	45
Postfarrow	28	29	29	27	31
Lactation	−7	−7	11	15	16
Daily lactation feed intake					
1st wk	4.71	4.68	5.17	4.94	5.11
2nd wk	5.62	5.58	5.46	4.45	5.11
3rd wk	6.06	5.81	5.75	5.02	5.21
ADFI	5.46	5.36	5.46	4.81	5.14

Abbreviations: SBM, soybean meal; RSB, raw soybeans; ISO, isonitrogenous; EWB, equal weight basis; wt., weight; ADFI, average daily feed intake.

[a] Isonitrogenous diets.

[b] RSB replaced SBM on ISO and EWB.

(Data from Crenshaw and Danielson 1985c and Danielson 1986.)

dams are fed lactation diets containing raw soybeans. Milk protein is not affected by the feeding of raw soybeans. Other researchers (Matzat et al. 1985; Yen and Pond 1986) have reported similar results.

Processing and Storage

Feeding raw or cooked soybeans as the only feedstuff has proven to be unsuccessful. It is essential that soybeans be properly processed to ensure maximum nutrient utilization. When swine are fed whole soybeans, the soybeans should be ground and blended with the other constituents of the diet. A complete diet with uniform particle size is recommended.

If soybeans are processed with a hammer mill, a 3.2-mm screen is satisfactory during cool weather, while a 4.8-mm screen may be needed during warm weather. Oil (fat) content of the raw soybeans, environmental temperature, and humidity dictate the screen size that works best.

As previously indicated, the fat or oil (18%) found in whole soybeans requires proper care and management during storage. If ground soybeans or the complete mixed diet containing soybeans are to be stored for any length of time, especially during warm weather, an antioxidant should be added to prevent rancidity, which could reduce palatability. If possible, soybeans should be ground just prior to blending with the other diet ingredients in order to maintain quality.

Proper storage of whole soybeans starts at harvest. Soybeans should be properly dried and stored at a moisture not to exceed 12%. Eliminate as much foreign material as possible to facilitate proper storage. Avoid long-term storage of soybeans.

Soybean Meal

Today, most soybean meal is derived during the solvent-extraction process of oil extraction. This method has replaced the expeller and hydraulic-press methods formerly used in soybean oil production.

A chemical solvent such as commercial hexane is used in the solvent-extraction process. The solvent is recovered from the oil by distillation and used again. Because it contains less oil, the meal is less susceptible than the untreated bean to rancid conditions.

Properly processed soybean meal is an excellent source of protein. However, if the soybean meal is undercooked, the antigrowth factors may not be destroyed or deactivated. Feeding undercooked soybean meal reduces the average daily gain and feed conversion in growing pigs. Likewise, if soybean meal has been overcooked, the antigrowth factors are destroyed, but the availability of the essential amino acids, particularly lysine, are reduced substantially.

Limestone is sometimes added to soybean meal for improved flowability. Soybean meal that includes excessive foreign material should not be fed to pigs because foreign material usually does not provide any nutritional benefits and toxicity could occur.

Roasted Soybeans (Whole Cooked Soybeans)

Proper heat application deactivates the antigrowth factors in raw soybeans. Raw soybeans contain the trypsin inhibitor in an active form, which retards normal growth of pigs, thus it is referred to as an antigrowth factor. The trypsin inhibitor is enzymatic in property.

Deactivation of the trypsin inhibitor is accomplished with dry pulsating heat (a combination of radiant and infrared) from the gas shield of the machine, conduction through the bean, convection between the beans, and direct flame impingement.

As the beans are intermittently subjected to the heat source, the hammering effect

Table 35.6 Cooked Whole Soybeans as a Protein Supplement for Growing-Finishing Swine

Performance and Carcass Criterion	*Soybean Meal*	*Cooked Whole Soybeans*
Avg. daily gain (kg)	0.84	0.85
Avg. daily feed (kg)	2.83	2.68
Feed/gain ratio	3.36	3.15
Carcass length (cm)	76.02	76.56
Backfat (cm)	3.23	3.30
Longissimus muscle area (cm^2)	28.69	29.61
Ham and loin (%)	37.31	38.12
Iodine no.	63.0	70.5
Carcass firmness[a]	4.0	3.2

[a]Firmness scores increase with hardness (1 to 5).
(Data from Wahlstrom et al. 1971.)

of the pulsating heat into the interior of the bean slightly darkens the hull. The actual cooking is accomplished within the bean itself by the bean's moisture content. Boiling the moisture within the bean deactivates both the urease and lipoxidase and at the same time cracks the outer hull of the bean without rupturing the oil cells which could, over an extended time, diminish bean quality.

The process destroys both the urease and lipoxidase at about the same temperature, which is sufficiently below the temperature required to adversely alter the first-limiting amino acid, lysine. Therefore the deactivation of the inhibitor occurs without changing the structure of the protein or binding it by a chemical reaction that might make it resistive to digestion.

Proper cooking of soybeans destroys or deactivates the trypsin inhibitor and also increases the availability and value of protein by making the sulfur-containing amino acids more readily available. Cooking also improves the palatability of soybeans for pigs.

Roasted or whole cooked soybeans have little effect on rate of gain, but improvement in feed efficiency as high as 7% may be observed due to the higher fat content of the whole soybeans, which produces a more energy-dense diet (Table 35.6). Improvements in feed efficiency may be offset by the lower protein content of whole soybeans; whole cooked soybeans average about 37% protein, whereas soybean meal usually contains 44% or 48.5% protein (Table 35.1), depending upon whether or not the hulls are retained in the meal. Whole cooked soybeans may be used to replace soybean meal or other sources of protein in swine diets (Danielson and Crenshaw 1985; Danielson 1988).

Although the carcass fat from pigs fed whole soybeans is softer, research reported at several experiment stations in the United States (Anderson 1971 as summarized by Wahlstrom et al. 1971) indicates that whole cooked soybeans can be fed at 22% of a corn-based diet with no adverse effects on pig performance, carcass criteria, or consumer acceptance of pork (Table 35.6).

Table 35.7 Summary of Growing-Finishing Pig Performance When Diets Were Supplemented With Soybean Meal, Cooked (Roasted), or Extruded Soybeans on an Isonitrogenous Basis (105 d)

	Dietary Treatment					
	SBM		*RSB*		*ESB*	
Criteria	*(1) Pellet*	*(2) Meal*	*(3) Pellet*	*(4) Meal*	*(5) Pellet*	*(6) Meal*
ADG (kg)	0.84^{c}	$0.77^{a,b}$	0.80^{b}	0.74^{a}	0.79^{b}	$0.78^{a,b}$
ADFI (kg)	$2.58^{b,c}$	2.59^{c}	2.35^{a}	2.38^{a}	2.28^{a}	$2.40^{a,b}$
F/G	$3.06^{a,b}$	3.39^{c}	2.95^{a}	$3.20^{b,c}$	2.88^{a}	$3.06^{a,b}$
Backfat (cm)	2.24^{a}	2.21^{c}	2.41^{a}	2.34^{a}	2.29^{a}	2.26^{a}

(Abbreviations: SBM, soybean meal; RSB, roasted soybeans; ESB, extruded soybeans; ADG, average daily gain; ADFI, average daily feed intake; F/G, feed/gain.
[a,b,c]Means in same row with different superscripts differ significantly ($P < .05$.).

Extruded Soybeans

The extrusion of soybeans can be accomplished in several ways. The method of preconditioning the soybeans for the actual extrusion process may vary, depending on the equipment that is used. Some methods employ steam, others water, and still others friction to establish the heat needed for the extrusion process.

Like roasted soybeans, if extrusion procedures are inadequate for trypsin inhibition or urease deactivation, there probably will be decreased pig performance. Properly extruded soybeans can be successfully used to supplement growing-finishing pig diets (Table 35.7; Danielson 1988).

Raw soybeans have been successfully used to replace soybean meal in swine gestation-lactation diets, serving as a suitable protein and energy source. Heating by cooking, roasting, or extrusion is essential to secure favorable nutritional value of raw soybeans in diets of starting, growing, and finishing pigs.

REFERENCES

Anderson, W. 1971. *Feedstuffs* 43:13.
Chiba, L.I., et al. 1985. *J. Anim. Sci.* 61:763.
Combs, G.E., et al. 1967. *J. Anim. Sci.* 26:1067.
Combs, G.E., and H.G. Wallace. 1969. *Report of the 14th Annual Swine Field Day.* Gainesville, FL: University of Florida.
Crenshaw, M.A., and D.M. Danielson. 1983. *J. Anim. Sci.* 57(Suppl. 1):93.
Crenshaw, M., and D. Danielson. 1985a. *1985 Nebraska Swine Report.* p. 27. Lincoln: University of Nebraska.
Crenshaw, M.A., and D.M. Danielson. 1985b. *J. Anim. Sci.* 60:725.
Crenshaw, M.A., and D.M. Danielson. 1985c. *J. Anim. Sci.* 60:163.
Danielson, D.M. 1988. *Professional Animal Scientist* 4:4.
Danielson, M. 1986. *Proceedings of the International Pig Veterinary Society Congress.* p. 415. Barcelona, Spain.
Danielson, M., and M. Crenshaw. 1985. *1985 Nebraska Swine Report.* p. 29. Lincoln: University of Nebraska.
Doty, H.O. 1965. *Economic Research Service Bulletin 228.* Washington, DC: USDA.
Hanke, H.E., et al. 1972. *J. Anim. Sci.* 35:958.
Hooks, R.D., V.W. Hays, and V.C. Speer. 1967a. *J. Anim. Sci.* 26:908.
Hooks, R.D., V.W. Hays, and V.C. Speer. 1967b. *J. Anim. Sci.* 26:908.
Hooks, R.D., et al. 1965. *J. Anim. Sci.* 24:894.
Jensen, A.H., et al. 1970. *J. Anim. Sci.* 31:1023.
Jensen, A.H., et al. 1971. *Illinois Pork Industry Day Report AS6-658B.* p. 6. Urbana: University of Illinois.
Jimenez, A.A., et al. 1963. *J. Anim. Sci.* 22:471.
Matzat, P.D., E.R. Miller, and M.G. Hogberg. 1985. *Michigan State Report on Swine Research* 469:19. East Lansing: Michigan State University.
Mease, J. 1804. *Willich's Domestic Encyclopedia. First American Edition.* Vol. 5 p. 13. Philadelphia.
Morse, W.J. 1950. "History of soybean production." In: *Soybeans and Soybean Products.* Vol. 1. pp. 3–59. Morksley, K.S. (Ed.). New York: Interscience Publishers, Inc.
Moser, B.D., and A.J. Lewis. 1981. *Pig News Information.* 2:265.

Nagata, T. 1959. *Proc. Crop Sci. Soc. Jpn* 28:79.
Nagata, T. 1960. *Mem. Hyogo Univ. Agr.* 3 Ser. 4:63.
Newman, C.W., et al. 1987. *Nutr. Rep. Int.* 36:319.
NRC. 1979. *Nutrient Requirements of Swine.* 8th ed. Washington, DC: National Academy of Sciences.
NRC. 1988. Nutrient Requirements of Swine. 8th ed. Washington, DC: National Academy of Sciences.
Osborne, T.B., and L.B. Mendel. 1917. *J. Biol. Chem.* 52:369.
Robison, W.L. 1930. *Ohio Agricultural Experiment Station Bulletin 452.* Columbus: Ohio State University.
Sheppard, S., et al. 1967. *J. Anim. Sci.* 26:1478.
USDC. 1988. *Statistical Abstract of the United States.* Washington, DC: U.S. Department of Commerce–Bureau of Census.
Wahlstrom, R.C., G.W. Libal, and R.J. Burns. 1971. *J. Anim. Sci.* 32:891.
Yen, J.T., and W.G. Pond. 1986. *U.S. Meat Animal Research Center. Swine Research Progress Report* 2:56. Clay Center, NE.
Yen, J.T., T. Hymowitz, and A.H. Jensen. 1974. *J. Anim. Sci.* 38:304.
Yen, J.T., A.H. Jensen, and J. Simon. 1977. *J. Nutr.* 107:156.
Young, L.G. 1967. *Can. J. Anim. Sci.* 47:227.
Young, L.G. 1969. *J. Anim. Sci.* 29:150.
Young, L.G., et al. 1970. *Can J. Anim. Sci.* 50:717.

Chapter 36

Utilization of Cereal Grain By-products in Feeding Swine

P.J. Holden and D.R. Zimmerman

Many of the by-products of cereal grains cannot be used for human foods. Animal agriculture serves a useful function by utilizing these feedstuffs and converting them into "value added" animal products. The group includes products of the flour milling, distilling, brewing, and dry- and wet-corn milling industries. In general, these by-products have higher concentrations of fiber, crude protein, and minerals than their parent grains, because much of the starchy fraction has been removed.

High-fiber feedstuffs are poorly digested by monogastric animals. Therefore, the energy densities of many grain by-products are low for swine. Some by-products are concentrated sources of crude protein, but in general, the quality of the protein is poor because of deficiencies of lysine, threonine, and tryptophan. In addition, the digestibility by pigs of the amino acids in grain by-products is low relative to that in most protein supplements (see Chapter 19). Phosphorus is the mineral of most economical value in grain by-products. Its availability, however, is poor relative to that from inorganic phosphorus sources.

Because of low availability of some nutrients and poor protein quality in grain by-products, much of the supply of each of these by-products is used in feeds for ruminants. Their use in swine diets requires careful formulation if economical benefits are to be obtained.

MARKET AVAILABILITY OF GRAIN BY-PRODUCTS

The amounts of grain by-products used in livestock feed are considerable and have remained relatively stable in recent years (Table 36.1). The data do not differentiate utilization by species. In the United States, production of some of these by-products is considerably greater than domestic utilization, and therefore, the export market is large. If the United States were to lose this export market, more by-product would be available domestically.

Table 36.1 Quantity of Grain By-Products Fed in Selected Years in the United States (1000 Metric Tons)

	Year				
Feedstuff	*1972*	*1976*	*1980*	*1984*	*1988*
Brewers' dried grains	361	269	290	142	110
Distillers dried grains	428	339	453	807	970
Corn gluten feed and meal	1235	941	763	1876	1320
Rice millfeed	442	546	706	456	580
Wheat millfeed	4327	4351	4638	5084	5789

(Data from *Feed Situation* [1974] FDS-225, *Feed—Outlook and Situation Report* [1985] FDS-297, and [1988] FDS-308.)

FEEDING VALUE

Feeding values of feedstuffs for swine are determined largely by the usable energy, protein (lysine), and phosphorus contents. Because corn, soybean meal (SBM), and dicalcium phosphate are the primary sources of energy, lysine, and phosphorus, respectively, in U.S. swine diets, prices of these feedstuffs largely determine the dietary costs of energy, lysine, and phosphorus. Feeding value in dollars can be calculated using nutrient analyses of feedstuffs and local prices of corn, SBM, and dicalcium phosphate. Table 36.2 contains estimates of the feeding value of grain by-products when corn costs $97/metric ton, SBM (44%) costs $198/metric ton, and dicalcium phosphate costs $247/metric ton. The table also includes relative values of the products when corn is assigned a feeding value of 100%.

The data in Table 36.3 are ratios of the average yearly costs of brewers' dried grains (BDG), corn gluten feed, and distillers dried grains with solubles to the average cost of corn. The ratios were adjusted for the relative feeding values in Table 36.2. These ratios indicate that only in 1974 and 1984 were by-products economical to feed as a replacement for corn. These ratios are based on average yearly prices for the United States and do not necessarily apply at all times and in all localities.

Because of the low energy density and low lysine content, the grain by-products should not completely replace grains and protein supplements in swine diets. Table 36.4 gives suggested maximum dietary inclusion rates.

DESCRIPTION AND EXPERIMENTAL EVALUATION OF GRAIN BY-PRODUCT INGREDIENTS*

Brewers' Dried Grains

"The dried extracted residue of barley malt alone or in mixture with other cereal grains or grain products resulting from the manufacture of wort or beer and may contain pul-

*The following statements within quotation marks were taken from the Association of American Feed Control Officials (AAFCO) (1987).

Table 36.2 Feeding Value of Grain By-product Relative to Corn Based on Metabolizable Energy, Digestible Lysine, and Available Phosphorus[a]

Source	*ME (kcal/kg)*	*Digestible Lysine (%)*	*Available Phosphorus (%)*	*Feeding Value ($/metric ton)*	*Relative Value (%)*
Corn	3420	0.22	0.04	97.00	100
Dicalcium phosphate	—	—	18.50	247.00	—
Soybean meal, 44% CP	3220	2.61	0.23	198.00	—
Brewers' dried grains	1900	0.64	(0.17)[b]	78.30	81
Corn gluten feed	2695	0.32	0.58	90.00	93
Corn gluten meal, 41%	3880	(0.68)	0.13	129.80	134
Corn hominy feed	3310	(0.31)	(0.17)	99.80	103
Distillers dried grains with solubles (corn)	3335	(0.61)	0.47	117.40	121
Rice bran (unextracted)	3065	(0.49)	0.34	98.60	102
Wheat bran	2155	0.45	0.41	79.60	82
Wheat middlings	2965	0.54	0.40	104.00	107
Wheat shorts	2865	0.64	0.36	110.50	109

[a] Calculations based on prices ($/metric ton) for corn, dicalcium phosphate, and soybean meal of $97, $247, and $198, respectively. Available nutrients based on data by Knabe et al. (1986a, 1986b), LaRue et al. (1987), and Cromwell (1989). Analyses are on an as-fed moisture basis.

[b] Values in parentheses are author's estimates.

Table 36.3 Ratios of Costs of Selected Grain By-products Adjusted for Differences in Feeding Value[a]

Year	*DDGS*	*BDG*	*CGF*
1973	1.0	1.3	1.0
1974	0.9	1.0	0.8
1975	1.0	1.2	1.0
1976	1.4	1.8	1.5
1977	1.3	1.5	1.3
1978	1.3	1.5	1.5
1979	1.2	1.5	1.5
1980	1.2	1.3	1.1
1981	1.3	1.3	1.3
1982	1.2	1.4	1.3
1983	1.2	1.2	1.0
1984	0.8	0.8	0.8
1985	1.1	1.1	1.2
1986	1.7	1.8	1.9
1987	1.5	1.8	1.7

Abbreviations: DDGS, distillers dried grain with solubles (corn); BDG, brewers' dried grains (barley); CGF, corn gluten feed.

[a] [(By-product price − corn price) − by-product relative value in Table 36.2, 100. Prices from Feed Yearbook (1989) FDS-309.]

Table 36.4 Suggested Maximum Dietary Inclusion Rates of Grain By-products

	(%)			
Grain By-product	*Gestation*	*Lactation*	*Starter*	*Grower-Finisher*
Brewers' dried grains	40	5	0	5
Corn gluten feed	90	5	0	5
Corn gluten meal	5	5	5	2
Corn hominy feed	80	80	10	60
Distillers dried grains with solubles (corn)	40	5	5	20
Rice bran (unextracted)	30	5	5	20
Wheat bran	30	10	0	5
Wheat middlings	30	10	5	20
Wheat shorts	30	10	5	20

verized dried spent hops in an amount not to exceed 3%, evenly distributed.'' The product is a bulky, low-energy feed containing 13% to 16% crude fiber. It has about 25% crude protein of low quality, being low in lysine, threonine, and tryptophan. Because of its low energy concentration, it cannot be used in significant amounts in diets of growing and lactating swine, but it can be used in gestation formulations.

Growing-finishing pigs were fed up to 23% (Young and Ingram 1968) or 15% (Cromwell et al. 1979) brewers' dried grains (BDG) in diets without depression in rate of gain. However, in both reports, the feed:gain ratio increased with each increasing level of BDG. Wahlstrom and Libal (1976) successfully fed gestating sows diets containing up to 40% BDG when lysine levels were held at 0.50%. BDG has the same amino acid limitations as barley grain; lysine and threonine being first- and second-limiting for pig growth. Knabe et al. (1986a) and LaRue et al. (1987) have reported ileal apparent digestibilities for lysine, threonine, and tryptophan of 68%, 67%, and 71%, respectively.

Corn Gluten Feed

''The part of the commercial shelled corn that remains after extraction of the larger part of the starch, gluten and germ by the processes employed in the wet milling manufacture of corn starch or syrup. It may or may not contain fermented corn extractives and/or corn germ meal.'' Corn gluten feed (CGF) is often pelleted to increase its density and improve handling qualities. It has about 80% the metabolizable energy (ME) value of corn. It can be used at low levels ($\leq$5%) in growing-finishing diets and can supply most of the energy in gestation diets. It contains 20% crude protein of rather poor quality. The levels of lysine and tryptophan are low and poorly digestible.

The earliest reported use of CGF in pig diets was by Evvard (1920). He noted reduced feed intake when CGF was fed in combination with tankage. Geurin et al. (1951) demonstrated differences in protein quality of corn by-products. Corn germ meal, but not corn gluten meal, supported growth similar to that obtained with whole eggs, milk, or soybean meal. Growth with corn gluten meal was poor, and corn solubles did not support any growth. Yen et al. (1971) demonstrated that up to 30% CGF supported good performance if it replaced corn on an equal weight basis, but not if it replaced both corn and soybean meal on an isonitrogenous basis. If, however, both lysine and tryptophan were added, the growth was similar to an isonitrogenous corn-soybean meal diet. Harmon et al. (1975a) evaluated condensed fermented corn solubles with germ meal and bran as a protein source. It was found limiting in lysine and tryptophan. In a second publication by Harmon et al. (1975b), it was found that the product could effectively supply about 30% of the pig's lysine need. Knabe et al. (1986b) and LaRue et al. (1987) have shown that the amino acids in CGF are quite resistant to digestion, with ileal apparent digestibilities for lysine, threonine, and tryptophan of 41%, 46%, and 32%, respectively.

Because of the poor protein quality in CGF, it should be considered primarily as an energy source, even though it is a relatively fibrous feedstuff. Cornelius et al. (1977) estimated a ME value corrected for nitrogen (MEn) of 3790 kcal/kg of dry matter, and Ewan (unpublished data) estimated an ME of 3780 and net energy (NE) of 2040 kcal/kg of dry matter. This net energy value is 79% that of corn grain. Jones and Easter (1986) demonstrated that finishing pigs performed equally on diets ranging from 0% to 30% CGF if supplemented with tryptophan and if diets were isocaloric, assuming the ME value of CGF was 75% that of corn.

Zimmerman and Honeyman (1986) fed diets containing 0%, 25%, and 50% CGF to finishing pigs, keeping the lysine level constant. Increasing CGF levels did not affect daily feed intake, but rate of gain and feed efficiency were decreased, reflecting the decreased energy concentration of diets. Feeding CGF also reduced the dressing percentage at slaughter. Because of its relatively low energy concentration, CGF may be used to greatest advantage in diets of gestating sows. Honeyman and Zimmerman (1986) have successfully used CGF as the primary energy source in diets of pregnant sows. Because of a good export demand for CGF, it is usually not an economical energy replacement for corn (Table 36.3).

Corn Gluten Meal

"The dried residue from corn after removal of the larger part of the starch and germ, and the separation of the bran by the process employed in the wet milling manufacture of cornstarch or syrup or by the enzymatic treatment of the endosperm. It may contain fermented corn extractives and/or corn germ meal." It is sold as two products, containing 40% protein or 60% protein. The protein is of limited value in swine diets because of its low content of lysine and tryptophan. It is, however, a rich source of sulfur amino acids. The ingredient is usually not an economic source of nutrients for swine diets because of its demand as a pigmentation source for poultry.

Distillers Dried Grains with Solubles

The product "obtained after removal of ethyl alcohol by distillation from the yeast fermentation of a grain or a grain mixture by condensing and drying at least three-fourths of the solids of the resultant stillage by methods employed in the grain distilling industry. The predominant grain shall be declared as the first word of the name.'' Grains used include barley, corn, rye, sorghum, and wheat. Corn distillers dried grains with solubles (DDGS) contains 27% crude protein and an ME concentration of 3335 kcal/kg of air-dry diet.

DDGS is used as a source of energy, protein, and phosphorus in pig diets. If the lysine requirement is met, 20% corn DDGS can be included in growing-finishing diets with no depression in rate of gain and feed efficiency (Wahlstrom et al. 1970; Harmon 1975; Cromwell et al. 1983). A level of 44% DDGS was successfully utilized in gestation diets (Thong et al. 1978).

Newman and Gras (1983) fed up to 15% barley distillers grains to growing-finishing pigs with no effect on rate of gain. Feed efficiency was depressed at levels above 5% of the diet. Salo (1978) successfully used low levels of wheat distillers grains in pig diets. Peters et al. (1971) determined an MEn of 3340 kcal/kg of dry matter for corn DDGS. The phosphorus in corn DDGS is well-utilized as indicated by metatarsal breaking strength of pigs fed up to 40% DDGS (Cromwell et al. 1983). These pigs received most of their dietary phosphorus from DDGS.

Hominy Feed

''A mixture of corn bran, corn germ and part of the starchy portion of either white or yellow corn kernels or mixtures thereof, as produced in the manufacture of pearl hominy, hominy grits or table meal, and must contain not less than 4% crude fat.'' The crude protein concentration in hominy feed is 10%.

It is a relatively energy-rich grain by-product as indicated by ME and NE values of 3850 and 2290 kcal/kg dry matter, respectively (Stanley and Ewan 1982). Peo et al. (1987) observed that it can replace all of the corn in 16% protein grower and 14% protein finisher diets with no change in performance of pigs.

Rice Bran

''The pericarp or bran layer and germ of the rice, with only such quantity of hull fragments, chipped, broken, or brewers' rice, and calcium carbonate as is unavoidable in the regular milling of edible rice. It must contain not more than 13% crude fiber. When calcium carbonate exceeds 3% (Ca 1.2%), the percentage must be declared in the brand name.'' The fat in rice bran oxidizes rapidly and will become rancid and unpalatable in 2 or 3 days. Its value is proportional to the amount of rice hulls included. It can be used at up to 20% of the diet or to replace 30% of the corn.

Rice Bran, Solvent Extracted

''It is obtained by removing part of the oil from rice bran by the use of solvents and must contain not less than 14% crude protein and not more than 14% crude fiber.''

This product contains considerably less energy than the unextracted product, but it does not have the rancidity problem.

Rice bran may or may not contain a relatively high level of fat. Robles and Ewan (1982) evaluated the energy contribution of a rice bran containing 10.8% ether extract. For young pigs, the ME and NE concentrations were 3710 and 2030 kcal/kg dry matter, respectively. Hew et al. (1982) reported a phosphorus availability in rice bran of only 25%.

Wheat Middlings

"Consists of fine particles of wheat bran, wheat shorts, wheat germ, wheat flour, and some of the offal from the 'tail of the mill.' This product must be obtained in the usual process of commercial milling and must contain not more than 9.5% crude fiber." Midds comprise the layer of the wheat kernel just inside the outer bran covering, endosperm particles, bran particles, ground weed seeds, and other nonwheat materials. The appearance is that of a brownish, finely ground meal. Specifications for midds are usually of the order of 10% to 14% minimum protein, 3% minimum fat, 9.5% maximum fiber, and 2965 kcal/kg of ME. It is commonly added at low concentrations to all types of swine diets, except starter feeds. Its feeding value is 8% to 10% greater than corn and can compose up to 30% of a gestation diet.

Other Wheat Mill Feed Products

Wheat bran consists of the outer covering of the wheat kernel together with small amounts of flour and finely ground weed seeds. It has 13.5% to 15% minimum protein, 2.5% minimum fat, and 12% maximum fiber. It is a bulky product that has traditionally been used in sow diets as a laxative feed. *Wheat mill* run is a blend of bran and midds as produced in a mill. It has 14% to 16% minimum protein, 3% minimum fat, and 9.5% maximum fiber. *Wheat shorts* contain primarily wheat midds plus more flour than midds. It has 14% to 16% minimum protein, 3.5% minimum fat, and 7% maximum fiber. *Wheat red dog* contains more flour than the other mill feeds. It has 13.5% to 15% minimum protein, 2% minimum fat, and 4% maximum fiber. It has been used as an ingredient in weanling pig diets.

These products are similar except for fiber content and can replace up to 30% of the diet for gestating sows and 5% to 20% for growing-finishing pigs. Wheat bran is often added at 5% to 10% of lactation diets for its laxative effect.

Many experiments have been reported that evaluated wheat middlings, wheat shorts, and "pollard" as ingredients in swine diets. Except for starter pigs (Erickson et al. 1985), levels of up to 30% of the diet are well-tolerated. Energy evaluations (Frape et al. 1969; Patience et al. 1977a; Pals and Ewan 1978; Young 1980) indicated that digestible energy (DE) and ME values of wheat middlings are somewhat variable, and less than corn. Pals and Ewan (1978) found a very low NE value (910 kcal/kg of dry matter) for young pigs.

In performance trials with growing-finishing pigs (Beames and Natoli 1968; Hanrahan and O'Grady 1970; Patience et al. 1977a; Erickson et al. 1985), the inclusion of increasing levels of wheat by-product in diets resulted in an increase in feed intake, a poorer feed efficiency, and little, if any, effect on rate of gain. At relatively high levels of wheat middlings the amino acid balance and calcium and phosphorus utilization may limit growth. Patience et al. (1977b) indicated that lysine and threonine were growth-limiting amino acids in wheat shorts. Knabe et al. (1986a) and LaRue et al. (1987) indicated that the ileal digestibilities of amino acids in wheat middlings were intermediate; lysine 72%; threonine, 59%; and tryptophan, 70%. Hew et al. (1982) reported the phosphorus availability from wheat pollard was 55%. Erickson et al. (1977) and Collings et al. (1979) reported that wheat middlings adversely affected calcium and phosphorus absorption in pigs. When the phosphorus contribution of wheat middlings was considered in diet formulation, increasing levels of wheat middlings in the diets of growing-finishing pigs linearly decreased metatarsal bone ash (Erickson et al. 1985).

SUMMARY

Judicious use of grain by-products in swine diets may be cost-effective at times. It is imperative, however, to consider the content and availability of critical nutrients (i.e., energy, lysine, and phosphorus) when formulating swine diets that include grain by-products.

REFERENCES

AAFCO. 1987. *Official Publication.* Charleston, WV: Association of American Feed Control Officials, West Virginia Department of Agriculture.
Beames, R.M. and W.J. Natoli. 1969. *Aust. J. Exp. Agric. Anim. Husb.* 9:594.
Collings, G.F., et al. 1979. *J. Anim. Sci.* 49:528.
Cornelius, S.G., B.G. Harmon, and J.P. Totsch. 1977. *J. Anim. Sci.* 45:482.
Cromwell, G.L. 1979. *Proceedings of the Distillers Feed Research Council.* p. 40. Cincinnati: Distillers Feed Research Council.
Cromwell, G.L. 1989. *Proceedings, Meat and Milk Production Symposium.* Des Moines, IA: Pitman-Moore, Inc.
Cromwell, G.L., H.J. Monegue, and T.S. Stahly. 1979. *J. Anim. Sci.* 49(Suppl. 1):93.
Cromwell, G.L., et al. 1983. *J. Anim. Sci.* 57(Suppl. 1):49.
Erickson, J.P., et al. 1977. *Michigan State University Swine Research Report.* 363:89.
Erickson, J.P., et al. 1985. *J. Anim. Sci.* 60:1012.
Evvard, J.M. 1920. *Proc. Amer. Anim. Prod.* 1918:70.
Feed Situation. 1974. USDA Economic Research Service. FDS-225.
Feed—Outlook and Situation Report. 1985. USDA Economic Research Service FDS-297.
Feed-Outlook and Situation Report. 1988. USDA Economic Research Service FDS-308.
Feed Yearbook—Situation and Outlook Report. 1989. USDA Economic Research Service FDS-309.
Frape, D.C., J. Wilkinson, and L.G. Chubb. 1969. *Anim. Prod.* 11:429.
Guerin, H.B., et al. 1951. *J. Anim. Sci.* 10:607.

Hanrahan, T.J., and J.F. O'Grady. 1970. *Irish J. Agric. Res.* 9:335.
Harmon, B.G. 1975. *Proceedings 30th Distillers Feed Conference.* 30:23. Cincinnati, Distillers Feed Research Council.
Harmon, B.G., et al. 1975a. *J. Anim. Sci.* 40:242.
Harmon, B.G., et al. 1975b. *J. Anim. Sci.* 40:247.
Hew, V.G., G.L. Cromwell, and T.S. Stahly. 1982. *J. Anim. Sci.* 55(Suppl. 1):277.
Honeyman, M.S., and D.R. Zimmerman. 1986. *J. Anim. Sci.* 63(Suppl. 1):120.
Jones, R.W., and R.A. Easter. 1986. *J. Anim. Sci.* 63(Suppl. 1):120.
Knabe, D.A., et al. 1986a. *J. Anim. Sci.* 63(Suppl. 1):279.
Knabe, D.A., et al. 1986b. *J. Anim. Sci.* 63(Suppl. 1):278.
LaRue, D.C., D.A. Knabe, and T.D. Tanksley. 1987. *J. Anim. Sci.* 65(Suppl. 1):126.
Newman, C.W., and P.W. Gras. 1983. *J. Anim. Sci.* 47(Suppl. 1):260.
NRC. 1988. *Nutrient Requirements of Domestic Animals. Nutrient Requirements of Swine.* Ninth Revised Ed. Washington, DC: National Academy of Science–National Research Council.
Pals, D.A., and R.C. Ewan. 1978. *J. Anim. Sci.* 46:402.
Patience, J.F., L.G. Young, and I. McMillan. 1977a. *J. Anim. Sci.* 45:1294.
Patience, J.F., et al. 1977b. *J. Anim. Sci.* 45:1302.
Peo, E.R., Jr., J.D. Hancock, and A.J. Lewis. 1987. *J. Anim. Sci.* 65(Suppl. 1):314.
Peters, R.A., et al, 1971. *J. Anim. Sci.* 33:1153.
Robles, A., and R.C. Ewan. 1982. *J. Anim. Sci.* 55:572.
Salo, M.L. 1978. *J. Scient. Agric. Soc. Finland* 50:291.
Stanley, D.L., and R.C. Ewan. 1982. *J. Anim. Sci.* 54:1175.
Thong, L.A., et al. 1978. *J. Anim. Sci.* 46:674.
Wahlstrom, R.C., and G.W. Libal. 1976. *J. Anim. Sci.* 42:871.
Wahlstrom, R.C., C.S. German, and G.W. Libal. 1970. *J. Anim. Sci.* 30:532.
Yen, J.T., et al. 1971. *J. Anim. Sci.* 33:987.
Young, L.G. 1980. *J. Anim. Sci.* 51:1113.
Young, L.G., and R.H. Ingram. 1968. *Can. J. Anim. Sci.* 48:83.
Zimmerman, D.R., and M. Honeyman. 1986. *ISU Swine Research Report—1986. AS-5808.* Ames, IA: Iowa State University.

PART VII

Techniques in Swine Nutrition Research

Chapter 37

Computer Modeling for Diet Optimization

D.P. Dyer, Jr.

During the past several decades, mathematical and computer modeling have played an increasingly important role in animal agriculture as well as in biological science in general. An area of practical application has been that of livestock nutrition. In this chapter the application of the modeling process to the problem of swine diet formulation is discussed.

A mathematical model uses equations and other quantitative relationships to represent a natural process. Mathematical models generally provide a simplification of the actual processes they emulate, but they can be quite complex themselves. Frequently, these models are not tractable without computers.

Modeling is an iterative process. To an initial, simple model, successive layers of complexity and refinements are added in an attempt to make the model more realistic and hence more useful. In the examples that follow, the iterative nature of the modeling process is demonstrated by a series of models used to formulate a protein-vitamin-mineral supplement for a hypothetical feed mill. Initially, a linear programming model is employed to develop a least-cost formula for the supplement. In the second step, a nonlinear component is added to the model and the supplement is reformulated to give the least cost of gain. Finally, the implications of adding a stochastic (random) element to the model are examined.

LINEAR PROGRAMMING IN DIET FORMULATION

Let us suppose that a feed mill wishes to make a protein-vitamin-mineral supplement that can be combined with corn to produce a diet for finishing swine. The finishing diet will be composed of 17.5% supplement and 82.5% corn. Table 37.1 shows the nutrient levels in corn and in potential ingredients of the supplement. The specification for the complete feed and the corresponding specifications for the protein-vitamin-mineral supplement are shown below.

Table 37.1 Cost and Nutrient Profile for Ingredients Used in Sample Formulations

Ingredient	*Ingredient Cost ($/kg)*	*Manufacturer and Distributor Cost ($/kg)*	*ME (Mcal/kg)*	*Protein*	*Calcium*	*Phosphorus*	*Salt*
				%			
44% CP soybean meal	0.1960	0.1323	3.090	44.0	0.30	0.60	0
48% CP soybean meal	0.2105	0.1323	3.485	48.0	0.30	0.60	0
Salt	0.0287	0.1323	0	0	0	0	100
Vit-TM premix	0.6504	0.1323	0	0	12.00	0	0
Mono-dicalcium phosphate	0.2646	0.1323	0	0	16.00	21.00	0
Limestone	0.0198	0.1323	0	0	38.00	0	0
Corn	0.0761	—	3.325	8.6	0.01	0.25	0

Abbreviations: ME, metabolizable energy; CP, crude protein; Vit-TM, vitamin-trace mineral.

	Complete Feed	Supplement
Minimum protein	13.65%	37.46%
Minimum calcium	0.64%	3.61%
Minimum phosphorus	0.50%	1.68%
Minimum salt	0.32%	1.83%
Minimum vitamin-trace mineral premix	0.25%	1.43%

Typically, the feed mill will attempt to formulate the supplement to satisfy the nutrient and ingredient restrictions at the lowest cost per unit of supplement. This process is called "least-cost formulation." As both cost and nutrient levels are linear functions of the ingredient levels, least-cost formulation belongs to a set of optimization problems known as linear programming (LP). In 1947, the Simplex Method was developed by a team under G.B. Dantzig to solve LP problems (Dantzig 1982). Since then, numerous modifications and refinements of the original Simplex Method have been proposed. It is not the purpose of this chapter to detail the mechanics of solving LP problems. It is sufficient to note that commercial programs are available and that almost every introductory operations research textbook presents a step-by-step description of the Simplex Method or one of its variants.

For this example, it will be assumed that all of the ingredients in Table 37.1, except corn, are available to make the protein-vitamin-mineral supplement. Because the corn is to be mixed with the supplement at the farm, no additional manufacturing and distribution cost is shown for it.

Least-cost formulation of the supplement produces the following result:

Composition of Supplement (No. 1)

48% crude protein soybean meal	78.05%
44% crude protein meal	0%
Salt	1.83%
Vitamin-trace mineral premix	1.43%
Mono-dicalcium phosphate	5.76%
Limestone	12.93%

Nutrient Levels in Complete Feed

Protein	13.65%
Calcium	1.10%
Phosphorus	0.50%
Salt	0.32%

The cost of supplement (including manufacturing and transportation costs) is \$0.3242/kg and the corresponding complete feed cost is \$0.1195/kg. However, the calcium level in the complete feed is 1.10%, substantially higher than the minimum requirement of 0.64%. Many nutritionists would regard this high level of calcium and the resulting high calcium:phosphorus ratio as undesirable. The reason for the high calcium level is that in meeting the nutrient requirements, the LP algorithm used as little as possible of the more expensive ingredients. The remaining "space" in the formula was filled with the least expensive ingredient available, which in this case was limestone. The high level of limestone results in a high level of calcium.

There is a tendency for LP to fill formulas with low-cost combinations of ingredients that may not be wise nutritionally. This problem can sometimes be circumvented by putting additional restrictions on ingredient or nutrient levels. The present example can be improved by placing additional restrictions on calcium and salt in the supplement. When the maximum calcium and salt levels in the supplement are restricted to be 3.61% and 1.83%, respectively, least-cost formulation produces the following supplement:

Composition of Supplement (No. 2)

48% CP soybean meal	0%
44% CP soybean meal	85.15%
Salt	1.83%
Vitamin-trace mineral premix	1.43%
Mono-dicalcium phosphate	5.56%
Limestone	6.04%

Nutrient Levels in Complete Food

Protein	13.65%
Calcium	0.64%
Phosphorus	0.50%
Salt	0.32%

This formula is better than the first one. However, it is still slightly disturbing that 44% CP soybean meal rather than 48% CP soybean meal was used even though the ingredient cost per unit of protein and energy is greater for 44% CP soybean meal than for 48% CP soybean meal; for example, \$0.1960/0.44 = \$0.445 is greater than \$0.2105/0.48 = \$0.439.

NONLINEAR PROGRAMMING

Many of the complications and inefficiencies associated with least-cost ration formulation and LP can be avoided by using nonlinear programming (NLP) or, equivalently, nonlinear optimization methods.

In the past, nonlinear optimization techniques have received relatively little attention by the feed industry and by livestock producers. This is partly due to the increased computational requirements of nonlinear optimization and to the fact that the algorithms involved were neither as well understood nor as widely available as the simplex algorithm and its variants. The lack of attention to nonlinear methods has also been partly because these methods require a much more explicit specification of the effects of nutrients. In addition, feed tag labeling conventions have frequently been developed specifically for linear programming and least-cost formulation and consequently they are somewhat cumbersome to use with the more general optimization methods. However, as computer power becomes less expensive, as nonlinear optimization techniques become more accessible, and as swine nutrition becomes better understood, nonlinear optimization will become increasingly important in swine diet formulation.

There are a variety of nonlinear optimization techniques available. Both the Nelder-Mead (1965) and the Hooke and Jeeves (1961) algorithms are fairly robust general purpose procedures suitable for situations involving a small to medium number of ingredients. The SUMT method of Fiacco and McCormick (1968) can be useful when there are numerous constraints on nutrient and ingredient levels. Simulated anealization (Bohachevsky et al. 1986) may have some promise for very complex feed formulation problems. In some cases, it is useful to combine linear and nonlinear techniques: often the Simplex algorithm can be used to provide a starting point for a nonlinear optimization or sometimes a nonlinear function may be suitably approximated by a piecewise linear function. As was indicated, nonlinear optimization techniques require explicit specification of nutrient response functions. To illustrate a nonlinear optimization we will use a model (Balsbaugh and Dyer, unpublished data) that relates swine performance to the protein and energy in corn-soybean meal finishing diets. The model is defined as follows:

P = % Crude protein in the complete feed
E = Metabolizable energy (Mcal/kg) in the complete feed
F/G = Feed conversion efficiency, feed per unit weight gain

$$\mathrm{F/G} = \frac{\exp\,[-5.954\mathrm{R} + 26.549\mathrm{R}^2]}{0.0004714\mathrm{P} + 0.070605\mathrm{E}}$$

where R is defined as

$$\mathrm{R} = \frac{0.006676\mathrm{P} + \mathrm{E}}{3.2524\mathrm{P} - 7.0\mathrm{E}}$$

This model predicts feed conversion efficiency based on the protein and energy level in a corn-soybean meal diet. It is applicable only to those types of diets in which the minimum vitamin and mineral levels are approximately the same as indicated in the initial example for LP.

In the previous example, LP was used to find a supplement that had a use rate of 17.5% and satisfied the specified constraints at the least possible cost per unit of feed. However, feed cost relative to the weight gained by the pigs is a more appropriate measure of economic performance than is the cost of feed alone. Feed cost itself is a linear function of the ingredient use rates and as such it is a candidate for a minimization using LP techniques. On the other hand, the preceding model illustrates that feed conversion and consequently, feed cost of gain, are nonlinear functions of the ingredient use rates. When NLP is used to minimize cost of gain (subject to the same use of rate and nutritional constraints as supplement No. 1), the following supplement is obtained:

Composition of Supplement (No. 3)

48% CP soybean meal	85.15%
44% CP soybean meal	0%
Salt	1.83%
Vitamin-trace mineral premix	1.43%
Mono-dicalcium phosphate	5.56%
Limestone	6.04%

Nutrient Levels in Complete Feed

Protein	14.25%
Calcium	0.64%
Phosphorus	0.50%
Salt	0.32%

The LP method (after restrictions on excess calcium and salt were added) did not use 48% CP soybean meal in supplement No. 2. However NLP did use 48% soybean meal. In fact, in this simple example, the supplement formulated by NLP is essentially the same as that formulated by LP except that 48% soybean meal has been substituted for 44% soybean meal. As a consequence, NLP produced a complete diet with a protein content approximately 0.5% higher than LP. An economic comparison of the "optimum" diets produced by LP and NLP is as follows:

	Complete Feed Cost ($/kg)	*Cost of Gain ($/kg)*
LP (optimum: supplement No. 2)	0.1196	0.3825
NLP (optimum: supplement No. 3)	0.1218	0.3772

Thus, LP produced a diet with a lower feed cost; however, NLP produced a diet with a lower cost of gain.

STOCHASTIC SIMULATION

Both LP and NLP methods contain the implicit assumption that a given formulation inevitably results in an exactly specified protein level, feed cost, feed efficiency, etc. That is, they assume that by knowing the formula and use rate for the supplement, the exact protein level and cost of the complete feed can be determined. They also assume that the feed efficiency and cost of gain that would result from employing that particular formulation can be predicted exactly. For these models, the input variables completely determined the output variables; consequently, they are referred to as "deterministic" models.

In reality, the actual protein level or cost of gain cannot be determined exactly. There will inevitably be small random errors made in mixing the supplement or in combining the supplement with the corn. The nutrient levels in the actual ingredients may vary somewhat from the values shown in Table 37.1. The pigs may not perform exactly as expected due to weather, disease, or a variety of other factors. A model that specifically incorporates one or more of these random components is referred to as a "stochastic" model.

Stochastic models are frequently much more difficult to handle mathematically than are deterministic models. Some may elude even concerted efforts at analytical solution. Consequently, stochastic models are often resolved by computer "simulation" rather than by direct mathematical manipulation.

Stochastic simulation as used here refers to simulated repeated sampling of the random variables in a stochastic model. For some relatively simple discrete random variables, exhaustive sampling may be possible; however, more commonly random sampling (based on computer-generated random numbers) is used.

It may be useful to illustrate how a simple stochastic element can be added to the preceding model for F/G. That model was developed in a research setting using ingredients that were weighed out carefully. However, in actual practice, it is unlikely that all producers are willing to invest the effort required to assure this level of accuracy in their on-farm mixing. By chance the supplement will sometimes be included at a higher level than intended, and as a consequence the protein in the complete food will be higher than anticipated. On the other hand, the inclusion rate will sometimes be lower than expected, and as a result the protein will be low. To get a useful evaluation of a particular supplement formula, it is necessary to take these mixing errors into account. One way of doing this is to look at the projected performance of the given supplement across several selected inclusion levels, some a little below and some a little above the targeted rate. By taking the average projected cost of gain across several diets representing the various simulated inclusion level errors, a useful overall evaluation of the supplement formula will emerge.

For the purpose of illustration it will be assumed that inaccuracy in combining the supplement and corn introduces an error into the diet protein level that is normally distributed and has a standard deviation of 0.8%. (This standard deviation appears to be roughly consistent with the data presented by Nichols [1986] in a study of the accuracy of on-farm feed mixing and delivery.) As this is a relatively "simple" simulation, it was actually conducted by exhaustive sampling of a discrete approximation to the specified normal distribution.

Table 37.2 shows the effect of adding a stochastic element to the model for F/G. This table compares the formulation giving the optimum cost of gain under the deterministic versus the stochastic model for various costs of 48% CP soybean meal. (The cost of 44% CP soybean meal, the other ingredients, and manufacturing and transportation are held constant.) For example, when 48% CP soybean meal has an ingredient cost of $0.2227/kg, the optimum supplement under the deterministic model will have 64.82% 44% CP soybean meal and 20.33% 48% CP soybean meal, whereas the optimum supplement under the stochastic model has 0% 44% CP soybean meal and 85.15% 48% soybean meal. In this example, adding a stochastic element to the model put a small additional premium on the value of 48% CP soybean meal vis-à-vis 44% CP soybean meal.

Table 37.2 Amount of 44% Crude Protein and 48% Crude Protein Soybean Meal in the Optimal[a] Supplement

Ingredient Cost[b] of 48% CP Soybean Meal	*Deterministic Model*		*Stochastic Model*	
	44% CP SBM (%)	*48% CP SBM (%)*	*44% CP SBM (%)*	*48%CP SBM (%)*
≤0.2194	0	85.15	0	85.15
0.2205	2.35	82.80	0	85.15
0.2216	34.98	50.17	0	85.15
0.2227	64.82	20.33	0	85.15
0.2238	85.15	0	0	85.15
0.2249	85.15	0	21.01	64.14
0.2260	85.15	0	40.64	44.51
0.2271	85.15	0	58.73	26.42
0.2282	85.15	0	75.46	9.69
≥0.2293	85.15	0	85.15	0

Abbreviations: CP, crude protein; SBM, soybean meal.

[a] Optimal = lowest average feed cost of gain.

[b] Ingredient cost expressed as dollars per kilogram. Cost of ingredients other than 48% CP soybean meal were held constant at levels shown in Table 37.1.

In an effort to keep the preceding examples relatively simple, they were necessarily left incomplete. They do, however, illustrate concepts and potential economic benefits of the more general computer simulation and optimization techniques.

REFERENCES

Bohachevsky, I.O., M.E. Johnson, and M.L. Stein. 1986. *Technometrics* 28:209.
Dantzig, G.B. 1982. *Operations Res. Lett.* 1:43.
Fiacco, A.V., and G.P. McCormick. 1968. *Nonlinear Programming, Sequential Unconstrained Minimization Techniques.* New York: John Wiley.
Hooke, R., and T.A. Jeeves. 1961. *J. Assoc. Comp. Mach.* 8:212.
Nelder, J.A., and R. Mead. 1965. *Comput. J.* 7:308–313.
Nichols, S. 1986. *Accuracy of On-Farm Feed Mixing and Delivery Systems. Swine Day.* Sept. 4. Lafayette, IN: Purdue University.

Chapter 38

Statistical Techniques for the Design and Analysis of Swine Nutrition Experiments

D.K. Aaron and V.W. Hays

Statistical techniques should be considered as research tools that can produce meaningful, reliable, and unbiased results when properly applied to situations for which they are designed. However, no statistical technique can protect against poor planning, inaccuracies in the data, unsound analysis, or incorrect interpretation. High-quality research requires proper planning and careful execution of experiments, correct application of statistical techniques, and finally, interpretation of results by one who understands not only the statistical techniques, but also the field to which they are applied.

The objectives of this chapter are to (1) review some basic statistical techniques that are useful in the design and analysis of swine nutrition experiments, (2) provide some guidelines for interpretation and presentation of results, and (3) examine the role of the statistician in experimentation. The statistical techniques to be discussed are not new and generally are no different from those used in other fields of biological research; therefore, basic biometrical texts are recommended as references, for example, Cochran and Cox (1957), Gill (1978a,b), Snedecor and Cochran (1980), Steel and Torrie (1980), Lentner and Bishop (1986), and Damon and Harvey (1987). Also, it is assumed that readers will be familiar with the basic features of experimental design and analysis, and with commonly used statistical terms.

DESIGN OF EXPERIMENTS

Planning and Pre-experiment Protocol

In planning experiments, the first consideration must be the availability of resources in terms of financial support, personnel, animals, equipment, and time. Then, within the restrictions imposed by the available resources, experiments should be designed to obtain unbiased estimates of treatment effects, treatment differences, and experimental error. Also, experiments should be designed and replicated in such a way that treatment effects will be estimated with adequate precision to detect differences, if they truly exist, at the desired probability level.

Careful planning and organization before an experiment is initiated can maximize the amount of information gained from the resources utilized. Also, careful planning will help protect against statistical problems associated with violation of the basic principles of experimental design. Mark Twain once observed that "Statistics are like garbage, one should have in mind what is to be done with the stuff before collecting it!" Likewise, researchers should have specific objectives in mind and should know how those objectives are to be resolved before experiments are initiated and data are collected.

As part of the pre-experiment protocol, six pertinent questions should be addressed. First, what is to be accomplished by the experiment? Objectives of the experiment should be stated definitely and concisely in terms of questions to be answered, hypotheses to be tested, or effects to be estimated. Second, how many treatments or treatment combinations are to be included in the experiment? The success of the experiment depends on the careful selection of treatments, the evaluation of which will resolve the initial objectives. Third, what is the experimental unit (an individual, a litter, a pen, etc.)? Also, what measurements will be made on the experimental units (how, when, where)? Correct definition of the experimental unit is important because it is the variation among experimental units treated alike that provides the unbiased estimate of error for evaluating treatment effects. Fourth, how are the treatments or treatment combinations to be assigned to the experimental units? The randomization procedure used for assigning treatments to experimental units determines the structure of the experimental design and provides the mechanism that allows researchers to draw valid conclusions from the results. Fifth, how many times does each treatment need to be observed; that is, how much replication is necessary? The number of replications must be large enough to estimate treatment effects with the precision necessary to detect differences, if they truly exist, at the desired probability level. Finally, and perhaps most importantly, can the resulting experimental design be analyzed? Also, can the desired comparisons be made? Sources of variation and appropriate degrees of freedom should be written out as part of the pre-experiment protocol. Planned comparisons should be specified during this stage as well. Unfortunately, if too little time is spent in the planning stage of the experiment, researchers may find that no valid comparisons can be made, or that those that can be made do not resolve the objectives stated initially.

FUNDAMENTALS OF ALL EXPERIMENTS

Randomization

Randomization refers to the assignment of treatments to experimental units so that all units have an equal chance of receiving a treatment. Randomization prevents systematic bias from being introduced into an experiment and ensures that estimates of treatment means and differences, as well as experimental error, are unbiased. As experimental designs are simply plans to be used for assigning treatments to experimental units, the manner in which the randomization is accomplished is the key to the type of design. Design structures are addressed later in this chapter.

Replication

Replication refers to the assignment of more than one experimental unit to the same treatment or treatment combination. Each replication of a treatment is an independent observation; thus, each replication involves a different experimental unit. The basic function of replication is to provide an estimate of experimental error. In general, increasing the number of replications results in a more accurate estimate of experimental error and more precise estimates of treatment effects. For a particular experiment, the number of replications depends on the magnitude of the difference to be detected, the precision required, and the variability of the experimental material. Improving the precision of experiments by increasing the number of replications is discussed in a later section.

STRUCTURES OF ALL EXPERIMENTS

Treatment Structure

All experiments consist of two basic structures (Milliken and Johnson 1984). The first is the treatment structure and consists of the set of treatments or treatment combinations that have been selected for evaluation. The term *treatment* refers to those factors (either qualitative or quantitative) to be compared as measured by their effect on given response traits. It may be used to denote imposed or controllable factors such as types or levels of protein in the diet or uncontrollable factors such as sexes or breeds of pigs (Gill 1978a). The most common types of treatment structures are the one-way classification and the factorial arrangement.

The one-way treatment classification consists of a set of ''t'' treatments, which may be structured (those treatments having a gradient or grouped composition) or unstructured (those treatments that are unrelated). Observations are classified only on the basis of the one set of treatments or source of variation. As an example of a one-way treatment classification, consider comparing growth rates of pigs fed two types of corn (normal and high-lysine). The two groups (normal, high-lysine) are referred to as classes of the main classification, type of corn. This is the simplest type of treatment structure.

The factorial treatment arrangement consists of a set of treatment combinations constructed by combining the classes (or levels) of two or more different types of treatments (often called factors). Every class (or level) of one factor occurs in combination with every class (or level) of each other factor in the experiment. Factorial treatment arrangements provide information about each factor included in the experiment and also information about interactions among the different factors. Suppose that the normal and high-lysine corn of the previous example had each been stored by two different methods, dry and high-moisture. Thus, each of the two types of corn occurs in combination with each of the two storage methods, giving four treatment combinations in all. With this 2 × 2 factorial treatment arrangement, observations are classified by both type of corn and storage method. Experiments involving factorial treatment arrangements are often referred to as "factorial" experiments; however, it should be emphasized that factorial refers to the treatment structure and not the design structure of the experiment. A factorial treatment structure may be used with any of the general design structures.

Design Structure

The second structure common to all experiments is the design structure. This refers to the method of grouping experimental units into homogeneous groups or blocks; that is, the way in which the randomization is restricted. One of the primary objectives in choosing a design structure is to reduce experimental error. There are three general types of design structures: (1) completely randomized (CR), (2) randomized complete block (RCB), and (3) Latin square (LS). Most other design structures can be considered to be modifications of these three. The treatment structures previously described can be used in conjunction with any of the three general design structures.

The CR design is the simplest design structure possible because treatments (or treatment combinations) are assigned to experimental units completely at random. Thus, randomization is not restricted, and the only criterion for grouping experimental units is treatment. Use of this design is appropriate when experimental units are relatively homogeneous (uniform), or when there are no identifiable criteria for arranging the units into more homogeneous groups. Although the CR design provides the maximum number of degrees of freedom for estimating experimental error, it is often inefficient. In many cases, there are identifiable sources of variation among the experimental units other than treatments. However, because randomization is unrestricted in the CR design, all variation among experimental units except that due to treatments is included in the experimental error. When other sources of variation can be identified, it may be possible to group experimental units so that the variation among units within a group is less than among units in different groups. Design structures that take advantage of this grouping will exclude variation among groups from the experimental error and, as a result, increase the precision of the experiment.

In the RCB design, experimental units are arranged in homogeneous groups (blocks) on the basis of a single extraneous source of variability; that is, there is one restriction on the randomization. The extraneous source of variability may be a management factor such as time or location (e.g., different farms, buildings, sites within a single building, etc.) or an animal factor such as litter, breed, or sex. Treatments are assigned randomly to experimental units within a block, and an independent randomization is carried out for each block. Every treatment occurs the same number of times, usually once, within each block and each block contains each treatment; therefore, each block is complete with respect to the whole set of treatments. The objective of the RCB design is to have experimental units within a block as uniform as possible with regard to the blocking factor so that observed differences within blocks will be due largely to treatments. Ideally, variation not due to treatments is minimized within blocks and maximized among blocks. The variation among blocks is then arithmetically removed from the experimental error, thus improving the precision of the experiment. If there is no appreciable variability among blocks, the RCB design will not increase the precision of detecting treatment differences over that of the CR design. In fact, if the reduction in experimental error does not compensate for the loss in error degrees of freedom, blocking may actually reduce the power of the experiment. Also, as block size increases, variability within blocks not brought about by treatments tends to increase as well, causing a larger experimental error. Finally, an important assumption of the RCB design is that block and treatment effects are additive; that is, there is no interaction between blocks and treatments. Violation of this assumption results in an inflated experimental error and inaccurate estimates of treatment differences.

The LS design arises from blocking in two different ways; that is, there are two restrictions on the randomization. This double blocking makes it possible to remove two independent, extraneous sources of variability from the experimental error. Generally, rows and columns are the terms used to refer to the two blocking factors. They may refer to the sequence in which treatments are applied or to the spatial distribution of experimental units. Often in swine nutrition experiments, columns refer to pigs and rows refer to time periods. Each row and each column are a complete replicate or block. As a result, randomization is more complicated than in the RCB design. Treatments are randomly allotted to experimental units such that each treatment occurs once and only once in each row and once and only once in each column. The number of rows, columns, and treatments must be equal, and this is a major disadvantage associated with the LS design. The most commonly used squares range from 5×5 to 8×8. Squares smaller than 5×5 provide few degrees of freedom for estimating experimental error, while squares larger than 8×8 may encounter the same problem as the RCB design in that experimental error may increase with the size of the square.

More than one square can be used in the same experiment to increase degrees of freedom for estimating error. Since there are many possible configurations of squares, it is necessary to select the one(s) to be used by some random method. One method of randomization is presented by Cochran and Cox (1957). Use of the LS design will result in more precise estimates of treatment means and differences than the RCB design only when there is appreciable variation associated with the second blocking factor. Also, an important assumption of the LS design is that rows and columns do not interact with each other or with treatments. Violation of this assumption will result in an inflated experimental error and inaccurate estimates of treatment effects.

In addition to the three general design structures (CR, RCB, and LS), two other design structures are often useful in swine nutrition experiments. These are split-plot (SP) and repeated measures (RM) designs. Sometimes RM designs are referred to as "split-plots in time," although "repeated measures" is a more accurate term. These two designs have identical structures, and both involve more than one size of experimental unit. However, the RM design differs from the SP design in that the former involves a stage where there is no randomization of treatment levels and the latter involves randomization at all stages.

The basic SP design involves assigning treatments of one factor to main plots according to the randomization procedure for either a CR, RCB, or LS design. The treatments of the second factor are assigned randomly to subplots within each main plot. This design usually sacrifices precision in estimating the average effects of the main plot treatments, but it often improves the precision for comparing the average effects of the subplot treatments as well as the interaction. This occurs because the experimental error for main plots is usually larger than the experimental error used to compare subplot treatments. Also, the number of degrees of freedom available for experimental error is usually smaller for main plot comparisons than for subplot comparisons.

The primary advantage of the SP design is that it enables factors that require relatively large amounts of experimental material and factors that require small amounts to be combined in the same experiment. If the experiment is planned to investigate the first factor, so that large amounts of material are going to be used anyway, the second factor often can be included at little extra cost, and some additional information obtained. Sometimes in factorial experiments, the nature of the experimental material or the operations involved simply makes it difficult to handle all treatment combinations in the same manner, and an SP design is required. As an example, consider an experiment investigating the effects of environmental temperature and diet on growth performance of pigs. Two temperatures (10 °C and 35 °C) and three corn-based diets (normal corn, normal corn plus lysine, and high-lysine corn) are used in the experiment. Temperatures are randomly allotted to main plots consisting of environmental chambers (the larger experimental unit), and diets are randomly allotted to subplots consisting of either individually or group-fed pigs (the smaller experimental unit) within each main plot.

The RM design is appropriate for experiments in which treatments are assigned to animals according to the randomization procedure of the CR, RCB, or LS design, and animals are measured for trend at several sampling times (i.e., nonrandom repeated sampling). For example, suppose that an experiment is conducted to evaluate the effect of increasing levels of growth hormone on pig performance. Hormone levels are assigned to pigs completely at random, and serum hormone levels are measured on each pig at several sampling times. Thus, time of sampling is one of the factors in the treatment structure of the experiment. By measuring the same animal at several different times, the animal is essentially "split" into parts (time periods), and the response is measured on each part. The animal is the larger experimental unit (which corresponds to the main plot), and the time period is the smaller experimental unit (which corresponds to the subplot). However, since the levels of time cannot be assigned at random to the time periods, time is considered as a nonrandom repeated factor. Also, the variability associated with repeated measures on the same animal can be assumed to be less than the variability associated with measures among different animals. Gill and Hafs (1971) have presented a detailed discussion of appropriate statistical techniques for experiments that involve repeated measurements in animals.

METHODS OF IMPROVING PRECISION OF DESIGNED EXPERIMENTS

The precision (sensitivity) of an experiment refers to its ability to detect true treatment differences at a given significance level (Little and Hills 1978). Generally, the smaller the variability among experimental units treated alike, the more precise the experiment will be in detecting treatment differences. Also, as the number of replications increases, the variance of the difference between two means decreases, and the precision of the experiment increases. Therefore, statistical techniques used to improve the precision of an experiment involve either an increase in the number of replications or a reduction in the magnitude of the experimental error. In some cases, refinement of nonstatistical techniques, such as procedures for administration of treatments or collection of data, may improve precision more than statistical techniques. The discussion here will be limited to improving precision by statistical means.

Increasing the number of replications is probably the statistical technique first thought of as a means of improving precision of designed experiments. Although additional replications generally will improve the precision with which treatment means and differences are estimated, the extent of improvement declines as the number of replications increases. For example, if a difference in rate of gain of 40 g/day can be detected with four replicates, an experiment of approximately sixteen replicates will be needed to detect half this difference, or 20 g/day, because the standard errors are in the ratio of 2:1 (assuming the same variance). However, if the difference is halved again, to 10 g/day, approximately sixty-four replicates will be necessary to detect this difference.

The number of replications needed depends on the magnitude of the difference to be detected, the desired precision, and the variability of the experimental material. For a specific situation, this number can be estimated using procedures described by Cochran and Cox (1957). Estimates of the number of replications needed to detect differences of various sizes at several levels of variability and selected significance levels (1%, 5%, 10%) are presented for sow reproduction experiments and growing-finishing pig experiments in Tables 38.1 and 38.2, respectively. In both tables, estimates are based on an 80% chance of obtaining a significant result.

For the sow reproduction experiments (Table 38.1), a CR design with two treatments was assumed because it is common to assign treatments completely at random to individually fed sows. For the growing-finishing pig experiments (Table 38.2), an RCB design with four treatments was assumed because this design is commonly applied in such experiments. In both cases, the estimates of error available in the literature are based largely on these designs (CR in sow experiments and RCB in growing-finishing pig experiments). Although estimates of the number of replications are presented for various levels of experimental error (expressed as the coefficient of variation) and differences of several sizes (expressed as percent of the mean of the experiment), levels selected are within realistic ranges. The average coefficients of variation for total number of pigs born, number of live pigs at birth, and number of live pigs at 21 days are 28%, 29%, and 36%, respectively (Hays and Aaron, unpublished results). These values are based on five different estimates involving 7925 litters. Among these five studies, the estimates ranged from 26 to 28, 28 to 33, and 29 to 39 for the three repro-

Table 38.1 Estimated Number of Replications Needed in Sow Reproduction Experiments[a]

Significance Level (%)[c]	*Average Coefficient of Variation*[d]	*Expected Difference in Litter Size (% Mean)*[b]					
		2	*4*	*6*	*8*	*10*	*12*
1	40	9343	2336	1039	584	374	260
	35	7154	1788	795	448	287	199
	30	5256	1314	584	329	211	146
	25	3650	913	406	229	146	102
	20	2336	584	260	146	94	67
5	40	6280	1570	698	393	252	175
	35	4808	1202	533	301	193	134
	30	3533	883	393	221	142	99
	25	2453	614	273	154	99	69
	20	1570	393	175	99	63	45
10	40	4946	1237	550	310	252	138
	35	3787	947	421	237	152	106
	30	2782	696	310	174	112	78
	25	1932	483	215	121	78	55
	20	1237	310	138	78	50	36

[a] Assumes a CR design with two treatments, two-tailed test of significance, and an 80% chance of detecting a significant result (i.e., probability of accepting the null hypothesis when it is false is 20%).

[b] A 10% difference in litter size represents approximately 1 and 0.8 live pigs at birth and weaning, respectively.

[c] Probability of rejecting the null hypothesis when it is true.

[d] Average coefficient of variation = (pooled standard deviation/square root of the mean) × 100.

ductive traits, respectively. The average coefficients of variation for rate of gain and feed efficiency are approximately 4.5% and 4%, respectively (Hays and Aaron, unpublished results). These are based on data combined from several experiments and involve 3425 group-fed pigs (four to eight pigs per group).

Realistically, the prospective improvement in precision, as the number of replications is increased, must be balanced with increases in cost and time. As research is expensive, it is important not to replicate more than is necessary. At the same time, experiments with inadequate replication are of little value.

Another factor that affects the precision of an experiment is the choice of experimental unit. The experimental unit may be an individual animal, a litter, or a pen of animals. It is the smallest unit receiving a single treatment, provided that two such units could receive different treatments. As indicated earlier, correct definition of the experimental unit is important because it is the variation among experimental units treated alike that provides the unbiased estimate of error for evaluating treatment effects. Failure to recognize the appropriate experimental unit, and to replicate it, is a common error in animal experiments. This error often occurs because pen effects are ignored when animals are treated in groups. For example, if a single diet (treatment) is fed to a pen of pigs, the pen is the experimental unit and replication involves increasing the

Table 38.2 Estimated Number of Replications (Blocks) Needed in Growing-Finishing Experiments[a]

Significance Level (%)[b]	*Average Coefficient of Variation*[c]	*Expected Difference in Rate of Gain or Feed Efficiency (% Mean)*					
		2.5	*5.0*	*7.5*	*10.0*	*12.5*	*15.0*
1	15.0	842	211	97	54	35	25
	12.5	583	146	67	38	25	18
	10.0	374	97	43	25	17	12
	7.5	210	54	25	15	10	7
	5.0	97	25	12	7	5	4
	2.5	25	7	4	3	3	3
5	15.0	565	141	64	36	23	17
	12.5	393	99	44	26	17	12
	10.0	252	64	29	17	11	8
	7.5	142	36	17	10	7	5
	5.0	64	17	8	5	4	3
	2.5	17	5	3	3	2	2
10	15.0	445	111	51	29	19	13
	12.5	309	73	35	20	13	10
	10.0	198	51	23	13	9	7
	7.5	112	29	13	8	6	4
	5.0	51	13	7	4	3	3
	2.5	13	4	3	2	2	2

[a] Assumes an RCB design with four treatments, single degree of freedom comparisons, two-tailed test of significance, and an 80% chance of detecting a significant result (i.e., probability of accepting the null hypothesis when it is false is 20%).

[b] Probability of rejecting the null hypothesis when it is true.

[d] Average coefficient of variation = (pooled standard deviation/square root of the mean) × 100. For growing-finishing pigs (group-fed, 4 to 8 pigs/group), values range from 2.5% to 10%; for very young pigs, values range from 7.5% to 15%.

number of pens per treatment. Increasing the number of pigs per experimental unit will increase precision up to a point, but if a given number of pigs can be fed individually, precision may be increased more by using the individual pig as the experimental unit and having more replications than by using the same number of pigs in fewer experimental units. Treating pigs individually maximizes the use of animals, but maximizing the efficiency of total resources may necessitate grouping pigs. Also, pigs treated individually may or may not respond to treatment in the same manner as pigs treated in groups.

Although the number of replications and the choice of experimental unit are both important factors, the primary statistical technique used to improve precision of designed experiments is to group experimental units into homogeneous groups or blocks; that is, to choose an efficient design structure. General design structures and their roles in improving precision were discussed in the preceding section. Generally, as experimental error is reduced, efficiency is increased. Thus, the more efficient the design structure, the more precise the experiment will be for estimating treatment effects. Relative efficiencies of the basic designs can be estimated using procedures described in the references suggested earlier. Basically, estimates of relative efficiency involve comparison of the relative size of the error term, with and without the blocking components included.

Another statistical technique for improving precision of designed experiments is to take additional measurements on the experimental units. These additional measurements are referred to as *auxiliary variables* or *covariates.* Suppose that in the experiment designed to compare growth rates of pigs fed two types of corn (normal and high-lysine) there is considerable variation in weight from pig to pig at the start of the experiment. Treatment effects may be estimated with more precision if differences associated with initial weight are removed from the total variability in growth rate. As discussed earlier, blocking is one way this can be accomplished; however, in some cases use of a covariate will be more effective in reducing experimental error and at the same time will preserve more degrees of freedom for estimating error. Generally, the use of a covariate will be most effective when the primary and auxiliary variables are closely related in a linear manner, or if the auxiliary variable is responsible for a large portion of the total variation in the primary variable. Also, the use of an auxiliary variable as a covariate may allow the use of another factor for blocking. As an example, a littermate set of pigs may serve as a factor for blocking and initial weight or age may be used as a covariate.

ANALYSIS OF DATA

Analysis of Variance and Hypothesis Testing

The analysis of variance (Fisher 1935) is a powerful and efficient statistical technique for partitioning the total variability within an experiment into orthogonal components resulting from recognizable sources of variation. There are three general components of the analysis of variance: (1) a component representing the treatment structure, (2) a component representing the design structure (blocks, rows, columns, etc.), and (3) a component resulting from unknown or uncontrollable causes generally referred to as the experimental error. The first two components are sometimes referred to collectively as the model component. Once the treatment and design structures have been specified, the statistical model and its associated analysis of variance also have been specified. Thus, the time to ask, "How should the data be analyzed?" is before, not after, data have been collected. Unfortunately, often this question is asked too late.

Analysis of variance plans (sources of variation and degrees of freedom) for the three general design structures (CR, RCB, and LS) and an SP design are shown in Tables 38.3 and 38.4, respectively. Plans for the general design structures (Table 38.3) are based on an experiment involving four treatments and four replications, giving a total of sixteen experimental units. The plan for the SP design (Table 38.4) is based on an experiment with two levels of factor A (main plot treatment), three levels of factor B (subplot treatment), and five replications. Levels of factor A are assigned to main

Table 38.3 Analysis of Variance Plans for the Three General Design Structures[a]

Design Structure					
CR		*RCB*		*LS*	
Source of Variation	*df*	*Source of Variation*	*df*	*Source of Variation*	*df*
				Rows	3
		Blocks	3	Columns	3
Treatments	3	Treatments	3	Treatments	3
Experimental error	12	Experimental error	9	Experimental error	6
Total	15		15		15

Abbreviations: CR, completely randomized; RCB, randomized complete block; LS, Latin square.

[a]Assumes an experiment involving four treatments and four replications, giving a total of sixteen experimental units.

Table 38.4 Analysis of Variance Plan for a Split-Plot Design[a]

Source of Variation	*df*
Main plot analysis	
Factor A (environmental temperature)	2−1 = 1
Main plot error (error A)[b]	2(5 − 1) = 8
Main plot total	(2)(5) − 1 = 9
Subplot analysis	
Factor B (diet)	3 − 1 = 2
A × B interaction	(2 − 1)(3 − 1) = 2
Subplot error (error B)[c]	2(5 − 1)(3 − 1) = 16
Subplot total	(2)(5)(3 − 1) = 20
Total	(2)(3)(5) − 1 = 29

[a]Based on an experiment with two levels of factor A, three levels of factor B, and five replications. Levels of factor A are assigned to main plots according to the randomization procedure for the completely randomized design.

[b]Error term for testing factor A.

[c]Error term for testing factor B and the A × B interaction.

plots according to the randomization procedure for the CR design. If factor A refers to environmental temperature (10 °C and 35 °C) and factor B refers to diet (normal corn, normal corn plus lysine, and high-lysine corn), then this experiment corresponds to the SP example presented earlier. Although not presented here, the analysis of variance plan for an RM design would be similar to that of an SP design. In a typical RM design, the main plot portion of the analysis would be an ‘‘among animals’’ analysis, and the subplot portion of the analysis would be a "within animals" analysis with time as the subplot treatment.

One of the primary functions of the analysis of variance is to test hypotheses about the equality of treatment means and the presence of interactions among the treatment factors. Generally, hypotheses are stated in a form that is believed to be untrue (null hypotheses) and data from the experiment are used to reject or disprove this hypothesis. In this way, the null hypothesis acts as a base from which an alternate hypothesis may deviate. For the swine nutrition experiment described previously, a null hypothesis might be stated as, "The growth rate of pigs fed the normal corn diet is equal to the growth rate of pigs fed the high-lysine corn diet." The corresponding alternate hypothesis might be, "The growth rate of pigs fed the high-lysine corn diet is greater than the growth rate of pigs fed the normal corn diet." Evidence in favor of the alternate hypothesis is found by rejecting or disproving the null hypotheses.

The decision to reject the null hypothesis in favor of the alternate is based on a statistical test of significance, in this case an F test, which has some measure of confidence associated with it, based on the laws of probability. This measure of confidence is the chosen probability of rejecting the null hypothesis when it is really true and is referred to as the probability of a type I error. The most commonly chosen probability levels are $P < .10$, $P < .05$, $P < .01$, and $P < .001$. The choice of the level of probability should be based on the relative consequences of rejecting the null hypothesis when it is true (type I error) and accepting the null hypothesis when it is false (type II error).

Another basic function of the analysis of variance is to estimate the residual variability among experimental units treated alike. Throughout this chapter, this has been referred to as the experimental error. Sometimes this quantity is referred to as an estimate of the "common" variance. As indicated previously, the experimental error includes variation from all uncontrolled sources of variation. It may be a result of naturally inherent differences among experimental units, faulty experimental techniques, and other extraneous variation such as variation resulting from using an incomplete statistical model for the analysis. With proper experimental design and careful experimental technique, the two latter components should be negligible. The magnitude of the experimental error provides a measure of the precision of the experiment for evaluating treatment effects.

Each time an analysis of variance is conducted, certain assumptions about the data are made. The first major assumption involves the experimental error terms and is really a series of assumptions. The error terms are assumed to be normally and independently distributed with zero mean and a common (homogeneous) variance. Violations of these assumptions may affect both probability levels and precision; however, minor violations are usually not serious. As a precaution though, assumptions should be checked to ensure that major violations do not exist in the data being analyzed.

The first of this series of assumptions, that of normality, does not affect the estimation of treatment means and differences; however, it can be critical to probability statements and hypothesis tests. Fortunately, means from all but very small samples are at least approximately normally distributed. Also, the F test of the hypothesis of treatment effects is not greatly affected by moderate departures from normality. In experiments from which data are obviously nonnormal, transformations (e.g., square root for data consisting of counts of rare events, arc sine for data expressed as percentages or proportions, and logarithmic for data where standard deviations are proportional to means) will ensure approximate normality for the transformed variable (Little and Hills 1978).

The second of this series of assumptions, that of independence, is usually not a problem if proper randomization has been followed. Exceptions are experiments that involve repeated measurement. Ignoring the correlation of errors induced by the non-random, repeated measurement is a common mistake made in experiments in which animals are measured at several different times. When this correlation is ignored, inferences about the repeated factor (time) may be distorted.

The last of this series of assumptions, that of a common or homogeneous variance, is the one most frequently violated in animal experiments. In these types of experiments, it is not unusual for the mean and variance to be related; that is, groups with large means tend to have large variances and those with smaller means tend to have smaller variances. A typical example of heterogeneity of variances is found in experiments dealing with effects of dietary copper levels on liver copper stores. As the dietary level of copper increases from a low level (approximately 10 ppm) to a high level (approximately 250 ppm), the mean and the variance of liver copper stores remain low up to a point and then increase rapidly at the higher levels. Although the F test is only slightly affected by mild departures from homogenous variances, it is always advisable to check this assumption. Several test procedures for homogeneity of variances are available. Two of the most commonly used are Hartley's maximum F test (Hartley 1950) and Bartlett's test statistic (Bartlett 1957). Both of these procedures are described in detail by Gill (1978a). In cases where the experimental error is heterogeneous, the error component can be divided into components that are homogenous as described by Cochran and Cox (1957).

The second major assumption is that the three general components of an analysis of variance are additive. For example, in a RCB design, an experimental observation may be thought of as being made up of the overall mean plus a treatment effect plus a block effect plus a random error effect. Note that all the terms are added; thus the term *additivity.* This implies that a treatment effect is the same for all blocks and that the block effect is the same for all treatments; that is, blocks and treatments are independent. This was one of the assumptions made earlier about the RCB design.

The final major assumption associated with the analysis of variance is that treatments or treatment combinations are randomly assigned to experimental units within a homogenous group. As discussed earlier, randomization prevents systematic bias from being introduced into an experiment and ensures that estimates of treatment means and differences, as well as experimental error, are unbiased. Often, this last assumption is not stressed as much as it should be.

Designed Comparisons Among Treatment Means

Designed comparisons (sometimes referred to as planned F tests) should be based on the initial objectives of the experiment and identified during the planning stage. Carefully selected comparisons can answer as many independent questions as there are degrees of freedom for treatments. Contrary to popular belief, a significant overall F test for treatments is not a prerequisite for partitioning degrees of freedom into single degree of freedom contrasts. In fact, Chew (1976) stressed that the overall F test need not and should not be carried out at all. In comparing t treatments with (t − 1) degrees of freedom, the overall F test is averaged over (t − 1) orthogonal contrasts. If only one of these (t − 1) contrasts is significant, the overall F test is weakened by the (t − 2) nonsignificant contrasts and as a result may give a nonsignificant overall F value.

There are two types of designed comparisons among treatment means: (1) class comparisons (orthogonal contrasts) and (2) trend comparisons (orthogonal polynomials). Class comparisons are used when a set of treatments consists of several qualitative classes. For comparisons of this type, orthogonal F tests are the most sensitive of techniques for comparing means. This technique enables researchers to answer specific, meaningful questions about treatment effects in a way that is both simple and powerful. Methods of constructing orthogonal coefficients and calculations for component sums of squares are outlined in Little and Hills (1978).

Trend comparisons are used when the set of treatments consists of quantitative levels of some factor, that is dose-response experiments. For comparisons of this type, regression analysis or curve fitting is the most appropriate technique. Using orthogonal polynomials, treatment sums of squares and degrees of freedom are partitioned into linear and curvilinear regression components. If the levels are equally spaced and replicated, the computations for obtaining the linear, quadratic, cubic, etc., components are simple. For further details about polynomial coefficients and computations, readers should refer to one of the biometrics references cited at the beginning of this chapter.

Use and Misuse of Multiple Comparison Procedures

Whenever possible, specific contrasts should be planned before the experiment is conducted rather than selecting comparisons after the data have been collected. This will help guard against ambiguous comparisons and will ensure maximum sensitivity for comparisons that are meaningful. For the few situations in which an experiment consists of a set of treatments that are unrelated, unstructured, or undifferentiated by prior experience or theory (e.g., experiments to evaluate different varieties of feedstuffs), all possible pairwise comparisons among the observed treatment means may be appropriate. Several pairwise multiple comparison procedures (Duncan's Multiple Range Test, Tukey's Honestly Significant Difference, Student-Newman-Kuels' Test, Fisher's Least Significant Difference) are available for such cases. Of these procedures, Fisher's Least Significant Difference is the test recommended when comparisons each involve only two of the treatment means. Carmer and Walker (1985) presented an excellent review of the properties of these and other multiple comparison tests.

There are three specific situations where pairwise multiple comparisons should not be used: (1) comparing treatments to a control, (2) comparing treatments factorial in nature, and (3) comparing levels of a quantitative factor (dose-response experiments). In the first situation, the goal is to detect treatments that are different from a standard or a control and the problem is to compare the mean of each treatment group with the mean of the control group. A more appropriate procedure than any of the pairwise multiple comparison procedures is Dunnett's *t*-like test (Dunnett 1955). In the second situation, the effects and relationships of the factors used in the experiment can best be evaluated by partitioning the treatment sum of squares into main effects and interactions. This approach provides the experiment with the most powerful method of evaluating interaction effects or main effects if the interaction is absent or weak. Pairwise multiple comparison techniques provide no direct tests for these effects. In the third situation, the objective should be to characterize the nature of the response (linear or some degree of curvilinear) to the level or dose of treatment imposed. In this case, orthogonal polynomials (regression analysis) should be used. As pointed out by Chew (1978), if the linear regression is significant, no pairwise multiple comparison procedure is necessary because all treatments are significantly different in their effects.

INTERPRETATION AND PRESENTATION OF RESULTS

Partitioning Treatment Effects

Although the purpose of an experiment is to answer specific questions, often results are presented and interpreted with little reference to either the initial objectives of the experiment or the treatment structure. This is especially true of dose-response and factorial experiments (Little 1981).

As indicated earlier, dose-response experiments measure the response to quantitative levels of some treatment factor, for example, concentrations of dietary protein, levels of growth hormone, percentages of oats in the diet. The objective of these types of experiments is to characterize the nature of the response curve. This can be stated in one simple question: What is the relationship between dose level and response? Orthogonal polynomials can be used to answer this question. This is the correct approach regardless of whether the overall treatment effect was significant or not.

In some cases, orthogonal polynomials were used in the analysis; however, when results have been presented in manuscripts, superscripts indicating statistical significance among all possible pairs of means have been used to summarize results. This dual approach is neither correct nor useful. A more meaningful method of summarization would be to show the partitioned treatment sum of squares and the percentages of the variability among responses accounted for by linear and curvilinear components. If there is evidence of a significant linear relationship, pairwise tests of significance are unnecessary and, in fact, provide no useful information. Even if the observed difference between two levels is determined to be "nonsignificant" by a pairwise test, the regression already implies that an increment in dosage may be expected to effect a response.

Experiments involving factorial treatment structures constitute the second class of experiments that frequently is interpreted and presented poorly. For these types of experiments, the logical questions are: What is the effect of each factor? Does the response to one factor depend on the class (or level) of another factor, or in other words, are there any interactions?

In factorial experiments, when the factors are not independent (interaction is present), considerable caution must be exercised in drawing conclusions about the overall main effects. The presence of the interaction means that the response to different classes (or levels) of one factor changes (in either rank or magnitude) according to the class (or level) of another factor. If the interaction is one of rank, treatment combination (subclass) means should be presented instead of main effect means. If the interaction is one of magnitude, the interaction should be acknowledged, but main effect means may still provide meaningful information. Graphs are often an effective means of summarizing the results of factorial experiments.

Statistics in Manuscripts

When experimental results are reported in scientific manuscripts, the statistical methods should be summarized in a clear, concise manner that can be easily understood. Obviously, the biology should be emphasized, but a clear account of the way the experiment was conducted and how the results were analyzed assures readers that proper design and analysis were used. Ashton and McMillan (1981) presented a useful list of suggestions for the presentation of statistics in scientific manuscripts.

Stating only the computer software package used to analyze the data is not, in itself, a sufficient description of the statistical analysis. User's manuals for computer software packages generally are not adequate references for statistical methods. Analysis of standard designs should be described by name and size. For a factorial experiment in an RCB design, an adequate description of the analysis might be, "Data were analyzed as a randomized complete block design with a 2 × 3 factorial arrangement of treatments in five blocks." Also, the experimental unit should be defined. In cases in which the usual experimental error is not the term used for testing treatment differences, such as in SP or RM designs, the error term that was used should be identified. Finally, contrasts used to answer specific questions should be identified. If the contrasts were nonorthogonal, the test procedure should be referenced as well.

Significance levels associated with specific tests provide measures of reliability and should be identified in text, tables, and figures. The most commonly reported significance levels are $P < .10$, $P < .05$, $P < .01$, and $P < .001$. An alternative is to state exact probabilities for each comparison and let the reader decide what to reject; however, this tends to clutter a paper with numerous probability levels. Whatever level of significance is chosen by researchers, the choice should be based on the relative consequences of rejecting the null hypothesis when it is true (type I error) and accepting the null hypothesis when it is false (type II error). Since significance is implied when a probability statement is utilized; it is redundant to use any form of the word *significance* in the same sentence.

Regardless of the method of presentation or whether the results are statistically significant, some measure of residual variation (e.g., error mean square, pooled standard deviation, pooled standard error, coefficient of variation) should be reported with treatment means. Giving results of significance tests does not eliminate the need to present some measure of variability. As pointed out by Morse and Thompson (1981), this is so for several reasons. First, a measure of residual variability (experimental error) is required if a reader wants to consider a hypothesis other than the stated one or to combine subsets of published results with those from other sources. Second, a measure of the inherent variability in the experimental material will be valuable for researchers designing similar experiments. Third, a measure of variability will give an idea of the precision and power of the experiment. Fourth, estimation of treatment effects is often as important as hypothesis testing, and reliability of such estimates can be assessed if some measure of variability is presented.

Generally, either a pooled standard deviation (square root of the error mean square) or a pooled standard error (pooled standard deviation divided by the square root of the number of replications) will suffice. Unless there is heterogeneity of variances, standard errors should not be presented for individual means. In some situations, researchers may choose to report the coefficient of variation (pooled standard deviation multiplied by 100 and divided by the mean); however, use of the coefficient of variation generally is confined to giving a subjective measure of the efficiency of the experimental techniques or to comparing the relative variation among experiments.

ROLE OF THE STATISTICIAN IN EXPERIMENTATION

Including a statistician as a member of a research team will circumvent many potentially serious statistical problems. The statistician's role should begin during the planning stage of the experiment. Later, the statistician can be involved in data analysis, and finally, in interpretation and presentation of results. It is beneficial for the statistician on the team to have some training and expertise in the research field of interest. Likewise, it is beneficial for other team members to have some biometrical training in order to comprehend the potentials as well as the limitations of statistics as a research tool. Obviously, the degree to which a statistician is needed in the experiment will depend on the biometrical training of the primary researcher. If approached as a cooperative effort, the association between biologists and statistician can be of mutual benefit. As pointed out by Van Vleck and Henderson (1965), although statistical techniques should be considered as research tools, the statistician is not such a tool. As an active member of the research team, the statistician's contribution should be recognized just as any other team member's contribution would be recognized.

REFERENCES

Ashton, G.C., and I. McMillan. 1981. *A Medley of Statistical Techniques for Researchers.* Dubuque, IA: Kendall/Hunt Publishing Co.
Bartlett, M.S. 1937. *J.R. Stat. Soc.* 4(Suppl.):137.
Carmer, S.G., and W.M. Walker. 1985. *J. Agron. Ed.* 14:19.
Chew, V. 1976. *Hortscience* 11:348.
Cochran, W.G., and G.M. Cox. 1957. *Experimental Designs.* 2d ed. New York: John Wiley and Sons.
Damon, R.A., Jr., and W.R. Harvey. 1987. *Experimental Design. ANOVA, and Regression.* New York: Harper and Row.

Dunnett, C.W. 1955. *J. Am. Statist. Assoc.* 50:1096.
Fisher, R.A. 1935. *The Design of Experiments.* London: Oliver and Boyd, Ltd.
Gill, J.L. 1978a. *Design and Analysis of Experiments in the Animal and Medical Sciences.* Vol. 1. Ames, IA: Iowa State University Press.
Gill, J.L. 1978b. *Design and Analysis of Experiments in the Animal and Medical Sciences.* Vol. 2. Ames, IA: Iowa State University Press.
Gill, J.L., and H.D. Hafs. 1971. *J. Anim. Sci.* 33:331.
Hartley, H.O. 1950. *Biometrika* 37:308.
Lentner, M., and T. Bishop. 1986. *Experimental Design and Analysis.* Blacksburg, VA: Valley Book Co.
Little, T.M. 1981. *Hortscience* 16:19.
Little, T.M., and F.J. Hills. 1978. *Agricultural Experimentation.* New York: John Wiley and Sons.
Milliken, G.A., and D.E. Johnson. 1984. *Designed Experiments.* Vol. 1 of *Analysis of Messy Data.* New York: Van Nostrand Reinhold Co.
Morse, P.M., and B.K. Thompson. 1981. *Can. J. Plant. Sci.* 61:799.
Snedecor, G.W., and W.G. Cochran. 1980. *Statistical Methods.* 7th ed. Ames, IA: Iowa State University Press.
Steel, R.G.D., and J.H. Torrie. 1980. *Principles and Procedures of Statistics.* 2d ed. New York: McGraw-Hill Book Co.
Van Vleck, L.D., and C.R. Henderson. 1965. *J. Anim. Sci.* 24:559.

Chapter 39

Digestion and Metabolism Techniques in Pigs

L.G. Young, A.G. Low, and W.H. Close

Several textbooks provide excellent information regarding the many procedures and problems facing individuals who wish to conduct digestibility and metabolism studies in swine. These include *The Evaluation of Feeds Through Digestibility Experiments,* by Schneider and Flatt (1975), *Animal and Human Calorimetry,* by McLean and Tobin (1987), and *Protein Metabolism in Farm Animals,* by Bock et al. (1989).

Some of the techniques and problems applicable to swine will be described in this chapter, but space does not allow the detailed discussions found in the above references.

In a classical digestion study, the difference between the intake of a feedstuff or nutrient and the fecal excretion of the undigested portion of that feedstuff or nutrient is measured. This involves quantifying feed intake and feces output of the specific component. A balance or metabolism study, in addition to the above, also involves quantifying the excretion of the component of concern or its derivative in urine and gases. The subject becomes more complex if one considers the products of conception during pregnancy, milk in the lactating sow, or heat output in a balance study.

QUANTIFYING EXCRETIONS AND SECRETIONS

In the case of a digestibility study with growing pigs, one needs to measure the intake of the component of concern and the amount in the feces resulting from that intake. This can be achieved either by the use of indicators or total collection.

Use of Indicators

An indicator is a nontoxic, nonabsorbable, nonessential inert substance that remains with the feed material as it passes through the digestive tract and is readily measured.

Ferric oxide or chromic oxide uniformly mixed in the diet at 0.1% to 1% are frequently used. The formula for calculating percent digestibility by this method is:

$$\% \text{ Digestibility of nutrient} = 100 - 100 \cdot \frac{\% \text{ Indicator in feed} \times \% \text{ nutrient in feces}}{\% \text{ Indicator in feces} \times \% \text{ nutrient in feed}}$$

The use of this method does not require weighing of the feed fed or feces produced or close confinement of the animal in a digestion crate.

Some other indicators that have been evaluated include dysprosium (Kennelly et al. 1980) and rare earth elements (Pond et al. 1986). When using indicators, care must be taken to prevent possible coprophagy and recycling of the indicator, as may occur in pigs housed in pens.

Total Collection

Theoretically, determination of the total amount of the component ingested and the amount excreted in the feces from the feed ingested should provide the most accurate assessment of digestibility. However, two major problems arise: (1) there must be quantitative collection of feces without loss or contamination with urine, hair, or sloughed skin and (2) the animal has to be suitably adapted so that the feces originate solely from the test feed.

Where total collection is practiced, the pig is confined to an individual digestion crate. The crate can be designed so that it is fully adjustable to accommodate pigs of different sizes. It also should be designed so that all of the feces fall into a tray behind the pig rather than through a perforated floor onto a screen. Males are normally used to facilitate the separate collection of urine and of feces. However, gilts fitted with urinary catheters may be used. The use of smooth sides on the digestion crates may reduce skin sloughing.

Indigestible markers, ferric oxide or chromic oxide, are frequently used in an attempt to identify feces originating from the test feed. The marker is mixed with a small amount of diet fed at the initiation of the experimental period. The process is repeated after the last meal is administered at the end of the experimental period. It is assumed that the marker progresses through the digestive tract with a minimum of mixing with other digesta. Thus, feces collected between the appearance of the first marker and the appearance of the second marker are assumed to originate from the meals fed between the administration of the two markers. Since pigs may defecate only once or twice in a 24-hour period, the use of markers may aid in exclusion of feces originating from meals not administered in the experimental feeding period. When using markers, a preliminary period of 3 to 4 days followed by a collection period of 4 to 5 days may suffice. The actual collection of feces may not start until 1 or 2 days after the marker is fed. Markers containing chromium should be used cautiously due to possible toxicity.

An alternative to using markers is to increase the length of the preliminary period before collection is initiated and to extend the collection period. In this system, feces collection begins at the same time as the experimental feeding period starts and ceases when the experimental feeding period stops, usually after 5 to 7 days. Obviously, the first feces collected will have originated from meals fed prior to the initiation of the experimental feeding period. In this system, it is important to maintain a constant feeding level from late in the preliminary period until the end of the collection period, otherwise errors will be introduced due to variable intake and excretion. Timing of collections at the start and end of the collection period are important and subject to error due to the variable patterns of defecation. The larger the animal and the lower the level of feeding, the greater the problem becomes. Thus, where markers are not used, the longer the preliminary and collection periods, the lower the variability among pigs.

The foregoing applies to digestion studies. Metabolism studies, in which quantitative collection of urine is required, introduce additional factors. Identification of urine originating from a specific meal is difficult, especially with urine accumulation in the bladder and periodic voiding. Urine is usually collected quantitatively starting at or soon after the initial meal and ceasing at or soon after the last meal in the experimental period.

Quantitative collection of urine uncontaminated by feces is difficult. With male pigs, metabolism crates that allow adjustment of separate feces and urine collection trays should be used. Metabolism crates equipped with mesh flooring through which both feces and urine drop do not provide completely separate collection. Urinary catheters can be used in the female pig (Calvert et al. 1985) but may introduce urinary infections. A reliable mechanical system of separating urine and feces in female pigs has been described (Low 1977). Separate collection of urine and feces may not be required in some metabolism work such as the determination of metabolizable energy.

DIGESTIBILITY OF INGREDIENTS AND NUTRIENTS

The digestibility of dry matter, nitrogen, energy, fat, carbohydrate, minerals, crude fiber, cellulose, hemicellulose, acid detergent fiber, neutral detergent fiber, and non-starch polysaccharides is frequently determined. However, the digestibility of vitamins is not usually measured.

$$\text{Digestibility} = 100 \cdot \frac{\text{Quantity of nutrient in feed} - \text{Quantity of nutrient in feces}}{\text{Quantity of nutrient in feed}}$$

Because of secretions of enzymes, bile, and sloughing of cells lining the intestinal tract, as well as microbial activity, only part of the protein or fat found in the feces may be from the test material. Thus, digestibilities determined without correcting for the above fecal losses (endogenous losses) are referred to as measures of apparent digestibility. In the case of nitrogen, an estimate is frequently made of the fecal nitrogen not originating from the diet by feeding a protein-free diet, that is the endogenous or metabolic fecal nitrogen, and this is deducted from the total fecal nitrogen to give a "true" nitrogen digestibility.

The digestibility of ingredients that cannot be fed alone is determined by the addition method. One of two systems is frequently used:

1. Add to or substitute for a test ingredient. A basal diet is fed and the digestibility determined with a group of animals. Simultaneously, another group of animals is fed the basal diet plus a known quantity of the test ingredient and the digestibility is determined. The digestibility of the test ingredient can then be determined by difference.
2. Substitute the test ingredient for a component in the basal diet. If this is done at more than one level of substitution, it may be possible to estimate the digestibilities of two or three feedstuffs simultaneously (Young et al. 1977).

The possibility arises of "associative effects" of feedstuffs when the digestibility of the total diet is not the sum of the digestibility of its several individual ingredients. Determination of digestibility by difference assumes that there are no associative effects.

NUTRIENT BALANCE

In addition to accounting for loss of nutrients in feces and urine, balance studies are sometimes conducted to evaluate loss of nutrients from the body via (1) other excretions, such as gases, (2) secretions, such as milk, (3) products of conception, or (4) retention of nutrients, such as protein, fat, and minerals.

Open and closed respiration calorimetry to measure energy exchange are discussed in *Fire of Life* (Kleiber 1961) and more recently by McLean and Tobin (1987). Energy balance may also be evaluated through conventional metabolism trials in association with slaughter techniques (Sharma et al. 1977; McNutt and Ewan 1984).

Estimation of milk secretion by sows poses a challenge. Some investigators have designed and used milking machines (Miller 1981). Others (Noblet and Etienne 1986; Speer and Cox 1984; Lewis et al. 1978) have used the weigh-suckle-weigh technique, the deuterium dilution method (Pettigrew et al. 1987), or the estimation of milk yield from differences in body composition of the piglets over the experimental period (Mullan et al. 1989). It is also important to determine the composition of the milk, and samples may be drawn by hand after injection of oxytocin (Noblet and Etienne 1986). However, milk composition may be affected by the stage of lactation as well as the extent to which the mammary glands are emptied.

FEED INTAKE

The level of feeding used will be influenced by the objectives of the experiment and the nature of the diets. In general, feeding at a constant high plane without feed refusal may be desirable. Accumulation of refusals (orts) creates more work, both physical and analytical, and may introduce possible errors, as the orts must be weighed and analyzed to account for possible changes in moisture content, sorting, soiling, and contamination with saliva. Level of feed intake may have an effect on some measures of the digestibility of protein, fat, and energy because of changes in the relative proportions of endogenous microbial and dietary contributions to the feces as well as differences in the rate of passage through the digestive tract. However, intake may have a considerable effect on the balance (retention) of both nitrogen and energy (Willis and Maxwell 1984; Haydon et al. 1984; McNutt and Ewan 1984). Usually, a higher proportion of dietary nitrogen is retained at low protein intakes whereas dietary energy retention frequently increases as intake increases.

NITROGEN AND AMINO ACID DIGESTIBILITY AND METABOLISM

Readers are referred to recent reviews on this subject (Low 1982; Sauer and Ozimek 1986; Low and Zebrowska 1989) and to Chapter 19 in this text.

Apparent digestibility of dietary nitrogen and amino acids is influenced by the endogenous nitrogen from sloughed intestinal mucosal cells, digestive enzymes, and microbial activity in the gut. True digestibility of nitrogen and amino acids has been calculated by deducting the endogenous portion from the total amount in the feces; thus, true digestibility tends to be higher than apparent digestibility. Four methods have been used to estimate endogenous excretion of nitrogenous products:

1. Feeding a nitrogen-free diet and determining the amount of nitrogen or amino acids in the feces.
2. Feeding a number of levels of the nutrient and regressing the fecal level of the nutrient to a zero dietary intake.
3. Feeding a completely digestible protein.
4. Transforming lysine to homoarginine (Hagemeister and Erbersdobler 1985).

These methods may underestimate endogenous losses (Sauer and Ozimek 1986).

Protein and amino acids may be synthesized and/or degraded in the gut of the pig through the action of the microflora. The effect of this microbial activity is not considered in determining the apparent or true digestibilities of these nutrients by the fecal analysis method. In addition, some ammonia and amino acids may be absorbed from the hindgut and may not contribute to the animal's nutrient requirement. Any nitrogen absorbed from the large intestine can be assumed to have no nutritional value (Zebrowska 1973). For these reasons, it is entirely erroneous to measure digestible amino acids in feces.

To avoid some of these problems, amino acid digestibility estimates have been made using digesta sampled near the ileocecal junction rather than feces, using various types of ileocecal cannulas (Low and Zebrowska 1989). However, problems may be encountered using some of these techniques, including blockage of the cannula when fibrous feedstuffs are fed (using re-entrant cannulas), obtaining representative samples of digesta leaving the ileum (using single cannulas), and the necessity of surgery.

Another technique involves ileorectal anastomosis. Some of the possible implications of this technique include altered sites and patterns of mineral and water absorption and modified digesta flow rates (Low and Zebrowska 1989).

Neither of the above techniques appear to eliminate the microbial effect from the measurements, since some microbial activity occurs in the stomach and small instestine (Millard and Chesson 1984).

A nylon bag technique has been proposed for rapid determination of protein digestibility in small samples of feedstuffs (Sauer et al. 1983). The technique involves enclosing the sample in small nylon bags, in vitro, predigestion to simulate gastric digestion, and introducing it via a duodenal cannula to allow passage through the intestinal tract. The bags are separated from the feces, and the disappearance of nitrogen is determined. The system may provide comparative values of protein digestibility of individual feedstuffs. This method is not suitable for readily soluble feedstuffs and is subject to loss of bags as well as the effects of the microflora previously mentioned. In addition, the bags must be fabricated with suitable mesh to prevent loss of insoluble material from the bag yet allow ready transfer of digestive enzymes through it.

Nitrogen balance is a measure of the net consequences of nitrogen ingestion, digestion, absorption, metabolism, excretion, and secretion. It may be estimated by measuring the difference between intake and excretion plus secretion or by measuring the accumulation of nitrogen in the body from a given nitrogen intake (Just et al. 1982). Either system presents problems in obtaining representative samples for analysis. Just et al. (1982) suggested that the first method tends to overestimate the amount retained by as much as 20% as compared with the chemical analysis of the body. In comparing different sources of protein, it may be necessary to use semipurified diets with the protein of interest as the only source of nitrogen. In addition, a constant level of protein intake should be maintained, since both level of intake and protein "quality" will affect nitrogen balance. Also, nitrogen retention may be affected by the previous level of intake and the quality of protein, which may influence the labile pool of amino acids in the body.

FIBER AND DIGESTION

Various sources of fiber have been added to pig diets to make them isoenergetic or for other purposes. Frequently, these sources of fiber have been considered to be inert with respect to supplying nutrients or altering digestion. There is now ample evidence to indicate that this is not the case. Fiber may be digested in the hindgut with the production of volatile fatty acids, which can contribute to the energy requirement of the pig (Longland et al. 1988). Other implications of dietary fiber have been reviewed by Low and Zebrowska (1989), including the effect on amino acid digestion and absorption and on endogenous nitrogen production.

ENERGY DIGESTION AND METABOLISM

The determination of the digestible and metabolizable energy content of feedstuffs tends to be less complicated and less influenced by factors than is the determination of protein and amino acid digestibility. However, microbial activity in the gut may result in some overestimation of the energy value of high-fiber feeds due to the production of volatile fatty acids, typical mixtures of which may provide less energy than that derived from an equivalent weight of dietary starch.

Energy balance becomes a much more complex area for study due to the need to determine the energy produced as heat, expired gases, and energy content of other body excretions and secretions (McLean and Tobin 1987).

Modern computer-operated whole body calorimeters for pigs are very expensive, but these are necessary in order to obtain a more complete understanding of energy requirements and utilization. The developments in animal calorimetry are catalogued in the various reports of the Symposia on the Energy Metabolism of Farm Animals (European Association for Animal Production).

SUMMARY

There is no one ideal system or technique for conducting digestion and metabolism experiments with pigs. Different techniques may be applied depending on the information required. In many cases, relatively simple techniques may suffice. In other cases, more elaborate techniques may be justified. Whatever the case, the investigator must be aware of the limitations of the techniques used and interpret the results accordingly. Similarly, those reading the research reports of others must be aware of the limitations of the techniques used.

REFERENCES

Bock, H.D., et al. 1989. *Protein Metabolism in Farm Animals.* Oxford, England: Oxford University Press.

Calvert, C.C., N.C. Steele, and R.W. Rosebrough. 1985. *J. Anim. Sci.* 61:595–602.

Hagemeister, H., and H. Erbersdobler. 1985. *Proc. Nutr. Soc.* 44:133A.

Haydon, K.D., D.A. Knabe, and T.D. Tanksley, Jr. 1984. *J. Anim. Sci.* 59:717–724.

Just, A., J.A. Fernandez, and H. Jorgensen. 1982. "Nitrogen balance studies and nitrogen retention." In: *Digestive Physiology in the Pig.* Laplace, J.P., T. Corring, and A. Rérat. (Eds.). pp. 111-121. Les Colloques de l'INRA No. 12. Paris: Institut National de la Recherche Agronomique.

Kennelly, J.J., F.X. Aherne, and M.J. Apps. 1980. *Can. J. Anim. Sci.* 60:441–446.

Kleiber, M. 1961. *The Fire of Life.* New York: John Wiley & Sons.

Lewis, A.J., V.C. Speer, and D.G. Haught. 1978. *J. Anim. Sci.* 47:634–638.

Longland, A.C., et al. 1988. *Proc. Nutr. Soc.* 47:102A.

Low, A.G. 1977. *J. Sci. Food Agric.* 28:980–982.

Low, A.G. 1982. *Livestock Prod. Sci.* 9:511–520.

Low, A.G., and T. Zebrowska. 1989. "Digestion in pigs." In: *Protein Metabolism in Farm Animals.* pp. 53–121. Oxford, England: Oxford University Press.

McLean, J.A., and G. Tobin. 1987. *Animal and Human Calorimetry.* Cambridge, England: Cambridge University Press.

McNutt, S.D., and R.C. Ewan. 1984. *J. Anim. Sci.* 59:738–745.

Millard, P., and A. Chesson. 1984. *Br. J. Nutr.* 52:583–594.

Miller, E.R. 1981. *Michigan Agricultural Experiment Station Report of Swine Research 437.* p. 179. East Lansing: University of Michigan.

Mullan, B.P., W.H. Close, and D.J.A. Cole. 1989. "Predicting nutrient responses of the lactating sow." In: *Recent Advances in Animal Nutrition.* Haresign, W., and D.J.A. Cole (Eds.). pp. 229-243. London: Butterworths.

Noblet, J., and M. Etienne. 1986. *J. Anim. Sci.* 63:1888-1896.

Pettigrew, J.E., et al. *Livestock Prod. Sci.* 16:163-174.

Pond, W.G., et al. 1986. *J. Anim. Sci.* 63:1140-1149.

Sauer, W.C., H. Jorgensen, and R. Berzino. 1983. *Can. J. Anim. Sci.* 63:233-237.

Sauer, W.C., and L.S. Ozimek. 1986. *Livestock Prod. Sci.* 15:367-387.

Schneider, H., and W.P. Flatt. 1975. *The Evaluation of Feeds Through Digestibility Experiments.* Athens, GA: The University of Georgia Press.

Sharma, V.D., L.G. Young, and G.C. Smith. 1971. *Can. J. Anim. Sci.* 51:761-770.

Speer, V.C., and D.F. Cox. 1984. *J. Anim. Sci.* 59:1281-1285.

Willis, G.M., and C.V. Maxwell. 1984. *J. Anim. Sci.* 58:647-656.

Young, L.G., G.C. Ashton, and G.C. Smith. 1977. *J. Anim. Sci.* 44:765-771.

Zebrowska, T. 1973. *Roczn. Nauk rohr.* 95B(3):85-90.

Chapter 40

Techniques for Measuring Body Composition of Swine

R.G. Shields, Jr.

The lack of a nondestructive, inexpensive accurate measurement technique has limited body composition measurement in animal research. Additionally, there has been relatively little commercial incentive to raise lean animals (Topel 1986) and so there has not been much demand for this type of information. This situation is likely to change. As vertical coordination continues and exogenous agents that alter the composition of gain are approved, compensation for lean, uniform animals is likely to increase.

THE IMPORTANCE OF BODY COMPOSITION MEASUREMENT

Body composition measurement can be an important adjunct in most swine nutrition experiments. Body weight changes alone can be misleading during growth and reproduction. Whittemore and co-workers (1980) reported that sows lost an estimated 8 kg subcutaneous fat while gaining 22 kg in live weight through two reproductive cycles. Similar effects have been noted on the immediate postweaning period (Whittemore et al. 1981; Fenton et al. 1985). Body weight changes provide no information about the composition of gain (or loss) or about changes in gastrointestinal contents (Reid et al. 1963).

The main applications for body composition measurement are in experiments to determine nutrient requirements and availabilities. Daily requirements for any nutrient are dependent on the level of production, the composition of that nutrient in the product, and the efficiency with which the absorbed nutrients can be used for productive functions. Dietary quantities necessary to meet requirements for maintenance and growth are then a function of feed intake and nutrient availability within the selected ingredients. Requirements will be altered by factors that influence any of the above factors, including body composition. Energy requirements of swine are generally stated in terms of either digestible energy (DE) or metabolizable energy (ME), unlike ruminants, in which the net energy system is used. Development of a net energy system for swine will require estimates of energy deposition in the empty body. Deductive modeling applications make assumptions about maximum lean tissue growth rates and limitations to lean and fat deposition rates imposed by dietary nutrient content (Whittemore 1986). As interest in altering the composition of growth continues to increase, the use of some form of body composition measurement in swine nutrition experiments is likely to increase.

BODY COMPOSITION METHODOLOGY

There are several different methods of estimating body composition, and this makes it difficult to compare the results of different experiments. A scheme showing the various techniques is presented in Figure 40.1. Postmortem techniques include methods such as chemical analysis, carcass measurements, and specific gravity determinations. Live animal methods encompass subjective scoring, linear measurements, indirect estimations of body water and lean body mass, and cross-sectional imaging.

Postmortem Methods

Chemical analysis of the empty (ingesta-free) body or physical separation into muscle, fat, and bone usually form the basis against which all new methods of estimating body composition are compared. Chemical analysis is typically used in experiments concerned with nutrient partitioning or availability, while physical separation is generally used when the primary goal is to examine the effects of treatment on carcass value. Smith and Pearson (1985) have attempted to relate results obtained in these two types of studies by developing a series of regression equations. Further work in this area will be of considerable value.

Both chemical analysis and physical separation are time-consuming, prohibiting the use of large numbers of animals. Additionally, the chemical assay procedure results in the loss of saleable product. The analysis of sample joints has been evaluated as a method of reducing the loss of product. This method can discern large treatment differences (McMeekan 1941), but it is not thought to be precise enough to predict individual animal composition (Timon and Bichard 1965). Oslage and Farries (1962) described a technique involving chemical analysis of the sawdust collected from cross-sectional sawing of a frozen carcass. Recent evaluations of this procedure (Shields and Mahan 1983a; Shields et al. 1983a) have been promising and indicate that the method could allow some carcass salvage value. Near infrared reflectance has been evaluated as a method to save chemical assay time and costs, and initial studies with ground

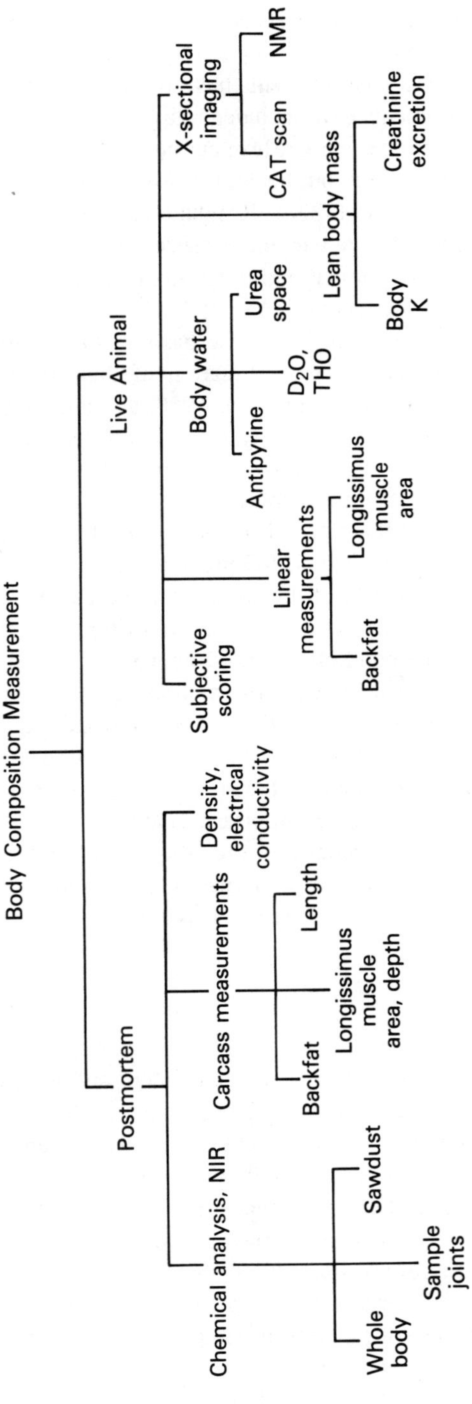

FIGURE 40.1 *Body composition measurement techniques.*

mouse (Eisen et al. 1984), bovine (Roberts et al. 1987), and swine (George et al. 1987) tissue have been encouraging.

Several different carcass measurements have been evaluated as indicators of carcass composition. Measurements have included retail cut weights, dressing percentage, carcass length, longissimus muscle area, lean cut percentage, and backfat depth. Most have been of low predictive value, but backfat measurement has shown some promise (Mersmann 1982a; Shields et al. 1983a). Residual standard deviations for estimating carcass water, protein, and fat from backfat measurements were 3.5%, 3.5%, and 1%, respectively. Measurement of backfat and longissimus muscle area have been used to estimate muscle quantity in pigs (Fahey et al. 1977; Edwards et al. 1981; Prince et al. 1981; Grisdale et al 1984), and they form the basis of the National Pork Producers Council (NPPC) (1976) equations for estimation of this criterion. Optical density probes (Kempster et al. 1981; Chizzolini et al. 1988) and total body electrical conductivity (TOBEC) measurement are currently being evaluated for rapid, simultaneous measurement of backfat and longissimus muscle area (or depth).

Specific gravity (SG) techniques exploit the density difference between lean and fat tissue. An important advantage of SG methods is that there is no loss of saleable product. The history and theory behind SG procedures were reviewed by Pearson et al. (1968). Between 36% and 90% of the variation in fat content in swine growth and reproduction studies has been associated with SG differences (Brown et al. 1951; Doornebal et al. 1962; Adam and Smith 1964; Joblin 1966; Shields and Mahan 1983a; Shields et al. 1983a). The residual standard deviation of percentage fat estimation of approximately 4% is too high for predictive purposes in individual animals. SG procedures assume that the body is composed of a fat and a fat-free component of different and constant densities (Keys and Brozek 1953). This assumption is probably incorrect.

A major drawback of all postmortem measurements is that they can be performed only once on a given animal. A procedure that allows repeated measurements on the same animals with a low error of estimation may be preferrable to postmortem techniques when expected animal-to-animal variation is high.

Live Animal Methods

Visual conformation assessment is the most convenient and least costly in vivo measurement procedure, but because of its subjective nature, attempts to use this method have been largely unsuccessful (Kempster and Evans 1979a; 1981). Energy and nitrogen balance studies have also been used; although quantitative, these techniques measure intake and loss rather than deposition. They have been criticized for overestimating retention because of short trial duration and difficulties in absolute measurement of intake and output (Wallace 1959). Several live animal methods that measure deposition rather than balance are listed below. Unfortunately, most of these techniques directly measure only one chemical component, and they rely heavily on predictable relationships between components to estimate overall composition.

Several linear measurements, including shoulder height, neck circumference, body length, and foreleg and hindleg length and width were evaluated by Houseman and McDonald (1976). Measurement repeatability was low, probably because of a lack of anatomical measurement standardization. Close relationships should not have been expected because shape bears little relationship to body composition. As mentioned previously, backfat and longissimus muscle area have been used to estimate muscle quantity in swine carcasses, and ultrasonic measuring devices appear to have high repeatability and accuracy for measuring loin and fat depth in the live animal when measured over the midback and loin (Mersmann 1982a). Real-time ultrasonics with multiple transducers can actually create an image of the loin muscle in the live animal (Moore et al. 1985).

Fortin and Elliot (1985) found that backfat measurements reflected changes in subcutaneous rather than total fat stores, so factors that influence distribution of fat stores may reduce the accuracy of ultrasonic measurement. The relatively high standard error of estimate for ultrasonic measurements must be weighed against the fact that they are inexpensive and repeated measurements on the same animal are possible. They are quite useful in studies involving large numbers of animals where general composition trends are of interest.

In contrast to the linear measurements listed above, body water estimation using tracer dilution techniques has shown promise for estimation of composition in the individual animal. To provide valid data, a tracer must equilibrate rapidly and completely in all body water compartments, must be transformed or excreted slowly from these compartments, and must be capable of being measured accurately in body fluids (Hansard 1963). Several substances including antipyrine and its derivatives, urea, and hydrogen isotopes have been used successfully to measure body water. Others have failed to meet one or more of the above criteria.

Antipyrine (1,5-dimethyl-2-phenyl-3-pyrazolone) and its derivatives were evaluated in the 1950s. Although antipyrine binds to body proteins and is soluble in lipid tissue (Keys and Brozek 1953), antipyrine was used to measure total body water, while N-acetyl-4-amino antipyrine measured a space roughly equivalent to empty body water (Reid et al. 1957, 1958). The difference between these two quantities is roughly equivalent to gastrointestinal water, a large and variable body water compartment in ruminants. Subsequent studies revealed much higher precision for hydrogen isotope measurement (Garrett et al. 1959; Hansard 1963; Panaretto and Till 1963), thus reducing further application of antipyrine and its derivatives.

Urea dilution has been investigated more thoroughly in ruminants than nonruminants. The low cost of the tracer and ease of measurement make urea dilution particularly attractive. Initial acceptance was slow because it was felt that urea was not evenly distributed in body fluids (Keys and Brozek 1953). Positive relationships between urea space and body water have been noted in several ruminant (Preston and Kock 1953; Kock and Preston 1979; Meissner et al. 1980; Hammond et al. 1984; Bartle et al. 1983, 1987), horse (Lawrence et al. 1986), and swine (Stansbury et al. 1985; Chiba et al. 1987) studies. Jones and co-workers (1982), however, failed to find a close relationship.

A portion of this inconsistency may be because urea is normally present in the body in variable amounts, and as the infused urea is not labeled, relatively large tracer doses must be administered to increase the pool size (Trenkle 1986). The influence of this factor on body urea kinetics is unknown. Incorporation of preinfusion urea level has improved accuracy of estimation for this technique (Bartle et al. 1983). Most studies have involved blood urea measurement at a particular time postinfusion, and this may cause some inaccuracies in studies involving animals with markedly different water turnover rates, such as pregnant and lactating sows. Acceptance of this methodology will require further validation.

Hydrogen isotopes have been the most thoroughly researched body water tracers. Both deuterium oxide (D_2O, ^2H_2O) and tritiated water (TOH, ^3H_2O) cross barriers at the same rate as water and distribute evenly in body fluids (Pinson 1952), making them ideal tracers. These two compounds have been used to quantitatively estimate body water in many species, including swine (Wood and Groves 1963; Groves and Wood 1965; Flynn et al. 1968; Houseman et al. 1973; Shields et al. 1983b, 1984; Ferrell and Cornelius 1984; Rudolph 1984). Correlation coefficients have been quite high (above 0.9) and residual coefficients of variation, low (below 5%) in studies evaluating animals with a wide range of fatness. The advent of a measurement procedure accurate to within 1 ppm (Byers 1979), its adaptation to automatic sampling (Ferrell and Phillips 1980), and the fact that it is a stable isotope have encouraged preference for deuterium oxide over tritiated water.

Two major concerns expressed regarding the deuterium oxide dilution procedure are its overestimation of body water and the difficulty in quantitation of ingesta water and that contributed by conceptus products. Pinson (1952) proposed that deuterium oxide overestimated body water by 0.5% to 2%, based on isotope exchange with hydrogen atoms not attached to carbon. Panaretto (1963) modified this factor to 3% to additionally account for exchange with hydrogen atoms of newly synthesized compounds and for vapor losses during the equilibration period. Overestimations as high as 24% have been reported in studies dealing with growing beagle dogs (Sheng and Huggins 1971). Although studies with suckling pigs have suggested similar values for deuterium oxide space and total body water (Shields et al. 1983b; Rudolph 1984), those conducted with growing-finishing and reproducing swine have reported overestimations of 18% to 20% (Shields et al. 1983b, 1984). The source of this overestimation remains to be identified.

As the main concern of body composition studies is to measure changes in body stores, methods are needed to partition ingesta and conceptus water from empty (growth) or maternal (reproduction) body water. Interference from ingesta water is a greater problem in ruminants, where the quantity of gastrointestinal water is large and variable, but it can pose a problem in nonruminants also. The variable influence of conceptus products and mammary tissue water has prevented widespread application of the deuterium oxide dilution procedure for reproducing animals.

Two- (Byers 1978) and three- (Odwongo 1984) compartment models have been evaluated to differentiate between body stores and exogenous water, but studies with cattle (Arnold et al. 1985; Arnold and Trenkle 1986) and swine (Shields et al. 1983b, 1984) have failed to find improvements in these models over the one-compartment approach, perhaps resulting from lack of ability to relate water compartments to anatomical locations (Russell and Reed 1987). Shields et al. (1984) found that maternal body water measurement in gestating sows could be improved substantially by including day of gestation in the estimation equation.

Table 40.1 contains several regression equations for estimating empty or maternal body water in growing or reproducing swine, respectively. Studies with swine up to conventional slaughter weight (Shields et al. 1983b; Ferrell and Cornelius 1984) yielded similar regression equations, while those for heavier animals resulted in equations that were quite different and less accurate (Shields et al. 1983b). Incorporation of pig type improved accuracy of estimation in the Ferrell and Cornelius (1984) study, and it is possible that leanness influences the tracer-solute relationship. Work evaluating the deuterium oxide dilution procedure is continuing at several research facilities.

Direct determination of muscle or body protein using body potassium measurement, creatinine excretion, neutron activation analysis, and ^{51}Cr-labeled red blood cells has also been evaluated in body composition studies. The first two have been researched more extensively and discussions will therefore be focused on them.

Potassium estimation using whole body counting (^{40}K) or isotope dilution (^{42}K) has been used extensively in body composition research. Excellent reviews of the techniques are those of Ward and Johnson (1972) and Shebaita (1975). Both techniques capitalize on the presence of potassium as the major intracellular cation. Whole body counting involves the measurement of gamma radiation emitted by body ^{40}K content (Shebaita 1975), and it is particularly attractive because no injections or chemical analyses are involved. Equipment expense and inconsistent results (Preston et al. 1968; Krzywicki et al. 1974) have limited application of this technique. The latter effect may result from difficulties in correction for animal geometry and instrument calibration differences. Isotope dilution using ^{42}K has also experienced difficulty in acceptance because it measures exchangeable rather than total potassium. The isotope does not equilibrate with potassium in bone and other extracellular tissues and adjustments for species, age, and sex are necessary.

Table 40.1 Comparison of Regression Equations to Predict Empty (or Maternal) Body Water from Deuterium Oxide Space

Regression Equation	*No. of Pigs*	*Description*	R^2	*Reference*
EBW = 2.6 + 0.87 D_2O	24	Growth (84 kg)	—	Houseman et al. 1973
EBW = 1.5 + 0.77 D_2O	56	Growth (6.4–109 kg)	0.99	Shields et al. 1983b
EBW = 10.6 + 0.61 D_2O	25	Growth (109–145 kg)	0.60	Shields et al. 1983b
EBW = 1.7 + 0.78 D_2O	60	Growth (5–92 kg)	0.93	Ferrell and Cornelius 1984
MBW = 4.2 + 0.82 D_2O − 0.19 d gest + 0.0004 d gest	46 2	Gestation (0–105 d)	0.96	Shields et al. 1984
MBW = 3.85 + 0.66 D_2O	16	Lactation (5–25 d)	0.67	Shields et al. 1984

Abbreviations: EBW, empty body water; MBW, maternal body water; d. gest., days postcoitum.

Measurement of creatinine excretion should, in theory, be proportional to muscle mass, because creatinine is a waste product formed following dephosphorylation of phosphocreatine to creatine in muscle (Novak 1963). Aulstad (1970) found large variations in creatinine excretion both between and within days, resulting in inconsistent results. This has prevented further investigation of this technique.

Direct estimation of fat in the live animal would be extremely valuable, since it is the most variable chemical component in the body. Griffin and co-workers (1982) were successful in using plasma triglyceride concentration as a selection criterion in broiler breeding programs, but studies evaluating it as a direct estimator of body fat (Bartov et al. 1974; Mirosh et al. 1980) have provided less optimistic results.

X-ray computer assisted tomography (CAT scanner) and nuclear magnetic resonance (NMR), used extensively in human medicine, have been used to provide cross-sectional imaging of the live pig. The former method had its first animal application in Norway and uses x-ray transmission through tissues and numerous detectors. Based on the variable radiation transmitted through different types of tissues, the computer can reconstruct a cross-sectional image of the body. An excellent review of this method was prepared by Leymaster (1986). The latter method depends on the electromagnetic energy released after exposure to a strong magnetic field and is currently being evaluated extensively at Rowett Research Institute (M. Fuller, personal communication). Both methods may be cost prohibitive for routine use in swine nutrition studies but have extremely broad application.

Although all body composition techniques have certain drawbacks, refinement of existing techniques and development of new methodology will continue as the need for this type of information increases.

COMPOSITIONAL CHANGES DURING GROWTH AND REPRODUCTION

Changes in Body Composition During Growth

The accretion of chemical components during growth represents variable contributions of cell multiplication, cell enlargement, and incorporation of materials from the environment (Brody 1945). Numerous studies, beginning with those of Lawes and Gilbert (1861), have evaluated changes in chemical composition that occur during growth. McMeekan (1940) related these chemical changes to the sequential development of bone, muscle, and fat tissue. Although the general relationships remain today, genetic progress has shifted tissue growth curves. Clausen (1953) found maximum muscle deposition rate was obtained by 70 to 80 kg live weight, while later studies by Oslage (1965) and Doornenbal (1971) failed to show a plateau or decline in muscle growth rate throughout the growth period studied (up to 130 kg). Carcass fatness at a given weight has continued to decrease in response to selection pressure. Shields et al. (1983c) found 30% fat in 110-kg pigs, compared with 37% in a previous study by Doornenbal (1972). The accretion patterns of chemical components in the former study are presented in Figure 40.2.

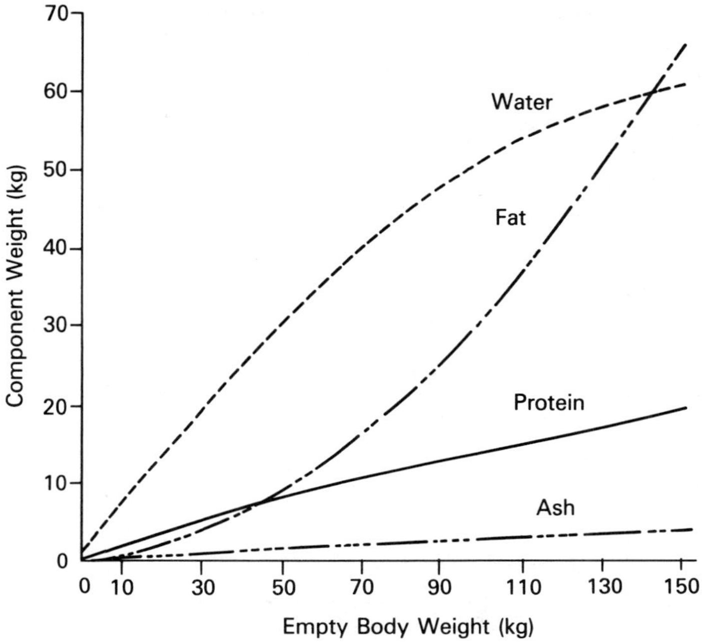

(Adapted, by permission, from Shields et al. 1983c.)

Figure 40.2 *Accretion of chemical components in swine from birth to 145 kg.*

In addition to the absolute quantities of muscle, fat and bone, chemical component relationships within the fat-free body have changed during years of selection. Moulton (1923) proposed the concept of "chemical maturity," a point at which the fat-free body becomes constant in composition. The water content of the fat-free body falls rapidly during fetal growth (Moulton 1923) and continues to decline during the postnatal period (Moulton 1923; Reid et al. 1955, 1968; Shields et al. 1983c). Changes in the composition of the fat-free body during postnatal swine growth are depicted in Figure 40.3. No evidence of chemical maturity was found in studies by Reid et al. (1955) during cattle growth or by Shields et al. (1983c) during swine growth. In the latter study, the water:protein ratio fell from 8:1 at birth to 4.5:1 at weaning to approximately 3.5:1 at market weight. A portion of this effect may be attributed to the fact that the water content of fat tissue decreases with age (Wood 1984). The relative proportions of protein and ash also change during postnatal swine growth. Protein:ash ratio was 3:1 in the neonatal pig but 5:1 in pigs of weaning age and older.

Changes in Body Composition During the Reproductive Cycle

Body composition changes during the reproductive cycle are biphasic in nature, with deposition of all tissues occurring during the first two thirds of pregnancy, and a reduc-

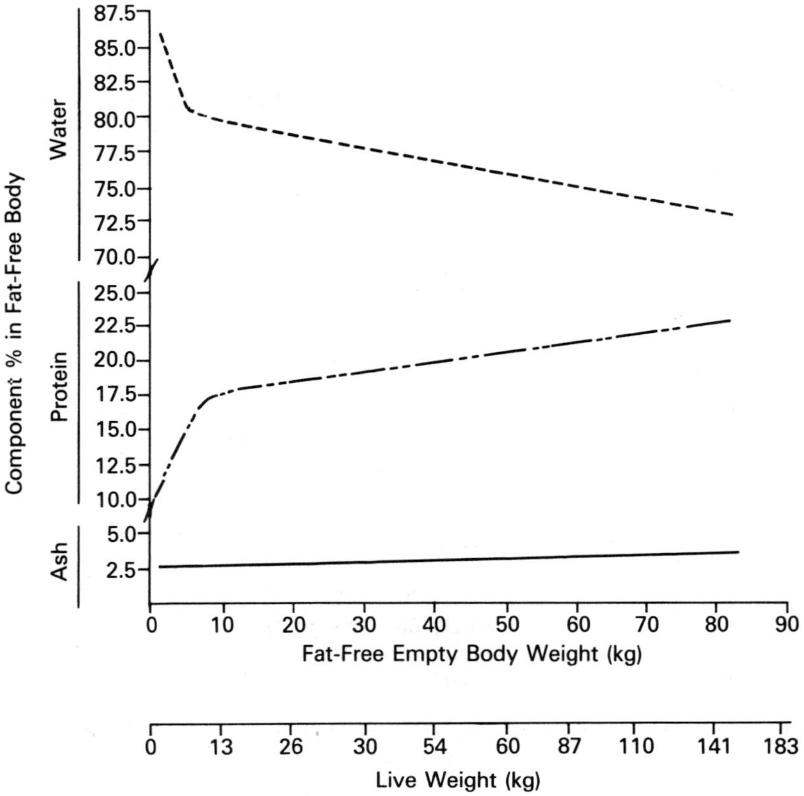

(Reprinted, by permission, from Shields et al. 1983c.)

FIGURE 40.3 *Changes in body composition (fat-free basis) of growing swine from birth to 145 kg.*

tion in deposition rate or mobilization beginning in the last third of pregnancy when fetal demands increase. Mobilization of body tissues continues through the initial stages of lactation, and deposition occurs again in the later stages of lactation if early weaning is not practiced (Naismith 1966; Johnson 1973; Whittemore et al. 1980; Shields and Mahan 1983b; Close et al. 1984; Robinson 1986). Tissue depletion (mostly water) is again observed during the postweaning period and appears to be related to sow lactation feed (energy) intake (Zoiopoulos et al. 1983). At the end of pregnancy, some studies have reported a net accretion of maternal tissue (Salmon-Legganeur and Rerat 1962; Heap and Lodge 1967), whereas others have not (Howell et al. 1977; Lodge et al. 1979; DeWilde 1980; Shields and Manan 1983b; Close et al. 1985). The presence or absence of this ''pregnancy anabolism'' appears to be related to sow parity and gestation feeding level.

Lactation provides a drain on sow body stores. The extent of this drain depends on nutrient intake and milk production demands. Although it is possible for sows to complete a lactation period with the same body stores with which they began (Shields and Mahan 1983b; Shields et al. 1985), this is unusual in breeds that have high milk production capacity and relatively low feed intakes (Whittemore et al. 1980; Whittemore 1985). Sow nutrient partitioning between milk production and the maintenance of body stores can differ widely among sow groups, and it is influenced by energy and protein intakes (Brendemuhl et al. 1986).

Chemical component relationships have received a great deal of attention in sow studies because of the well-recognized pregnancy hydration that occurs in humans (Hytten 1969; Robertson 1969), sheep (Robinson et al. 1978), cattle (Degen and Young 1980), rats (Kanto and Clawson 1980), and swine (Shields and Manan 1983b). This hydration represents a combination of additional blood volume (Elsley et al. 1966) and weight increases in the uterus and mammary tissue. Little evidence of maternal hydration was evident in first-litter sows when the contribution of reproductive tissue was removed (Shields and Mahan 1983b). The dry, fat-free maternal body consistently contained a 5:1 ratio of protein to ash in this study, a composition similar to that listed previously for growing-finishing pigs.

FACTORS INFLUENCING COMPOSITIONAL PATTERNS

Several factors, including weaning age, genetic background, sex, growth modulators, temperature, and diet can alter the composition of swine growth. A brief description of their influence follows. Many of these are also discussed in several previous chapters of this text.

Weaning Age

Age at weaning can have profound short-term effects on body composition. Pigs weaned at 2 weeks of age lose 25% to 30% of their fat stores in the initial week postweaning, resulting in a 40% to 50% reduction compared with unweaned counterparts (Whittemore et al. 1978; Fenton et al. 1985). The water:protein ratio was also elevated (4.93 versus 4.74) in the earlier weaned pigs. In contrast, pigs weaned at 5 weeks of age experience a 15% to 20% increase in fat stores during the initial week postweaning. Whittemore and co-workers (1981) have suggested that when postweaning gains fall below 193 g/day, lipid is catabolized to support gains of more essential tissues. Compensation for these initial body composition differences is generally complete by the time the pig leaves the nursery (Seve 1982; Fenton et al. 1985). Weaning age (lactation length) probably has an effect on sow body composition, but further research is necessary to quantitate these effects.

Breed and Sex Differences

Genetic selection can have profound effects on body composition (Bereskin and Davey 1976). Selection for rate of gain alone generally results in increased fatness (Biondini et al. 1968). Breed differences are known to exist, with Hampshire, Duroc, Large White, Landrace, and Gloucester Old Spots having progressively increasing amounts of fat (Goenga and Carden 1979; Wood et al. 1979; Smith and Pearson 1986). Several studies have also reported differences in fat distribution among depots (Goenga and Carden 1979; Kempster and Evans 1979b; Jones et al. 1980; Richmond and Berg 1982).

Sex also influences body composition at a given weight. Boars have less fat, more water and protein, and similar ash content as compared with gilts at conventional slaughter weights (Davies et al. 1980; Campbell et al. 1985). Gilts, in turn, are leaner than barrows (Reid et al. 1968; Bereskin and Davey 1976; Kempster and Evans 1979; Shields et al. 1983c) with differences becoming apparent between 54 and 73 kg body weight (Shields et al. 1983c; Just et al. 1984). At similar carcass fat weights, boars are approximately 40 kg heavier than barrows (Knudson et al. 1985). At similar slaughter weights, barrows have 6 kg more fat (chemically determined) than gilts (Shields et al. 1983c) and 6.5 kg more fat than boars (Knudson et al. 1985). Martin et al. (1972) additionally reported sex differences in fat distribution.

Repartitioning Agents

Evaluation of various agents that alter normal nutrient partitioning is one of the most exciting areas of swine research because such agents can enhance genetic selection effects. Excellent reviews of these agents were prepared by Mersmann (1987) and Ricks (1988). Two products that seem to have most immediate industry application are beta-adrenergic agonists (repartitioning agents) and porcine somatotropin. A review article by McKeith (1987) suggested that somatotropin administration during the finishing period increased carcass muscle and decreased fat 12% to 13%, about twice the amount observed when beta-agonists are fed. However, the water:protein ratio in muscle remained unchanged (Boyd et al. 1987). The magnitude of response at a particular dosage is affected by pig genotype (Kanis et al. 1988) and sex (Steele et al. 1987).

Temperature

Phillips and MacHardy (1982) stated that the composition of gain is influenced in a predictable manner by the interaction of energy intake and temperature. Below the lower critical temperature, maintenance energy needs increase (Holmes and Close 1977; Noblet et al. 1985) while ration digestibility decreases (Phillips et al. 1982). The composition of gain is fairly uniform across temperatures when pigs are fed high-energy diets (Stahly et al. 1981; Coffey et al. 1982; Phillips and MacHardy 1982; Noblet et al. 1985), while leaner gains are evident at low temperatures when low-energy diets are fed (Coffey et al. 1982; Phillips and MacHardy 1982).

Diet Amount and Composition

Diet can influence composition of gain during all phases of production. Fat (Pettigrew 1981), fructose (Kanurek and Orthen-Gambill 1982; White et al. 1984), and 1,3-butanediol (Stahly et al. 1985) supplementation to sow diets and maternal feed restriction (Ezekwe 1981) have been investigated as methods to alter pig body stores at birth and/or survival to weaning. During the postweaning period, widening the energy:protein ratio by lowering dietary protein percentage (Wyllie et al. 1969; Zimmerman and Khajarern 1973; Hogberg and Zimmerman 1979) or supplementing fat without corresponding protein addition (Clawson et al. 1962; Leibbrandt et al. 1975; Bartov 1979) results in reduced water and protein and increased body fat at similar body weights. Campbell et al. (1984) hypothesized that when diets are deficient in protein, muscle deposition rate is linearly related to protein intake, whereas when diets contain adequate amounts of protein, deposition of protein is related to energy rather than protein intake.

Restricting only energy intake either through feed restriction or by increasing dietary fiber levels results in increased body water and protein content and decreased fat at a common slaughter weight (Just 1984). These results help explain why European feeding systems generally result in leaner hogs at a common slaughter weight (Whittemore 1984).

Diet can also influence sow body stores. Feeding a low-protein (5% versus 14%) diet during gestation resulted in a 60% reduction in protein and a 100% increase in fat deposition rate (Shields et al. 1985). During lactation, previous gestation and current lactation diets both influence body stores (Salmon-Legagneur and Rerat 1962; Shields et al. 1985). When lactation intake is low, consumption of all nutrients is reduced, and both muscle and fat stores will be depleted unless milk production is reduced (Chigaru and Topps 1981; Brendemuhl et al. 1986).

Sows have an amazing capacity to deplete body stores to support milk production. A 75% loss of fat stores has been reported when dietary energy is severely restricted (O'Grady et al. 1975). Large quantities of protein reserves can also be drained and restored rapidly (Allison and Wannemacher 1965; Paquay et al. 1972; Botts et al. 1979). Feeding a 5% protein diet throughout one reproductive cycle resulted in a drain of approximately 20% in all chemical components (Shields et al. 1985).

Compensatory Growth

For the purpose of this discussion, compensatory growth is defined as differential rate and composition of growth (compared with other animals of equal weight) after nutritional insult. Comparisons of body composition at equal age and weight provide different conclusions regarding treatment effects (Buhlinger et al. 1978). Animals previously deprived of protein exhibit a greater accumulation of water and protein and lower fat retention when nutritionally adequate diets are fed (Zimmerman and Khajarern 1973; Wyllie and Owen 1978; Hogberg and Zimmerman 1979; Campbell and Biden 1978). If low-protein diets are fed, those deprived previously will deposit protein at a faster rate (Campbell and Dunkin 1983a).

Animals previously restricted in energy intake deposit both protein and fat at a greater rate (per unit of body weight) when energy intake is again sufficient to meet nutrient needs (Campbell and Dunkin 1983b). The ability to completely compensate for a period of nutritional inadequacy will depend on the animal weight at the time of restriction, the degree and length of time the restriction is imposed, and the effective environmental temperature.

SUMMARY

Body composition measurement can be a valuable addition to swine growth, reproduction, and nutrient partitioning studies. Cost and inconvenience have been the primary factors limiting widespread use of this parameter. In vivo techniques that allow repeated measurements on the same animal have the most widespread application in nutrition experiments. Defining chemical component relationships is critical when using indirect methods to estimate body composition. Several factors, including stage of growth or reproduction, weaning age, genetic background, sex, growth modulators, temperature, and diet, can alter these relationships.

REFERENCES

Adam, J.L., and W.C. Smith. 1964. *Anim. Prod.* 6:97.
Allison, J.B., and R.W. Wannemacher. 1965. *Am. J. Clin. Nutr.* 16:445.
Arnold, R.N., and A. Trenkle. 1986. *J. Anim. Sci.* 63:1400.
Arnold, R.N., E.J. Hentges, and A. Trenkle. 1986. *J. Anim. Sci.* 60:1188.
Aulstad, D. 1970. *Acta Agric. Scand.* 20:65.
Bartle, S.J., J.R. Males, and R.L. Preston. 1983. *J. Anim. Sci.* 56:410.
Bartle, S.J., et al. 1987. *J. Anim. Sci.* 64:1024.
Bartov, I. 1979. *Fed. Proc.* 38:2627.
Bartov, I., J. Bornstein, and B. Lipstein. 1974. *Br. Poult. Sci.* 15:107.
Bereskin, B., and R.J. Davey. 1976. *J. Anim. Sci.* 42:43.
Biondini, P.E., T.M. Sutherland, and L.H. Haverland. 1968. *J. Anim. Sci.* 27:5.
Botts, R.L., R.W. Hemken, and L.S. Bull. 1979. *J. Dairy Sci.* 62:433.
Boyd, R.D., et al. 1987. *Proceedings of the Maryland Nutrition Conference.* p. 58.
Brendemuhl, J.H., A.J. Lewis, and E.R. Peo, Jr. 1986. *J. Anim. Sci.* 63(Suppl. 1):263.
Brody, S. 1945. *Bioenergetics and Growth.* New York: Reinhold Publishing Corp.
Brown, C.J., J.C. Hillier, and J.A. Whatley. 1951. *J. Anim. Sci.* 10:97.
Buhlinger, C.A., et al. 1978. *Growth* 42:225.
Byers, F.M. 1978. *Fed. Proc.* 37:410 (Abstr.).
Byers, F.M. 1979. *Anal. Biochem.* 98:208.
Campbell, R.G., and R.S. Biden. 1978. *Anim. Prod.* 27:223.
Campbell, R.G., and A.C. Dunkin. 1983a. *Anim. Prod.* 36:415.
Campbell, R.G., and A.C. Dunkin. 1983b. *Anim. Prod.* 36:435.
Campbell, R.G., M.R. Taverner, and D.M. Curic. 1984. *Anim. Prod.* 38:233.
Campbell, R.G., M.R. Taverner, and D.M. Curic. 1985. *Anim. Prod.* 40:497.
Chiba, L.I., A.J. Lewis, and E.R. Peo, Jr. 1987. *J. Anim. Sci.* 65(Suppl. 1):139.

Chigaru, P.R., and J.H. Topps. 1981. *Anim. Prod.* 32:95.
Chizzolini, R., et al. 1988. *Meat Sci.* 22:33.
Clausen, H. 1953. "The improvement of pigs." The George Scott Robertson Memorial Lecture. Queen's University, Belfast.
Clawson, A.J., et al. 1962. *J. Anim. Sci.* 21:62.
Close, W.H., J. Noblet, and R.P. Heavens. 1984. *Livest. Prod. Sci.* 11:517.
Close, W.H., J. Noblet, and R.P. Heavens. 1985. *Br. J. Nutr.* 53:267.
Coffey, M.T., et al. 1982. *J. Anim. Sci.* 54:95.
Davies, A.S., G. Pearson, and J.R. Carr. 1980. *J. Agric. Sci. (Camb.)* 95:251.
Degen, A.A., and B.A. Young. 1980. *J. Agric. Sci. (Camb.)* 95:1.
DeWilde, R.O. 1980. *Livest. Prod. Sci.* 7:497.
Doornenbal, H. 1971. *Growth* 35:281.
Doornenbal, H. 1972. *Growth* 36:185.
Doornenbal, H., G.H. Wellington, and J.R. Stouffer. 1962. *J. Anim. Sci.* 21:464.
Edwards, R.L., et al. 1981. *J. Anim. Sci.* 52:703.
Eisen, E.J., et al. 1984. *J. Anim. Sci.* 58:1181.
Elsley, F.W.H., et al. 1966. *Anim. Prod.* 8:391.
Ezekwe, M.O. 1981. *J. Anim. Sci.* 53:1504.
Fahey, T.J., et al. 1977. *J. Anim. Sci.* 44:8.
Fenton, J.P., et al. 1985. *J. Anim. Sci.* 60:190.
Ferrell, C.L., and S.G. Cornelius. 1984. *J. Anim. Sci.* 58:903.
Ferrell, C.L., and F.P. Phillips. 1980. *J. Anim. Sci.* 51(Suppl. 1):358.
Flynn, M.A., et al. 1968. In: *Body Composition in Animals and Man.* Reid, J.T. (Ed.). pp. 480–491. Washington, DC: National Academy of Sciences.
Fortin, A., and J.I. Elliot. 1985. *J. Anim. Sci.* 61:158.
Garrett, W.N., J.H. Meyer, and G.P. Lofgreen. 1959. *J. Anim. Sci.* 18:116.
George, S.A., et al. 1987. In: *Manipulating Pig Production.* Barnett, J.L., et al. (Eds.). p. 154. Werribee, Australia: Australasian Pig Science Assn.
Goenga, P.R., and A.E. Carden. 1979. *J. Agric. Sci. (Camb.)* 93:271.
Griffin, H.D., C.C. Whitehead, and L.A. Broadbent. 1982. *Br. Poult. Sci.* 23:15.
Grisdale, B., et al. 1984. *J. Anim. Sci.* 58:335.
Groves, T.D.D., and A.J. Wood. 1965. *Can. J. Anim. Sci.* 45:14.
Hammond, A.C., T.S. Rumsey, and G.L. Haaland. 1984. *Growth* 48:29.
Hansard, S.L. 1963. *Ann. N. Y. Acad. Sci.* 110:229.
Heap, F.C., and G.A. Lodge. 1967. *Anim. Prod.* 9:237.
Hogberg, M.G., and D.R. Zimmerman. 1979. *J. Anim. Sci.* 49:472.
Holmes, C.W., and W.H. Close. 1977. In: *Nutrition and Climatic Environment.* Haresign, W., H. Swan, and D. Lewis (Eds.). pp. 51–73. London: Butterworths.
Houseman, R.A., and I. McDonald. 1976. *J. Agric. Sci. (Camb.)* 87:499.
Houseman, R.A., I. McDonald, and K. Pennie. 1973. *Br. J. Nutr.* 30:149.
Howell, F.D.B., et al. 1977. *Anim. Prod.* 25:281.
Hytten, F.E. 1969. *J. Reprod. Fertil.* 9(Suppl. 9):1.
Joblin, A.D.H. 1966. *N.Z. J. Agric. Res.* 9:227.
Johnson, C.L. 1973. *J. Endocrinol.* 56:37.
Jones, S.D.M., et al. 1980. *Can. J. Anim. Sci.* 60:223.
Jones, S.D.M., et al. 1982. *Can. J. Anim. Sci.* 62:371.
Just, A. 1984. *J. Anim. Sci.* 58:740.
Kanarek, R.B., and N. Orthen-Gambill. 1982. *J. Nutr.* 112:1546.
Kanis, E.K., et al. 1988. *J. Anim. Sci.* 66(Suppl. 1):296.
Kanto, U., and A.J. Clawson. 1980. *J. Nutr.* 110:1829.
Kempster, A.J., and D.G. Evans. 1979a. *Anim. Prod.* 28:87.
Kempster, A.J., and D.G. Evans. 1979b. *J. Agric. Sci. (Camb.)* 93:349.
Kempster, A.J., and D.G. Evans. 1981. *Anim. Prod.* 33:313.
Kempster, A.J., et al. 1981. *Anim. Prod.* 33:319.

Keys, A., and J. Brozek. 1953. *Physiol. Rev.* 33:245.
King, R.H., E. Speirs, and P. Eckerman. 1986. *Anim. Prod.* 43:167.
Knudson, B.K., et al. 1985. *J. Anim. Sci.* 61:797.
Kock, S.W., and R.L. Preston. 1979. *J. Anim. Sci.* 48:319.
Krzywicki, H.J., et al. 1974. *Am. J. Clin. Nutr.* 27:1380.
Lawes, J.B., and J.H. Gilbert. 1861. *J. R. Agric. Soc. England* 21:1.
Lawrence, L.M., et al. 1986. *J. Anim. Sci.* 63(Suppl. 1):233.
Leibbrandt, V.D., et al. 1975. *J. Anim. Sci.* 40:1070.
Leymaster, K.A. 1986. *J. Anim. Sci.* 63(Suppl. 2):89.
Lodge, G.A., D.W. Friend, and M.S. Wolynetz. 1979. *Can. J. Anim. Sci.* 59:51.
Martin, A.H., et al. 1972. *J. Anim. Sci.* 35:534.
McKeith, F. 1987. *University of Illinois Pork Industry Conference.* p. 69. Urbana, IL: University of Illinois Press.
McMeekan, C.P. 1940. *J. Agric. Sci. (Camb.)* 30:276.
McMeekan, C.P. 1941. *J. Agric. Sci. (Camb.)* 31:1.
Meissner, H.H., J.H. van Staden, and E. Pretorius. 1980. *S. Afr. J. Anim. Sci.* 10:165.
Mersmann, H.J. 1982a. *J. Anim. Sci.* 54:268.
Mersmann, H.J. 1982b. *J. Anim. Sci.* 54:276.
Mersmann, H.J. 1987. *Prog. Food Nutr. Sci.* 11:175.
Mirosh, L.W., et al. 1980. *Poult. Sci.* 59:945.
Moore, K., et al. 1985. *University of Missouri Swine Research Report.* p. 44. Columbia, MO: University of Missouri Press.
Moulton, C.R. 1923. *J. Biol. Chem.* 57:79.
Naismith, D.J. 1966. *Metabolism* 15:582.
Noblet, J., J. LeDividich, and T. Bikawa. 1985. *J. Anim. Sci.* 61:452.
Novak, L.P. 1973. *Ann. N. Y. Acad. Sci.* 110:545.
NPPC. 1976. *Procedures to Evaluate Market Hogs.* Des Moines, IA: National Pork Producers Council.
Odwongo, W.O., H.R. Conrad, and A.E. Staubus. 1984. *J. Nutr.* 114:2127.
O'Grady, J.R., et al. 1975. *Anim. Prod.* 20:257.
Oslage, H.J. 1965. *Heft* 40:65.
Oslage, H.J., and F.E. Farries. 1962. *Atschr. Tierphysiol. Tiernahr. Futtermittelkd.* 17:343.
Panaretto, B.A. 1963. *Aust. J. Agric. Res.* 14:944.
Panaretto, B.A., and A.R. Till. 1963. *Aust. J. Agric. Res.* 14:926.
Paquay, T., R. DeBaere, and A. Lousse. 1972. *Br. J. Nutr.* 27:27.
Pearson, A.M., R.W. Purchas, and E.P. Reineke. 1968. In: *Body Composition in Animals and Man.* Reid, J.T. (Ed.). pp. 153–169. Washington, DC: National Academy of Sciences.
Pettigrew, J.E., Jr. 1981. *J. Anim. Sci.* 53:107.
Phillips, P.A., and F.V. MacHardy. 1982. *Can. J. Anim. Sci.* 62:109.
Phillips, P.A., B.A. Young, and J.B. McQuitty. 1982. *Can. J. Anim. Sci.* 62:95.
Pinson, E.A. 1952. *Physiol. Rev.* 32:123.
Preston, R.L., and S.W. Kock. 1973. *Proc. Soc. Exp. Biol. Med.* 143:1057.
Preston, R.L., et al. 1968. In: *Body Composition in Animals and Man.* Reid, J.T. (Ed.). pp. 413–427. Washington, DC: National Academy of Sciences.
Prince, T.J., et al. 1981. *J. Anim. Sci.* 53:663.
Reid, J.T., C.C. Balch, and R.F. Glascock. 1958. *Br. J. Nutr.* 12:43.
Reid, J.T., C.C. Balch, and M.J. Head. 1957. *Nature* 179:1034.
Reid, J.T., G.H. Wellington, and H.O. Dunn. 1955. *J. Dairy Sci.* 38:1344.
Reid, J.T., et al. 1963. *Ann. N.Y. Acad. Sci.* 110:327.
Reid, J.T., et al. 1968. In: *Body Composition in Animals and Man.* Reid, J.T. (Ed.). pp. 19–44. Washington, DC: National Academy of Sciences.
Richmond, R.S., and R.T. Berg. 1982. *Can. J. Anim. Sci.* 62:587.
Ricks, C.A. 1988. *Proceedings of the Maryland Nutrition Conference* p. 67.
Roberts, C.A., et al. 1987. *J. Anim. Sci.* 65:278.

Robertson, E.G. 1969. *J. Reprod. Fertil.* 9(Suppl. 9):27.
Robinson, J.J. 1986. *Proc. Nutr. Soc.* 45:71.
Robinson, J.J., et al. 1978. *J. Agric. Sci. (Camb.)* 91:291.
Rudolph, B.C. 1984. Use of deuterium oxide as an estimator of milk intake and body composition of nursing pigs and the effect of oxytocin administration to the dam on early lactation performance. Ph.D. diss., University of Kentucky, Lexington, KY.
Russell, R.W., and R.B. Reed. 1987. *J. Anim. Sci.* 64:1010.
Salmon-Legagneur, E., and A. Rerat. 1962. In: *Nutrition of Pigs and Poultry.* Morgan, J.T., and D. Lewis (Eds.). pp. 207–223. London: Butterworths.
Seve, B. 1982. *Livest. Prod. Sci.* 9:603.
Shebaita, M.K. 1975. *World Rev. Anim. Prod.* 11:83.
Sheng, H.P., and R.A. Huggins. 1971. *Proc. Soc. Exp. Biol. Med.* 137:1093.
Shields, R.G., Jr., and D.C. Mahan. 1983a. *J. Anim. Sci.* 57:604.
Shields, R.G., Jr., and D.C. Mahan. 1983b. *J. Anim. Sci.* 57:594.
Shields, R.G., Jr., D.C. Mahan, and F.M. Byers. 1983b. *J. Anim. Sci.* 57:66.
Shields, R.G., Jr., D.C. Mahan, and F.M. Byers. 1984. *J. Anim. Sci.* 59:1239.
Shields, R.G., Jr., D.C. Mahan, and V.R. Cahill. 1983a. *J. Anim. Sci.* 57:55.
Shields, R.G., Jr., D.C. Mahan, and P.L. Graham. 1983c. *J. Anim. Sci.* 57:43.
Shields, R.G., Jr., D.C. Mahan, and P.F. Maxson. 1985. *J. Anim. Sci.* 60:179.
Smith, W.C., and G. Pearson. 1985. *Meat Sci.* 14:29.
Smith, W.C., and G. Pearson. 1986. *N.Z. J. Exp. Agric.* 14:43.
Stahly, T.S., G.L. Cromwell, and H.J. Monegue. 1985. *J. Anim. Sci.* 61:1485.
Stahly, T.S., G.L. Cromwell, and J.R. Overfield. 1981. *J. Anim. Sci.* 53:1269.
Stansbury, W.F., R.L. Preston, and L.F. Tribble. 1985. *Texas Tech. Swine Day Report, Agricultural Sciences Technical Report No. T-5-186.* p. 34.
Steele, N.C., R.G. Campbell, and T.J. Caperna. 1987. *Proceedings of the Cornell Nutrition Conference for Feed Manufacturers.* p. 15. Ithaca, NY: Cornell University Press.
Timon, V.M., and M. Bichard. 1965. *Anim. Prod.* 7:173.
Topel, D.G. 1986. *J. Anim. Sci.* 63:633.
Trenkle, A. 1986. *J. Anim. Sci.* 63(Suppl. 2):96.
Wallace, W.M. 1959. *Fed. Proc.* 18:1125.
Ward, G.M., and J.E. Johnson. 1972. In: *Isotope Studies on the Physiology of Domestic Animals.* pp. 3–18. Vienna: International Atomic Energy Agency.
White, C.E., et al. 1984. *J. Anim. Sci.* 59:141.
Whittemore, C.T. 1984. *J. R. Agric. Soc. England* 145:126.
Whittemore, C.T. 1985. *S. Afr. J. Anim. Sci.* 15:97.
Whittemore, C.T. 1986. *J. Anim. Sci.* 63:615.
Whittemore, C.T., A. Aumaitre, and I.H. Williams. 1978. *J. Agric. Sci. (Camb.)* 91:681.
Whittemore, C.T., M.F. Franklin, and B.S. Pearce. 1980. *Anim. Prod.* 31:183.
Whittemore, C.T., et al. 1981. *Anim. Prod.* 32:203.
Wood, A.J., and T.D.D. Groves. 1963. *Ann. N. Y. Acad. Sci.* 110:349.
Wood, J.D. 1984. In: *Fats in Animal Nutrition.* Wiseman, J. (Ed.). pp. 407–435. London: Butterworths.
Wood, J.D., G.A. Lodge, and D. Lister. 1979. *Anim. Prod.* 28:371.
Wyllie, D., and J.B. Owen. 1978. *J. Agric. Sci. (Camb.)* 90:69.
Wyllie, D., et al. 1969. *J. Anim. Sci.* 29:433.
Zimmerman, D.R., and S. Khajarern. 1973. *J. Anim. Sci.* 36:189.
Zoiopoulos, P.E., J.H. Topps, and P.R. English. 1983. *Br. J. Nutr.* 50:163.

Chapter 41

Surgical Techniques

J.T. Yen

CARE AND USE OF SWINE IN EXPERIMENTAL SURGERY

It cannot be overemphasized that routine care and management of pigs for experimental surgery should carefully adhere to the regulations specified in the Animal Welfare Act and its amendments. These regulations have been summarized and published in a recent report by U.S. Congress, Office of Technology Assessment (1986). The Consortium for Developing a Guide for the Care and Use of Agricultural Animals in Agricultural Research and Teaching (1988) has also published the first edition of a guide that provides information on the requirements and recommendations for operating institutional animal facilities and programs concerning animals residing in simulated or actual production agricultural settings. If the surgically prepared pigs are used as models for humans in biomedical research projects, the care and use of these animals should follow the requirements and recommendations given by the *Guide for the Care and Use of Laboratory Animals,* published by National Institutes of Health (1985).

PREPARATION FOR ASEPTIC SURGERY

The use of rigid aseptic technique in swine surgery is mandatory. The common misconception that pigs are not especially susceptible to postsurgical infection is a fallacy arising from the short-term use of the surgically prepared animal, and from the fact that casualties in the operated animal are soon forgotten. The routine, indiscriminate administration of antibiotics to the animal following surgery tends to cover the trails of poor technique.

The preparation for aseptic surgery includes at least four areas: sterilization of instruments and supplies needed to perform surgery; aseptic preparation of the surgical site on the animal; aseptic preparation of the surgeon and assistants; and aseptic draping of the animal. Detailed information and general principles regarding the preparation for aseptic surgery in swine are readily available and can be found in textbooks, such as that by Swindle (1983), on basic surgical exercises with pigs and those on large animal surgery by Knecht et al. (1987) and Oehme (1988).

PRESURGICAL CARE OF THE ANIMAL

To obtain meaningful information from surgically prepared swine, the animals need to be trained properly, so their normal physiological functions and behavior will not be altered under the experimental conditions. For experiments in which pigs have to be housed individually in specially designed cages or crates for continuous infusion and repeated sampling, stepwise training of the pigs seems to be the most proper approach. In our studies with pigs having their portal vein, ileal vein, and systemic artery cannulated chronically, the animals were first housed in individual cylindrical metabolism cages approximately 4 weeks. They were then moved into individual pens, measuring 1.2 × 1.2 m, and trained to adapt to rectangular crates designed for infusion and sampling study. Usually within 3 to 4 days, the animals were well adapted and were willing to enter the rectangular crates, consume their daily feed allowance, and rest inside the crates until they were put back into the pens (Yen and Killefer 1987).

Before surgery, the pigs should be fasted for at least 12 hours to prevent vomiting or severe gaseous gastrointestinal distention (Thurmon and Benson 1987; Swindle 1983). Water should be available to the pigs until the time of surgery with the exception of upper gastrointestinal tract surgery, in which case, water should be withheld for at least 6 hours (Swindle 1983).

ANESTHESIA

It is beyond the scope of this chapter to provide detailed information regarding anesthesia in swine. Individuals interested in the principles and techniques of anesthesia should consult textbooks and references of veterinary anesthesia such as those by Short (1987), Thurmon (1986), Hall and Clarke (1983), and Riebold et al. (1982). Several excellent overviews of anesthesia in swine have also been published by Thurmon and Benson (1987), Riebold and Thurmon (1988), and Swindle (1983). A list of dosages of selected preanesthetics, intramuscular and intravenous injectable general anesthetics, and inhalation anesthetics for swine is given in Table 41.1. For our swine surgery, the pig is physically restrained by a nose snare. The anesthesia is induced by intravenous injection of sodium thiopental (15 mg/kg body weight in 2.5% solution) into the anterior vena cava. Care is taken to avoid perivascular injection of thiopental. Additional thiopental is administered to the pig through an indwelling cannula in the ear vein after the animal becomes immobilized. The anesthesia during the surgery is maintained with 1% to 2% vaporized halothane in oxygen (22 to 44 ml/kg/minute) by a close-circuit anesthetic machine through a nose cone.

Table 41.1 Dosage of Selected Agents in Swine Anesthesia

Drug	*Dosage*
Preanesthetics	
Acetylpromazine	0.11–0.22 mg/kg IM
Atropine	0.06–0.08 mg/kg IM
Azaperone	2.0–8.0 mg/kg IM
Glycophyrrole	0.01 mg/kg IM or IV
Promazine	0.4–1.0 mg/kg IM
IM anesthetics	
Ketamine	20 mg/kg
Ketamine:acetylpromazine	22:1.1 mg/kg
Ketamine:xylazine	20:2 mg/kg
Ketamine:xylazine:oxymorphone	4:4:0.15 mg/kg
IV anesthetics	
Pentobarbital	25–30 mg/kg
Thiamylal	6–18 mg/kg
Thiopental	10–20 mg/kg
Inhalant anesthetics	
Halothane	4%–5% for induction 1%–2% for maintenance
Isoflurane	3%–4% for induction 1.5%–2% for maintenance

Abbreviations: IM, intramuscular(ly); IV, intravenous(ly).

MONITORING THE ANIMAL DURING AND AFTER SURGERY

Because ocular and pupillary reflexes are not reliable in anesthetized pigs (Riebold et al. 1982; Swindle 1983), the depth of anesthesia in pigs is best monitored by the degree of muscle relaxation and respiratory movement. A practial guide to muscle relaxation in pigs is the absence of withdrawal reflex of the legs when a pinch is applied between the hooves. In anesthetized pigs, the normal respiration rate is 10 to 25 per minute and heart rate is 80 to 130 per minute (Riebold et al. 1982). Loss of withdrawal reflex to painful stimulus and full, rhythmic respiration indicate the surgical plane of anesthesia. To minimize shock due to surgery trauma and to hasten recovery from surgery, the pig should be maintained on a continuous intravenous drip of a dextrose-electrolyte solution during the surgery. A flow rate of 10 ml/kg/hour has been recommended by Swindle (1983). The rate should be increased if blood loss occurs.

After surgery, the incision should be covered with gauze and protected with bandage or adhesive tape to avoid contamination of the wound. The animal should be monitored daily for appetite, bowel movement, urinary output, and behavior. Post-operative administration of antibiotics to the animal is not necessary if strict aseptic surgery is conducted. The length of recovery after surgery depends on the type of surgery. The best indication of recovery is the restoration of normal appetite (Low 1980).

SURGICAL TECHNIQUES FOR SELECTED IN VIVO NUTRITION STUDIES

The objective of this section is to describe a few surgical techniques that are valuable for nutrition studies in the pig in vivo. Information about other surgical procedures in the pig has been published by Pond and Houpt (1978) and Swindle (1983).

Surgically prepared animals provide a powerful tool for investigating digestion and absorption of nutrients in swine. They are particularly useful for studies relating to the kinetics of digestion and absorption. However, certain alteration or destruction of tissues occurs as a consequence of surgery. This raises the question concerning whether the surgically prepared animals function normally or not. The use of surgically prepared pigs indicates an intensive type of research and limits the number of animals that can be employed for the experiment. The maximum length of the experiment is dictated by the length of cannula patency.

Nutrient Digestibility

The digestibility of a nutrient in swine is traditionally estimated by the disappearance of the nutrient from the gastrointestinal tract (GIT). Simple and re-entrant cannulas placed in the GIT have been used to measure the disappearance of a nutrient in conscious swine. A great number of publications exist concerning cannula designs and surgical techniques on the GIT in pigs. Low (1980) provided a critical review of the methodology of GIT cannulation. A review of the application of ileum-cannulated pigs for determining amino acid digestibility was published recently by Sauer and Ozimek (1986). An example of placing a simple ileal cannula in 30- to 35-kg pigs has been described by Gargallo and Zimmerman (1980). A laparotomy incision is made in the right abdominal wall 4 cm below the transverse process of the fifth lumbar vertebra. The terminal ileum is located using the cecum as anatomical reference. A longitudinal incision is made on the antimesenteric surface 10 cm cranial to the ileocecal junction. The cannula is inserted into the lumen of the ileum. A pursestring suture is placed around the barrel of the cannula. The cannula is exteriorized through a stab wound made through the right body wall. It is essential that the flanges of the cannula bring the ileum in close contact with the body wall so good adhesion can take place. A simple T-cannula for ileal cannulation in preweaned pigs has also been described by Walker et al. (1986).

Most techniques for re-entrant cannulation of pigs are similar to that described by Markowitz et al. (1964) in dogs. To bypass the resistance of the ileocecal valve and to allow a more normal flow of digesta through the externally connected cannulas, re-entrant ileocecal cannulation is more appropriate (Easter and Tanksly 1973). After locating the ileocecal junction, the terminal ileum is transected 15 to 20 cm cranial from the ileocecal junction. The caudal end of the ileum is closed by the Parker-Kerr oversew technique. A longitudinal incision is made on the antimesenteric surface of the ileum near the closed end and a pursestring suture is placed around the incision. The ileal cannula is inserted into the lumen of the ileum and the ileum is drawn snuggly around the barrel of the cannula. A second pursestring suture is placed 1 cm from the first suture to invert the edges of the secretory mucosa. The cecal cannula is inserted into the lumen of the cecum through a stab wound made in the longitudinal band of the cecum near the ileocecal junction. The ileal cannula is exteriorized through a stab wound in the right abdominal wall 4 to 5 cm caudal to the last rib and 15 cm to the dorsal midline. The cecal cannula is exteriorized 15 cm ventral to the location of the ileal cannula. The two cannulas are connected externally with polyvinyl chloride tubing.

An alternative technique for the ileal cannulation is the ileorectal anastomosis (Green et al. 1987; Bengala-Friere et al. 1988). The method allows the digesta to bypass the large intestine and be excreted via the anus for collection. The technique involves making a 15-cm laparotomy incision in the ventral abdominal wall 15 cm caudal to the base of the sternum and dextral to the midline. The terminal ileum is transected 10 cm cranial to the ileocecal junction. The caudal end of the ileum is closed using a pursestring suture and then reinforced by an oversew suture. The open cranial end of the cut ileum is packed with gauze to prevent digesta contamination and tissue drying. The descending colon is located. A 3-cm longitudinal incision is made on the antimesenteric surface of the colon 12 cm cranial to the anus. The open cranial end of the ileum is sutured on the colon over the incision to form a T-shaped ileocolonic junction. The colon loop immediately cranial to the newly formed junction is then transected 2 cm cranial to the junction. The two transected ends are closed with the pursestring and oversew sutures. The colon is then isolated completely from the rest of the GIT. A 2-cm longitudinal incision is made on the antimesenteric surface of the isolated colon 5 cm cranial to the caudal end of the colon. A simple T-cannula is inserted into the lumen of the colon and a pursestring suture is placed around the barrel of the cannula. The cannula is exteriorized through a stab wound in the left dorsal flank 15 cm caudal to the last rib to allow products of residual fermentation to escape from the isolated colon.

Net Portal Nutrient Absorption

Concentration difference of a nutrient between the efferent (portal) and afferent (systemic arterial) blood of the GIT reflects the net uptake from, or loss to, the GIT and is a more critical measurement of nutrient availability than is the disappearance of a nutrient from the GIT (Rerat et al. 1980, 1984a,b). By multiplying concentration differences of a nutrient between the portal and arterial blood by the simultaneously determined portal blood flow rate, the net nutrient absorption into the portal vein per unit of time can be estimated (Rerat et al. 1980, 1984a,b).

Techniques have been developed to collect blood samples from the portal vein and the systemic artery and measure portal vein blood flow in conscious swine (Rerat et al. 1980; Yen and Killefer 1987). The principles for quantifying the net portal absorption as adopted by Rerat et al. (1980) and by Yen and Killefer (1987) are similar. However, the techniques for cannulating blood vessels and for estimating the portal vein blood flow rate are different between the two laboratories. A constant infusion of p-aminohippuric acid into the ileal vein was used by Yen and Killefer (1987) to provide an indicator-dilution method for estimating the portal vein blood flow rate, whereas an electromagnetic probe was used by Rerat et al. (1980).

As described by Yen and Killefer (1987), to cannulate the portal and ileal vein in pigs weighing 29 to 55 kg, a 15- to 20-cm incision is made 2 to 3 cm behind and parallel to the last rib on the right side of the animal. The portal vein is brought toward the incision by inserting the fingers into the space between the pig's portal vein and posterior vena cava. A puncture is made in the portal vein cranial to the gastroduodenal vein. The cannula (polyurethane tubing, 1.68 mm inside diameter [i.d.], 2.41 mm outside diameter [o.d.]) is inserted into the portal vein toward the hilum of the liver. It is secured to the vein by suturing the nylon mesh bonded on the cannula to the connective tissue and outer sheet of the vein. Through the same incision, the terminal ileum is brought toward the incision and the ileal vein is located. The polyurethane ileal cannula (0.65 mm i.d., 1.02 mm o.d.) is inserted into the ileal vein cranially through a puncture in the vein. It is secured to the vein in a fashion similar to that for the portal vein cannula. The two cannulas are exteriorized and exit 2 to 3 cm dorsal and cranial or caudal to the incision for the portal vein cannula or ileal vein cannula, respectively. The incision is then closed.

The carotid artery is the preferred source of systemic arterial blood over the abdominal aorta , which is used as the back-up source. To cannulate the carotid artery, a 7- to 8-cm ventral midline incision is made over the larynx. Muscles of ventral neck are separated and a 3- to 4-cm segment of carotid artery is exposed. Three ligatures are placed loosely around the artery, two caudally and one cranially from the intended puncture site. The polyurethane cannula (1.68 mm i.d., 2.41 mm o.d.) is inserted into the artery through a puncture on the artery and toward the aorta, so the tip of the cannula will be located in the brachiocephalic trunk. The three ligatures are tied. The cannula is further secured by tying the remaining strands of the caudal ligature to the nylon mesh of the cannula and suturing the nylon mesh to the adjacent connective tissue. The cannula is exteriorized to the right side of the neck before the incision is closed.

The distal end of each cannula is tunneled subcutaneously and exteriorized 2 to 3 cm lateral to the dorsal midline. Cannulas are anchored to the skin by cannula collars. The cannulas are fitted with needle adaptors, filled with heparinized saline, and capped with plugs. The adapters and plugs are wrapped with elastic tape to prevent damage.

Rerat et al. (1980) have described a method of placing an electromagnetic flow probe to measure portal vein blood flow and for cannulating the portal vein in pigs weighing 41 to 63 kg. To place the flow probe, a 20-cm incision is made along the right upper lateral region of the abdomen, behind the last rib. The portal vein between the convergence of mensenteric veins and its entrance into the hepatic hilum is exposed. A 1- to 1.5-cm peritoneal tunnel is made between the portal vein and the mesentery. The probe is placed around the portal vein, and the opening of the tunnel is closed. The probe wire is fastened to the parietal peritoneum and then exteriorized near the upper angle of the margins of the incision. To cannulate the portal vein, a pursestring suture is prepared on the portal vein between the flow probe and the liver. A hole in the center of the pursestring suture is made with a special needle containing the cannula over two thirds of its length. The needle will split lengthwise into two parts and yet is hinged to permit opening. The cannula is pushed inside the portal vein and the needle is withdrawn, opened, and removed from the cannula. The pursestring suture is tightened and the cannula is thus fastened directly in the portal vein. The cannula is exteriorized through an abdominal wound at the top of the right side of the body along the edge of the lumbar muscles.

Bajjalieh et al. (1981) also described procedures for placing an electromagnetic blood flow probe around the portal vein in 12- to 15-kg pigs. A mechanical, hydraulically activated sample needle is attached to the portal vein for obtaining blood samples. A cannula is placed in the vena cava for sampling systemic blood. Rerat et al. (1980) showed that the concentrations of reducing sugars and amino acids in the pig are lower in the vena cava blood than in the arterial blood. Thus, a systematic error would exist if the porto-venal instead of porto-arterial difference were used for estimating net portal absorption.

Salivary Secretion

The saliva in a pig's mouth is a composite contributed by all salivary glands (Moran 1982). The salivary glands of the pig consist of three major pairs of glands (parotid, mandibular, and sublingual) and small glands of the oral cavity such as buccal, labial, and lingual glands (Nickel et al. 1973). The number and various locations of salivary glands make it almost impossible to cannulate all the glands for a complete collection of saliva. Corring (1980) reported the use of an esophageal fistula to study the entire saliva collected during consumption of feed. However, no description of surgical procedures was given. Techniques for preparing esophageal fistulas in ruminants have been reviewed by Daugherty (1981) and may be useful to individuals interested in fistulating the esophagus of the pig. Denny and Messervy (1972) have described surgical techniques for the translocation of the parotid salivary duct and the cannulation of the parotid and submandibular saliva ducts in the pig. The translocation of the salivary duct provides a longer period for saliva collection than does the cannulation but can only be used for the parotid salivary duct.

To translocate the parotid salivary duct in a 1-year-old pig, a 12-cm skin incision is made over the ventral border of the lower jaw, beginning on a level with the eye and ending on a level with the ear. The subcutaneous fat and platysma muscle are incised to expose the mandibular part of the parotid gland, which is attached to the masseter muscle by a fascial sheet. The parotid duct lies dorsally within the fascial sheet. A 5-cm segment of the parotid duct is isolated. The duct is severed and its anterior end is brought out through the skin incision. The sheet of fascia is re-attached to the masseter muscle and the incision of subcutaneous fat and platysma muscle is closed. A 1-cm longitudinal incision is made in the end of the parotid duct and the edge of the duct is sutured to the skin and the incision closed. Parotid saliva can be collected 2 days after surgery and for up to 2 months.

To cannulate the parotid duct, the duct is exposed as for translocation. A 2-cm length of the parotid duct is isolated. Through an incision in the duct, a 1.5-mm cannula is inserted caudally for 14 cm and secured by two ligatures tied around the duct.

The fascial sheet is re-attached to the masseter muscle and the cannula is anchored to the fascia to avoid kinking. The cannula is exteriorized through the subcutaneous tissue to exit 8 cm behind the ear. It is then anchored to the neck with a collar of adhesive tape.

For the cannulation of the submandibular duct, a 12-cm incision is made cranial to the angle of the jaw and parallel to the vertical ramus. The platysma muscle is incised and retracted caudally along with the adherent parotid gland to show a sheet of fascia attached to the caudal border of the vertical ramus. The fascia is incised and retracted to expose the submandibular salivary gland and its duct, which is cranial to the gland. A 7-cm segment of the duct is isolated, severed cranially, and brought out through the incision. A 1.5-cm cannula is inserted into the lumen of the duct and secured to the duct by two ligatures. The cannula is exteriorized to exit behind the ear and anchored to the neck.

Gastric Secretion

Gastric secretion in the pig has been studied with the use of a Heidenhain pouch or gastric cannula. Because both the pH and pepsin activity of the gastric secretion obtained from a Heidenhain pouch are significantly lower than those from a gastric cannula, the use of a Heidenhain pouch to study the gastric secretion has been questioned (Corring 1980). Besides permitting study of gastric secretion, gastric cannulas also provide a convenient tool for administering a gastric load.

A technique for gastric cannulation in the pig has been described by Abel and Buck (1967). A 13-cm anterioventral laparotomy is made caudal to the twelfth rib. The stomach is located, and two intestinal clamps that have been covered with surgical tubing are used to isolate the portion of the stomach intended for cannulation. Around the intended incision site, a pursestring suture is placed. An incision with the length equal to the diameter of the cannula and parallel to the greater curvature of the stomach is made. The flange of the cannula is inserted into the lumen of the stomach. After inverting the stomach wall, the pursestring suture is tied off around the cannula and a second pursestring suture is placed peripheral to the first one. The cannula is exteriorized through a second abdominal incision, dorsal to the first one and between the distal ends of the last two ribs. The stomach is pulled up against the abdominal peritoneum, and the washer of the cannula is positioned to hold the cannula in place.

Gastric cannulas can also be prepared with the technique described by Decuypere et al. (1977). The technique employs two types of cannulas made of disposable plastic syringes. For pigs weighing 3 to 10 and 10 to 20 kg, syringes of 2- and 5-ml capacity, respectively, are used as the insertion cannulas. Depending on the size of the animal, syringes of 5- or 10-ml capacity are used as the replacement cannulas. For gastric cannulation, a 5- to 7-cm midline incision is made cranial to the navel. A pursestring suture is placed in the lateroventral fundus region of the stomach. The insertion cannula is inserted into the stomach through an incision in the center of the suture. The stomach is drawn around the barrel of the cannula after the stomach wall is properly inverted.

The cannula is placed in the cranial end of the midline incision and the incision is closed. The first replacement cannula is installed 7 to 8 days after surgery. If necessary, the animal is sedated or anesthetized. The insertion cannula is removed. The internal washer of the replacement cannula is introduced through the fistula and into the stomach. The barrel of the replacement cannula with its external washer in place is then inserted, and the internal washer is pulled on the barrel. By knotting the nylon strings that thread through the internal and external washers, the cannula is secured against the abdominal wall.

This technique described by Decuypere et al. (1977) can also be adapted for duodenal, ileal, and cecal cannulations in the pig. Bjornhag and Jonsson (1984) have also described one type of replaceable gastrointestinal cannula for 12- to 40-kg pigs.

Pancreatic Secretion

The exocrine pancreatic secretion in the pig can be collected by direct cannulation of the pancreatic duct (Pekas 1965; Corring et al. 1972) or a duodenal pouch (Zebrowska et al. 1983; Hee et al. 1985). Direct cannulation allows collections for ≤ 45 days (Corring et al. 1972; J.T. Yen and A.H. Jensen, unpublished data), whereas a duodenal pouch may allow the collection to last several months (Corring 1980). However, the secretion collected from a duodenal pouch may be contaminated with duodenal secretions, and the technique is more stressful to the animal due to the transection of the duodenum.

Corring (1974) demonstrated that the exocrine pancreatic secretion in the pig is regulated by a negative feedback mechanism. To avoid hypersecretion and to obtain a normal physiological response in the pancreatic secretion, it is imperative that the collected pancreatic secretion should be returned to the duodenum of the animal. The re-introduction of the pancreatic secretion also prevents dehydration, acidosis, and eventual death in the pig (Wass 1965).

A method for direct cannulation of the pancreatic duct and re-introduction of the pancratic secretion into the duodenum in 4-week-old pigs has been described by Pekas (1965). A 10-cm incision is made parallel to the caudal-ventral margin of the rib cage on the right side of the animal. A rubber cannula (size, French 8) with a polyethylene nipple (PE 90) is inserted into the pancreatic duct toward the pancreas and 1 to 2 mm from the duct's entrance into the intestine. A slightly larger rubber cannula is inserted into the duodenum in the area adjacent to the entrance of the pancreatic duct. The duodenum cannula is secured to the duodenum with a pursestring suture. The two cannulas are exteriorized, 15 cm apart and through stab wounds, to the back of the body and behind the last rib. A one-way valve, which allows a flow only from the pancreas to the duodenum and thus prevents the duodenal-pancreatic reflux, is used to connect the two cannulas. The ends of the one-way valve are secured to the skin of the pig by intradermal sutures. A two-way stopcock at the entrance of the one-way valve provides a simple means of collecting the pancreatic secretion.

Corring et al. (1972) have described another method for re-entrant cannulating the pancreatic duct and duodenum in the pig weighing 35 to 45 kg. A 15-cm incision is made parallel to and behind the last rib on the right side of the animal. A 5-mm segment of the pancreatic duct is exposed. A polyethylene cannula (1.2 mm i.d., 1.7 mm o.d.) with two polyethylene cuffs bonded to its proximal end is inserted into the duct and toward the pancreas for 1 to 2 cm. The cuff closest to the tip of the cannula is also inserted, and a ligature is placed between the two cuffs and toward the pancreas to tie off the duct around the cannula. The cannula is further fixed to the duodenum at the second cuff by a ligature. The duodenal cannula (1.5 mm i.d., 2.0 mm o.d.) is then inserted into the duodenum near the entrance of the pancreatic duct with the first polyethylene cuff remaining in the lumen of the duodenum. The duodenal cannula is also secured to the duodenum by the cuff with two ligatures. The two cannulas are exteriorized to the right side of the body. The part of the duodenum where two cannulas are attached is brought up against the peritoneum. The incision is closed and the cannulas are anchored to the skin. The two cannulas are connected so as to immediately return the pancreatic secretion to the animal. Because no duodenal-pancreatic reflux has been noted, the one-way valve is not needed between the two cannulas. The pancreatic secretion can be collected continuously in a fraction collector with collection tubes maintained at 2 °C. After being sampled, the secretion is brought to 38 °C and re-introduced to the animal with a variable-rate peristaltic pump.

Techniques for collecting pancreatic secretion through a duodenal pouch in pigs weighing 30 kg have been described by Hee et al. (1985). A 15-cm incision is made parallel and caudal to the last rib on the right side of the animal. A 4- to 6-cm segment of the duodenum that receives the pancreatic duct is isolated. Two intestinal clamps are placed on the duodenum 2 to 3 cm caudal to the pancreatic duct. The duodenum is transected between the two clamps, and the cranial end is closed by a Parker-Kerr oversew to form the bottom of the pouch. Another pair of clamps is applied to the duodenum 2 to 3 cm cranial to the pancreatic duct. The duodenum is transected between the clamps and a pursestring suture is placed around the opening of the pouch. The draining arm of the silicon rubber cannula with its perforated basket at the tip is inserted and secured. After the remaining duodenum is anastomosed, the silicon rubber re-entrant arm of the cannula is inserted into the duodenum through the antimesenteric side 1 cm cranial to the anastomosis and secured by a pursestring suture. The draining and re-entrant arms are exteriorized and exit 15 cm apart and dorsal to the costochondral junction of the right side of the animal. They are connected by stainless steel tubing and secured to the body with rigid polyvinyl chloride washers and silicon rubber retaining rings. For collecting pancreatic secretion, the re-entrant cannula is disconnected and an extension tubing is attached. Pancreatic secretion is re-introduced to the animal by gravity flow.

Bile Secretion

To study bile secretion in the pig with little interruption of the enterohepatic circulation of bile salt, the bile has to be re-introduced to the animal. A bile-duct re-entrant cannulation technique in pigs of 25 to 30 kg has been described by Sambrook (1981). A 25-cm midline incision is made. After separating the bile duct from the adjacent tissue, an incision is made at the midpoint of the duct. An exit cannula and then entry cannula are inserted and ligated in place. The cannulas are made of 30-cm-long silicon rubber tubing (2 mm i.d., 4 mm o.d.) with a 2-cm-long rigid nylon tip. The bile duct is transected between the two cannulas. The two cannulas are sutured to the parietal peritoneum and exteriorized to the right flank of the animal. After suturing the entry cannula to the pylorus, the midline incision is closed. The two exteriorized cannulas are connected with curved stainless steel tubing and covered with adhesive tape. For bile flow measurement sampling, a small Perspex drop-chamber with a three-way stopcock is connected to the cannulas by silicon rubber tubing. A photoelectric counting system is used to record drops of bile.

Juste et al. (1983) have described an automated system in which bile is returned to the pig at a rate directly corresponding to its secretion rate. In the pig weighing 50 kg, a silicone rubber cannula (2.64 mm i.d., 4.88 mm o.d.) is inserted through an incision into the bile duct toward the liver and ligated in place. A second silicon rubber cannula (1.57 mm i.d., 3.18 mm o.d.) is inserted between the first cannula and the sphincter of Oddi and toward the duodenum without reaching the sphincter muscle. The two cannulas are exteriorized to the right flank of the animal. For measurement and sampling of bile, the exit cannula is connected to the plastic container of the automated system and the entry cannula to a peristaltic pump. The system also consists of a glass container having two platinum wire electrodes, an electronic relay, an electric stop valve, a recorder pen, a bile sampling tube, and two nitrogen caps. Bile is reintroduced automatically in a volume determined by the position of one of the two electrodes. The system records bile flow and continuously samples bile for analysis.

Gastrointestinal Lymph

Long-chain fatty acids absorbed from the GIT are transported by the lymphatic system. Cisterna chyli, the dilated sac at the lower end of the thoracic duct, receives lymph from the visceral and lumbar lymphatic trunks (Schummer et al. 1981).

Techniques for the cannulation of the cisterna chyli of the pig weighing 45 kg have been described by Manolas et al. (1983). A laparotomy is made 3 cm beneath and parallel to the costal margin and extends from the lateral end of the costal margin to the midline on the left side of the pig. An incision is made in the caudal peritoneum above the left kidney and 4 cm from the midline. A 5- to 10-cm cisterna chyli is exposed by pulling the left kidney toward the midline and separating the celiac aortic wall from the left psoas muscle with a very gentle blunt dissection. An incision is made in the lymph vessel wall and a T-shaped cannula (1.6 mm i.d., 2.7 mm o.d.) is inserted into the lumen of the cisterna chyli. The caudal peritoneum is closed after returning the left kidney to its normal position. The cannula is exteriorized below the left kidney and through the abdominal wall. In ten pigs so prepared, the cannula was found to be patent for only 2 to 7 days.

CONCLUSION

The information provided in this chapter regarding surgical techniques for selected in vivo nutrition studies in swine is very brief and should be used only as a guide. Furthermore, the techniques may have to be modified in most cases to accommodate the objectives of certain research, the availability of surgical equipment and supplies, the variation in the size of animals, and the unavoidable anatomical deviation among pigs even of the same breed, sex, and size. Nevertheless, the surgically prepared pig is an extremely valuable tool for nutrition research, and, in some cases, the use of such pigs is the only way to obtain certain types of nutritional data.

REFERENCES

Abel, M., and W.B. Buck. 1967. *Cornell Vet.* 57:383.
Bajjalieh, N.L., et al. 1981. *J. Anim. Sci.* 52:101.
Bengala-Freire, J., et al. 1988. *Livest. Prod. Sci.* 20:233.
Bjornhag, G., and E. Jonsson. 1984. *Livest. Prod. Sci.* 11:179.
Consortium for Developing a Guide for the Care and Use of Agricultural Animals in Agricultural Research and Teaching. March 1988. *Guide for the Care and Use of Agricultural Animals in Agricultual Research and Teaching.* 1st ed.
Corring, T. 1974. *Ann. Biol. Anim. Bioch. Biophys.* 14:487.
Corring, T. 1980. In: *Current Concepts of Digestion and Absorption in Pigs. Technical Bulletin 3.* Low, A.G., and I.G. Partridge (Eds.). pp. 136–150. Reading, England: National Institute for Research in Dairying.
Corring, T., A. Aumaitre, and A. Rerat. 1972. *Ann. Biol. Anim. Bioch. Biophys.* 12:109.
Daugherty, R.W. 1981. *Experimental Surgery in Farm Animals.* Ames, IA: Iowa State University Press.
Decuypere, J.A., et al. 1977. *J. Anim. Sci.* 46:463.
Denny, H.R., and A. Messervy. 1972. *Vet. Rec.* 90:650.
Easter, R.A., and T.D. Tanksley. 1973. *J. Anim. Sci.* 36:1099.
Gargallo, J., and D.R. Zimmerman. 1980. *Am. J. Vet. Res.* 41:618.
Green, S., et al. 1987. *J. Sci. Food Agric.* 41:29.
Hall, L.W., and K.W. Clarke. 1983. *Veterinary Anesthesia.* 8th ed. London: Bailliere Tindall.
Hee, J.H., et al. 1985. *Can. J. Anim. Sci.* 65:451.
Juste, C., T. Corring, and Y.L. Coz. 1983. *Lab. Anim. Sci.* 33:199.
Knecht, C.D., et al. 1987. *Fundamental Techniques in Veterinary Surgery.* 3rd ed. Philadelphia, PA: W.B. Saunders Co.
Low, A.G. 1980. In: *Current Concepts of Digestion and Absorption in Pigs. Technical Bulletin 3.* Low, A.G., and I.G. Partridge (Eds.). pp. 10–23. Reading, England: National Institute for Research in Dairying.
Manolas, K.J., et al. 1983. *Cornell Vet.* 73:333.
Markowitz, J., J. Archibald, and H.G. Downie. 1964. *Experimental Surgery.* 5th ed. Baltimore, MD: Williams and Wilkins, Co.
Moran, E.T., Jr. 1982. *Comparative Nutrition of Fowl and Swine—The Gastrointestinal Systems.* Guelph, Ontario: University of Guelph.
National Institutes of Health. 1985. *Guide for the Care and Use of Laboratory Animals. NIH Publication No. 85–230.* Bethesda, MD: National Institutes of Health.
Nickel, R., et al. 1973. *The Viscera of the Domestic Mammals.* New York: Springer-Verlag.
Oehme, F.W. (Ed.). 1988. *Textbook of Large Animal Surgery.* 2d ed. Baltimore, MD: Williams and Wilkins Co.

Pekas, J.C. 1965. *J. Appl. Physiol.* 20:1082.
Pond, W.G., and K.A. Houpt. 1978. *The Biology of the Pig.* pp. 203–237. Ithaca, NY: Cornell University Press.
Rerat, A.A., P. Vaissade, and P. Vaugelade. 1984a. *Br. J. Nutr.* 51:505.
Rerat, A.A., P. Vaissade, and P. Vaugelade. 1984b. *Br. J. Nutr.* 51:517.
Rerat, A., P. Vaugelade, and P. Villiers. 1980. In: *Current Concepts of Digestion and Absorption in Pigs. Technical Bulletin 3.* Low, A.G., and I.G. Partridge (Eds.). pp. 177–216. Reading, England: National Institute for Research in Dairying.
Riebold, T.W., D.O. Goble, and D.R. Geiser. 1982. *Large Animal Anesthesia.* Ames, IA: Iowa State University Press.
Riebold, T.W., and J.C. Thurmon. 1986. In: Vol. 1 of *Swine in Biomedical Research.* Tumbleson, M.E. (Ed.). pp. 243–254. New York: Plenum Press.
Sambrook, I.E. 1981. *J. Sci. Food Agric.* 32:781.
Sauer, W.C., and L. Ozimek. 1986. *Livest. Prod. Sci.* 15:367.
Schummer, A., et al. 1981. In: *The Circulatory System, the Skin and the Cutaneous Organs of the Domestic Mammals.* Vol. 3 of *The Anatomy of the Domestic Animals.* Nickel R., A. Schummer, and E. Seiferle (Eds.). New York: Springer-Verlag.
Short, C.E. 1987. *Principles and Practices of Veterinary Anesthesia.* Baltimore, MD: Williams and Wilkins.
Swindle, M.M. 1983. *Basic Surgical Exercises Using Swine.* New York: Praeger Publishers.
Thurmon, J.C. 1986. In: *Anesthsia.* Vol. 2, No. 3 of *The Veterinary Clinics of North America: Food Animals Practice.* Philadelphia: W.B. Saunders Co.
Thurmon, J.C., and G.J. Benson. 1987. In: *Principles and Practice of Veterinary Anesthesia.* Short, C.E. (Ed.). pp. 308–322. Baltimore, MD: Williams and Wilkins.
U.S. Congress, Office of Technology Assessment. 1986. *Alternatives to Animal Use in Research, Testing and Education.* Washington, DC: U.S. Government Printing Office.
Walker, W.R., G.L. Morgan, and C.V. Maxwell. 1986. *J. Anim. Sci.* 62:407.
Wass, W.M. 1965. *Vet. Rec.* 114:1106.
Yen, J.T., and J. Killefer. 1987. *J. Anim. Sci.* 64:923.
Zebrowska, T., A.G. Low, and H. Zebrowska. 1983. *Br. J. Nutr.* 49:401.

Index